ITS Textbook of Thyroid Disorders

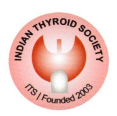

Editors

Sarita Bajaj
MD (Medicine) DM (Endocrinology) FRCP (London, Glasgow and Edinburgh)
Consultant Endocrinologist
Former Director-Professor and Head
Department of Medicine
MLN Medical College
Prayagraj, Uttar Pradesh, India

Rajesh Rajput
MD (Medicine) DM (Endocrinology) FRCP (Edinburgh) FACE FICP FIACM FISH FIMSA FRSSDI
Head
Department of Endocrinology
Kainos Superspeciality Hospital
Former Senior Professor and Head
Department of Endocrinology
Postgraduate Institute of Medical Sciences
Rohtak, Haryana, India

Foreword

Susan J Mandel

JAYPEE BROTHERS MEDICAL PUBLISHERS
The Health Sciences Publisher
New Delhi | London

Jaypee Brothers Medical Publishers (P) Ltd

Headquarters
EMCA House
23/23-B, Ansari Road, Daryaganj
New Delhi 110 002, India
Landline: +91-11-23272143, +91-11-23272703
+91-11-23282021, +91-11-23245672
E-mail: jaypee@jaypeebrothers.com

Corporate Office
Jaypee Brothers Medical Publishers (P) Ltd.
4838/24, Ansari Road, Daryaganj
New Delhi 110 002, India
Phone: +91-11-43574357
Fax: +91-11-43574314
E-mail: jaypee@jaypeebrothers.com

Overseas Office
JP Medical Ltd.
83, Victoria Street, London
SW1H 0HW (UK)
Phone: +44-20 3170 8910
Fax: +44(0)20 3008 6180
E-mail: info@jpmedpub.com

Website: www.jaypeebrothers.com
Website: www.jaypeedigital.com

© 2023, Jaypee Brothers Medical Publishers

The views and opinions expressed in this book are solely those of the original contributor(s)/author(s) and do not necessarily represent those of editor(s) or publisher of the book.

All rights reserved by the author. No part of this publication may be reproduced, stored or transmitted in any form or by any means, electronic, mechanical, photocopying, recording or otherwise, without the prior permission in writing of the publishers.

All brand names and product names used in this book are trade names, service marks, trademarks or registered trademarks of their respective owners. The publisher is not associated with any product or vendor mentioned in this book.

Medical knowledge and practice change constantly. This book is designed to provide accurate, authoritative information about the subject matter in question. However, readers are advised to check the most current information available on procedures included and check information from the manufacturer of each product to be administered, to verify the recommended dose, formula, method and duration of administration, adverse effects and contraindications. It is the responsibility of the practitioner to take all appropriate safety precautions. Neither the publisher nor the author(s)/editor(s) assume any liability for any injury and/or damage to persons or property arising from or related to use of material in this book.

This book is sold on the understanding that the publisher is not engaged in providing professional medical services. If such advice or services are required, the services of a competent medical professional should be sought.

Every effort has been made where necessary to contact holders of copyright to obtain permission to reproduce copyright material. If any have been inadvertently overlooked, the publisher will be pleased to make the necessary arrangements at the first opportunity.

Inquiries for bulk sales may be solicited at: jaypee@jaypeebrothers.com

ITS Textbook of Thyroid Disorders / *Sarita Bajaj, Rajesh Rajput*

First Edition: 2023

ISBN: 978-93-5696-114-2

Printed at: SDR Printers

CONTRIBUTORS

EDITORS

Sarita Bajaj MD (Medicine) DM (Endocrinology) FRCP (London, Glasgow and Edinburgh)
Consultant Endocrinologist
Former Director-Professor and Head
Department of Medicine, MLN Medical College
Prayagraj, Uttar Pradesh, India

Rajesh Rajput MD (Medicine) DM (Endocrinology) FRCP (Edinburgh) FACE FICP FIACM FISH FIMSA FRSSDI
Head
Department of Endocrinology
Kainos Superspeciality Hospital
Former Senior Professor and Head
Department of Endocrinology
Postgraduate Institute of Medical Sciences
Rohtak, Haryana, India

SECTION EDITORS

Section 1: Introduction
Sanjay Kalra MD DM
Consultant
Department of Endocrinology
Bharti Research Institute of Diabetes
and Endocrinology (BRIDE)
Karnal, Haryana, India

Section 2: Diagnosis of Thyroid Disorders
KAV Subrahmanyam DM (Endocrinology)
Professor and Head
Department of Endocrinology
Andhra Medical College
Visakhapatnam, Andhra Pradesh, India

Section 3: Hypothyroidism
Narendra Kotwal MD DNB MPhil DM
Professor
Department of Endocrinology
HQ MB AREA
Jabalpur, Madhya Pradesh, India

Section 4: Disorders of Thyroid Hormone Excess
SK Singh MD DM
Professor
Department of Endocrinology and
Metabolism, Institute of Medical
Sciences, Banaras Hindu University
Varanasi, Uttar Pradesh, India

Section 5: Goiter, Thyroid Nodules and Thyroid Cancer
Mahendra Kumar Garg MD (Medicine) DM (Endocrinology) FAMS FICP FUDA
Head, Department of Medicine and Endocrinology
All India Institute of Medical Sciences
Jodhpur, Rajasthan, India

Section 6: Thyroid Disorders in Women
Rakesh K Sahay MD DNB DM
Professor and Head
Department of Endocrinology
Osmania Medical College
Hyderabad, Telangana, India

Section 7: Thyroid Disorders in Children
Mala Dharmalingam MD DM FAMS FACE
Director and Head
Bangalore Endocrinology and Diabetes
Research Center
Bengaluru, Karnataka, India

Section 8: Thyroid Disorders in Special Situations
SK Wangnoo MD (Medicine) DM (Endocrinology) FRCP (London)
Senior Consultant Endocrinologist and
Diabetologist, Apollo Centre for Obesity,
Diabetes and Endocrinology (ACODE)
Indraprastha Apollo Hospital
New Delhi, India

Section 9: Miscellaneous Thyroid Disorders
Manoj Chadha MD DM (Endocrinology)
Consultant Endocrinologist
PD Hinduja Hospital
Mumbai, Maharashtra, India

CONTRIBUTING AUTHORS

Abhishek Krishna MS MCh (Endocrine Surgery)
Assistant Professor
Department of Endocrine Surgery
Sanjay Gandhi Postgraduate Institute of Medical Sciences
Lucknow, Uttar Pradesh, India

Abilash Nair MD (General Medicine) DM (Endocrinology)
Assistant Professor
Department of Endocrinology
Government Medical College
Thiruvananthapuram, Kerala, India

Ajay Tom Francis MBBS
Junior Resident, Department of Surgery
St John's Medical College Hospital
Bengaluru, Karnataka, India

Alok Sachan MD DM (Endocrinology)
Professor and Head
Department of Endocrinology and Metabolism, Sri Venkateswara Institute of Medical Sciences
Tirupati, Andhra Pradesh, India

Ameya Joshi MD DM (Endocrinology)
Consultant In Charge
Department of Endocrinology
Bhaktivedanta Hospital and Research Institute
Thane, Maharashtra, India

Amit Agarwal MS FRCS FACS FICS FNAMS
Director
Department of Endocrine and Breast Surgery, Medanta Hospital
Former Head
Department of Endocrine Surgery
Sanjay Gandhi Postgraduate Institute of Medical Sciences
Lucknow, Uttar Pradesh, India

A Mythili MD DM
Consultant Endocrinologist and Former Professor
Department of Endocrinology
Andhra Medical College
Visakhapatnam, Andhra Pradesh, India

Ananda Mohan Chakraborty MD
Senior Resident
Department of Endocrinology
Postgraduate Institute of Medical Education and Research
Chandigarh, India

Arun S Menon MD CCT (UK, Endocrinology) FRCP
Senior Consultant and Head
Department of Endocrinology
Lisie Hospital
Kochi, Kerala, India

Ashish Sehgal MD DM
Consultant Endocrinologist
Dr Ashish's Clinic
Karnal, Haryana, India

Ashu Rastogi MD DM
Associate Professor
Department of Endocrinology
Postgraduate Institute of Medical Education and Research
Chandigarh, India

Ashwin Valliyot MD (General Medicine)
Senior Resident
Department of Endocrinology
Government Medical College
Thiruvananthapuram, Kerala, India

Beatrice Anne MD DM (Endocrinology) SCE (UK)
Associate Professor and Head
Department of Endocrinology
NIMS Hospital, Punjagutta
Hyderabad, Telangana, India

Bharathi Kolla MD
Senior Resident 2nd Year
Ramaiah Medical College and Hospitals
Bengaluru, Karnataka, India

Chandrakant S Pandav MD MSc
President
Indian Coalition for Control of Iodine Deficiency Disorders
New Delhi, India

Chinnu Mariam MS
Senior Resident
Department of Surgery
St John's Medical College Hospital
Bengaluru, Karnataka, India

CS Bal MD DSc
Professor and Head
Department of Nuclear Medicine
All India Institute of Medical Sciences
New Delhi, India

Deep Dutta DM (Endocrinology) DNB (Endocrinology)
Director Endocrinologist
Department of Endocrinology
CEDAR Superspeciality Clinic
New Delhi, India

Gagan Priya MD DM (Endocrinology and Metabolism)
Senior Consultant
Department of Endocrinology
Fortis Hospital
Mohali, Punjab, India

Ganapathi Bantwal MD DM (Endocrinology) DNB (Endocrinology)
Professor and Head
Department of Endocrinology
St John's National Academy of Health Sciences
Bengaluru, Karnataka, India

Garima Gautam BDS MPH
Senior Research Officer
Indian Coalition for Control of Iodine Deficiency Disorders
New Delhi, India

Gazal Bakshi MD
DrNB Resident
Medanta – The Medcity
Gurugram, Haryana, India

Girish Jeer MD
Senior Resident
Centre for Community Medicine
All India Institute of Medical Sciences
New Delhi, India

CONTRIBUTORS

Gopinath N MD
Senior Resident
Department of Endocrinology
Gauhati Medical College
Guwahati, Assam, India

Himagirish K Rao MCh
Associate Professor
Department of Surgery
St John's Medical College Hospital
Bengaluru, Karnataka, India

Jubbin Jagan Jacob MD (Medicine)
DNB (Endocrinology) MNAMS FRCP
(Edinburgh)
Professor and Head
Department of Endocrinology
Christian Medical College and Hospital
Ludhiana, Punjab, India

K Neelaveni MD (General Medicine)
DM (Endocrinology)
Professor
Department of Endocrinology
Osmania Medical College and Osmania
General Hospital
Hyderabad, Telangana, India

Kripa Elizabeth Cherian MD DM
(Endocrinology) DNB (Endocrinology)
Associate Professor
Department of Endocrinology
Christian Medical College and Hospital
Vellore, Tamil Nadu, India

Krishna G Seshadri MBBS AB Certified
Senior Consultant Endocrinologist and
Diabetologist
Chennai Diabetes and Endocrine Clinic
Apollo Hospitals
Chennai, Tamil Nadu, India

Kunal Thakkar MD DM (Endocrinology)
Consultant Endocrinologist
Sterling Ram Krishna Speciality Hospital
Gandhidham, Gujarat, India

Kapil Yadav MD
Professor
Centre for Community Medicine
All India Institute of Medical Sciences
New Delhi, India

Leena Priyambada MD (Pediatrics)
PDCC (Pediatric Endocrinology)
Consultant Pediatric Endocrinologist
Rainbow Children's Hospital
Hyderabad, Telangana, India

Mayur Parkhi MD DNB DM MNAMS
Senior Research Associate
Department of Histopathology
Postgraduate Institute of Medical
Education and Research
Chandigarh, India

Mini G Pillai MD (General Medicine)
DNB MNAMS (Endocrinology)
Consultant Endocrinologist
Lakshmi Hospital
Kochi, Kerala, India

Mohd Ashraf Ganie MD DM FRCP
Professor
Department of Endocrinology,
Metabolism and Diabetes
Sher-i-Kashmir Institute of Medical
Sciences
Srinagar, Jammu and Kashmir, India

Ch. Mounika Anitha MD DM
(Endocrinology)
Assistant Professor
Department of Endocrinology
Andhra Medical College
Visakhapatnam, Andhra Pradesh, India

Nisha Bhavani MD DNB (Medicine)
DNB (Endocrinology) Fellowship in Pediatric
Endocrinology
Professor, Department of Endocrinology
Amrita Institute of Medical Sciences
Kochi, Kerala, India

Nitin Kapoor MD (Medicine) DM
(Endocrinology) ABBM (USA) Post Doc
Fellowship (Endocrinology) PhD (University of
Melbourne)
Professor and Acting Head (Unit 1)
Department of Endocrinology, Diabetes
and Metabolism
Christian Medical College
Vellore, Tamil Nadu, India
Baker Heart and Diabetes Institute
Melbourne, Victoria, Australia

Pallavi D Rao MRCP (UK)
PG Dip (D&E, London)
Consultant Endocrinologist
Centre for Diabetes and Endocrine
Care
Bengaluru, Karnataka, India

Parjeet Kaur MD DM
Associate Director
Department of Endocrinology and
Diabetes, Medanta – The Medicity
Gurugram, Haryana, India

Partha Pratim Chakraborty
MD (Medicine) DM (Endocrinology)
DNB (Endocrinology) MNAMS FACE FICP
FIACM
Assistant Professor
Department of Endocrinology and
Metabolism
Medical College
Kolkata, West Bengal, India

Paulami Deshmukh
3rd MBBS Student
SKN Medical College
Pune, Maharashtra, India

Pinaki Dutta MD DM
Professor
Department of Endocrinology
Postgraduate Institute of Medical
Education and Research
Chandigarh, India

PK Jabbar MD DNB (Medicine) DM DNB
(Endocrinology) FRCP
Professor and Head
Department of Endocrinology
Government Medical College
Director
Indian Institute of Diabetes
Thiruvananthapuram, Kerala, India

PK Pradhan MD DNB
Professor
Department of Nuclear Medicine
Sanjay Gandhi Postgraduate Institute of
Medical Science
Lucknow, Uttar Pradesh, India

Pradip Mukhopadhyay MD (Medicine) DM (Endocrinology)
Professor
Department of Endocrinology and Metabolism
Institute of Postgraduate Medical Education and Research
Kolkata, West Bengal, India

Pranab Dey MBBS MD MIAC FRC (Pathology)
Professor
Department of Cytology and Gynecological Pathology
Postgraduate Institute of Medical Education and Research
Chandigarh, India

Prasanna Kumar MD DM (Endocrinology)
Senior Consultant Endocrinologist
Centre for Diabetes and Endocrine Care
Bengaluru, Karnataka, India

Pramila Kalra MD DM (Endocrinology) FACE MAMS FRCP (Edinburgh)
Professor and Head
Department of Endocrinology
Ramaiah Medical College and Hospitals
Bengaluru, Karnataka, India

Rajat Gupta MD DM (Endocrinology and Metabolism)
Senior Consultant Endocrinologist
Alchemist Hospital
Panchkula, Haryana, India

Rajesh Rajput MD (Medicine) DM (Endocrinology) FRCP (Edinburgh) FACE FICP FIACM FISH FIMSA FRSSDI
Head, Department of Endocrinology
Kainos Superspeciality Hospital
Former Senior Professor and Head
Department of Endocrinology
Postgraduate Institute of Medical Sciences
Rohtak, Haryana, India

Rakesh K Sahay MD DNB DM
Professor and Head
Department of Endocrinology
Osmania Medical College
Hyderabad, Telangana, India

Rashi Agrawal MD (Pediatrics)
Senior Resident
Department of Endocrinology
Amrita Institute of Medical Sciences
Kochi, Kerala, India

Roma Pradhan MS MCh (Endocrine Surgery – SGPGIMS)
Associate Director
Department of Endocrine and Breast Surgery
Medanta Hospital
Former Head
Department of Endocrine Surgery
Dr Ram Manohar Lohia Institute of Medical Sciences
Lucknow, Uttar Pradesh, India

Sabaretnam Mayilvaganan MS MCh
Additional Professor
Department of Endocrine Surgery
Sanjay Gandhi Postgraduate Institute of Medical Sciences
Lucknow, Uttar Pradesh, India

Sailesh Kumar Bansiwal MD
Senior Resident
Department of Endocrinology and Metabolism
Sher-i-Kashmir Institute of Medical Sciences
Srinagar, Jammu and Kashmir, India

Sanjay Kalra MD DM
Consultant
Department of Endocrinology
Bharti Research Institute of Diabetes and Endocrinology (BRIDE)
Karnal, Haryana, India

Sanjay K Bhadada MD DM (Endocrinology and Metabolism) FAMS
Professor and Head
Department of Endocrinology
Postgraduate Institute of Medical Education and Research
Chandigarh, India

Sarita Bajaj MD (Medicine) DM (Endocrinology) FRCP (London, Glasgow and Edinburgh)
Consultant Endocrinologist
Former Director-Professor and Head
Department of Medicine
MLN Medical College
Prayagraj, Uttar Pradesh, India

Shakun Chaudhary MD DM
Assistant Professor
Department of Endocrinology
Dr Rajendra Prasad Government Medical College Kangra
Tanda, Himachal Pradesh, India

Shashank R Joshi MD DM FICP FACP (USA) FACE (USA) FRCP (London, Glasgow, and Edinburgh) (Padma Shri Awardee)
Consultant Endocrinologist
Joshi Clinic, Lilavati Hospital, Sir HN Reliance and Bhatia Hospitals
Mumbai, Maharashtra, India
Adjunct Faculty JSS Medical College, Mysore and Jaipur National University
Mysore, Karnataka, India
Chair, International Diabetes Federation, South East Asia
President Indian Academy of Diabetes
Past President Association of Physicians of India

Shruthi B MD DM (Endocrinology)
Assistant Professor
Department of Endocrinology and Metabolism, Sri Venkateswara Institute of Medical Sciences
Tirupati, Andhra Pradesh, India

Sindhu Sree Rallapalli MD DM (Endocrinology)
Senior Resident
Department of Endocrinology, Diabetes and Metabolism
Christian Medical College
Vellore, Tamil Nadu, India

Sonali Appaiah MD DM (Endocrinology)
Assistant Professor
Department of Endocrinology
St John's National Academy of Health Sciences
Bengaluru, Karnataka, India

Soumya S MD (Pediatrics) DNB (Pediatrics) DM (Endocrinology) DrNB (Endocrinology)
Consultant Endocrinologist
Indian Institute of Diabetes
Thiruvananthapuram, Kerala, India

Sphoorti P Pai MD DM (Endocrinology)
Consultant Endocrinologist
Nanjappa Multi-Specialty Hospital
Shimoga, Karnataka, India

Subhankar Chatterjee MD (Medicine)
Senior Resident
Department of Endocrinology
Medical College and Hospital
Kolkata, West Bengal, India

Sujoy Ghosh MD (Medicine) DM (Endocrinology) FRCP FACE
Professor
Department of Endocrinology
Institute of Postgraduate Medical Education and Research
Kolkata, West Bengal, India

Sunetra Mondal MD (Medicine) DM (Endocrinology)
Consultant
Department of Endocrinology and Metabolism, Healthworld Hospitals
Durgapur, West Bengal, India

Sunil Kumar Mishra MD (Medicine) DM (Endocrinology)
Senior Director
Division of Endocrinology and Diabetes
Medanta – The Medcity
Gurugram, Haryana, India

Surabhi Puri MD DNB
Senior Resident
Centre for Community Medicine
All India Institute of Medical Sciences
New Delhi, India

Sushil Kumar Gupta MD DNB DM
Professor
Department of Endocrinology
Sanjay Gandhi Postgraduate Institute of Medical Sciences
Lucknow, Uttar Pradesh, India

S Vageesh Ayyar MD (General Medicine) DM (Endocrinology) DNB (Endocrinology, Diabetes and Metabolism)
Endocrinologist and Professor
Department of Endocrinology
St John's Medical College and Hospital
Bengaluru, Karnataka, India

Subhankar Chowdhury DTM&H MD (Medicine) DM (Endocrinology) MRCP
Professor and Head
Department of Endocrinology and Metabolism
Institute of Postgraduate Medical Education and Research (IPGMER) and Seth Sukhlal Karnani Memorial (SSKM) Hospital
Kolkata, West Bengal, India

Thomas V Paul MD DNB (Endocrinology) PhD (Endocrinology)
Professor
Department of Endocrinology
Christian Medical College and Hospital
Vellore, Tamil Nadu, India

Tushar Bandgar MD DM (Endocrinology)
Professor and Head
Department of Endocrinology
Seth GS Medical College and KEM Hospital
Mumbai, Maharashtra, India

Uma Kaimal Saikia MD DM
Professor
Department of Endocrinology
Gauhati Medical College
Guwahati, Assam, India

Uma Nahar Saikia MD (Pathology) NAMS
Professor
Department of Histopathology
Postgraduate Institute of Medical Education and Research
Chandigarh, India

Vaishali Deshmukh MD DNB (Medicine–Gold Medalist) DM (Endocrinology)
Assistant Professor in Endocrinology
Sassoon General Hospital
Consultant and Head of Endocrinology
Deenanath Mangeshkar Hospital and Research Centre
Director, Deshmukh Clinic and Research Centre
Pune, Maharashtra, India

Vasundhara Rajput MBBS
Final Year Student
Kasturba Medical College
Manipal, Karnataka, India

Vijaya Sarathi MD DM (Endocrinology)
Professor and Head
Department of Endocrinology
Vydehi Institute of Medical Sciences and Research Center
Bengaluru, Karnataka, India

Vijay Singh MD
Senior Resident, Department of Nuclear Medicine, Sanjay Gandhi Postgraduate Institute of Medical Sciences
Lucknow, Uttar Pradesh, India

RV Jayakumar MD DM MNAMS FRCP
Senior Consultant
Department of Endocrinology
Aster Medcity and Caritas Hospital
Kochi, Kerala, India

FOREWORD

This comprehensive volume, which focuses on thyroidology, is a welcome addition to our medical libraries. It has been developed to provide practitioners with comprehensive and current information about thyroid diseases and the many manifestations of thyroid disorders in patients. The editors, who are members of the Indian Thyroid Society, have assembled these chapters with the primary care physician in mind, and they succeed in providing valuable learnings for the entire spectrum of learners, from specialist endocrinologists to the physicians in training and students at all levels.

Thyroid disorders are common. The organization of the material builds a foundation of knowledge, beginning with the intriguing history of the thyroid gland, and progression through its structural development and physiological function and regulation. To diagnose thyroid disorders, the next chapters then clearly outline the key testing modalities available to clinicians, focusing on evidence based usage.

Subsequent sections guide the learner through the common clinical scenarios of thyroid dysfunction, hypo- and hyperthyroidism, focusing on clinical approach, diagnosis, and treatment. However, thyroid dysfunction can have pleiomorphic manifestations in patients and rarer presentations of common disorders are also presented and discussed. Importantly, there are chapters devoted to hypo- and hyperthyroidism in pregnancy, and recommendations for optimal gestational care—a time when the clinician is actually responsible for two people, the mother and fetus, rather than one patient.

The sections on special situations and miscellaneous topics address clinical scenarios that range from the common (subclinical thyroid disease and thyroid nodules) to the uncommon (resistance to thyroid hormone and anaplastic thyroid cancer). Each topic is presented clearly, with review of recent literature, and a rational, evidence-based approach to the care of patients. Clinicians who are hospital based will find the information on nonthyroidal illness, drugs interference with thyroid function, and thyroid emergencies very relevant to their practices. Our most current knowledge of how COVID-19 affects the thyroid is also included.

The thoughtful, deliberate, and thorough coverage of each topic in this book makes it relevant to all interested learners in clinical practice. I congratulate the editors and the authors and I encourage the readers to explore this text in its fullness.

Susan J Mandel MD MPH
Chief, Division of Endocrinology, Diabetes, and Metabolism
Professor of Medicine, Perelman School of Medicine, University of Pennsylvania

PREFACE

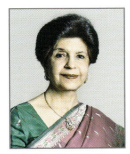
Sarita Bajaj

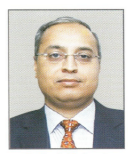
Rajesh Rajput

Advances in thyroid science and practice continue at a breathtaking rate and it is important to keep up with the progress in this field. The first edition of "*ITS Textbook of Thyroid Disorders*" retains the fundamental nature to provide a concise but comprehensive and fully updated treatise on thyroidology covering the breadth of thyroid practice, stressing the Indian perspective, highlighting new advances, and their potential to transform the established paradigms of prevention, diagnosis, and treatment.

There are very few books which are truly created with the working primary care physician in mind. Therefore, while this book is written by the leading endocrine and medical specialists we have taken pains to design the book to provide endocrinologists, family practitioners, internists, physicians in training, and students at all levels with what is needed to keep abreast to rapidly changing scientific foundations in clinical research, result, and evidence-based medical practice in thyroid health.

The chapters are written by clinicians and basic scientists from a variety of fields. The book makes abundant use of four-color illustrations, tabular material, and particularly algorithms for evaluating the functions of different systems and the diseases of those systems.

This textbook allows the reader to quickly identify and understand topics of interest which translates into very practical treatment planning. Our authors who are pioneers in the field of endocrinology present relevant pathophysiology with practical protocols for evaluation and treatment. The target audience continues to be any health professional who desires a rapid answer to any challenging question in thyroidology including endocrinologists, diabetologists, endocrine surgeons, general practitioners, and students of medicine.

The book is divided into nine sections arranging closely related subjects into clusters. There are a total of 38 chapters. *Section 1* commences with introduction to thyroid disorders, *Section 2* discusses the diagnostic approaches, *Section 3* highlights all aspects of hypothyroidism, *Section 4* encompasses disorders of thyroid hormone excess, *Section 5* elaborates the entire spectrum of goiter, thyroid nodules and thyroid cancer, *Section 6* focuses on thyroid disorders in women, *Section 7* is exclusively devoted to thyroid disorders in children while *Sections 8* and *9* address thyroid disorders in special situations and miscellaneous thyroid topics.

We were extremely fortunate to attract contributors who are renowned as authors and researchers, and who are most importantly consummate physicians. We thank all of them for their diligence, intellectual approach, and clinical acumen without which this volume would not have been possible. We would like to express our gratitude to all the authors and section editors who have balanced their many other obligations to prepare truly masterful presentations and for the large amount of work in reviewing and commenting on the chapters.

And although this book was written for clinicians, it is our hope that the millions of patients with thyroid disease will be the primary beneficiaries. It is therefore, with great humility that we have the distinct honor to be the editors of the first edition of the "*ITS Textbook of Thyroid Disorders*".

Sarita Bajaj
Rajesh Rajput

ACKNOWLEDGMENTS

Publishing *"ITS Textbook of Thyroid Disorders"* is in every way a collaborative effort. We are deeply indebted to the executive committee of Indian Thyroid Society, Dr Pramila Kalra, Dr Arun S Menon, Dr Shashank R Joshi, Dr Mohd Ashraf Ganie, Dr Himagirish K Rao, Dr Krishna G Seshadri, Dr Sujoy Ghosh, Dr Mini G Pillai, Dr PK Jabbar, Dr Sushil Kumar Gupta, and section editors—Dr Sanjay Kalra, Dr KAV Subrahmanyam, Dr Narendra Kotwal, Dr SK Singh, Dr Mahendra Kumar Garg, Dr Rakesh K Sahay, Dr Mala Dharmalingam, Dr SK Wangnoo, Dr Manoj Chadha who have each made major contributions in edition and writing chapters as well as for their considerable time, effort, and commitment to maintaining the high standards of the textbook. Special thanks to our patrons Dr RV Jayakumar and Dr Prasanna Kumar for their constant support and encouragement.

We have assembled an outstanding group of authors, all recognized as leaders in their field and we would like to thank them for taking the time away from their busy clinical schedules and other academic responsibilities to write these chapters.

We are immensely grateful to Dr Susan J Mandel for the Foreword.

We would also like to thank the editorial staff at Jaypee Brothers Medical Publishers (P) Ltd, New Delhi, India, for their patience, encouragement, and support. We particularly thank Ms Chetna Malhotra (Senior Director – Professional Publishing, Marketing and Business Development), Ms Pooja Bhandari (Production Head), Ms Nedup Bhutia Pillai (Team Leader – Print Publishing) and entire team who has contributed in a very significant way to the concepts, design, and preparation of the 1st edition of *"ITS Textbook of Thyroid Disorders."* Our special thanks to Shri Jitender P Vij (Group Chairman), Mr MS Mani (Group President), and Mr Ankit Vij (Managing Director) for their help in publishing this book.

CONTENTS

SECTION 1: INTRODUCTION

1. **History of the Thyroid** — 3
   Pallavi D Rao, Prasanna Kumar

2. **Anatomy of Thyroid Gland** — 8
   Sabaretnam Mayilvaganan, Vijaya Sarathi

3. **Physiology of Thyroid Gland** — 12
   Alok Sachan, Shruthi B

SECTION 2: DIAGNOSIS OF THYROID DISORDERS

4. **Clinical Evaluation of Thyroid** — 19
   Parjeet Kaur

5. **Laboratory Evaluation of Thyroid Functions** — 22
   Arun S Menon, RV Jayakumar

6. **Thyroid Imaging from an Endocrinologist's Perspective** — 29
   Ganapathi Bantwal, Sonali Appaiah

7. **Nuclear Imaging in Thyroid Disorders** — 43
   Vijay Singh, CS Bal, PK Pradhan

8. **Clinical and Pathological Aspect of Benign and Malignant Thyroid Nodules** — 57
   Uma Nahar Saikia, Pranab Dey, Pinaki Dutta, Mayur Parkhi, Ananda Mohan Chakraborty

SECTION 3: HYPOTHYROIDISM

9. **Hypothyroidism in Adults** — 89
   Sarita Bajaj

10. **Refractory Hypothyroidism** — 98
    Soumya S, PK Jabbar

11. **Hypothyroidism and Associated Comorbidities** — 103
    Sphoorti P Pai, S Vageesh Ayyar

SECTION 4: DISORDERS OF THYROID HORMONE EXCESS

12. **Clinical Evaluation and Manifestations of Thyroid Hormone Excess** — 113
    Mini G Pillai, Abilash Nair, Ashwin Valliyot

13. **Management of Thyroid Hormone Excess** — 119
    K Neelaveni, Beatrice Anne

14. **Rare Forms of Thyroid Hormone Excess** — 128
    Subhankar Chowdhury, Partha Pratim Chakraborty

15. **Thyroid-associated Orbitopathy** — 138
    Jubbin Jagan Jacob

SECTION 5: GOITER, THYROID NODULES AND THYROID CANCER

16. **Simple or Nontoxic Goiter** — 149
    Sushil Kumar Gupta, Sabaretnam Mayilvaganan

17. **Nodular Thyroid Disease** — 155
    Krishna G Seshadri

18. **Thyroid Carcinoma** — 172
    Gazal Bakshi, Sunil Kumar Mishra

19. **Surgery in Differentiated Thyroid Cancers** — 180
    Abhishek Krishna, Roma Pradhan, Amit Agarwal

20. **Surgery in Poorly Differentiated and Anaplastic Thyroid Carcinoma** — 188
    Himagirish K Rao, Chinnu Mariam, Ajay Tom Francis

SECTION 6: THYROID DISORDERS IN WOMEN

21. **Thyroid and Reproduction** — 197
    Gagan Priya

22. **Hypothyroidism and Pregnancy** — 206
    Rajesh Rajput, Ashish Sehgal, Vasundhara Rajput

23. **Thyroid Excess in Pregnancy** — 211
    Mohd Ashraf Ganie, Sailesh Kumar Bansiwal

SECTION 7: THYROID DISORDERS IN CHILDREN

24. **Congenital Hypothyroidism** — 219
    Sunetra Mondal, Pradip Mukhopadhyay, Sujoy Ghosh

25. Hypothyroidism in Children — 228
Rashi Agrawal, Nisha Bhavani

26. Hyperthyroidism in Children, Adolescents, and Neonates — 234
Leena Priyambada

27. Thyroid Nodules in Children — 243
Shakun Chaudhary, Ashu Rastogi

SECTION 8: THYROID DISORDERS IN SPECIAL SITUATIONS

28. Subclinical Hypothyroidism — 251
Pramila Kalra, Bharathi Kolla

29. Thyroid and Obesity: Coexisting Perplexity — 257
Sindhu Sree Rallapalli, Nitin Kapoor

30. Nonthyroidal Illness Syndrome — 262
Rakesh K Sahay, Ameya Joshi

31. Drugs and Other Substances Interfering with Thyroid Function — 265
Kunal Thakkar, Tushar Bandgar

32. Thyroid Emergencies — 272
A Mythili, Ch. Mounika Anitha

SECTION 9: MISCELLANEOUS THYROID DISORDERS

33. Thyroiditis — 281
Subhankar Chatterjee, Deep Dutta

34. Thyroid and Coronavirus Disease 2019 — 288
Vaishali Deshmukh, Paulami Deshmukh, Shashank R Joshi

35. Sustaining Elimination of Iodine Deficiency Disorders in India — 299
Kapil Yadav, Surabhi Puri, Girish Jeer, Garima Gautam, Chandrakant S Pandav

36. Thyroid and Bone — 307
Sanjay K Bhadada, Rajat Gupta

37. Thyroid Hormone Resistance — 310
Kripa Elizabeth Cherian, Thomas V Paul

38. Environmental Thyroid Disruptors — 315
Uma Kaimal Saikia, Sanjay Kalra, Gopinath N

Index — 319

SECTION 1

Introduction

CHAPTER 1

History of the Thyroid

Pallavi D Rao, Prasanna Kumar

INTRODUCTION

Goiters have been common all over the world. Since prehistoric times, they have been objects of curiosity. Through the years people have tried to study them, understand them, and find a cure for them. Goiters have been depicted in various paintings and mentioned in historical records through the ages. In this chapter, we look at the history of events in relation to thyroid disorders. Although we have been treating thyroid disorders with thyroxine, antithyroid medicines, and surgery for the last few decades only, physicians, healers, and philosophers over the years had been trying may a time to come up with explanations for disorders of the thyroid gland. Physicians all across the globe have tried various ointments or sea weeds or sponges in their practices independently through the ages. In this chapter, we look at the understanding of thyroidal illness and its treatment through the age, all across the globe.

PREHISTORIC AND ANCIENT TIMES

Enlarged thyroids are said to have been known in ancient China and India. It is one of the most common medical problems portrayed in ancient paintings. Chinese have described enlarged thyroids around 2700 BC and seem to have used burnt sponge and seaweed to treat it since 1600 BC.

Goiters have been portrayed in sculptures of the ancient Gandhara civilization, which date back to the 1st or 2nd century AD. In *Ayurveda*, goiters have been described in detail as galaganda. Thyroid diseases are classified into three types: (1) *Vataja* (hyperthyroidism), (2) *Kaphaja* (hypothyroidism), and *Medaja* (thyroid cyst). The symptoms of these diseases have been described in detail in *Ayurvedic* medicine and correlate with those described by modern medicine. Charaka said that ingesting adequate quantities of milk, rice, barley, green grams, sugarcane juice, and cucumber would prevent hypothyroidism. His belief was that consuming sour foods would aggravate thyroid diseases. Various herbs have been used over the ages and still continue to be prescribed for all sorts of thyroid problems. *Guggulu* (*Commiphora mukul*), a herb is used to increase basal metabolic rate in hypothyroid patients. *Punarnava* (*Boerhaavia diffusa* Linn), which is a diuretic, is prescribed to reduce the swelling in thyroid diseases.

To treat hyperthyroid patients, bugleweed (*Lycopus virginicus*), gypsywort (*Lycopus europaeus*), water horehound (*Lycopus lucidus* or *Lycopus americanus*), gromwell (*Lithospermum ruderale*), and European gromwell (*Lithospermum officinale*) are used. Ancient Indian physicians also recognized pitting and nonpitting edema, and facial and pedal edema. However, they were of the opinion that the edema caused goiter, rather than an underactive thyroid gland leading to goiter.

The God Bes of ancient Egypt is usually depicted as a dwarf but it has not been conclusively determined whether he suffered from myxedematosis or achondroplasty. Also, Cleopatra has been depicted with what could be an enlarged thyroid.

In his book de Glandulis, Hippocrates (460–337 BC) seems to have mentioned the thyroid when he writes about the glands in the neck becoming tubercular and producing stroma when they are diseased. Also, in the Hippocratic writings of the 4th century BC, we come across the term "choiron". This term was used by Paul of Aegina, a 7th century Byzantine Greek physician and most probably signified goiter as well as the word Gongronema.

THE GRECO-ROMAN PERIOD (156 BC–AD 576)

During the Hellenistic and Roman periods, goiter was simply regarded as a deformity and was attributed to the drinking of snow water. At the time of the early Roman Empire two very famous though nonprofessional physicians, namely Celsus and Pliny described thyroid abnormalities.

Aurelius Celsus (25 BC–AD 50) differentiated between the various forms of tumors of the neck. He defined the enlargement of the neck as bronchocele, being fleshy and containing some sort of honey-like substance.

Gaius Plinius Secundus of Pliny (23 BC–AD 79) believed that goiter was caused by dirty water. The Chinese physician Tshui Chin-thi, in AD 85, differentiated between solid (malignant) neck tumors, which were incurable, and movable (benign) ones, which were curable.

Chinese alchemist Ko Hung around AD 340 recommended treatment of goiters with an alcoholic extract of seaweed. Goiter was described as being associated with certain mountainous regions in Chinese medicine from at least the 5th century AD onward.

THE BYZANTINE PERIOD (330–AD 1453)

Bsyzantine physicians in the 8th century had recognized exophthalmos with its associated symptoms of nervousness and changes in the mood. They had even mentioned that these people with eye problems, nervousness, and mood changes were unfit to work. Similarly Avicenna and Al-Jurjani, two Persian physicians from the 12th century, described that a swollen neck is closely associated with eye disease. They also have opined that both these diseases formed a single clinical entity, and were associated with increased appetite in which people did not feel full despite eating large quantities of food. They felt that weakness of the extraocular muscles to be the cause of protrusion of eyes.

Around 550, Aetios, a prominent physician of these times, described goitrous enlargement of the neck and apparently regarded exophthalmic goiter as a variety of aneurysm.

In 1110, a Persian doctor, Jurjani, associated exophthalmos with goiter. In AD 1170, Roger of Palermo prescribed ashes of sponges and seaweed to treat goiter. Marco Polo wrote about the province of Karkan as follows: "the inhabitants are in general afflicted with swellings in the legs and tumors in the throat occasioned by the quality of the water they drink".

During the 14th century, various doctors from various countries, including China and Italy treated goiters with products such as sea sponges, seaweeds, and mollusks. These were sometimes mixed with saltpeter or antimony.

THE RENAISSANCE TO THE PRESENT

Many physicians and surgeons across the globe over these years seem to have tried treating goiters with various products like powder of dried pig's glands, (Chinese Wang His in 1475) and ointments.

In 1656, the exact anatomical structure of the thyroid gland along with the other glands of the body was discovered by Thomas Wharton (1614–1673) a famous anatomist. He gave the thyroid its modern name in his book Adenographia. He explained that the glands primary function was to secrete. He was of the opinion that the thyroid gland was responsible for heating the thyroid cartilage, lubricate the neck, and also gave the round shape and to the neck and hence beautify the neck. The gland was named thyroid, because it looked very much like the shield shape of the thyroid cartilage of the larynx.

De Bordeu felt that each organ in the body gave off certain "emanations". These emanations were necessary as well as useful for the body. He noted that goiter was common in regions to the West of the Pyrenees mountains (between France and Spain). He also observed that larger thyroids were more commonly seen in women in comparison to men. Also, women seemed to suffer more frequently from ailments of the gland, in comparison to men. De Bordeu also associated goiter with changes in voice. In 1776, von Haller of Bern (Switzerland) described the thyroid along with the thymus and spleen, to be ductless glands which poured their special secretions into the bloodstream.

The German–Swiss alchemist and physician Paracelsus (1453–1541) attributed goiter to occur due to mineral impurities in drinking water, especially iron sulfide. He postulated a hereditary factor as well. Andreas Vesalius (1514–1564) described the thyroid gland in great detail, and B Eustachius (1520–1547) was the first to use the term isthmus for the part of the gland connecting the two lobes of the gland.

The two lobes of the thyroid gland and the isthmus were described by Morgagni, the founder of modern pathological anatomy. The pyramidal lobe, however, had been described earlier by Lalouette. Between 1772 and 1802, exophthalmos, palpitations, and goiter were described as being associated with goiters. Exophthalmic goiter was connected with "malady of the heart", protrusion of the eyes and "bronchocele" by Caleb Hillier Parry (1775–1822) in 1786. Even though he was unaware of the association of these three diseases, Giuseppe Flajani successfully cured a man with exophthalmos, goiter, and palpitations in 1802 by compressing the swelling in the neck of such a patient with vinegar and ammonia and he reported disappearance of the swelling within 4 months.

A remarkable discovery occurred at the beginning of the 19th century when iodine was discovered by Bernard Courtois (1771–1838) in Paris in the year 1811. The first person to use it to treat goiter was Coindet of Geneva. He prescribed hydriodate of potash or "tincture of iodine" to successfully treat thyroidal swelling. The toxic effects of iodine were also described as "constitutional iodism" by Rilliet of Geneva.

Subsequently, numerous physicians around the globe described treatment of goiters with iodine. In 1885, the edition of Hirsch's classic pathology text mentioned that goiter and cretinism had to be reckoned among the infective diseases and treating these disorders with iodine was recommended.

Eugen Baumann, a scientist in the 19th century, discovered that high levels of iodine were present in a precipitate that he obtained by boiling the thyroid glands of

1,000 sheep in dilute sulfuric acid. He named this precipitate "iodothyrin". This when used to treat patients with goiter and showed very good results.

In 1877, Theodor Billroth noted that iodine, although beneficial in the early stages of goiter, was in fact ineffective for the same in its established form. Fugen Bauman (1846–1896) in 1896, showed iodine was present in organic combination as a normal constituent of the thyroid gland. The first few years of the 19th century saw descriptions of the different types of goiters: cystic, hyperplastic, etc.

James Berry in London, at the beginning of the 20th century, described six types of goiter:
1. Parenchymatous, occurring in young people usually
2. Wolfer's fetal adenoma, usually small, solid, and encapsulated
3. Cystic adenoma
4. Fibrous
5. Malignant
6. Exophthalmic

G Crile in the US in 1910 wrote about three types of simple goiter: (1) hypertrophy, (2) hyperplasia, and (3) involution. Selwyn Taylor in London in the year 1953 described five stages in the evolution of the glandular problem.

Robert James Graves, the famous Irish physician, in 1835, wrote about palpitations and thyroid enlargement in some of his patients. Also in the mid-19th century in Merseburg, the German physician, Carl Adolph von Basedow, wrote about three of his patients who suffered from exophthalmos due to hypertrophy of the cellular tissue of the orbit, goiter, and palpitations. This syndrome subsequently came to be known as the Merseburg triad syndrome. However, history shows that older civilizations were well aware of this condition. Mentions of this disease are found in works of Aristotle and Xenophon from the 5th century BC.

Special credit should go to CH Parry who, in 1813, wrote "some connection between the malady of the heart and the bronchocele".

The first description of thyroid diseases as we know today was that of Graves' disease by Caleb Parry in 1786, but the pathogenesis of thyroid disease was not discovered until 1882–86. Thyroidectomy for hyperthyroidism was first performed in 1880, and antithyroid drugs and radioiodine therapy were developed in the early 1940s. Thomas Curling first described hypothyroidism (myxedema and/or cretinism) in 1850 and the cause and suitable treatment were established after 1883.

Myxedema and/or cretinism was described in detail and connection of these symptoms to dysfunction of the thyroid gland was made by Curling in 1850, Gull in 1873, and Ord in 1871. They described the differences between sporadic and endemic cretinism. Sir Horsley, between 1884 and 1886, when working on monkeys, found that thyroidectomy led to myxedema and cretinism in the animals.

Public health and study of thyroid disorders came together in the 19th century. In 1833, iodization of salt was suggested by Boussingault to prevent goiter. Chatin (1803–1901) proved in 1850 that iodine could prevent endemic goiter and cretinism. He correlated thyroid disorders with iodine deficiency. He also suggested supplementing iodine in drinking water and using mineral water springs. In 1835, Cahtin showed that use of salt sent from goiter-free regions in regions with endemic goiter reduced the incidence of goiter.

In 1907, David Marine (1880–1976), also known as the Nestor of Thyroidology, proved that iodine was necessary for thyroid function. He treated Graves' disease with iodine. 10 years later, he introduced prevention of goiter with iodine, by using low doses of iodine. In 1932, he wrote about cyanide goiter which developed due to consumption of thiocyanates found in plants of the genus Brassicaceae (cabbage, cauliflower, and turnip).

The first to use thyroid extract to treat were Horsley and Murray. Many were very sceptical about the use of sheep's thyroid in humans though. However, thyroid extract soon became an accepted part of medical practice.

Thyroid preparations were administered both orally and as injectables by various people as treatment. It was Adolf Oswald who identified thyroid colloid protein as thyroglobulin. In 1914, Kendall was able to isolate crystals of thyroxine. It took 3 tons of porcine thyroids to be able to make 33 g of pure thyroxine. More cost-effective methods of extraction were subsequently devised, which reduced the cost of manufacturing. It was in 1927 that synthetic thyroxine was made by Harington and Barger.

Triiodothyronine was discovered by gross and Pitt-Rivers in 1952. Next few years saw further advances in the study of thyroid disorders and in 1956, Roitt, Doniach, Campbell, and Hudson demonstrated autoantibodies to thyroid in Hashimoto's disease. This however, was 44 years after Hakaru Hashimoto (1881–1934) had described Hashimoto's thyroiditis as lymphoid infiltration of the thyroid.

Along with developments in the diagnosis, advancements in clinical thyroidology were also seen in the 20th century. Charles Mayo in 1907, first used the term hyperthyroidism for an over active thyroid gland. In the same year, Brissaud described thyroid infantilism. In 1931, Naffziger orbital decompression was performed to treat exophthalmos.

In 1911, Marine used iodine to treat Graves' disease. Iodine was also used for preoperative management of exophthalmic goiter by Plummer and Boothby in 1924. In the year 1943, radioactive iodine was used to treat Graves' disease, independently, by Hertz and Roberts, as well as Leblond.

Thiourea and thiouracil were used by Astwood in 1943 to treat Graves' disease. In 1949, methimazole was synthesized by Jones, Kornfeld, McLaughlin, and Anderson. In 1951,

Lawson, Rimington, and Searle synthesized carbimazole. Commercial synthesis of levothyroxine was successfully done in 1949.

Edward Kendall isolated the pure form of thyroxine in 1914, after 4 years of working at it. It took him another 3 years to isolate enough crystals of thyroxine to begin clinical trials on them. Believing it was an oxindole, he coined the term "thyroxin". This was later changed to thyroxine. Charles Harington synthetically prepared a compound by condensation of two molecules of diiodotyrosine after another few years in 1927. This compound was seen to have properties similar to that of thyroxine. This was how the exact structure of thyroxine was discovered.

Jack Gross and Rosalind Pitt-Rivers in 1952 detected the presence of a more potent thyroid hormone while using radioactive iodine and carrying out research on mice. This compound differed from thyroxine in having three iodine atoms instead of four. It was named "liothyronine". This was later changed to triiodothyronine.

SURGICAL TREATMENT OF THYROID DISEASE

Briefly referring to the surgical treatment of thyroid disease.

Early accounts of operations are unclear. In the Greco-Roman period, Aurelius Celsus clearly defined cystic goiters and recommended making an incision down to the cyst, which then to be bluntly dissected and removed. If that was not possible, he advised it be destroyed with caustics.

Aetios around the year 550 quoted a Greek surgeon, named Leonidas, who had recognized very early the importance of avoiding injury to the vocal nerves (recurrent laryngeal) during operations. Persian surgeon Ali Ibn Abbas in 990, dealt with surgery of the goiter in his treatise. Albucasis (1013-1106) successfully operated on a patient with what he described as elephantiasis of the throat, which was in fact a goiter.

In the 12th century, the Bamberg Surgery was published. In this book, removal of the goiter has been described in detail, in a manner similar to that being performed in modern times.

In 1656, Wharton named the gland "thyroid", because of the gland's proximity to the thyroid cartilage. Rare attempts were made at thyroidectomy early on, mainly to prevent suffocation due to goiter with little success. Mortality rate from the surgery was as high as 40%.

In the 14th century, the French surgeon Guy de Chauliac (1300-1370) reported goiter to be a local and hereditary disease, and recommended surgical removal of the thyroid gland.

Surgeons across the globe recommended surgical removal of the thyroid gland in the 15th century as did L Heister (1683-1758) the founder of scientific surgery in Germany and Ambroise Pare, a French barber surgeon in 1561.

The first known thyroidectomy was described by Wilhelm Fabricius in Geneva in the year 1646. Christian Albert Theodor Billroth also made significant contributions to thyroid surgery. The first well-documented partial thyroidectomy for a tumor of the thyroid was in 1789, by PS Dessault (1744-1795) in Paris. A few years later, in 1808, Guillaume Dupuytren (1777-1835) performed a total thyroidectomy for a tumor of the gland. In 1880, Ludwig Rehn (1847-1930) carried out the first successful removal of the thyroid gland for exophthalmic goiter.

Around the year 1850, thyroid surgery was performed for a few vital indications only, as the mortality rate from this surgery was often as high as 40%. The reason for death was usually uncontrollable bleeding or infection. Few European surgeons, including Emil Theodor Kocher and Billroth, started to improve surgery and report their results. Kocher innovated the use of silk sutures and asepsis in surgery apart from thyroid surgery. As a result, in 1883 mortality rate from Kocher's patients was only 13%.

Kocher, the Swiss surgeon was the most notable surgeon of the 20th century, and is also considered the father of thyroid surgery. He was awarded the Nobel Prize in Medicine or Physiology in 1909, for his work in thyroidology. He observed postoperative hypothyroidism in his thyroidectomy patients. Till date, he remains the only winner of the Nobel Prize for work done in thyroidology.

Also, around this time other complications from thyroid surgery were recognized. Particularly damage to the recurrent laryngeal nerve, causing hoarseness. It was soon understood that it was important to preserve this nerve during surgery. The complications of tetany and hypoparathyroidism, however, were not understood. Kocher in contrast to Billroth had a very neat and precise operating technique and worked in a relatively bloodless field. This was probably the reason he had less problems with postoperative tetany. Also well known to all thyroid surgeons is the "Kocher incision", a slightly curved transverse incision about 2 cm above the sternoclavicular joints.

CONCLUSION

Although the thyroid gland and treatment of its disorders have only recently been understood, we have all the scientists, physicians, and surgeons through the ages to thank for to get us to where we are right now. If not for all their experimentation and research, our understanding would not be the same. May be in the future, we will improve on our understanding and treatment protocols further in order to be able to replace the deficiency states much better, without many fluctuations in thyroid-stimulating hormone (TSH) levels and help our patients better.

SUGGESTED READINGS

1. Niazi AK, Kalra S, Irfan A, Islam A. Thyroidology over the ages. Indian J Endocrinol Metab. 2011;15(Suppl 2):S121-S126.
2. Kalra S. Endocrinology in Ayurveda: Modern Science, Ancient history. Indian J Endocrinol Metab. 2011. [In press].
3. Marketos S, Eftychiadis A, Koutras DA. Thyroid diseases in the Byzantine era. JR Soc Med. 1990;83:111-3.
4. Nabipour I, Burger A, Moharreri MR, Azizi F. Avicenna, the first to describe thyroid-related orbitopathy. Thyroid. 2009;19:7-8.
5. Rolleston HD. The endocrine glands with an historical review. London: H Milford; Oxford University Press; 1936. p. 142.
6. Rolleston HD. The Endocrine Organs in Health and Disease. London: H Milford; Oxford University Press; 1936. p. 16.
7. Medvei VC. A History of Endocrinology. Lancaster: MTP Press; 1982. pp. 289-96.
8. Coindet JF. Découverte d'un nouveau remède contre le goître. Ann Chim Phys. 1820;15:49-59.
9. Boussingault JB. Recherches sur la cause qui produit le goître dans les Cordilieres de la Nouvelle-Grenade. Ann Chim Phys. 1833;48:41-69.
10. Flajani G. Collezione d'osservazione e riflessioni di chirurgia. Sopra un tumor freddo nell anterior partedell collo detto bronchocele. Rome: Michele A Ripa Presso Lino Contedini; 1802. p. 270.
11. Rilliet F. Constititutional iodism. Bull Acad Med. 1859;25:382.
12. Hirsch A. Handbook of historical and geographical pathology. London: New Sydenham Society; 1985.
13. Kendall EC. Isolation of the Iodine Compound which Occurs in the Thyroid. J Biol Chem. 1919;39:125.
14. Harington CR, Barger G. Chemistry of Thyroxine. III. Constitiution and synthesis of thyroxine. Biochem J. 1927;21:169-83.
15. Roitt IM, Doniach D, Campbell PN, Hudson RV. Autoantibodies in Hashimoto's disease (lymphadenoid goiter). Lancet. 1956;2:820-1.
16. Hashimoto H. Zur Kenntnis der lympho matosen Verendering der Schilddruese (Struma lymphomatosa). Arch Klin Chir. 1912;97:219-48.
17. Kendall EC. The isolation in crystalline form of the compound containing iodine which occurs in the thyroid: Its chemical structure and physiological activity. Trans Assoc Am Physicians. 1915;30:420-9.
18. King TW. Observations in the Thyroid gland. Guys Hosp Rep. 1836;1:429-46.

CHAPTER 2

Anatomy of Thyroid Gland

Sabaretnam Mayilvaganan, Vijaya Sarathi

INTRODUCTION

The thyroid gland is the first endocrine organ to develop in a fetus which emphasizes its importance for optimal fetal development. Developmental anomalies of the thyroid gland (agenesis or ectopia) are the most common causes of *congenital hypothyroidism*. Thyroid surgeries are one of the commonly performed surgical procedures and are often associated with injury to recurrent laryngeal nerve and hypoparathyroidism. In-depth knowledge of anatomy of the thyroid gland, especially its structural relation to recurrent and superior laryngeal nerves and parathyroid glands is essential. This chapter reviews the pertinent anatomy and some embryological aspects of the thyroid which shall aid in the appropriate identification and preservation of these structures during safe thyroid surgery.

EMBRYOLOGY OF THYROID GLAND

The thyroid gland is derived from two main structures—primitive pharynx (medial anlage) and neural crest (lateral anlagen). The development of the thyroid gland begins by the late third week of gestation from the pharyngeal endoderm (first and second pharyngeal pouches) at the foramen cecum to form the medial anlage (thyroid bud) **(Fig. 1A)**. This is the source of follicular cells and gives rise to most of the thyroid gland. Thyroid bud starts migrating by the fourth week of gestation anterior to the pharyngeal gut along with it the thyroglossal duct **(Figs. 1B and C)**. By the fifth week, superior part of the thyroglossal duct degenerates and the thyroid gland acquires its rudimentary shape (two lateral lobes connected by an isthmus) **(Fig. 1D)**. Further descent till the level of cricoid cartilage occurs by the seventh week of gestation **(Fig. 1E)**. The distal part of the thyroglossal duct usually degenerates but may persist as pyramidal lobe **(Fig. 1E)**. The lateral anlagen, derived from the fifth pharyngeal pouch (ultimobranchial body), develops fifth week of gestation and migrate to fuse with medial anlage by 7–8 weeks of gestation **(Fig. 1E)**. It contains cells from neural crest and gives rise to parafollicular C cells that secrete calcitonin. Thyroid folliculogenesis begins by the tenth week of gestation and thyroid hormone synthesis by 12 weeks of gestation.

CONGENITAL ANOMALIES OF THYROID GLAND

Complete (aplasia) or partial (hypoplasia) congenital absence of the thyroid gland may result from defects in the development of thyroid gland. Failure to migrate during the developmental process may result in ectopic thyroid gland, most commonly just below the foramen cecum (lingual thyroid). Failure to involute the thyroglossal duct may result in its persistence as thyroglossal cyst. Thyroglossal cyst may rarely rupture and lead to a thyroglossal fistula.

THYROID GLAND SHAPE AND SIZE

A butterfly-shaped (shield-like) gland in the anterior part of the neck consists of two lateral lobes which are united

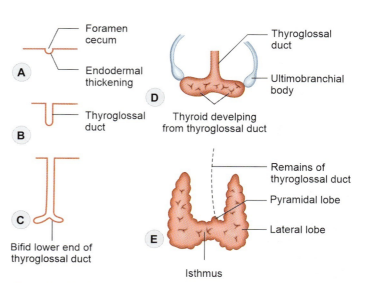

Figs. 1A to E: Embryogenesis of thyroid gland.

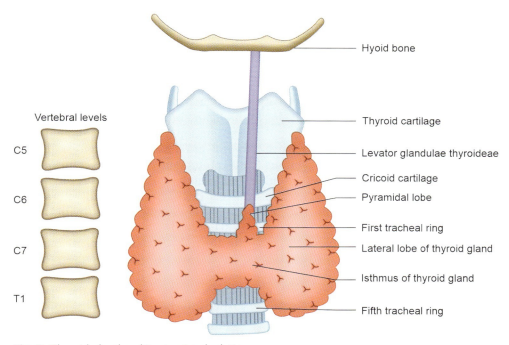

Fig. 2: Thyroid gland and its structural relations.

by an isthmus located anterior to the trachea and weighs ~15–25 g in adults. The lobe measures 4 cm × 2 cm × 3 cm and can be markedly altered in some thyroid diseases. The gland is covered by a thin capsule and the lobes are located between the trachea and larynx medially and carotid artery and sternocleidomastoid muscle laterally, overlying from the level C5 to T1 vertebra (**Fig. 2**). A prominence of the lateral edge of the thyroid lobe that stems from the fusion of the lateral and medical thyroid anlage is called the "tubercle of Zuckerkandl." The recurrent laryngeal nerve passes below the tubercle of Zuckerkandl and hence, caution should be executed to avoid potential injury to recurrent laryngeal nerve. The pyramidal lobe is the inferior portion of the thyroglossal duct and observed in ~50% of individuals. It is attached to the hyoid bone by a fibrous band (**Fig. 2**) and its length measures 1.4 cm in men and 2.5 cm in women, but the insertion of the pyramidal lobe varies widely. In patients requiring total thyroidectomy, it is important to identify and excise the pyramidal lobe with special caution not to leave residual thyroid tissue.

VASCULAR ANATOMY OF THE THYROID GLAND

The thyroid gland is one of the most vascular structures of the human body. It receives its blood supply from the superior and inferior thyroid arteries, and these are constant branches (**Fig. 3**). The superior thyroid artery is the first branch of the external carotid artery and provides most of the arterial supply (80%) to the thyroid gland. The inferior thyroid artery usually arises from thyrocervical trunk. A third vessel "thyroidea ima" may be present in up to 10%

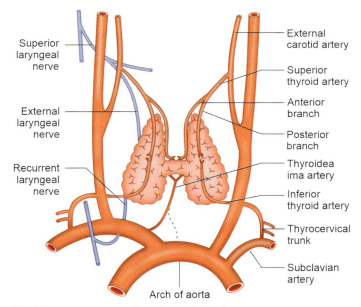

Fig. 3: Arterial supply of the thyroid gland.

of individuals and often replaces the inferior thyroid artery. The arteries extensively anastomose with each other over the surface of the thyroid gland. The inferior thyroid artery supplies both superior and inferior parathyroid glands. The thyridea ima artery could be a source of hemorrhage not only during thyroidectomy but also during tracheostomy as it is often unrecognized due to its infrequent occurrence and small size. The hemorrhage from thyroidea ima artery is often brisk and difficult to control as the severed artery may retract behind the sternum.

The venous drainage is usually by the superior, middle, and inferior thyroid veins **(Fig. 4)**. The number of veins is variable and can be up to five. Thyroid veins are a major source of hemorrhage during thyroid surgery and tracheotomy. Middle thyroid veins, most frequently on the right side, are short and stout and are a common source of hemorrhage when not ligated properly. Hence, these veins are ligated first during thyroidectomy.

The lymphatic drainage of the thyroid gland is extensive with the multidirectional flow and parallels venous drainage. The initial lymphatic drainage is to the perithyroid lymph nodes and subsequently, to prelaryngeal (Delphian), pretracheal and paratracheal lymph nodes (central lymph nodes and level IV nodes). Further drainage occurs to deep cervical and mediastinal lymph nodes. Hence, prophylactic central neck lymph node dissection is recommended in patients with a subgroup of patients with thyroid carcinomas which is often helpful to plan further steps in the management.

Nerves in Close Relation to the Thyroid Gland

Recurrent laryngeal nerve is injured in up to 20% of thyroidectomies. This nerve is identified in Simon's triangle formed by the esophagus medially, carotid artery laterally and inferior thyroid artery superiorly. The recurrent laryngeal nerve innervates the intrinsic muscles of the larynx and provides sensory innervations to the glottic area of the larynx. The recurrent laryngeal nerve has a longer course on the left side of the neck than on the right side. The nerve is nonrecurrent (directly arises from the cervical vagus nerve) in around 1% of the cases, more frequently on the right side than the left. This variant course often remains unrecognized during the surgery, thereby increasing the risk of iatrogenic injury during thyroid surgeries.

The right recurrent laryngeal nerve is anterior to and loops around the right subclavian artery and accompanies the right inferior thyroid artery. The left recurrent laryngeal nerve arises from the left vagus nerve, passes posterior to the ligamentum arteriosum in the thorax, ascends in the tracheoesophageal groove, and enters the larynx. It is both motor and sensory (55% motor and 45% sensory but distally 80% motor) and contains 2–4 times higher fibers to adductors that to abductors. It supplies the posterior cricoarytenoid, lateral cricoarytenoid, and interarytenoid muscles. It is usually deep to the inferior thyroid artery (40%).

The recurrent laryngeal nerve is closely related to the inferior thyroid artery near the base of the gland. It is important to identify the recurrent laryngeal nerve before the arterial branches are ligated. The relation of recurrent laryngeal nerve to the ligament of Berry (posterior suspensory ligament) varies; superficial, deep, passing-through, and splitting around the ligament. This relation may lead to stretching and injury of the recurrent laryngeal nerve during retraction of the thyroid gland on the medial side which should not be compelling.

The external branch of the superior laryngeal nerve (EBSLN) is purely a motor branch that supplies the cricothyroid muscle which controls the quality and pitch of the voice. It is in close relation with superior thyroid arteries and the superior pole of the thyroid which increases the risk of its injury during thyroid surgeries. Injury to EBSLN leads to significant morbidity, especially in teachers and professional singers. Hence, the nerve should be identified during thyroid surgeries to avoid accidental transection and excessive stretching. If the nerve is not identified, ligating superior thyroid arteries close to the thyroid gland minimizes the injury to EBSLN.

PARATHYROID GLANDS

Parathyroid glands are usually located in posterolateral relation to the thyroid gland. The superior parathyroid gland arises from the fourth branchial pouch and is located posterior to the recurrent laryngeal nerve. The inferior parathyroid is located anterior to the recurrent laryngeal nerve and arises from the third branchial pouch. Accidental excision of parathyroid glands and injury to their blood supply is not uncommon during thyroid surgeries and may lead to transient (14–60%) or permanent (4–11%) hypoparathyroidism. Hence, it is essential to identify each of the parathyroid glands during thyroid surgeries and perform meticulous dissection to preserve them and their vascularity. The capsular dissection of the thyroid, securing the blood supply close to the thyroid gland, rather than at the main trunks of the superior or inferior thyroid arteries, minimizes devascularization of the parathyroid glands.

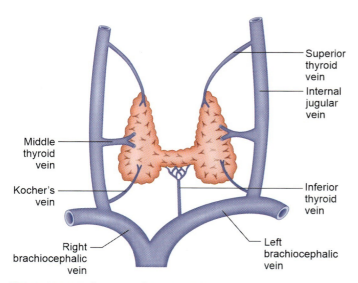

Fig. 4: Venous drainage of the thyroid gland.

CONCLUSION

Knowledge regarding the embryological aspects of the thyroid enhances the understanding of various congenital anomalies of the thyroid with clinical relevance. Knowledge of surgical anatomy is the cornerstone of successful thyroid surgery. Routine identification of all the known constant landmarks and caution to recognize anatomical variations will shorten the learning curve and reduce the complication rates in thyroid surgery and thereby enable to do safe thyroid surgery.

SUGGESTED READINGS

1. Bliss RD, Gauger PG, Delbridge LW. Surgeon's approach to the thyroid gland: surgical anatomy and the importance of technique. World J Surg. 2000;24(8):891-7.
2. Mohebati A, Shaha AR. Anatomy of thyroid and parathyroid glands and neurovascular relations. Clin Anatom. 2012;25(1):19-31.
3. Ranade AV, Rai R, Pai MM, Nayak SR, Krisnamurthy A, Narayana S. Anatomical variations of the thyroid gland: possible surgical implications. Singapore Med J. 2008;49(10):831-4.
4. Benvenga S, Tuccari G, Ieni A, Vita R. Thyroid gland: anatomy and physiology. Reference Module in Biomedical Sciences. Amsterdam: Elsevier; 2018. pp. 382-90.
5. Ellis H. Anatomy of the thyroid and parathyroid glands. Surgery (Oxford). 2007;25(11):467-8.
6. Policeni BA, Smoker WR, Reede DL. Anatomy and embryology of the thyroid and parathyroid glands. Semin Ultrasound CT MR. 2012;33(2):104-14.
7. Miller FR. Surgical anatomy of the thyroid and parathyroid glands. Otolaryngologic Clinics of North America. 2003;36(1):1-7.
8. Marine D, Lenhart CH. Pathological anatomy of exophthalmic goiter: the anatomical and physiological relations of the thyroid gland to the disease; the treatment. Arch Intern Med (Chic). 1911;8(3):265-316.
9. Rajini T, Ramachandran A, Savalgi GB, Venkata SP, Mokhasi V. Variations in the anatomy of the thyroid gland: clinical implications of a cadaver study. Anat Sci Int. 2012;87(1):45-9.
10. Sackett WR, Reeve TS, Barraclough B, Delbridge L. Thyrothymic thyroid rests: incidence and relationship to the thyroid gland. J Am Coll Surg. 2002;195(5):635-40.
11. Abbas G, Dubner S, Heller KS. Re-operation for bleeding after thyroidectomy and parathyroidectomy. Head Neck. 2001;23(7):544-6.
12. Rosenbaum MA, Haridas M, McHenry CR. Life-threatening neck hematoma complicating thyroid and parathyroid surgery. Am J Surg. 2008;195(3):339-43.
13. Morton RP, Mak V, Moss D, Ahmad Z, Sevao J. Risk of bleeding after thyroid surgery: matched pairs analysis. J Laryngol Otol. 2012;126(3):285-8.
14. Shaha AR, Jaffe BM. Practical management of post-thyroidectomy hematoma. J Surg Oncol. 1994;57(4):235-8.
15. Leyre P, Desurmont T, Lacoste L, Odasso C, Bouche G, Beaulieu A, et al. Does the risk of compressive hematoma after thyroidectomy authorize 1-day surgery? Langenbecks Arch Surg. 2008;393(5):733-7.
16. Park I, Rhu J, Woo JW, Choi JH, Kim JS, Kim JH. Preserving parathyroid gland vasculature to reduce post-thyroidectomy hypocalcemia. World J Surg. 2016;40(6):1382-9.
17. Sadowski SM, Fortuny JV, Triponez F. A reappraisal of vascular anatomy of the parathyroid gland based on fluorescence techniques. Gland Surg. 2017;6(Suppl 1):S30-7.
18. Lin DT, Patel SG, Shaha AR, Singh B, Shah JP. Incidence of inadvertent parathyroid removal during thyroidectomy. Laryngoscope. 2002;112(4):608-11.

CHAPTER 3

Physiology of Thyroid Gland

Alok Sachan, Shruthi B

INTRODUCTION

Thyroid gland is situated at the level of second and third tracheal rings, anterior to the trachea. It is of butterfly shape and due to its appearance like a shield similar to nearby thyroid cartilage of the larynx; in 1656, Thomas Wharton gave the name (thyreos in Greek means "shield"). The thyroid gland secretes two hormones: (1) thyroxine (T4) and (2) triiodothyronine (T3). This chapter deals with hypothalamic pituitary thyroid axis, thyroid hormone synthesis, secretion, and mechanisms of action.

HYPOTHALAMIC–PITUITARY–THYROID AXIS

Thyrotropin-releasing hormone (TRH), a 26-kD protein, is synthesized in hypothalamus, in median eminence and paraventricular nuclei. TRH hormone secretion occurs in a pulsatile manner. TRH production is under direct negative feedback control by thyroid hormones. High levels of thyroid hormone cause decrease production of TRH. Anterior pituitary gland, under the influence of both TRH and thyroid hormones produces thyroid-stimulating hormone (TSH). TSH is a 28-kD glycoprotein. It consists of two subunits, (1) alfa (α) and (2) beta (β). α subunit structure is shared by follicle-stimulating hormone, luteinizing hormone, and chorionic gonadotropin. β subunit structure is unique to TSH and responsible for biological action. Normal daily secretion of TSH is 15–30 µg/day, which is pulsatile in nature. Maximum secretion occurs in late evening, followed by decline in plasma TSH concentration during the rest of the night to achieve low daytime levels. Low levels of TRH in portal blood of pituitary decreases TSH concentration. Increase in T4 and T3 levels inhibits secretion of TSH **(Fig. 1)**. Hormones like somatostatin, dopamine, and glucocorticoids also regulate TSH secretion, all act as inhibitors of TSH secretion.

Thyrocyte structure and function: Thyroid follicle is a functional unit of thyroid gland. The wall of follicle is lined by thyrocytes or follicular cells, which are specialized epithelial

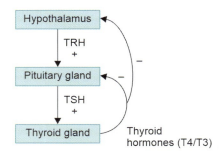

Fig. 1: Hypothalamic–pituitary–thyroid axis.
(TRH: thyrotropin-releasing hormone; TSH: thyroid-stimulating hormone)

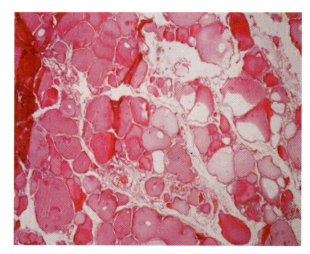

Fig. 2: Thyroid gland: follicular cells lining thyroid follicle filled with colloid.

cells. Follicular content is called colloid. Colloid is made up of thyroglobulin (Tg), a large glycoprotein and main storage form of thyroid hormone **(Fig. 2)**. Monitoring of Tg values is important part of differentiated thyroid cancer management. TSH acts on follicular cells through TSH receptor (TSHR), which is located on basolateral membrane of thyrocyte. TSHR is a transmembrane G protein-coupled receptor protein. Adenylyl cyclase stimulation following activation of TSHR mediates intracellular effects of TSH. Increased iodine uptake, followed by increased thyroid hormone production occurs in thyrocytes due to stimulatory effects of TSH.

Thyroid Hormones

Thyroid gland secrets two slightly different molecules, (1) T4 contains four iodine atoms and (2) T3 contains three iodine atoms **(Fig. 3)**. Thyroid hormones produced from thyroid gland under normal circumstances contains 90% T4 and 10% T3. Daily production of T4 is 80–100 µg and T3 is 30–40 µg.

Thyroid Hormone Synthesis and Secretion

Steps involved in synthesis of thyroid hormones are **(Fig. 4)**:
- *Uptake of iodine*: Trapping of iodide from blood is mediated by sodium/iodine symporter (NIS) at basolateral membrane of thyrocytes. Thyrocytes ability to concentrate iodide 20- to 40-fold above serum concentration is due to this active process. In diagnosis and management of thyroid cancers such as papillary and follicular carcinoma, radioactive iodine plays a major role. Thyroglobulin-elevated negative iodine scintigraphy (TENIS) is a condition which arises during the course of thyroid cancer management. Loss of expression of NIS in malignant thyroid cells results in TENIS. Use of radioactive iodine is limited in this condition.
- *Oxidation*: Peroxidase enzyme oxidizes iodine to I^0 or I^+.
- *Organification*: Iodination of tyrosine molecules in Tg results in formation of monoiodotyrosine (MIT) and diiodotyrosine (DIT). This organification occurs at the apical membrane of thyrocytes in the presence of key enzyme thyroid peroxidase (TPO). Regulation of selenoprotein TPO is complex.
  - *Wolff–Chaikoff effect*: Blockage of TPO activity during exposure to excess amounts of iodine causes hypothyroidism. This is the mechanism behind amiodarone-induced hypothyroidism.

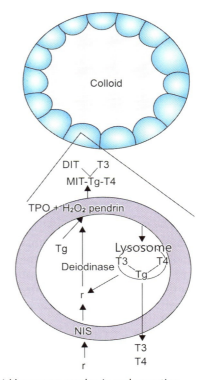

Fig. 4: Thyroid hormone synthesis and secretion.

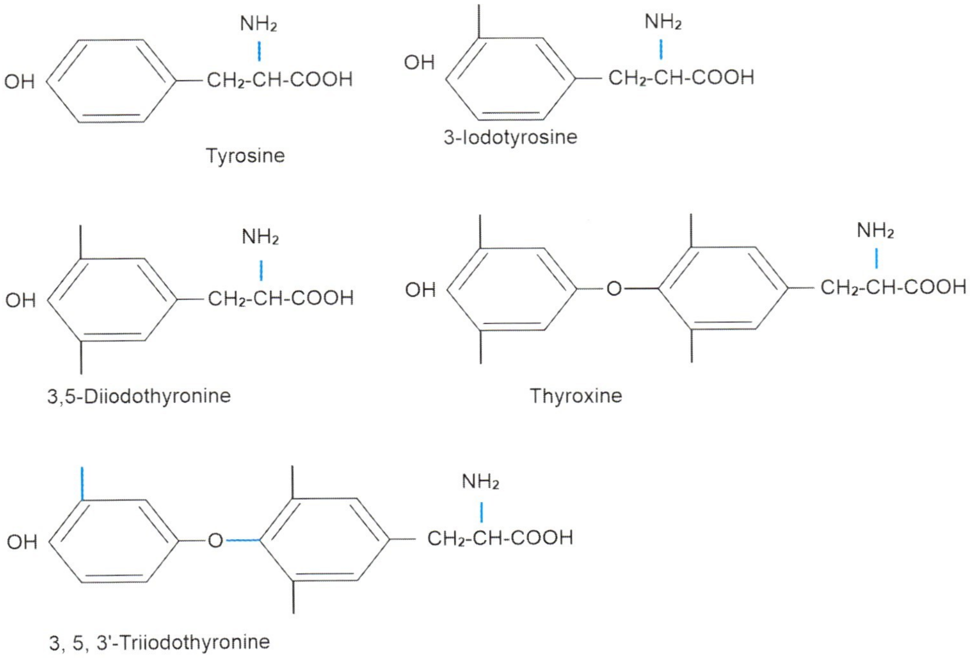

Fig. 3: Thyroid hormones structure.

○ *Jod–Basedow effect*: Escape from protective Wolff–Chaikoff effect causes this phenomenon. In this phenomenon following exposure to excess iodine, thyrocytes produce increased amounts of T4 and T3. Clinically, this process lead to thyrotoxicosis in subclinical autonomous functioning thyroid nodule.
- *Coupling*: One DIT molecule combines with an MIT molecule or another DIT molecule, this process results in formation of T3 and T4 respectively.
- *Release*: As and when required, colloid is taken up by the follicular cells. Enzymatic hydrolysis of Tg after endocytosis occurs and T3 and T4 are released into circulation.

THYROID HORMONES PERIPHERAL ACTIONS

Thyroid hormones circulate in blood mainly in the bound forms, bound to thyroid carrier proteins (>95% in bound form). Less than 1% of the circulating thyroid hormones circulate in free the unbound forms.

Thyroid carrier proteins: Main thyroid-binding proteins are thyroid-binding globulin (TBG), transthyretin (TTR), albumin, and lipoprotein. These proteins maintain levels of free thyroxine (FT4) and free triiodothyronine (FT3) within narrow limits for physiological actions of thyroid hormones on tissues. They also act as storage structures for thyroid hormones **(Table 1)**.

Mode of cell entry: For thyroid hormone, the main mode of target cell entry is through passive diffusion. Transporting proteins facilitates this process. Monocarboxylate transporters (MCT8 and MCT10) and the organic anion transporting polypeptide 1C1 (OATP1C1) play important roles in thyroid hormone transport into the cell. A mutation of MCT8 gene causes a rare disease, Allan–Herndon–Dudley syndrome. In this disease, characteristic features are presence of severe psychomotor retardation and elevated levels of serum T3.

T3 is the biological active hormone. Prohormone T4 is converted into its active form T3 by a group of selenoproteins called "deiodinases" **(Table 2)**. Consumptive hypothyroidism is a condition where D3 is over expressed in hemangiomas and results in hypothyroidism. This condition is due to excessive degradation of T3 and T4 by excessive D3. Half-life of T3 in circulation is 18 hours while T4 is 6.7 days.

Thyroid Hormone Action

Thyroid hormones act through a nuclear receptor. This receptor-mediated thyroid action is known as genomic. Inside the cell T3 binds to thyroid hormone receptor (TR), which dimerizes with the retinoid X receptor. After dimerization, it binds to the thyroid hormone response element (TRE) mediating its biologic effects. TREs are usually found in target genes in the promoter sequence. Ligand-dependent transcriptional activation of thyroid nuclear receptor is enhanced by large number of cofactors. These cofactors are coactivators and corepressors. Coactivators activate TR action, whereas corepressors suppress thyroid hormone action. Important among them are steroid receptor coactivator (SRC) complex and thyroid receptor-associated protein (TRAP). Nongenomic actions of thyroid hormones are also described, which are nonnuclear actions of thyroid receptors.

Thyroid hormone receptors: TR is of mainly two subtypes: (1) TRα and (2) TRβ. Further these subtypes have several isoforms with tissue specific function **(Table 3)**. T3 acts

TABLE 1: Thyroid carrier proteins.			
Serum-binding proteins	**Thyroid-binding globulin (TBG)**	**Transthyretin**	**Albumin**
Molecular weight	54 kD (TBG)	55 kD	66.5 kDa
Synthesis	Liver	Liver	Liver
Affinity	High affinity for T4 than T3	Lesser affinity compared to TBG	Lower affinity than TBG
Fraction of binding	75% of T4 80% of T3	10% of T4 5% of T3	12% of T4 15% of T3

TABLE 2: Types of deiodinases.			
Type	**Type 1 deiodinase (D1)**	**Type 2 deiodinase (D2)**	**Type 3 deiodinase (D3)**
Location	Cell membrane	Endoplasmic reticulum membrane	Cell membrane
Tissue	Liver, kidney, thyroid	Brown adipose tissue, heart, central nervous system, skeletal muscle	Skin, central nervous system, placenta
Action	T4 to T3, and T4 to the rT3	T4 to the active T3	T4 to the rT3
Deiodination site in thyroid hormones	Outer/inner ring	Outer ring	Inner ring
Substrate preference	rT3 > T4 > T3	T4 > rT3	T3 > T4
Half-life	>12 hours	40 minutes	12 hours

TABLE 3: Thyroid hormone receptors.

Thyroid hormone receptor isoforms	Tissue distribution	Able to bind T3
TRα1	Kidney, skeletal muscle, lungs, heart, testes, and brain	Yes
TRα2	Kidney, skeletal muscle, lungs, heart, testes, and brain	No
TRβ1	Kidney, thyroid, liver, and brain	Yes
TRβ2	Anterior pituitary, hypothalamus, and developing brain	Yes

on the TRα receptor in cardiac muscle to regulate heart rate. Another action mediated through the TRα receptor is resting energy expenditure in skeletal muscle. Regulation of cholesterol and lipoprotein metabolism in the liver is regulated through the TRβ1 receptor. Mutations of the *TRβ1* gene result in resistance to thyroid hormone. Novel drugs, called thyromimetics have been developed that bind preferentially to TRα or TRβ1. These thyromimetics are used in treatment of dyslipidemia, thyroid hormone resistance, and heart failure. TRβ1 selective agonist like resmetirom is in clinical trials for management of patients with hypercholesterolemia and nonalcoholic fatty liver disease.

CONCLUSION

Thyroid hormone synthesis, secretion, circulation, and mechanism of action involve many efficiently regulated steps. Hypothalamic–pituitary–thyroid axis maintains thyroid hormone secretion within normal limits. Knowledge of thyroid gland physiology is the cornerstone for management of thyroid disease.

SUGGESTED READINGS

1. Braverman LE, Cooper DS, Kopp P (Eds). Werner and Ingbar's The Thyroid: A Fundamental and Clinical Text, 11th edition. Philadelphia: Wolters Kluwer; 2020.
2. Ortiga-Carvalho TM, Chiamolera MI, Pazos-Moura CC, Wondisford FE. Hypothalamus-Pituitary-Thyroid Axis. Compr Physiol. 2016;6(3):1387-428.
3. Magner JA. Thyroid-stimulating hormone: biosynthesis, cell biology, and bioactivity. Endocr Rev. 1990;11(2):354-85.
4. Davies TF, Yin X, Latif R. The genetics of the thyroid stimulating hormone receptor: history and relevance. Thyroid. 2010;20(7):727-36.
5. Kleinau G, Krause G. Thyrotropin and homologous glycoprotein hormone receptors: structural and functional aspects of extracellular signaling mechanisms. Endocr Rev. 2009;30(2):133-51.
6. Engler D, Burger AG. The deiodination of the iodothyronines and of their derivatives in man. Endocr Rev. 1984;5(2):151-84.
7. Eng PH, Cardona GR, Fang SL, Previti M, Alex S, Carrasco N, et al. Escape from the acute Wolff-Chaikoff effect is associated with a decrease in thyroid sodium/iodide symporter messenger ribonucleic acid and protein. Endocrinology. 1999;140(8):3404-10.
8. Woeber KA. Iodine and thyroid disease. Med Clin North Am. 1991;75(1):169-78.
9. Mendel CM, Weisiger RA, Jones AL, Cavalieri RR. Thyroid hormone-binding proteins in plasma facilitate uniform distribution of thyroxine within tissues: a perfused rat liver study. Endocrinology. 1987;120(5):1742-9.
10. Grijota-Martínez C, Bárez-López S, Gómez-Andrés D, Guadaño-Ferraz A. MCT8 Deficiency: The Road to Therapies for a Rare Disease. Front Neurosci. 2020;14:380.
11. Sabatino L, Vassalle C, Del Seppia C, Iervasi G. Deiodinases and the Three Types of Thyroid Hormone Deiodination Reactions. Endocrinol Metab (Seoul). 2021;36(5):952-64.
12. Luongo C, Trivisano L, Alfano F, Salvatore D. Type 3 deiodinase and consumptive hypothyroidism: a common mechanism for a rare disease. Front Endocrinol (Lausanne). 2013;4:115.
13. Fondell JD, Guermah M, Malik S, Roeder RG. Thyroid hormone receptor-associated proteins and general positive cofactors mediate thyroid hormone receptor function in the absence of the TATA box-binding protein-associated factors of TFIID. Proc Natl Acad Sci USA. 1999;96(5):1959-64.
14. Ortiga-Carvalho TM, Sidhaye AR, Wondisford FE. Thyroid hormone receptors and resistance to thyroid hormone disorders. Nat Rev Endocrinol. 2014;10(10):582-91.
15. Saponaro F, Sestito S, Runfola M, Rapposelli S, Chiellini G. Selective Thyroid Hormone Receptor-Beta (TRβ) Agonists: New Perspectives for the Treatment of Metabolic and Neurodegenerative Disorders. Front Med (Lausanne). 2020;7:331.

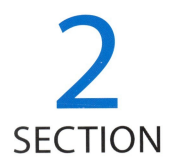

SECTION 2

Diagnosis of Thyroid Disorders

CHAPTER 4

Clinical Evaluation of Thyroid

Parjeet Kaur

INTRODUCTION

Assessment of any patient with thyroid disorder is incomplete without a good clinical evaluation. Despite advancement in diagnostics and imaging, making a clinical diagnosis based upon a thorough history and physical examination of the thyroid gland is the first step in the approach to thyroid disorders. This section reviews the historical cues and the characteristic physical findings needed to reach a clinical diagnosis in a patient with thyroid disorder.

HISTORY

Patients with thyroid disorders come to medical attention for several reasons. They may present with symptoms attributable to high or low plasma levels of thyroid hormones (thyrotoxicosis or hypothyroidism respectively). They may also present with neck swelling due to localized or generalized enlargement of the gland. Finally, patient may be referred for an abnormal thyroid function test found incidentally in general health check or in the tests ordered by other specialities.

Typical symptoms of thyrotoxicosis in adults are weight loss, anxiety or nervousness, tremulousness, increased sweating, palpitations, diarrhea, heat intolerance, muscular weakness, shortness of breath and oligomenorrhea. Manifestations of hyperthyroidism or thyrotoxicosis may be atypical in elderly and include, fatigue or weakness (apathetic hyperthyroidism), weight loss, chronic diarrhea, loss of appetite, refractory cardiac arrhythmias or heart failure.

The term thyrotoxicosis denotes increased plasma levels of thyroid hormones which can occur due to thyroiditis (due to release of prestored thyroid hormones) or overactive thyroid gland, i.e., hyperthyroidism. It is important to differentiate these two conditions as their management differs. Historical cues of subacute thyroiditis include a short history, a recent history of sore throat or upper respiratory tract infection, throat or mid line neck pain sometimes radiating to the ear. A lady presenting with thyrotoxic symptoms in postpartum period is most likely suffering from postpartum thyroiditis, which is a painless condition. Pointers which favor hyperthyroidism are—a relatively long history, overt symptoms, muscular weakness, neck swelling, and eye symptoms in the form of pain, redness, and bulging eyes. History of treatment of an "overactive" thyroid in the past, a family history of thyroid dysfunction and a coexisting autoimmune disorder also favor hyperthyroidism.

Typical symptoms of overt hypothyroidism in adults are fatigue, weight gain, depression, constipation, lethargy, dry skin, cold intolerance, voice change, menstrual irregularities, muscle cramps, and carpal tunnel syndrome. History of treatment of a thyroid condition may be present in the past. Patients with subclinical hypothyroidism often have nonspecific symptoms.

Thyroid enlargement (goiter) may occur in both hypo and hyperthyroidism. It may also occur in a patient with normal thyroid function (euthyroid patient). Patients can present with a generalized neck swelling (diffuse goiter) or neck mass (uninodular or multinodular goiter). In the presence of large or retrosternal goiter, they can present with compressive symptoms in the form of dysphagia, hoarseness of voice or breathing difficulty.

Patients referred for incidentally detected abnormal thyroid function test should be asked questions directed to uncover underlying thyroid problems. Ask: Have you noted a change in weight? Have you noticed a change in your skin or hair? Do you feel more uncomfortable in hot or cold weather? Has there been a change in your bowel habit (constipation or diarrhea)? Have you noticed any change in your mood? Do you get easily fatigued? Have you had any pain or discomfort in your neck? Have you ever received radiation treatments to the head or neck or undergone any thyroid surgery in the past? Have you taken thyroid medication? Have you suffered any thyroid problem in the past? Questions pertaining to typical symptoms of thyrotoxicosis and overt hypothyroidism should also be asked.

Drug history holds a significant importance in the clinical evaluation of thyroid. Intake of certain drugs can result in overt hypothyroidism (e.g., tyrosine kinase inhibitors) or thyrotoxicosis (e.g., amiodarone). There is a whole list of drugs which can interfere with thyroid function tests. Hence, it is important to note down all the drugs which patient is taking at present or has taken in the recent past.

PHYSICAL EXAMINATION

General Physical Examination

A clinical impression of an overt hypothyroidism or hyperthyroidism can be made the moment the patient walks into the clinician's room. A patient with overt hypothyroidism has puffy face, slowed speech with a thick low voice and looks pale with dry wrinkled skin. On the other hand, patient with hyperthyroidism looks nervous, hyperactive, with rapid speech, tremulousness, and stare. Careful physical examination can reveal many signs of hyper or hypothyroidism involving almost every organ system. These signs are enlisted in **Table 1**.

Eye Examination in a Patient with Hyperthyroidism

Eye signs such as stare (lid retraction) and lid lag represent sympathetic hyperactivity which occurs in thyrotoxicosis of any etiology. However, characteristic features of eye involvement in Graves' disease (Graves' ophthalmopathy) include exophthalmos, periorbital and conjunctival edema, and limitation of eye movement. Physical examination of the eyes of a patient with Graves' orbitopathy should include:
- Inspection of the conjunctivae and periorbital tissue, looking for conjunctival injection and edema (chemosis) and periorbital edema.
- Determination of the extent of closure of the upper and lower lids.
- Assessment of the range of motion of the eyes.
- Objective measurements of the degree of proptosis, using an exophthalmometer.
- Assessment of visual acuity, color vision and visual fields.

Severity of Graves' ophthalmopathy is commonly assessed using European Group of Graves' Orbitopathy (EUGOGO) classification and activity is assessed using a seven-point clinical activity score (CAS).

Thyroid Examination

Examination of the neck should be done with patient seated and neck relaxed.

Inspection

Following points should be noted on inspection:
- The presence of old surgical scars
- Distended veins
- Redness or fixation of the overlying skin
- Presence of any mass
- If a mass is noted then patient should be asked to swallow. Movement on swallowing is a characteristic of the thyroid gland.
- If a midline mass in addition to moving up with swallowing also rises further when the patient extends the tongue, is likely a thyroglossal duct cyst.
- *Pemberton sign*: This test is useful when a retrosternal goiter is suspected. Patient is asked to raise both arms raising both arms until they touch the sides of the head. This maneuver further narrows the thoracic inlet causing facial plethora and venous engorgement of the face and sometimes respiratory distress or even (rarely) syncope.

Palpation

Thyroid palpation can be performed with the physician facing the seated patient or standing behind the seated patient, palpating with the fingertips of both hands. Landmarks for examination of thyroid gland are depicted in **Figure 1**.
- *Facing the patient*: Thyroid isthmus is palpated just caudal to the cricoid cartilage with the use of gentle thumb pressure. To palpate the left lobe, examiner approaches the patient from the right and from the left to palpate the right lobe **(Fig. 2)**. Lobes are palpated with two or three fingers lateral to the trachea and medial to sternocleidomastoid (SCM) muscles. Palpation should be done in a circular, rubbing motion applying gentle pressure. Keeping the fingers stationary at various levels

TABLE 1: Signs of hyperthyroidism and hypothyroidism on examination.		
Organ system	**Hypothyroidism**	**Hyperthyroidism**

Face and neck	• Puffy face
	• Enlarged tongue
	• Hoarse voice
		• Eye signs:
		  ○ Stare
		  ○ Lid lag
		  ○ Lid retraction
		• Ophthalmopathy (seen in Graves' disease)
		  ○ Exophthalmos, periorbital, and conjunctival edema
		  ○ Ophthalmoplegia

Skin	• Dry, coarse, thick, cold and pale
	• Coarse and brittle hair
	• Thinning of lateral one-third of eyebrows
		• Warm and moist
		• Dermopathy (seen in Graves' disease):
		  ○ Hands—acropachy
		  ○ Legs—pretibial myxedema

Cardiovascular	• Bradycardia • Hypertension (diastolic)	• Tachycardia • Widened pulse pressure • Hypertension (systolic)
Neurological	Delayed tendon reflexes	Brisk reflexes

Clinical Evaluation of Thyroid

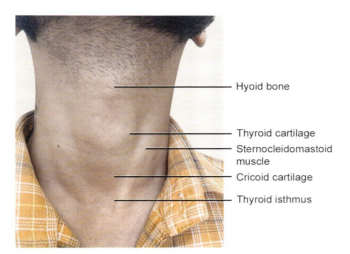

Fig. 1: Anatomical landmarks in the examination of the thyroid gland.

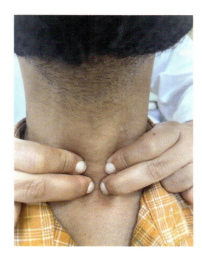

Fig. 3: Examination of the thyroid gland from behind the patient with simultaneous palpation of both thyroid lobes.

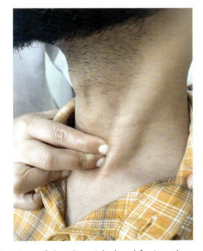

Fig. 2: Examination of the thyroid gland facing the patient showing palpation of left lobe with the fingers of the right hand.

of interest, patient is asked to swallow in order to move the thyroid beneath the fingers.
- *Standing behind the patient*: The head of the patient is tilted posteriorly enough to release the tension of the overlying structures and allow SCM muscles to displace slightly laterally. Place the fingers of both hands on the patient's neck localizing cricoid cartilage initially. Thyroid lobes are palpated with the tips of two or three fingers sliding them over the lobes with gentle but sufficient pressure to feel beneath the overlying structures and outlining the borders of both lobes **(Fig. 3)**.

Following points should be noted during palpation:
- The shape of the gland and its size. The size of the normal thyroid lobe is approximately the same size as the terminal phalanx of the patient's thumb.
- Consistency of the gland. The diffuse goiter of Graves' disease is softer than normal whereas gland of Hashimoto disease is firm.
- Any tender areas should be noted.
- Lower border of the goiter should be identified, if not palpable, may indicate retrosternal extension.
- If nodules are palpated, their size, shape, position, and consistency should be noted. A firm mass may indicate a cyst whereas a hard nodule goes in favor of malignancy.
- Regional lymph nodes should be palpated.

Auscultation

A systolic or continuous bruit can be heard over an enlarged gland which may confirm the increased vascularity, suggesting Graves' disease.

SUGGESTED READINGS

1. Ross DS, Burch HB, Cooper DS, Greenlee MC, Laurberg P, Maia AL, et al. 2016 American Thyroid Association Guidelines for Diagnosis and Management of Hyperthyroidism and other causes of Thyrotoxicosis. Thyroid. 2016;26(10):1343-421.
2. Chaker L, Razvi S, Bensenor IM, Azizi F, Pearce EN, Peeters RP. Hypothyroidism. Nat Rev Dis Primers. 2022;8(1):30.
3. Hennessey JV, Garber JR. Physical examination of the thyroid gland. In: Werner & Ingbar's the Thyroid: A Fundamental and Clinical Text, 12 edition. Philadelphia: Lippincott Williams & Wilkins; 2020. p. 259.
4. Bahn RS. Graves' Ophthalmopathy. N Engl J Med. 2010;362(8):726-38.
5. Boelaert K, Torlinska B, Holder RL, Franklyn JA. Older subjects with hyperthyroidism present with a paucity of symptoms and signs: a large cross-sectional study. J Clin Endocrinol Metab. 2010;95(6):2715-26.

CHAPTER 5

Laboratory Evaluation of Thyroid Functions

Arun S Menon, RV Jayakumar

INTRODUCTION

Thyroid hormones measurement is one of the most used hormonal tests in modern-day clinical practice. The methodologies have progressively evolved over the last five decades, from competitive immunoassays and competitive immunometric assays in 1970 and 1990s to the more recent introduction of liquid chromatography mass spectrometry. This has helped significantly in improving the sensitivity and specificity of these tests.

Both hypothyroidism and hyperthyroidism cause a variety of nonspecific symptoms and signs, making it difficult to make a clinical diagnosis without the aid of laboratory evaluation. The accuracy of these tests helps in ruling out thyroid disorders in a large proportion of patients presenting with such symptoms. The most encountered thyroid function abnormalities are subclinical hypothyroidism and subclinical hyperthyroidism which in many cases may not be the reason for the presenting symptoms. Hence, interpreting the thyroid function abnormalities and the correlating it with the clinical context, needs expertise. A physician also needs to develop skills to identify potential pitfalls of laboratory tests such as assay interference, drug effects, and the effect of nonthyroidal illness.

THYROID FUNCTION TESTS

The commonly used tests are thyroid-stimulating hormone (TSH), total tetraiodothyronine and total triiodothyronine (TT4 and TT3), free tetraiodothyronine and free triiodothyronine (FT4 and FT3), antithyroid peroxidase antibodies (TPOAb), antithyroglobulin antibodies (TgAb), and TSH receptor antibodies (TRAB). Measurement of thyroid hormone-binding proteins such as TTR, TBG, thyroxine-binding prealbumin (TBPA), thyroxine-binding albumin, and thyroglobulin are useful in certain special situations.

Thyroid-stimulating hormone is the most sensitive screening test as it is an excellent indicator of the thyroid status of a patient. Its secretion from the pituitary gland is determined by the plasma concentration of free thyroid hormones. Even small changes in serum thyroid function cause logarithmic amplifications of TSH secretion. The reference range of serum TSH by immunometric assays is 0.4–4.2 mU/L. Although extremely sensitive (third-generation chemiluminescent) TSH assays can detect levels as low as ≤0.004 mU/L, for clinical use a method that detects TSH values of ≤0.1 mU/L are considered sufficient. There is a diurnal variation for TSH with peak values between midnight and 4 am and a nadir in the afternoon. Hence, a morning test is desirable routinely. If TSH levels are found to be abnormal, then circulating TT3/FT3 and TT4/FT4 levels should be evaluated.

A normal TSH value is a sufficient indicator to stop further testing of thyroid function in most cases. However, one needs to be aware of the limitations of using TSH assay alone in certain clinical scenarios. When a pituitary or hypothalamic cause is suspected, both free T4 and TSH concentration should be measured concomitantly as TSH can be low, inappropriately normal, or minimally elevated at times. Thyrotropin-releasing hormone (TRH) test is sometimes used in such situations. Interpretation of TSH values in special situations such as pregnancy and intercurrent illness also needs careful consideration **(Table 1)**.

Thyroid-stimulating hormone testing should be routinely performed in certain specific situations. TSH test performed on a heel-prick blood specimen is an excellent

TABLE 1: Reference values of thyroid function test.	
Test	Range
TSH	0.5–4.2 mU/L
FT3	0.22–6.78 pmol/L
T4	58–140 nmol/L
FT4	10.3–35 pmol/L
T3	0.92–2.78 nmol/L

(FT3: free triiodothyronine; FT4: free thyroxine; TSH: thyroid-stimulating hormone; T3: triiodothyronine; T4: thyroxine)

screening test for congenital hypothyroidism (CH) at birth. All suspected cases of goiter should have TSH done as part of the evaluation. Pregnancy is another scenario where a TSH is essential at booking visit. Those patients with atrial fibrillation, dyslipidemia, osteoporosis, and infertility, should have a TSH measured at the time of presentation. Screening can be done by measuring serum TSH levels in suspected cases that are asymptomatic or have nonspecific thyroid dysfunction manifestations. The high-sensitivity TSH test should be performed in such cases as there is low pretest probability of disease as the negative predictive value of the test is very high; thus, a vast majority of the results come out negative. Serum TSH testing alone can also be used in follow-up of suspected cases of thyroid dysfunction who have not been started on any treatment. Although low TSH is sensitive in picking up hyperthyroidism, treatment on antithyroid drugs should never be initiated based on low TSH alone. Those being followed up on antithyroid medications should have their dose adjusted based on free T3 and free T4 along with TSH **(Table 2)**.

In case of altered TSH readings, a detailed history, physical examination including examination of thyroid gland, repeat TSH test, serum T3 and T4 level determination and imaging studies (as and when required) need to be carried out. Several patients with increased TSH levels are prescribed lifelong treatment with levothyroxine without clear-cut evaluation and no further follow-up or advice is provided. This leads to a lack of clarity in the long term, for treating physicians as well as the patient. Those patients with goiter or thyroid nodules and a raised TSH, should undergo further detailed evaluation including antithyroid antibodies, ultrasound imaging, and fine-needle aspiration cytology (FNAC) if required.

Free T3 and T4 levels are better markers in patients with abnormal TSH over TT3 and TT4, as T3 and T4 (>99%) are mostly bound to plasma proteins. A detectable or elevated serum TSH concentration in the presence of raised FT4 and/or FT3 is associated with some rarer clinical scenarios. The laboratory findings should be verified by repeat testing of serum samples and on confirmation other probable diagnosis which includes binding protein abnormalities like familial dysalbuminemic hyperthyroxinemia or assay-dependent antibody interference should be considered. Once the laboratory error or artifact has been ruled out, a "true" cause of the abnormal TSH should be considered. The possibilities are TSH-secreting pituitary tumor (TSHoma) or thyroid hormone resistance syndrome. Appearance of an elevated serum sex hormone-binding globulin (SHBG) and circulating free α-subunit support the presence of TSHoma. There might be altered secretion (hypo or hyper) of other pituitary hormones in TSHoma. Once the laboratory diagnosis is made then it can be confirmed by the pituitary imaging. The second cause of the inappropriately detectable TSH is thyroid hormone resistance which can be suspected from family history and can be confirmed by sequencing of the β-thyroid hormone receptor.

TABLE 2: Some causes of abnormal serum thyroid-stimulating hormone concentrations.	
Thyroid-stimulating hormones below normal	**Thyroid-stimulating hormone above normal**
Primary hyperthyroidism	Primary hypothyroidism
Pituitary/hypothalamic disease with central hypothyroidism (TSH unreliable)	Pituitary thyrotroph adenoma; pituitary resistance to thyroid hormone (central hyperthyroidism) (TSH unreliable)
	Generalized thyroid hormone resistance
Prolonged thyrotroph cell suppression after recent hyperthyroidism in euthyroid or hypothyroid patient	
Recent hyperthyroidism in euthyroid or hypothyroid patient	Thyrotoxicosis from overly rapid correction of severe hypothyroidism with parenteral T4
Old age	Old age
Drugs, e.g., glucocorticoids and dopamine	Drugs, e.g., amiodarone
Problems with T4 treatment—overdosage in treatment for fatigue or overweight, altered gastrointestinal absorption because of drugs or disease, altered T4 clearance because of drugs, patient compliance problems, prescription error, and testing too soon after T4 dose decrease	Problems with T4 treatment—underdosage based on misleadingly high TT4, altered gastrointestinal absorption because of drugs gastrointestinal absorption because of drugs gastrointestinal absorption because of drugs prescription error, testing too soon after T4 dose increase
Many severe systemic illnesses analytical precision limits (sick euthyroid state)	Recovery phase after severe systemic illness (sick euthyroid state)
Combination of pulsatile TSH secretion and analytical precision limits	Combination of pulsatile TSH secretion and analytical precision limits
	Antibody in patient serum against antibody in TSH assay, causing analytical artifact
	TSH assay, causing analytical artifact

(TSH: thyroid-stimulating hormone; T4: thyroxine; TT4: total thyroxine)

Total T3 and Total T4 are still commonly used tests but may not always give a true reflection of the thyroid status of an individual. The metabolically active form of thyroid hormones is the unbound form which is only a fraction of the total hormone level as most of it is bound to carrier proteins (TGB, TTR, and albumin). In some clinical conditions where there is an alteration of the amount of carrier proteins, the TT3 and TT4 may be elevated but the thyroid functional state (FT3 and FT4 level) will be in the normal limits. Such conditions include: (i) hereditary abnormalities of binding proteins—TBG deficiency or TBG excess, abnormal albumin levels and abnormal transthyretin (TTR) levels, (ii) acquired deficiency of binding proteins can be due to protein loss (e.g., nephrotic syndrome), impaired synthesis of proteins (chronic liver disease), (iii) alteration of carrier protein levels (use of anabolic steroids or androgens), (iv) drug-induced alterations in T4 binding to TBG such as with salicylates, phenytoin and phenylbutazone and oral contraceptive pills, and (v) the presence of T4 antibodies.

Radioimmunoassay measurement of total serum T4 levels is highly sensitive in reflecting the hyperthyroid (85–95%) and the hypothyroid status (80–90%) of patients.

T3 assessment is not done on a routine basis (only T4 is measured) in patients suspected of having thyroid disorders. In cases of hypothyroidism approximately 25% have low levels of T3. Free and TT3 are usually performed in patients suspected of having T3 thyrotoxicosis and in patients taking drugs that inhibit the peripheral conversion of T4 to T3 (dexamethasone, propranolol, propylthiouracil (PTU), amiodarone, and I-containing contrast media).

Testing both Thyroid-stimulating Hormone and Free Thyroxine

In cases where pituitary thyroid axis is not intact or unstable there is necessity to measure both TSH and FT4 serum levels. These situations include:
- Optimizing T4 therapy in newly diagnosed patients with hypothyroidism
- Diagnosing and monitoring thyroid disorders in pregnancy
- Monitoring patients with hyperthyroidism in the early months after treatment
- Diagnosis and monitoring treatment for central hypothyroidism
- End-organ thyroid hormone resistance
- Sick euthyroid state
- Thyroid-stimulating hormone-secreting pituitary adenomas
- Women with type 1 diabetes mellitus (T1DM) should have their thyroid function, including serum TSH, FT4, and TPOAb status, at established preconception, at booking when pregnant, and at 3 months postpartum.
- Possible subclinical hypothyroidism-on screening high serum TSH concentration with normal FT4, the test should be repeated after 3–6 months, along with measurement of serum FT4, after ruling out nonthyroidal illness and drug interference.

When acutely ill, patients may have mild to moderate high TSH values (<20 mIU/L) with FT3 and FT4 levels under normal limits. Similarly, such patients may have subnormal serum TSH with FT4 and serum T3 values in the normal range. These may not be due to intrinsic thyroid disease and hence should only be commenced on treatment after a close follow-up and repeat testing. It is best to estimate both serum TSH and FT4 together in all inpatient cases where sufficient clinical details are not available, so that a correct clinical decision can be made **(Table 3)**.

THYROID-SPECIFIC AUTOANTIBODIES

Antibodies against thyroid-specific antigens, thyroid peroxidase, thyroglobulin, and TSH receptors are routinely performed to diagnose autoimmune thyroid disorders. The techniques for antibody measurement have evolved from semiquantitative agglutination, complement fixation tests, and whole animal bioassays to specific ligand assays using recombinant antigens and cell culture systems transfected with the human TSH receptor. The diagnostic and prognostic value of autoantibodies is restricted due to the differences in sensitivity and specificity of current methods.

Thyroid Peroxidase Antibodies

Thyroid peroxidase antibodies enzyme, is a 100 kD glycosylated protein responsible for iodine oxidation and iodination of tyrosyl residues of thyroglobulin molecule. Thyroid peroxidase antibodies, also termed antimicrosomal antibodies (AMA), are detected using semiquantitative complement fixation and tanned erythrocyte hemagglutination techniques. TPOAb immunoassays or IMA based on purified or recombinant TPO have replaced older manual techniques.

An abnormally raised TPOAb can be seen in 90–95% of patients with autoimmune thyroid disease (AITD), atrophic thyroiditis or postpartum thyroiditis. Nearly 70–80% of patients with GD and 15–20% of "healthy" euthyroid cases also have raised anti-TPO antibodies. Thyroid peroxidase antibodies cause the destruction of thyroid tissue by playing the role of cytotoxic agent resulting in hypothyroidism in patients of Hashimoto's thyroiditis.

The TPOAb measurement can be used as a prognostic indicator for thyroid dysfunction. Hypoechoic ultrasound pattern appears first in Hashimoto's thyroiditis followed by TPO antibodies and later thyroid dysfunction sets in. The paradoxical absence of TPOAb in some patients with definite TSH abnormalities shows the suboptimal sensitivity and/or specificity of current TPOAb tests or nonautoimmune thyroid failure (atrophic thyroiditis). Repeated thyroid autoantibody measurements are not advised for assessing treatment for AITD, although fluctuations in levels might indicate changes in disease activity. Higher TPOAb

TABLE 3: Characterization of thyroid disorders according to results of thyroid function tests.												
Disorder	TSH	T4	T3	FT4	Tg	TBG	rT3	ATPO	ATG	TBII	TSI	TBA
Primary hypothyroidism	↑	↓	N or ↓	↓	N or ↓	N	↓	N or ↑	N or ↑	N or ↑	n	n or ↑
Transient neonatal hypothyroidism	↑	↓	↓	↓	N or ↓	N	↓	N	N	↑	n	↑
Hashimoto's thyroiditis hypothyroidism	↑	N or ↓	N or ↓	N or ↓	N or ↓	N	↓	↑	↑	n or ↑	n	n or ↑
Graves' disease	↓	↑	↑	↑	↑	N	↑	↑	↑	↑	↑	n or ↑
Neonatal Graves' disease	↓	↑	↑	↑	↑	N	↑	n or ↑	n or ↑	↑	↑	n or ↑
TSH deficiency	N or ↓	↓	↓	↓	↓	N	↓	n	N	n	n	n
Thyroid dyshormonogenesis	↑	↓	↓	↓	N, ↓ or ↑	N	↑	n	N	n	n	n
Thyroid hormone resistance	N or ↑	↑	↑	↑	↑	N	↑	n	N	n	n	n
TSH-dependent hyperthyroidism	↑	↑	↑	↑	↑	N	↑	n	N	n	n	n
T4 protein-binding abnormalities*	N	V	V	N	N	V†	V	n	N	n	n	n
Nonthyroidal illness	V	N or ↓	↓	V	N	N	N or ↑	n	N	n	n	n
Subacute thyroiditis†	↓ or ↑	↑ or ↓	↑ or ↓	↑ or ↓	↑ or ↓	N	↑ or ↓	n	n	n	n	n

*The spectrum of binding protein abnormalities includes increased or decreased TBG binding, increased or decreased transthyretin binding, and ↑ albumin binding.
†Subacute thyroiditis involves a transient period of hyperthyroidism followed by a transient hypothyroid state.
(ATPO: antithyroidperoxidase; ATG: antithyroglobulin; FT4: free thyroxine; TBA: TSH receptor-blocking antibody; TBG: thyroxine-binding globulin; TBII: TSH-binding inhibiting immunoglobulin; Tg: thyroglobulin; TSH: thyroid-stimulating hormone; TSI: thyroid-stimulating immunoglobulin; T3: triiodothyronine; T4: thyroxine; rT3: reverse T3; N: normal; n: negative; V: variable)
Courtesy: Reprinted from Disorders of Thyroid function, Quest Diagnostic Manual 3rd edition, Fisha DA, p. 268.

prevalence is found with aging and in autoimmune diseases such as T1DM and pernicious anemia. Presence of detectable antibodies in a euthyroid patient indicates that the patient is at higher risk of developing subclinical or overt hypothyroidism. Detectable level of TPOAb typically precedes the increased levels of TSH which is indicative of hypothyroidism. Reproductive complications (such as miscarriage, infertility, in vitro fertilization failure, fetal death, preeclampsia, preterm delivery, postpartum thyroiditis, and depression) have been linked with the presence of TPOAb.

■ Thyroglobulin Antibodies

Thyroglobulin is a large (600 kDa) glycoprotein consisting of dimers and containing on average 2–3 molecules of T4 and 0.3 molecules. Antithyroglobulin antibodies were the first thyroid antibodies to be recognized by tanned red cell hemagglutination methods in autoimmune thyroiditis patients. With time, laboratory techniques have evolved in parallel with TPOAb methodology from semiquantitative techniques to more sensitive enzyme-linked immunosorbent assay (ELISA) and RIA methods to latest chemiluminescent immunoassays. TgAb assays have bigger-inter method variability than that of the TPOAb tests.

Circulating Tg antibodies can be detected in about 10% of healthy young subjects and 15% of people >60 years of age. Hence the value of routinely testing TPOAb and TgAb for thyroid autoimmunity is doubtful. TgAb prevalence was 60–80% in Hashimotos thyroiditis and 50–60% in Graves' disease patients. Anti-Tg antibodies can cross the placenta barrier, but the effect on the neonate is unclear.

Current guidelines state that all sera must be prescreened for TgAb by a sensitive immunoassay technique prior to thyroglobulin testing. Consequently, TgAb is primarily used as an adjunct test for serum Tg estimation. Thyroglobulin autoantibodies are detected in estimated 20% of patients with differentiated thyroid carcinoma compared with 10% of normal subjects by the immunoassay methods. False positives are occasionally due to assay artifacts or illegitimate transcription whereas false negatives result may be seen in patients with metastatic disease.

■ Thyroid-stimulating Hormone Receptor Autoantibodies

Thyroid-stimulating hormone receptor antibodies is an antibody belonging to immunoglobulin G class that is primarily used to differentiate Graves' disease (GD) from other types of hyperthyroidism. There are two types of TSH receptor antibodies: Thyroid-stimulating autoantibodies (TSAb) that cause Graves' hyperthyroidism and thyroid blocking antibody (TBAb) which blocks receptor binding of TSH. Thyroid-stimulating hormone receptor antibodies tests are also a reliable indicator of fetal and neonatal thyroid pathology due to transplacental passage of maternal TRAb. They are useful in predicting recurrence of hyperthyroidism in GD after treatment with antithyroid drugs.

Although thyrotropin-binding inhibiting immunoglobulin (TBII) assays do not directly measure the stimulating antibodies, these tests have similar diagnostic sensitivity to the earlier available TSAb bioassays (70–95%) for diagnosing Graves' hyperthyroidism or detecting a relapse or response to therapy. However, the TBII tests are crucial for evaluating pregnant patients with a history of AITD, where there is a risk of transplacental passage of TRAb to the infant. The lack of specificity of the TBII methods is an advantage in such clinical situation as it can detect both stimulating and blocking antibodies that can produce transient hyper- or hypothyroidism, respectively, in the fetus and newborn. The cut-offs recommended are assay specific.

Thyroid-stimulating hormone receptor antibodies estimation may play a role in thyroid-associated ophthalmopathy (TAO), which appears to be exacerbated by radioiodine therapy. Since TRAb and other thyroid antibodies levels increase acutely significantly after radioiodine therapy its measurement prior to radioiodine therapy may be useful to predict risk of TAO. It is also useful in differentiating between type 1 and type 2 amiodarone induced thyrotoxicosis.

In pregnancy, TRAb can readily cross the placenta, stimulate fetal thyroid and cause thyrotoxicosis. Untreated fetal thyrotoxicosis is associated with both poor fetal (growth retardation, fetal congestive heart failure, and fetal hydrops) and maternal outcomes (preterm delivery, placental abruption, and preeclampsia). Measurement of TRAb is recommended among—(i) pregnant women with a past history of GD treated with radioactive iodine or surgery (check once in early pregnancy and once again between 18 and 22 weeks), (ii) patients on treatment for GD with ATD at the time of confirmation of pregnancy (check early in pregnancy), (iii) patients requiring ATD for GD through midpregnancy (repeat testing between 18 and 22 weeks), and (iv) pregnant women with previously elevated TRAb levels in midpregnancy (18–22 weeks) require repeat testing in the third trimester (repeat testing at 30–34 weeks). Values of TRAb >3 times the upper limit of normal anytime during pregnancy is considered to put the fetus at risk for thyrotoxicosis. While TRAb >3 times the upper limit of normal in the last trimester additionally increases the risk of neonatal thyrotoxicosis.

Thyroglobulin Levels

Thyroglobulin (Tg) is a glycoprotein molecule synthesized exclusively by the thyroid follicular cells, and used as a tumor marker in the management of patients with differentiated thyroid carcinomas (DTC). Immunometric assay (IMA) and RIA techniques are currently used to measure Tg. Assays for measuring serum Tg have improved since the first generation RIA although accurate measurement of serum Tg is still challenging. Currently, noncompetitive immunometric assay (IMA) is commonly used with the advantages of shorter incubation time, full automation, and higher sensitivity compared with the RIA. The presence of antithyroglobulin antibodies (TgAb) leads to over- or underestimation of Tg concentration and none of the commercially available assays are free from this interference. Liquid chromatography-tandem mass spectrometry (LC-MS/MS) is expected to overcome this interference but still requires further validation.

Calcitonin

Calcitonin is secreted by "C" cells of thyroid and is used as a tumor marker in medullary thyroid carcinoma. It is measured with chemiluminescent immunometric assays, which is highly specific and not affected by interfering substance such as procalcitonin, which is raised in many physiological and pathological conditions. It is used to screen multiple endocrine neoplasia 2, planning treatment, and follow-up after treatment for medullary thyroid carcinoma (MTC).

THYROID FUNCTION TESTS IN SPECIAL PATIENT POPULATIONS

Women with Type 1 Diabetes Mellitus

Type 1 diabetes mellitus in women raises their likelihood of developing postpartum thyroid dysfunction by three times. Women with T1DM should have their thyroid function (including TSH, FT, and TPOAb status) assessed at preconception, at the time of registration for pregnancy and at three months postpartum.

Patients with Diabetes

Patients with T1DM have high incidence of asymptomatic thyroid dysfunction and hence should have a yearly thyroid function test. In patients with type 2 diabetes mellitus, thyroid function should be assessed at diagnosis, however, annual thyroid function assessment may not be recommended.

Patients with Atrial Fibrillation, Hyperlipidemia, Osteoporosis, and Infertility

Patients presenting with atrial fibrillation, hyperlipidemia, subfertility, and osteoporosis should undergo serum TSH estimations as assessment of thyroid function because:
- Atrial fibrillation may be secondary to thyrotoxicosis in about 5–10% of patients.

- Osteoporosis may be secondary to hyperthyroidism and can be corrected by treating the underlying cause.
- Both hyper- and hypothyroidism may be contributing factors in menstrual cycle disorders, fetal loss, and infertility.

Women with a Past History of Postpartum Thyroiditis

These women have an increased long-term risk of developing hypothyroidism and relapse in subsequent pregnancies. Therefore, all women with a history of postpartum thyroiditis should be advised to have a yearly thyroid function test, and also prior to and at 6–8 weeks after the subsequent pregnancies.

Down Syndrome and Turner's Syndrome

Patients of Down's syndrome as well as Turner's syndrome are recommended to undergo thyroid function assessment annually, keeping in mind the high incidence of hypothyroidism seen in these patients.

Following Destructive Treatment for Thyrotoxicosis by either Radioiodine or Surgery

Patients who received radioiodine therapy or those who have undergone thyroidectomy should be screened indefinitely for the development of hypothyroidism or recurrence of hyperthyroidism. Assessment of thyroid function in these patients should be done 4–8 weeks after treatment, followed by quarter yearly assessments for the subsequent year and annually thereafter.

Post-neck Irradiation

Patients who undergo surgery or external radiation therapy of the neck, or both, for head and neck cancer (including lymphoma) have a high incidence (up to 50%) of hypothyroidism. The incidence is particularly high in patients who undergo surgery and receive high doses of radiation as the effect is dose-dependent. The onset of overt hypothyroidism due to surgery or irradiation is gradual and may precede subclinical hypothyroidism for many years. In such patients, thyroid function assessment should be carried out annually.

Patients Receiving Amiodarone and Lithium

Amiodarone therapy is associated with iodide-induced thyroid dysfunction (hypothyroidism or hyperthyroidism) as 200 mg tablet consists, 75 mg of iodine. Patients on amiodarone therapy should have thyroid function assessment at the time of initiation and thereafter every 6 months during treatment and till 12 months after cessation of therapy.

Lithium therapy (for bipolar disorder) is associated with mild to overt hypothyroidism in up to 34–16% of patients, respectively, which can occur abruptly even after years of cessation of therapy. Thyrotoxicosis can also occur due to long-term treatment with lithium but is relatively rare. Therefore, all patients on lithium therapy should have a thyroid function assessment before commencement of treatment and thereafter every 6–12 months during lithium therapy.

Treatment of Thyrotoxicosis with Antithyroid Drugs

Antithyroid drugs used in the management of thyrotoxicosis, carbimazole and PTU, decrease thyroid hormone secretion. Thyroid function assessment should be carried out every 1–3 months to determine whether stable hormonal concentrations have been reached when antithyroid therapy is instituted and annually thereafter if long term treatment is used.

Patients on Thyroxine Therapy

In patients undergoing T4 therapy regardless of the cause, long-term follow-up with annual measurements of serum TSH are recommended. This helps to check compliance, verify the dosage, and take account of variations in dosage requirements due to concomitant medications. In pregnant women, the dose may need to be increased by a minimum of 50 μg/day to maintain normal serum TSH levels. The TSH levels should be tested in each trimester.

ANALYTICAL VARIATIONS AND ASSAY INTERFERENCES

- *Heterophil antibodies*: The presence of these antibodies in serum can lead to falsely high or low TFTs. Heterophile antibodies are antibodies induced by external antigens (heterophile antigens) that cross-react with self-antigens. The best-known heterophile antibodies are human antimouse antibodies (HAMA), which can react with the mouse monoclonal antibodies that are used in many immunometric assays, such as in TSH estimation where if they are present, they may lead to erroneously high or low values of TSH. Various approaches are being developed to deal with this issue with varying degrees of success, including the use of chimeric antibody combinations and blocking agents to neutralize the effects of HAMA.
- *Macro-TSH* is a rare condition where serum contains antibodies against TSH (anti-TSH Ig) which binds to TSH and neutralizes its activity, but leaves open epitope to interact with assay antibodies leading to spuriously high TSH value. This can be identified by the following methods—serial dilution which will show an increase in TSH levels with dilution in presence of macro TSH, polyethylene glycol precipitation which will bring TSH levels down if antibodies are removed, and gel filtration

chromatography which will demonstrate the high molecular weight of anti-TSH antibodies.
- *Drug interference*: Both in vitro and in vivo interferences occur occasionally. The presence of heparin in the blood sample can cause stimulation of lipoprotein lipase and inhibit T4 binding to serum protein. Furosemide can inhibit thyroid hormone binding and cause a low T4 result.
- *Biotin (Vitamin B7)* easily binds to hormones and can affect measurement of TSH or FT4/FT3. A falsely low TSH with raised FT4 and T3 mimicking that seen in thyrotoxicosis may be observed.

FUTURE DIRECTIONS

For last 50 years, immunoassays have been the mainstay for thyroid function testing. Although the high sensitivity, ease of use and reduced cost of equipment has been the advantages, reduced selectivity, lack of reproducibility and assay time has been limitations. Liquid chromatography-mass spectrometry (LC-MS) with its selectivity, high sensitivity and reproducibility will slowly start to replace the existing RIA especially with further technological advances.

CONCLUSION

- Thyroid function tests are the most common endocrine tests done worldwide and its use is only going to increase in the future due to rise in thyroid disorders and increased awareness among physicians and patients.
- Thyroid disorders have diverse clinical manifestations and hence an astute physician should have a low threshold to perform thyroid function tests when clinically relevant.
- Testing TFT aids in making the right clinical decision whether it be instituting the right treatment or close follow-up.
- The enhanced sensitivity and specificity of TSH assays have greatly improved the assessment of thyroid function tests. Since TSH levels change dynamically in response to the alterations of T3 and T4, TSH serves as an accurate screening test in most scenarios.
- When hypothyroidism is suspected, an FT4 estimate is appropriate because TT3 and FT3 tests have inadequate sensitivity and specificity.
- When hyperthyroidism is suspected, the combination of an FT4 estimate and a total- or FT3 estimate provides the most complete assessment of the severity of hyperthyroidism and identifies cases of "T3-toxicosis," i.e., a selective increase of the serum T3 concentration.
- From time to time, a deviation from the typically observed pattern of thyroid function tests might arise. Interpretation of such tests requires a deeper understanding of factors that could influence it including assay interference.

SUGGESTED READINGS

1. Joshi SR. Laboratory evaluation of Thyroid function. J Assoc Physicians India. 2011;59(Suppl):14-20.
2. British Thyroid Association. (2006). UK guidelines for the use of thyroid function tests. [Online] Available from http://www.acb.org.uk/docs/TFTgudelinefinal.pdf [Last accessed January, 2023].
3. Werner SC, Ingbar SH, Braveman LE, Utiger RD. Werner & Ingbar's The Thyroid: A Fundamental and Clinical Text, 9th edition. Philadelphia: Lippincott Williams & Wilkins; 2013. pp. 279-97.
4. Ross DS, Cooper DS, Mulder JE. (2022). Laboratory assessment of Thyroid function. [Online] Available from https://www.uptodate.com/contents/laboratory-assessment-of-thyroid-function [Last accessed January, 2022].
5. Garg MK, Mahalle N, Hari Kumar K. Laboratory evaluation of thyroid function: Dilemmas and pitfalls. Med J DY Patil Univ. 2016;9:430-6.
6. Tapper MA, Francis CA, Dilworth LL, McGrowder DA. Evaluating thyroid function in the clinical laboratory. Thyroid Res Pract. 2017;14(3):118-21.
7. Feldt-Rasmussen U, Klose M, Feingold KR, Anawalt B, Boyce A, Chrousos G, et al. Clinical Strategies in the Testing of Thyroid Function. In: Endotext [Internet]. South Dartmouth (MA): MDText.com, Inc; 2000.

CHAPTER 6

Thyroid Imaging from an Endocrinologist's Perspective

Ganapathi Bantwal, Sonali Appaiah

INTRODUCTION

The thyroid is one of the largest of the endocrine organs. Thyroid gland dysfunction and anatomic abnormalities of thyroid are one of the most common endocrine diseases. Thyroid gland imaging helps in diagnosis, treatment, follow-up, and assessing prognosis of thyroid diseases such as thyroid nodule, goiter, thyroiditis, and thyroid cancer.

NORMAL THYROID IMAGING

Normal Anatomy

The normal thyroid is made up of two lobes joined by a thin band of tissue, the isthmus, and weighs about 15–20 g. The thyroid resides in the midline of the lower neck, anterolateral to the larynx and trachea at approximately the level of the second and third tracheal rings. Each lobe is approximately 2–2.5 cm in thickness and width at its largest diameter and is approximately 4 cm in length, while the isthmus is approximately 0.5 cm thick, 2 cm wide, and 1–2 cm high. The individual lobes normally have a pointed superior pole and a poorly defined blunt inferior pole that merges medially with the isthmus. The gland is bordered laterally by the common carotid arteries and sternocleidomastoid muscles, anterolaterally by the jugular veins, anteriorly by strap muscles, and posteriorly by the longus colli muscles. The thyroid is attached to the larynx and trachea posteriorly.

Ultrasonography is generally the first choice and the most sensitive imaging modality for evaluation of thyroid, and is usually done with high-frequency sonography (using 7–13 MHz transducer). The ultrasound (US) appearance (**Fig. 1**) of a healthy thyroid parenchyma is usually homogeneous, bright, and slightly hyperechoic with little identifiable internal architecture. Thyroid tissue is more echogenic than muscle but less echogenic than fat. The common carotid artery and internal jugular vein appear sonolucent. The air-filled trachea in the midline gives a characteristic curvilinear reflecting surface, with an associated reverberation artifact.

On computed tomography (CT), the thyroid gland appears brighter [80–100 Hounsfield units (HUs)] because of the high concentration of iodine in the thyroid gland, resulting in greater attenuation than surrounding structures. The thyroid gland is isointense on T1, slightly hyperintense on T2, shows homogenous signal intensity relative to the surrounding neck musculature, and enhances homogenously postcontrast on magnetic resonance imaging (MRI).

The thyroid gland is uniquely able to take up iodine, from the environment and to concentrate it thousands of times. This phenomenon allowed the use of radioiodine (^{123}I, ^{131}I) and technetium pertechnetate (technetium-99m; ^{99m}Tc) isotopes in thyroid imaging (**Table 1**). Here, the normal thyroid appears as a bilobed structure connected by a thin isthmus (**Fig. 2**). Tracer distribution is fairly homogeneous. Asymmetry is common, with the

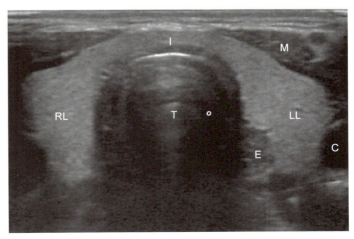

Fig. 1: Ultrasonography of a normal thyroid gland. Parenchyma is homogeneous, bright, and slightly hyperechoic with respect to the surrounding muscles.

(C: common carotid artery; E: esophagus; I: isthmus; LL: left lobe; M: muscles; RL: right lobe; T: trachea)

Source: Andrioli M, Valcavi R. Sonography of Normal and Abnormal Thyroid and Parathyroid Glands. Front Horm Res. 2016;45:-15.

SECTION 2

DIAGNOSIS OF THYROID DISORDERS

TABLE 1: Radionucleotides used in thyroid imaging.

Radionucleo-tides	Half-life	Route of administration	Principal gamma energy (keV)
^{123}I	13.2 hours	Oral	159
^{131}I	8.1 days	Oral	364
^{99m}Tc	6 hours	Intravenous	140

(^{123}I: iodine-123; ^{131}I: iodine-131; ^{99m}Tc: technetium pertechnetate isotope)

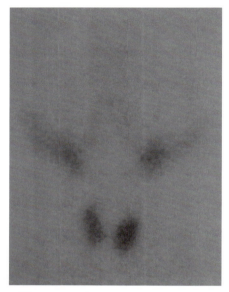

Fig. 2: Normal ^{99m}Tc scan of the thyroid gland.

right lobe usually larger than the left. Under conditions of euthyroidism with normal iodine intake, the maximum uptake of ^{99m}Tc is 0.5–2.0% of the administered activity, while the radioiodine uptake is 25–50% 24 hours after the administration of the diagnostic activity.

There is homogenous tracer uptake in both lobes with thin midline isthmus.

THYROID IMAGING IN CONGENITAL PRIMARY HYPOTHYROIDISM

Congenital primary hypothyroidism (CH) is the most common endocrine disorder in infants with recent studies showing an incidence of 1 in 1,500 live newborns. This includes thyroid dysgenesis which represents 80–85% of all cases with CH, with phenotypic spectrum of thyroid dyshormonogenesis (TD) ranging from athyreosis, hypoplasia, and hemiagenesis to ectopic thyroid without function. The rest 15–20% are caused by inherited defects in one of the steps of thyroid hormone synthesis known as TD. In neonates with CH both scintigraphy and ultrasound should be considered, however, there should not be delay in the initiation of treatment for the same. In such instances, scintigraphy can be done within 7 days of initiation of treatment.

Ultrasound in Congenital Primary Hypothyroidism

Ultrasound is useful to detect the absence or presence of thyroid gland, the structure, size, and echogenic texture of a thyroid gland. Ultrasound is highly observer-dependent and it cannot always detect lingual and sublingual thyroid ectopy.

Ultrasound also helps to prevent the incorrect diagnosis of athyreosis in conditions where there is an absence of uptake on scintigraphy in spite of eutopic thyroid gland. This is seen in conditions like the presence of maternal thyroid-stimulating hormone (TSH) receptor blocking antibodies, L-T4 treatment resulting in suppression of TSH, excess iodine due to exposure (e.g., from antiseptic preparations) and presence of sodium/iodide symporter (NIS) or TSH receptor inactivating mutations.

Thyroid Scintigraphy in Congenital Primary Hypothyroidism

Radionucleotides like 1–2 MBq of iodine-123 (^{123}I) or 10–20 MBq of technetium-99m (^{99m}Tc) are used for scintigraphy. Since, it is less expensive, quicker to use and widely available ^{99m}Tc is generally preferred over ^{123}I. However, since iodine (^{123}I) is preferentially taken up by the thyroid gland it gives a clearer scan than ^{99m}Tc.

Scintigraphy can facilitate the diagnosis of:
- Athyreosis—seen as absence of uptake **(Fig. 3)**
- Hypoplasia of a gland in situ—seen as hemithyroid or smaller sized thyroid gland in situ
- Ectopic thyroid—seen as uptake at a point along the route of normal embryological descent **(Figs. 4A and B)**

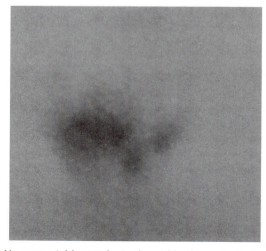

Fig. 3: No appreciable uptake in thyroid bed or ectopic location in the neck with normal background activity in a ^{99m}Tc scintigraphy done in child with congenital hypothyroidism suggestive of thyroid agenesis.

- *Dyshormonogenesis*—seen as a normal or large size thyroid gland in situ with or without abnormally high levels of uptake **(Fig. 5)**.

Perchlorate Discharge Test

Iodine-123 scan can be combined with perchlorate discharge test to evaluate the cause of dyshormonogenesis in patients with eutopic thyroid gland. In the perchlorate discharge test, 200–1,000 mg potassium perchlorate is given orally after ^{123}I uptake scan followed by repeat ^{123}I uptake scan after 30 minutes to 1 hour. More than 10% decrease in radioactivity is suggestive of iodine organification defect. The probable mutations causing dyshormonogenesis can be differentiated as in the **Flowchart 1**.

IMAGING IN THYROIDITIS

The inflammation of the thyroid, i.e., thyroiditis, causes follicular changes in its parenchyma. As a result, on ultrasonography, the gland loses its uniform and bright ultrasonographic appearance. The different types of thyroiditis usually present with specific ultrasonographic features **(Table 2)**. Clinical presentation varies in different types of thyroiditis ranging from hypothyroidism in Hashimoto's thyroiditis to hyperthyroidism in subacute and painless thyroiditis.

Hashimoto's Thyroiditis

It is the most common cause of hypothyroidism in adults in developed nations. It is also the most common cause of acquired hypothyroidism in children in iodine sufficient

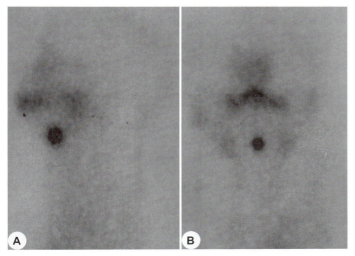

Figs. 4A and B: Lateral and anterior view ^{99m}Tc scintigraphy in congenital hypothyroidism with ectopic uptake at the upper neck midline at the level of submandibular gland suggestive of ectopic sublingual thyroid gland.

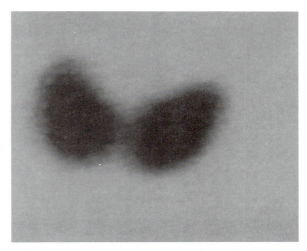

Fig. 5: Enlarged gland with increased uniform radioisotope uptake in ^{99m}Tc scintigraphy done in a child with congenital hypothyroidism suggestive of dyshormonogenesis.

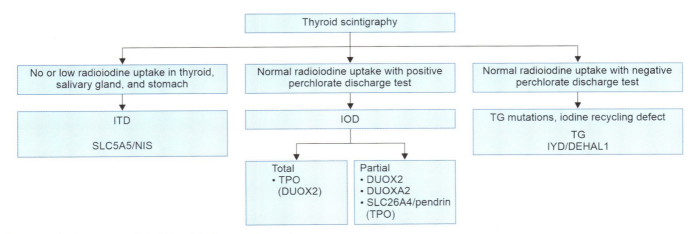

Flowchart 1: Diagnosis of etiology of dyshormonogenesis.
[DEHAL1: iodotyrosine dehalogenase 1 (IYD)/D1; DUOX2: dual oxidase2; DUOXA2: dual oxidase maturation factor A2; ITD: iodine transport defect; IOD: iodine organification defect; partial IOD: 10–90% of radioiodine washout after perchlorate intake, total IOD: >90% of radioiodine washout after perchlorate intake; PDS: pendrin (SLC26A4); SCL5A5/NIS: sodium-iodide symporter; TPO: thyroid peroxidase; TG: thyroglobulin]
Source: Szinnai G. Genetics of normal and abnormal thyroid development in humans. Best Pract Res Clin Endocrinol Metab. 2014;28(2):133-50.

SECTION 2
DIAGNOSIS OF THYROID DISORDERS

TABLE 2: Ultrasonographic features in different types of thyroiditis.	
Type of thyroiditis	Ultrasonographic features of thyroid
Acute thyroiditis (Fig. 6)	Thyroid is edematous with diffusely decreased echogenicity, sometimes bearing a focal abscess. Abscesses are seen as ill-defined hypoechoic, heterogeneous masses with internal debris and bright echoes from gas
Subacute thyroiditis (granulomatous and De Quervain's) (Fig. 7)	Focal patchy areas of marked hypoechogenicity, with irregular borders, which may elongate along the long-axis of the gland. They may be unilateral, bilateral or migrate over time
Tubercular thyroiditis	Round heterogeneously hypoechoic nodule or as an anechoic lesion (abscess) with internal echoes and ill-defined irregular borders
Hashimoto's thyroiditis (Fig. 8)	Hypoechoic and heterogeneous—mild and diffuse lymphocytic infiltration
	Pseudomicronodules—due to more discrete areas of lymphocytic infiltration, and forming localized hypoechoic (subcentimetric) pseudonodules
	"Swiss cheese" or "honeycomb" pattern—very little fibrotic parenchyma separates the hypoechoic pseudomicronodules
	Pseudomacronodules—large pseudonodules
	Markedly hypoechoic—when parenchyma completely replaced by lymphocytes
	Hyperechoic bands—due to fibrous bands
	Hyperechoic and heterogenous—late stage of the disease when the fibrosis is diffuse and the thyroid may appear hyperechoic
	Speckled (very rare)—numerous punctate densities scattered throughout the parenchyma
Painless thyroiditis (postpartum/silent thyroiditis)	Hypoechogenicity similar to other forms of autoimmune thyroid diseases, but with less fibrosis and hypoechogenicity
Riedel's thyroiditis	Enlarged diffusely hypoechoic gland with fibrous septations and hypovascularity. In contrast to Hashimoto's thyroiditis, there may be carotid artery encasement, compression of adjacent structures, and invasion of bordering muscles and mediastinum

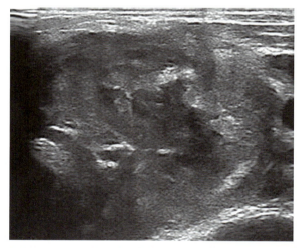

Fig. 6: Ultrasonography thyroid in acute thyroiditis. Ill-defined, hyperechoic, heterogeneous abscess is seen in the left thyroid lobe.
Source: Andrioli M, Valcavi R. Sonography of Normal and Abnormal Thyroid and Parathyroid Glands. Front Horm Res. 2016;45:1-15.

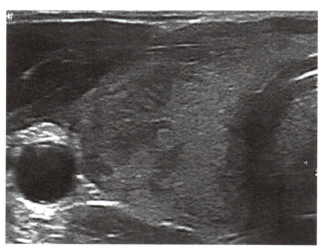

Fig. 7: Ultrasonography thyroid in subacute thyroiditis. Focal hypoechoic areas with ill-defined margins seen in the right lobe.
Source: Andrioli M, Valcavi R. Sonography of Normal and Abnormal Thyroid and Parathyroid Glands. Front Horm Res. 2016;45:1-15.

areas. The most common clinical manifestations of Hashimoto thyroiditis (HT) are goiter and hypothyroidism. The sonographic appearance of HT varies depending on the length and severity of the disease **(Table 2)**. Enlarged lymph nodes with reactivity features are almost invariably present in HT. The vascularity of HT is variable, ranging from avascular to hypervascular. Usually seen in the paratracheal and pretracheal space (level VI), and near the isthmus. Lymph nodes tend to appear rounded, with a variable presence of a hilum.

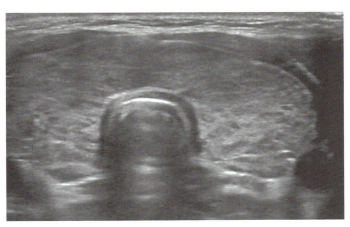

Fig. 8: Ultrasonography appearance in Hashimoto's thyroiditis. Enlarged predominantly hyperechoic thyroid gland with diffusely heterogeneous parenchyma. Hyperechoic fibrous strands separating poorly defined hypoechoic regions making a "Swiss cheese" or "honeycomb" pattern.
Source: Andrioli M, Valcavi R. Sonography of Normal and Abnormal Thyroid and Parathyroid Glands. Front Horm Res. 2016;45:1-15.

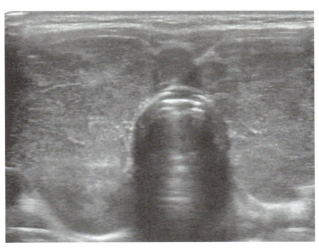

Fig. 9: Ultrasonographic appearance of Graves' disease (GD). The thyroid gland is typically enlarged, diffusely heterogeneous and hyperechoic.
Source: Andrioli M, Valcavi R. Sonography of Normal and Abnormal Thyroid and Parathyroid Glands. Front Horm Res. 2016;45;1-15.

IMAGING IN HYPERTHYROID DISORDERS

Hyperthyroidism has a prevalence of 1–2% in women and 0.1–0.2% in men. The most common causes are Graves' disease (GD) and toxic multinodular goiter, caused due to increased production of thyroid hormone by the gland. Thyroiditis can result in passive release of thyroid hormone from damaged follicles, resulting in thyrotoxicosis. Thyroid imaging with US and thyroid scintigraphy helps to diagnose etiology of hyperthyroidism.

IMAGING IN GRAVES' DISEASE

Graves' disease is a multisystem autoimmune disease characterized by the presence of TSH receptor antibody (TSHR-Ab). These antibodies stimulate the TSH receptor causing hypertrophy of the thyroid gland. The gland becomes more vascular and increases the production of thyroid hormones. GD and HT are both autoimmune diseases with similar ultrasonographic features. Since transition between the two clinical forms occurs in some patients, they probably represent the different ends of the clinical spectrum.

Ultrasound in Graves' Disease

On US the thyroid gland is enlarged in GD, with diffuse hypoechogenicity, and inhomogeneous echotexture with numerous tiny hypoechoic foci around 2–3 mm in size. However, but its heterogeneity and hypoechogenicity not as pronounced as seen in HT. Hyperechoic thyroid gland may be seen in few cases **(Fig. 9)**. The hypervascularity of the thyroid gland gives a characteristic appearance called the "thyroid inferno," which can be seen qualitatively in color Doppler as a diffuse increase in flow though the thyroid parenchyma. In GD there is a marked increase in the peak systolic velocity of the infrathyroidal artery. This could help to distinguish Graves' from other cause of hyperthyroidism like subacute thyroiditis or amiodarone-induced thyrotoxicosis type 2.

Thyroid Scintigraphy in Graves' Disease and Other Causes of Hyperthyroidism

The evaluation of regional thyroid function and identification of autonomous thyroid nodules is possible only with thyroid scintigraphy. Scintigraphy helps to visualize the differential accumulation of radionuclides (^{123}I or ^{131}I or ^{99m}Tc) in the thyroid cells and thus provides distribution of active thyroid tissue, or a functional thyroid map for differential diagnosis **(Table 3)**. ^{131}I thyroid uptake is not recommended for routine diagnostic use unless low-uptake thyrotoxicosis is suspected or for dosimetric appraisal before therapy with ^{131}I.

A diffuse increased radioisotope uptake in thyroid gland is suggestive of GD **(Fig. 10)**; a "cold" or poorly visualized gland **(Fig. 11)** is seen in conditions such as subacute thyroiditis, iatrogenic thyrotoxicosis; focal increased uptake in toxic adenoma; while multinodular localization is most likely toxic multinodular goiter **(Figs. 12A and B)**. The diagnosis of GD does not exclude the presence of thyroid nodules. Hyperthyroidism of autoimmune origin with the presence of focal cold lesions is known as Marine–Lenhart syndrome **(Fig. 13)**. The cancer risk in cold nodules is higher (15–19%) in GD than other thyroid nodules, and thyroid cancer in GD are clinically more aggressive.

SECTION 2
DIAGNOSIS OF THYROID DISORDERS

TABLE 3: Differential diagnosis of hyperthyroidism depending on the radioisotope uptake in thyroid gland.

Normal/increased radioisotope uptake	Near absent radioisotope uptake
Graves' disease	Painless (silent) thyroiditis
Toxic multinodular goiter	Subacute thyroiditis
Toxic adenoma	Amiodarone-induced thyroiditis
Trophoblastic disease	Iatrogenic thyrotoxicosis
TSH secreting pituitary adenoma	Factitious ingestion of thyroid hormone
Resistance to thyroid hormone (T3 receptor mutation)	Struma ovarii
	Acute thyroiditis
	Extensive metastases from follicular thyroid cancer

(TSH: thyroid-stimulating hormone; T3: triiodothyronine)

IMAGING OF THYROID NODULE/NODULAR THYROID GOITER AND THYROID MALIGNANCIES

A thyroid nodule is defined as discrete lesions within the thyroid gland, radiologically distinct from surrounding thyroid parenchyma. On physical examination (i.e., neck palpation), the prevalence of thyroid nodule in iodine-sufficient populations is approximately 5%, reaching up to 68% of the general population. The reported prevalence is about 65% with ultrasonography, 15% with CT or MRI, and 1–2% with 18-fluorodeoxyglucose positron emission tomography (18-FDG-PET).

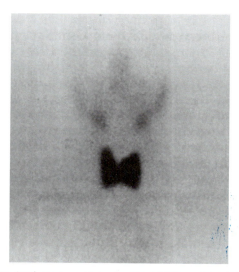

Fig. 10: Avid tracer uptake by thyroid in comparison to salivary gland in ^{99m}Tc scintigraphy of thyroid in Graves' disease.
Source: Meier DA, Kaplan MM. Radioiodine Uptake and thyroid scintiscanning. Endocrinol Metab Clin North Am. 2001;30(2):291-313.

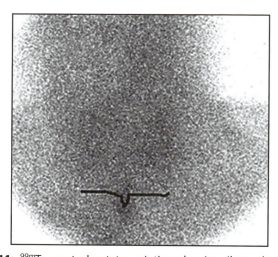

Fig. 11: ^{99m}Tc pertechnetate scintigraphy in silent thyroiditis showing poor tracer uptake.
Source: Garberoglio S, Testori O. Role of Nuclear Medicine in the Diagnosis of Benign Thyroid Diseases. Front Horm Res. 2016,45;1-15.

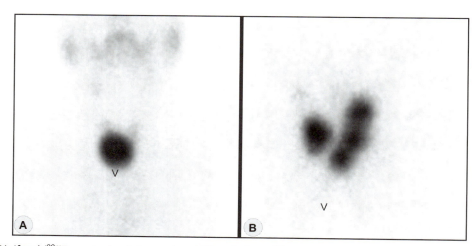

Figs. 12A and B: (A) Unifocal (^{99m}Tc-pertechnetate scan) and (B) multifocal (^{123}I-iodide scan) thyroid autonomy.
Source: Giovanella L, Ceriani L, Treglia G. Role of isotope scan, including positron emission tomography/computed tomography, in nodular goitre. Best Pract Res Clin Endocrinol Metab. 2014;28(4):507-18.

Around 10% of patients who present with thyroid nodules are at risk of malignancy. The rate of malignancy ranges from between 5 and 13% of patients with ultrasound, CT, or MRI-detected incidentalomas, and increases to 55% in case of focal uptake on the positron emission tomography (PET) scan and an increased maximum standardized uptake value.

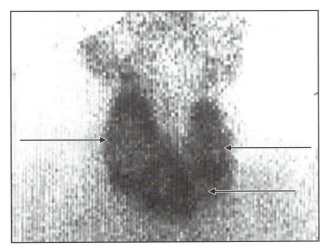

Fig. 13: Marine–Lenhart syndrome. ^{99m}Tc-pertechnetate image shows an enlarged thyroid with diffusely increased radiotracer trapping, as in Graves' disease. However, within the gland are distinct cold nodules (arrows).
Source: Intenzo M, dePapp AE, Jabbour S, Miller JL, Kim SM, Capuzzi DM. Scintigraphic manifestations of thyrotoxicosis. Radiographics. 2003;23(4):857-69.

Ultrasound of Thyroid Nodule/Nodular Thyroid Goiter

Sonography is the primary tool used for initial cancer risk stratification of thyroid nodules and for subsequently deciding whether to order a fine-needle aspiration (FNA) biopsy. It is indicated when thyroid is palpated on examination or when incidentally detected in other radiological study. Based on ultrasonographic features the thyroid nodules can be classified **(Table 4)** as low risk or benign, intermediate risk or moderately suspicious **(Figs. 14A to F)**, and high risk or suspicious thyroid nodules **(Figs. 15A to F)** as per American Thyroid Association (ATA) and other professional groups. Further evaluation by FNA biopsy is determined based on the scoring systems and the size of the nodule.

Ultrasonographic color and spectral Doppler imaging determines the vascular pattern of thyroid and helps to further determines the character of the nodule. Exclusively central vascular pattern is suggestive of malignancy, while a predominantly perinodular pattern is seen in benign nodule.

Ultrasonographic evaluation of the anterior cervical lymph node compartments (central and lateral) should be performed whenever thyroid nodules are detected. Ultrasonographic features of cervical lymph nodes predictive of metastasis include hyperechogenicity, microcalcifications, cystic aspect, peripheral vascularity, and round shape.

TABLE 4: The American Thyroid Association (ATA) sonological scoring system for thyroid nodule.			
ATA sonographic scoring system	**Sonographic pattern of nodule**	**Risk of malignancy**	**Fine needle aspiration size cut-off (largest dimension)**
Benign	Purely cystic	<1%	Not indicated
Very low suspicion	• Spongiform/partially cystic nodules • Without any ultrasound features defining low, intermediate, or high-suspicion patterns	<3%	When ≥20 mm or observation
Low suspicion	• Isoechoic/hyperechoic solid or partially cystic nodule with eccentric solid area • Without microcalcifications, irregular margin, extrathyroidal extension, and taller than wide shape	5–10%	≥15 mm
Intermediate-suspicion	• Hypoechoic solid nodule with smooth margins • Without microcalcifications, extrathyroidal extension, or taller than wide shape	10–20%	≥10 mm
High-suspicion	Solid hypoechoic nodule or solid hypoechoic component of partially cystic nodule with ≥1 of the following: • Irregular margins (infiltrative and microlobulated) • Microcalcifications • Taller than wide shape • Rim calcifications with small extrusive soft tissue • Extrathyroidal extension	>70–90%	≥10 mm

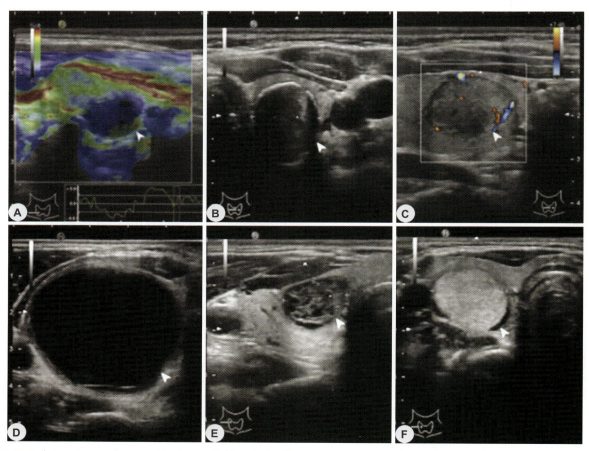

Figs. 14A to F: Indeterminate ultrasound features: (A) Elevated stiffness at elastography (red indicates soft tissues, blue hard tissues, and green intermediate values of stiffness). (B) Complete rim calcification. (C) Slightly hypoechoic nodule with intranodular vascularization (the mean flow velocity is converted into a color scale—flow toward the transducer is represented in red, while away from the transducer is depicted in blue). (D) Low-or very-low suspicion US features—pure cyst. (E) Spongiform nodule with >50% of the nodule volume composed of microcystic spaces. (F) Solid hyperechoic nodule. The arrows indicate the thyroid nodule. The gray scale graphically represents the shades of gray that can be provided by the ultrasound equipment.
Source: Durante C, Grani G, Lamartina L, Filetti S, Mandel SJ, Cooper DS. The diagnosis and management of thyroid nodules: a review. JAMA. 2018;319(9):914-24.

The ultrasonographic features of thyroid carcinoma in a thyroid nodule includes the presence a solid mass which is hypoechoic, taller than wide, with absent halo sign, irregular margins, microcalcifications, increased intranodular vascularity, and presence of metastasis in the cervical lymph nodes.

Ultrasound Elastography

Malignant lesions are often associated with changes in the mechanical properties of a tissue. Ultrasound elastography is a dynamic technique, based upon the principle that the (benign) softer parts of tissues deform easier than the harder (malignant) parts under compression by an external force. This elasticity can be assessed by measuring the degree of distortion of the US beam.

With the combined autocorrelation method (CAM), US elastographic measurements can be performed during the US examination, using the same real-time instrument and the same probe. Obese patients, those with multinodular goiters and coalescent nodules, cystic or partially cystic nodules, nodules having calcified shell or patients in whom the nodule is posterior or inferior are not candidates for elastography.

Ultrasound elastography was initially reported as highly predictive of benign or malignant disease. However, more recent reports suggest that elastographic cancer risk assessment may be inferior to gray scale ultrasound, with positive predictive values of around 30–40% only.

Thyroid Scintigraphy in Nodular Thyroid Goiter and Thyroid Malignancy

Autonomous nodules rarely harbor malignancy, and current clinical guidelines suggest refraining from FNA of hyperactive nodules diagnosed by thyroid scan with either ^{99m}Tc-pertechnetate or ^{123}I. Most thyroid carcinomas appear as areas of poor isotope uptake on scans, known as cold nodules. This is due to the inefficient trapping and

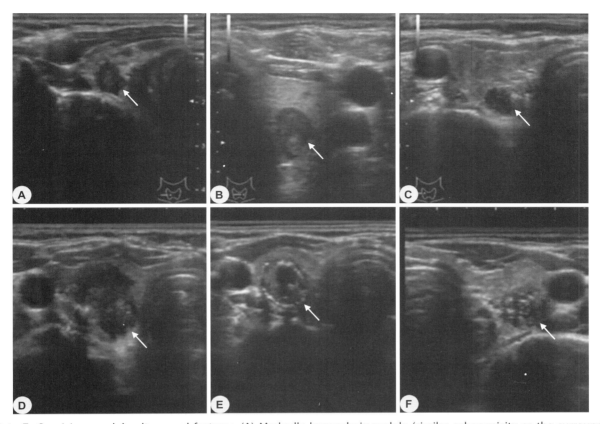

Figs. 15A to F: Suspicious nodule ultrasound features. (A) Markedly hypoechoic nodule (similar echogenicity as the surrounding strap muscles) with irregular margins. (B) Taller-than-wide hypoechoic nodule. (C) Markedly hypoechoic nodule with regular margins. (D) Hypoechoic nodule with infiltrative margins and suspicious extrathyroidal extension. (E) Multiple interruptions in calcific rim with evidence of extrusive tissue (echogenicity is difficult to interpret because of acoustic shadowing of the calcific rim). (F) Hypoechoic solid nodule with microcalcifications and irregular margins. The arrows indicate the thyroid nodule. The gray scale graphically represents the shades of gray that can be provided by the ultrasound equipment.
Source: Durante C, Grani G, Lamartina L, Filetti S, Mandel SJ, Cooper DS. The diagnosis and management of thyroid nodules: a review. JAMA. 2018;319(9):914-24.

organification of iodine by the thyroid cancer cells. Although almost all thyroid cancers are cold nodules, most of these nodules are benign (i.e., 90–95%) and this greatly reduces the specificity of a thyroid scan.

A thyroid scan is generally carried out when nodules occur in people with subnormal TSH levels. The AACE and ETA suggest to consider performing scintigraphy to exclude autonomy for thyroid nodules even if TSH is normal in iodine deficient regions.

Postoperatively in follicular cell thyroid cancers, ^{131}I whole-body scanning (WBS) is used to detect residual local disease and functioning distant metastases **(Figs. 16A and B)**. It is performed after the administration of larger activities of radioiodine, for diagnosis (1–5 mCi ^{131}I or 1–5 mCi ^{123}I), or more commonly for therapy (≥30 mCi ^{131}I). To ensure optimal uptake by thyroid cells, serum TSH level should be greater than an empirically determined level of 25–30 mU/L or by withholding levothyroxine treatment is for 3 to 4 weeks or intramuscular injections of recombinant human TSH (rhTSH) (0.9 mg for 2 consecutive days, with ^{131}I administered 1 day after the second injection).

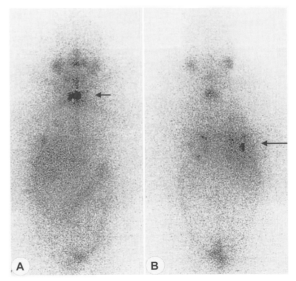

Figs. 16A and B: Post-therapy whole-body scan. After 7.4 GBq (200 mCi) of ^{131}I, WBS done in a woman with papillary thyroid carcinoma after total thyroidectomy showed uptake in thyroid bed (short arrow) and pulmonary metastasis (long arrow).
Source: Haugen BR, Lin E C. Isotope Imaging for metastatic thyroid cancer. Endocrinol Metab Clin North Am. 2001;30(2):469-92.

Computed Tomography and Magnetic Resonance Imaging in Nodular Thyroid Goiter and Thyroid Malignancy

Computed tomography is less sensitive than US for detecting and characterizing thyroid nodule. CT and MRI of the thyroid provide excellent anatomic detail of structures in the head and neck and is largely limited to presurgical evaluation. They are useful for the evaluation of substernal goiter **(Fig. 17)**, to assess caudal extension and compression of surrounding structures **(Figs. 18 and 19)**. It is necessary for staging thyroid malignancy, assessing lymph node metastasis, locoregional extension, and distant hepatic or pulmonary metastatic disease. CT should be performed without intravenous (IV) contrast material in follicular thyroid cancer, as it contains iodine. Use of iodine containing contrast will result in suppression of subsequent iodine uptake into thyroid tissue, necessitating a 4–6 weeks delay before either radioiodine scintigraphy or therapy can be done. In a patient with hyperthyroidism, iodine contrast could also lead to thyroid storm.

Magnetic resonance imaging demonstrates heterogeneity of the thyroid gland in multinodular goiter. Lymph nodes with metastasis often demonstrate hyperenhancement on T1-weighted images owing to the presence of colloid and thyroglobulin. MRI may better delineate aerodigestive axis involvement as compared with CT scan **(Figs. 19A and B)**. It is superior to CT for the detection of brain metastases. It is also useful for evaluation of axial bone metastases from thyroid cancers such as follicular

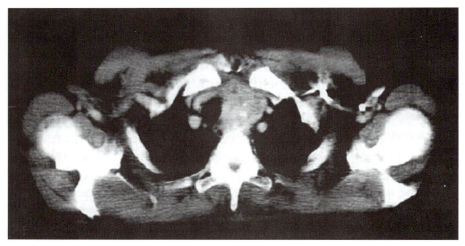

Fig. 17: Computed tomography (CT) image of substernal goiter containing calcifications and displacing the trachea to the right.
Source: Jennings A. Evaluation of substernal goiters using computed tomography and MR Imaging. Endocrinol Metab Clin North Am. 2001;30(2):401-14.

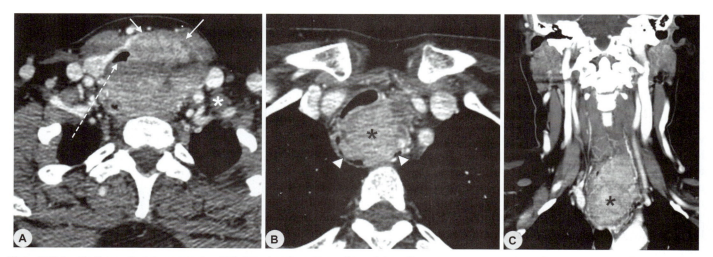

Figs. 18A to C: Computed tomography (CT) imaging in a case of Hürthle cell carcinoma. Axial (A and B) and coronal (C) postcontrast CT images of the neck show a large invasive mass centered in the left thyroid lobe with invasion of the strap muscles (arrows) as well as mucosal luminal invasion of the trachea (dashed arrow). The mass demonstrates caudal extension to the upper mediastinum (*) with gross intraluminal esophageal invasion (arrowheads).
Source: Calle S, Choi J, Ahmad S, Bell D, Learned KO. Imaging of the thyroid: Practical approach. Neuroimag Clin N Am. 2021;31(3):265-84.

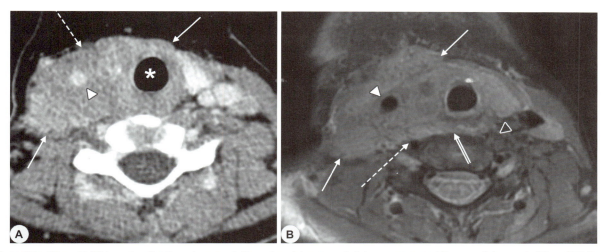

Figs. 19A and B: CT and MRI imaging findings in a medullary thyroid cancer. Axial postcontrast CT scan of the neck (A) and T2 fat-saturated axial MR image (B) show an invasive mass in the right thyroid lobe (arrows) with obliteration of the internal jugular vein, and circumferential encasement/invasion of the right common carotid artery (white arrowheads). CT image (A) illustrates circumferential involvement of the trachea by hypodense tumor (*) and invasion of the strap muscles anteriorly (dashed arrow). MR imaging (B) delineates how the mass posteriorly abuts the right vertebral artery (dashed arrow) and ventral vertebral body (double arrow) with invasion of the prevertebral musculature on the right and preservation on the left (black arrowhead).
(CT: computed tomography; MRI: magnetic resonance imaging)
Source: Calle S, Choi J, Ahmad S et al. Imaging of the thyroid- Practical approach. Neuroimag Clin N Am.2021;31:265-84.

and medullary thyroid cancer (MTC), which are poorly visualized on bone scintigraphy. For liver metastasis in MTC, the sensitivity of contrast-enhanced MRI is better than that of three-phase contrast-enhanced CT.

Diffusion-weighted imaging (DWI) of MRI has been shown to be helpful in differentiating benign and malignant nodules. The apparent diffusion coefficient (ADC) values of benign thyroid nodule are higher than for malignant nodule. Another sensitive method in differentiating thyroid carcinoma from benign follicular lesion is the MR spectroscopy using long echo-time. Here, no choline peak is seen in normal thyroid tissue and benign follicular lesions. Raised choline/creatinine ratio is seen in almost all carcinomas, with values varying from 1.6 in a well-differentiated thyroid cancer to 9.4 in anaplastic thyroid cancer.

Single-photon Emission Computed Tomography

Scintigraphy images of the distribution of radioiodine in the human body are poor in anatomical localization. This is overcome in single-photon emission computed tomography (SPECT-CT)/MRI by the use of hybrid cameras that integrate a nuclear medical detector unit with a CT or MRI scanner in one gantry. This allows the exact localization of foci of radioiodine uptake and thus has the potential to differentiate reliably between uptake in metastases of thyroid cancer and that in organs physiologically accumulating this tracer **(Figs. 20A to F)**. The resultant increase in diagnostic accuracy varies between 31 and 47.6%, mainly attributable to the ability to better differentiation between thyroid remnants and cervical lymph node metastasis.

Limitations of Single-photon Emission Computed Tomography

The limitations of SPECT-CT include:
- Lymph node metastasis in the central compartment of the neck may falsely be interpreted as thyroid remnants
- Microscopic disease may also escape detection by hybrid imaging
- Reactive enlarged lymph nodes seen after surgery are picked up.

F18-fluorodeoxyglucose-PET (^{18}F-FDG-PET) CT

It is a hybrid imaging system that combines a PET camera with a multislice spiral-CT/MRI in one gantry. [^{18}F]Fluorodeoxyglucose (^{18}F-FDG) is not taken up by normal thyroid gland, but is taken up by both dedifferentiated thyroid carcinoma and inflammatory process in thyroid gland. It remains trapped in these cells because of its inability to undergo glycolysis. In the case of dedifferentiation, DTC and its deposits may lose NIS expression and thus the ability to concentrate radioiodine, with an upregulation of the key proteins of glucose metabolism resulting in FDG uptake by thyroid. This is called the flip-flop phenomenon.

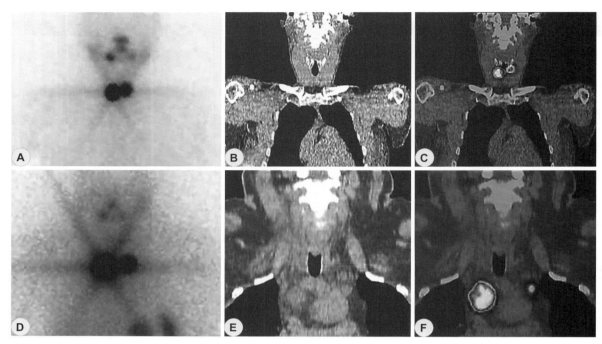

Figs. 20A to F: SPECT/CT imaging in two patients with papillary DTC obtained at radioiodine ablation 4 weeks post total thyroidectomy. First patient (A to C), second patient (D to F). Planar ^{131}I scintigraphies (A and D) disclose two foci of radioiodine accumulation in both subject. In the first patient, SPECT/CT fusion image (C) and low-dose CT (B) helps localize these foci to the thyroid bed so a diagnosis of benign thyroid remnants was made. In second patient, the foci of radioiodine uptake correspond to mediastinal lymph node metastasis visible clearly on the low-dose CT image (E).
(DTC: differentiated thyroid cancer; SPECT/CT: single-photon emission computerized tomography)
Source: Schmidt D, Kuwert T. Hybrid molecular imaging of differentiated thyroid carcinoma. Front Horm Res. 2016;45:37-45.

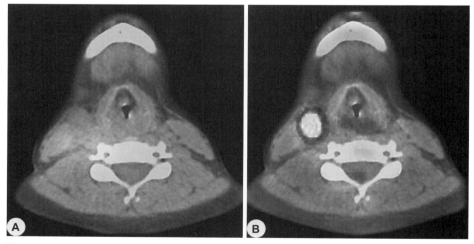

Figs. 21A and B: The ^{18}F-FDG-PET/CT fusion image (B) obtained in a 15-year-old female with a pT3mpN1 papillary differentiated thyroid cancer with elevated serum thyroglobulin levels but absence of tracer uptake seen in ^{131}I-SPECT/CT fusion image (A). The ^{18}F-FDG-PET fusion imaging (B) shows a FDG avid lymph node metastasis that has no radioiodine accumulation.
Source: Schmidt D, Kuwert T. Hybrid molecular imaging in differentiated thyroid carcinoma. Front Horm Res. 2016;45:37-45.

Fluorodeoxyglucose-positron emission tomography/computed tomography (FDG-PET/CT) has to be considered in the following situations:
- Disease localization in a Tg-positive patients (i.e., Tg levels >10 ng/mL) with no abnormality detected on routine diagnostic imaging **(Figs. 21A and B)**.
- Initial staging and follow-up of cases with poorly differentiated, anaplastic and Hurtle cell thyroid cancers.
- In patients with known distant metastases—here high FDG uptake in large metastases indicates a high risk for disease-specific fatality and poor response to ^{131}I therapy.

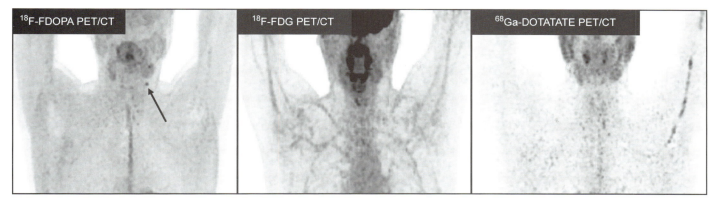

Fig. 22: Mapping of the metastatic lymph nodes in medullary thyroid carcinoma. Asymptomatic patient after thyroidectomy for medullary thyroid carcinoma and elevated calcitonin level (54 pg/mL) was evaluated for possible neck lymph node metastases. Ultrasound of the neck showed several suspicious lymph nodes (not shown). One of the lymph nodes (black arrow) was found to be positive on only ^{18}F-FDOPA PET/CT, while ^{18}F-FDG PET/CT and ^{68}Ga-DOTATATE PET/CT were negative.
Source: Kushchayev SV, Kushchayeva YS, Tella SH, Glushko T, Pacak K, Teytelboym OM. Medullary Thyroid Carcinoma: An Update on Imaging. J Thyroid Res. 2019;2019:1893047.

- For post-treatment response measurement following local or systemic therapy.
- Prognostication and determination of the disease extent in high-risk groups.

^{18}F-FDOPA PET/CT

The ^{18}F-FDOPA PET is the best method for detection of whole-body MTC metastasis/recurrence, with a sensitivity of 79–100%. It has higher patient-based sensitivity (64% vs. 48%, respectively) and lesion-based sensitivity (72% vs. 52%, respectively) as compared to ^{18}F-FDG PET for the evaluation of metastatic/recurrent MTC. It is the most suitable modality for the detection of liver metastases, small metastatic lymph nodes (about 6 mm), which are not detected by ^{18}F-FDG **(Fig. 22)**, and also to detect MTC metastases in uncommon locations.

Somatostatin Receptor Scintigraphy

^{111}In-octreotide which has high affinity for somatostatin receptor-2 (SST-R-2), forms a stable complex with ^{68}Ga using 1,4,7,10-tetraazacyclododecane-1,4,7,10-tetraacetic acid (DOTA) as a universal chelator and has been used in MTC. But it is a poor nuclear imaging with detection rates between 20 and 64%.

A meta-analysis studying the diagnostic efficacy of SST-analogs PET versus PET/CT (comprising ^{68}Ga-DOTATATE, ^{68}Ga-DOTALAN, and ^{68}Ga-DOTANOC) in evaluation of patients with recurrent MTC revealed a suboptimal detection rate of 64% (according to patient-based analysis); this increased to 83% for patients with calcitonin >500 ng/L. In recurrent MTC, the diagnostic efficacy of somatostatin receptor (SSTR) analogs PET or PET/CT is generally lower than ^{18}F-FDOPA PET/CT. SST analogs PET nevertheless detects 100% of the bone metastases in MTC as compared to only 44% of osseous lesions identified on bone scan.

CONCLUSION

Thyroid imaging has evolved from initial radionucleotide thyroid imaging to advanced techniques such as SPECT-CT and PET-CT. Ultrasound continues to be the primary and efficient method for evaluation of most thyroid diseases. Advances in US imaging, CT, and MRI have further improved evaluation of thyroid pathologies.

SUGGESTED READINGS

1. Salvatore D, Cohen R, Kopp A P, Larsen PR. Thyroid pathophysiology and diagnostic evaluation. In: Melmed S, Auchus R J, Goldfine AB, Koenig RJ, Rosen CJ (Eds). Williams textbook of Endocrinology; 14th edition. Philadelphia, PA: Elsevier; 2020. pp. 332-63.
2. Andrioli M, Valcavi R. Sonography of Normal and Abnormal Thyroid and Parathyroid Glands. Front Horm Res. 2016;45:1-15.
3. Hegedus L. Thyroid ultrasound. Assessment of thyroid function and disease. Endocrinol Metab Clin North Am. 2001;30(2): 339-60.
4. Warren Frunzac R, Richards M. Computed Tomography and Magnetic Resonance Imaging of the Thyroid and Parathyroid Glands. Front Horm Res. 2016;45:16-23.
5. Miemer DA, Kaplan MM. Radioiodine uptake and thyroid scintiscanning. Endocrinol Metab Clin North Am. 2001;30(2):291-313,viii.
6. Garberoglio S, Testori O. Role of Nuclear Medicine in the Diagnosis of Benign Thyroid Diseases. Front Horm Res. 2016;45:24-36.
7. Persani L. Congenital Hypothyroidism with Gland in situ is more Frequent than Previously Thought. Front Endocrinol (Lausanne). 2012;3:18.
8. Szinnai G. Genetics of normal and abnormal thyroid development in humans. Best Pract Res Clin Endocrinol Metab. 2014;28(2):133-50.
9. Grasberger H, Samuel Refetoff. Genetic causes of congenital hypothyroidism due to dyshormonogenesis. Curr Opin Pediatr. 2011;23(4):421-8.

10. Brabant G, Frank K, Ranft U, Schuermeyer T, Wagner TO, Hauser H, et al. Physiological regulation of circadian and pulsatile thyrotropin secretion in normal man and woman. J Clin Endocrinol Metab. 1990;70(2):403-9.
11. Dayal D, Prasad R. Congenital hypothyroidism: current perspectives. Res Rep Endocrine Disorder. 2015;17(5):91-102.
12. Zois C, Stavrou I, Kalogera C, Svarna E, Dimoliatis I, Seferiadis K, et al. High prevalence of autoimmune thyroiditis in schoolchildren after elimination of iodine deficiency in northwestern Greece. Thyroid. 2003;13(5):485-9.
13. Zdraveska N, Kocova M. Hashimoto Thyroiditis in Childhood – Review of the Epidemiology, Genetic Susceptibility and Clinical Aspects of the Disease. Access Maced J Med Sci. 2012;5(3):336-45.
14. Hollenberg A, Wiersinga MW. Hyperthyroid Disorders. In: Melmed S, Auchus R J, Goldfine AB, Koenig RJ, Rosen CJ (Eds). Williams textbook of Endocrinology, 14th edition. Philadelphia, PA: Elsevier; 2020. pp. 364-403.
15. Vitti P, Rago T, Mancusi F, Pallini S, Tonacchera M, Santini F, et al. Thyroid hypoechogenic pattern at ultrasonography as a tool for predicting recurrence of hyperthyroidism after medical treatment in patients with Graves' disease. Acta Endocrinol (Copenh). 1992;126(2):128-31.
16. Bogazzi F, Bartalena L, Brogioni S, Burelli A, Manetti L, Tanda ML, et al. Thyroid vascularity and blood flow are not dependent on serum thyroid hormone levels: studies in vivo by color flow Doppler sonography. Eur J Endocrinol. 1999;140(5):452-6.
17. Erdogan MF, Anil C, Cesur M, Başkal N, Erdoğan G. Color flow Doppler sonography for the etiologic diagnosis of hyperthyroidism. Thyroid. 2007;17(3):223-8.
18. Gharib H, Papini E, Paschke R, et al. American Association of Clinical Endocrinologists, Associazione Medici Endocrinologi, and European Thyroid Association medical guidelines for clinical practice for the diagnosis and management of thyroid nodules. Endocr Pract. 2010;16(Suppl 1):1-43.
19. Meller J, Becker W. The continuing importance of thyroid scintigraphy in the era of high-resolution ultrasound. Eur J Nucl Med. 2002;29(Suppl 2):S425-38.
20. Charkes ND. Graves' disease with functioning nodules (Marine-Lenhart syndrome). J Nucl Med. 1972;13(12):885-92.
21. Haugen BR, Alexander EK, Bible KC, Doherty GM, Mandel SJ, Nikiforov YE, et al. 2015 American Thyroid Association Management Guidelines for Adult Patients with Thyroid Nodules and Differentiated Thyroid Cancer: The American Thyroid Association Guidelines Task Force on Thyroid Nodules and Differentiated Thyroid Cancer. Thyroid. 2016;26(1):1-133.
22. Mazzaferri EL. Management of a solitary thyroid nodule. N Engl J Med. 1993;328(8):553-9.
23. Guth S, Theune U, Aberle J, Galach A, Bamberger CM, et al. Very high prevalence of thyroid nodules detected by high frequency (13 MHz) ultrasound examination. Eur J Clin Invest. 2009;39(8):699-706.
24. Russ G, Leboulleux S, Leenhardt L, Hegedüs L. Thyroid incidentalomas: epidemiology, risk stratification with ultrasound and workup. Eur Thyroid J. 2014;3(3):154-63.
25. Brito JP, Morris JC, Montori VM. Thyroid cancer: zealous imaging has increased detection and treatment of low risk tumours. BMJ. 2013;347:f4706.
26. Sharma SD, Jacques T, Smith S, Watters G. Diagnosis of incidental thyroid nodules on 18F-fluorodeoxyglucose positron emission tomography imaging: are these significant? J Laryngol Otol. 2015;129(1):53-6.
27. Durante C, Grani G, Lamartina L, Filetti S, Mandel SJ, Cooper DS. The diagnosis and management of thyroid nodules: A review. JAMA. 2018;319(9):914-24.
28. Kerr L. High resolution thyroid ultrasound: The value of color Doppler. Ultrasound Q. 1994;12:21-43.
29. Ophir J, Alam SK, Garra B, Kallel F, Konofagou E, Krouskop T, et al. Elastography: ultrasonic estimation and imaging of the elastic properties of tissues. Proc Inst Mech Eng H. 1999;213(3):203-33.
30. Rago T, Vitti P. Role of thyroid ultrasound in the diagnostic evaluation of thyroid nodules. Best Pract Res Clin Endocrinol Metab. 2008;22(6):913-28.
31. Moon HJ, Sung JM, Kim EK, Yoon JH, Youk JH, Kwak JY. Diagnostic performance of gray-scale US and elastography in solid thyroid nodules. Radiology. 2012;262(3):1002-13.
32. Azizi G, Keller J, Lewis M, Puett D, Rivenbark K, Malchoff C. Performance of elastography for the evaluation of thyroid nodules: a prospective study. Thyroid. 2013;23(6):734-40.
33. Filletti S, Tuttle RM, Leboulleaux S, Alexander EK. Nontoxic diffuse goiter, nodular thyroid disorders, and thyroid malignancies. In: Melmed S, Auchus R J, Goldfine AB, Koenig RJ, Rosen CJ (Eds). Williams textbook of Endocrinology, 14th Edition. Philadelphia, PA: Elsevier; 2020. pp. 433-78.
34. Giraudet AL, Vanel D, Leboulleux S, Aupérin A, Dromain C, Chami L, et al. Imaging medullary thyroid carcinoma with persistent elevated calcitonin levels. J Clin Endocrinol Metab. 2007;92(11):4185-90.
35. Bozgeyik Z, Coskun S, Dagli AF, Ozkan Y, Sahpaz F, Ogur E. Diffusion-weighted MR imaging of thyroid nodules. Neuroradiology. 2009;51(3):193-8.
36. King AD, Yeung DK, Ahuja AT, Tse GM, Chan AB, Lam SS, et al. In vivo 1H MR spectroscopy of thyroid carcinoma. Eur J Radiol. 2005;54(1):112-7.
37. Schmidt D, Kuwert T. Hybrid molecular imaging in differentiated thyroid carcinoma. Front Horm Res. 2016;45:37-45.
38. Ruf J, Lehmkuhl L, Bertram H, Sandrock D, Amthauer H, Humplik B, et al. Impact of SPECT and integrated low-dose CT after radioiodine therapy on the management of patients with thyroid carcinoma. Nucl Med Commun. 2004;25(12):1177-82.
39. Aide N, Heutte N, Rame J-P, Rousseau E, Loiseau C, Henry-Amar M, et al. Clinical relevance of single-photon emission computed tomography/computed tomography of the neck and thorax in postablation (131)I scintigraphy for thyroid cancer. J Clin Endocrinol Metab. 2009;94(6):2075-84.
40. Mustafa M, Kuwert T, Weber K, Knesewitsch P, Negele T, Haug A, et al. Regional lymph node involvement in T1 papillary thyroid carcinoma: a bicentric prospective SPECT/CT study. Eur J Nucl Med Mol Imaging. 2010;37(8):1462-6.
41. Verbeek HHG, Plukker JTM, Koopmans KP, de Groot JW, Hofstra RM, Muller Kobold AC, et al. Clinical relevance of 18F-FDG PET and 18F-DOPA PET in recurrent medullary thyroid carcinoma. J Nuclear Med. 2012;53(12):1863-71.
42. Romero-Lluch AR, Cuenca-Cuenca JI, Guerrero-Vazquez R, Martínez-Ortega AJ, Tirado-Hospital JL, Borrego-Dorado I, et al. Diagnostic utility of PET/CT with 18F-DOPA and 18F-FDG in persistent or recurrent medullary thyroid carcinoma: the importance of calcitonin and carcinoembryonic antigen cutoff. Eur J Nucl Med Mol Imaging. 2017;44(12):2004-13.
43. Skoura E. Depicting medullary thyroid cancer recurrence: The past and the future of nuclear medicine imaging. Int J Endocrinol Metab. 2013;11(4):e8156.
44. Treglia G, Tamburello A, Giovanella L. Detection rate of somatostatin receptor pet in patients with recurrent medullary thyroid carcinoma: A systematic review and a meta-analysis. Hormones (Athens). 2017;16(4):362-72.
45. Castroneves LA, Filho GC, de Freitas RM, Salles R, Moyses RA, Lopez RVM, et al. Comparison of 68Ga PET/CT to other imaging studies in medullary thyroid cancer: superiority in detecting bone metastases. J Clin Endocrinol Metab. 2018;3(9):3250-9.

CHAPTER 7

Nuclear Imaging in Thyroid Disorders

Vijay Singh, CS Bal, PK Pradhan

INTRODUCTION

The thyroid gland in the anterior neck is inferior to the thyroid cartilage and weighs roughly 15–20 g **(Fig. 1A)**. The thyroid gland consists of two lobes, each having superior and inferior poles, an isthmus, and frequently a pyramidal lobe that develops from either the isthmus or the medial portion of either lobe. The pyramidal lobe develops along the distal thyroglossal duct; therefore, it is located along the midline of the isthmus. Similarly, thyroid tissue may be ectopically placed anywhere along its embryonic migratory track, i.e., as a lingual thyroid near the root of the tongue, inside a vestigial midline thyroglossal duct cyst, or more caudally within the mediastinum. The thyroid gland is under the control of the hypothalamic-pituitary axis; the tasks of the gland include iodine trapping, the production and storage of hormones, and the subsequent release of hormones into the circulation are all depicted in **Figure 1B**. This capacity to trap iodine is not unique to the thyroid gland since trapping also happens in the salivary glands, gastrointestinal mucosa, and breast, but none of these other tissues can utilize the trapped iodine to synthesize thyroid hormones.

RADIOPHARMACEUTICALS

Technetium as pertechnetate ($^{99m}TcO_4$) and two isotopes of iodine (I-123 and I-131) are the radionuclides most frequently employed for thyroid imaging. Other radioisotopes of iodine are less suitable because of disproportionate half-lives,

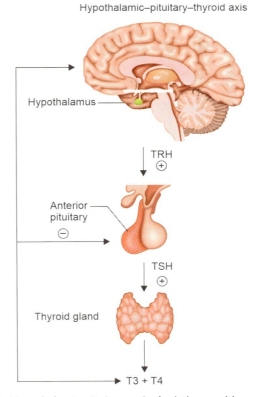

Fig. 1B: Hypothalamic-pituitary axis depicting positive and negative feedback mechanism.
(TRH: thyrotropin-releasing hormone; TSH: thyroid stimulating hormone; T3: triiodothyronine; T4: tetraiodothyronine)

Fig. 1A: Anatomical relation of the thyroid gland with hyoid bone, larynx, trachea, and adjacent muscular structures.

TABLE 1: Characteristics of various radionuclides employed for thyroid imaging.			
Properties	^{99m}Tc	^{123}I	^{131}I
Uptake mechanism	NIS, then washout	NIS + organification	NIS + organification
Photon energy	γ 140 keV	γ 159 keV	γ 364 keV + β
Recommended activity for adults	20–74 MBq (0.6–2 mCi)	7,4–25 MBq (0.2–0.6 mCi)	1.85–7.4 MBq (0.05–0.2 mCi)
Recommended activity for children	1–5 MBq/kg (0.015–0.07 mCi/kg)	0.1–0.3 MBq/kg (0.003–0.01 mCi/kg)	0.025–0.1 MBq/kg (0.0004–0.0016 mCi/kg)
Administration	IV	PO or IV	PO or IV
Start of acquisition	15–30 minutes	6–8 hours	24 hours

(I: iodine; IV: intravenous; keV: kiloelectron volt; MBQ: megabecquerel; mCi: millicurie; NIS: sodium iodide symporter; PO: per oral; Tc: technetium)

photon energies, or an excessive absorbed radiation dose from particulate emissions. The sodium-iodide symporter (NIS) is responsible for iodine uptake in the thyroid gland, first described by Kaminsky et al., in 1993. Technetium is administered intravenously, while iodine is given by oral route.

Technetium-99m

Technetium-99m is generally administered intravenously as ^{99m}TcO4 Na (sodium pertechnetate) acquired from a molybdenum-technetium generator. The benefit of ^{99m}Tc includes the high accessibility in the nuclear medicine department, the low energy of the γ-photons (140 keV), and the somewhat short half-life (6 hours). At a lesser cost, it is feasible to employ substantially greater activity than I-131 to get more accurate images in a shorter amount of time. ^{99m}Tc is iodomimetic, which means it is carried and trapped into thyroid cells in the same manner as iodine isotopes by NIS (sodium/iodide cotransporter). After intravenous injection, the maximum concentration of ^{99m}Tc-pertechnetate occurs 15–20 minutes later. The rise in ^{99m}Tc activity in the thyroid coincides with the increase in intravenous I-123 activity in the early phase. The dynamics of iodine absorption to thyroid tissue are reflected in the proportion of ^{99m}Tc accumulated in thyrocytes. However, after 15–30 minutes, the curve of thyroid ^{99m}Tc activity approaches a peak and subsequently drops, but iodine absorption continues to rise. This is because, unlike iodine, ^{99m}Tc-pertechnetate does not go through the organification process and can be easily removed from the thyrocytes.

Iodine Isotopes

Iodine-123

The physical properties of I-123 are quite similar to those of ^{99m}Tc; it is a pure γ-emitter with a low energy photon (159 keV) and a short half-life (13 hours). I-123's specificity and persistence of accumulation in the thyroid are due to its organification, which allows delayed acquisitions and comprehensive monitoring of iodine kinetics in thyroid tissue. Compared to ^{99m}Tc, I-123 provides more detailed pictures with a clear distinction of thyroid tissue from surrounding tissues, resulting in better visualization of retrosternal thyroid tissue and the thyroid gland when thyroid uptake is poor. In addition, the thyroid's actual iodine turnover may be determined, while ^{99m}Tc uptake is only a proxy parameter. However, since I-123 is synthesized using a cyclotron and has exorbitant prices, it is not readily accessible for routine use in many institutions.

Iodine-131

Iodine-131 is the radioactive isotope of iodine employed most often; it has a half-life of 8.1 days and emits both β and γ-radiation. Gamma rays—it produces have a greater energy level (364 keV) than those produced by ^{99m}Tc and I-123, allowing them to be used for diagnostic purposes. As a consequence of this, the use of I-131 scintigraphy should be restricted to the following—the monitoring of treatment in patients who have differentiated thyroid cancer; the imaging of ectopic thyroid (such as retrosternal or lingual thyroid and struma ovarii); dosimetric pretreatment evaluations and kinetic studies in dishormonogenetic pathologies. The characteristics of various nuclides for visualizing the thyroid gland are outlined in **Table 1**.

INSTRUMENTATION

After radiotracer administration, the patient becomes the source of emission. To capture these emissions (γ, β-negative, and β-positive) and electronically convert them into photons, parametric images, statistics, and molecular information, multiple devices have been investigated, including the following:

- *Gamma scintillation probe*: Nonimaging device used for uptake measurement.
- *The rectilinear scanner*: The earliest imaging technology, is no longer in use.
- *Gamma camera planar scanner*: Because of its ability to create segmental two-dimensional (2D) photos,

whole-body reconstructions, and dynamic acquisitions; it is one of the nuclear medicine equipment that is used the most often for the diagnosis of benign thyroid disorder.

- *Single-photon emission computed tomography (SPECT) scanner*: A three-dimesional (3D) tomographic instrument employing γ camera data from numerous predictions, it may be recreated in multiple planes **(Fig. 2A)** and computed tomography (CT)-assisted.
- The positron emission tomography-computed tomography (PET-CT) scanner is a CT-assisted positron emission tomography **(Fig. 2B)**.

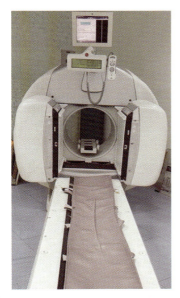

Fig. 2A: Single-photon emission computerized tomography (SPECT)/computed tomography (CT) scanner.
Courtesy: Nuclear medicine department, SGPGIMS, Lucknow, Uttar Pradesh, India.

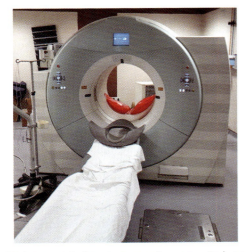

Fig. 2B: Positron emission tomography-computed tomography scan (PET/CT) scanner.
Courtesy: Nuclear medicine department, SGPGIMS, Lucknow, Uttar Pradesh, India.

IMAGING IN BENIGN THYROID DISORDERS

Thyroid Scan

Thyroid scintigraphy is considered a molecular imaging procedure given the active transport of $^{99m}TCO4^-$/I-131 by sodium iodide symporter (NIS) transporter, and it visualizes the location of active thyroid tissue in addition to the morphological information gained through ultrasonography. Consequently, the overall indications for scintigraphy are comprehensive and encompass both a solitary thyroid nodule and multinodular goiter. In addition to evaluating the amount of retrosternal goiter (where ultrasound cannot view the lower pole of the thyroid gland), the test is also employed in cases with suspected ectopic thyroid. Scintigraphy is employed to select the biopsy site in the goiter where no nodule is dominant. Only thyroid scintigraphy permits the evaluation of regional thyroid function and the detection of autonomously functioning thyroid nodules (AFTNs).

I-123 or ^{99m}Tc is the most often utilized radionuclides in scintigraphy, under American Association of Clinical Endocrinologists/Associazione Medici Endocrinology/European Thyroid Association (AACE/AME/ETA) criteria. I-131 thyroid uptake is not suggested for regular diagnostic usage unless low-uptake thyrotoxicosis is suspected or for dosimetric assessment before therapy with I-131.

Planar images are obtained by placing the patient in a sitting or recumbent position at a predetermined period (typically 15–120 minutes) after iodine injection. A marker is placed over the sternal notch to establish anatomical landmarks. As an iodine analog, ^{99m}Tc-pertechnetate is delivered to thyroid cells in the same manner as iodine isotopes, i.e., via the NIS symporter system. After 15–20 minutes of intravenous injection, ^{99m}Tc-pertechnetate accumulates at a maximum level. In this early phase, the increase in thyroid ^{99m}Tc activity parallels the increase in intravenous I-123 activity. The proportion of ^{99m}Tc that accumulates in thyrocytes reflects the kinetics of iodine absorption by thyroid tissue. After 15–30 minutes, however, the thyroid ^{99m}Tc activity curve approaches a plateau and gradually drops while the iodine uptake continues to increase. This is because ^{99m}Tc-pertechnetate does not undergo organification (like iodine does) and is therefore, washed out of the thyrocytes.

As many cases of unexpected radioiodine uptake have been recorded, the clinician should be aware of physiological and pathological uptake when interpreting thyroid scintigraphy. Even though the exact mechanisms are not fully understood, several hypotheses have been proposed, including the following:

- The expression of functional NIS in normal tissues, including the thymus, breast, salivary glands, and gastrointestinal system, as well as in various malignancies, both benign and malignant.

- Radioiodinated thyroid hormones and their metabolic breakdown.
- The retention of radioiodinated bodily fluids or contamination of other body fluids (such as saliva, tears, blood, urine, exudate, transudate, gastric, and mucosal secretions).
- The retention of radioiodine and its uptake in inflammatory tissue.
- Thyroid metastases.

Furthermore, activity in vascular systems can result in poor image quality when uptake is limited, which is why I-123 scintiscans have higher diagnostic power than ^{99m}Tc. In addition, the physician must be aware of coexisting conditions that can influence the diagnosis, such as:
- History of thyroid-related disorders.
- Ultrasonography (US) image or report.
- Current thyroid function test [free triiodothyronine (T3), free thyroxine (T4), and thyroid-stimulating hormone (TSH)].
- Pharmacological interventions, in particular, iodine-containing medicines, thyroid hormones, and antithyroid medications (amiodarone, disinfectant, and expectorant drugs).

A thyroid scan report should include the following:
- The location of thyroid tissue (normal, ectopic, and retrosternal goiter).
- The size and structure of the gland (symmetry of the gland lobes, ultimately the pyramidal lobe).
- Tracer distribution in the thyroid, increasing foci, or reduced tracer accumulation (warm, warm, or hypofunctioning nodules), by a physical examination of the throat.
- An evaluation of the ratio of the thyroid to the background—lower ratio is a functional representation of depression in thyroid absorption or impaired renal function.
- An evaluation of the ratio of the thyroid to the salivary glands—if the ratio is <3, it may be related to iodine contamination, hypotrophy, or inflammation.

Patient Preparation for Thyroid Scintigraphy

Thyroid scintigraphy usually does not require any prior patient preparation.
- If the patient is taking thyroid hormone replacement therapy or iodine, the study should be performed 4–6 weeks after cessation of these medications **(Table 2)**.
- Female patients who are pregnant or breastfeeding should notify the nuclear medicine physician before undergoing a diagnostic test. However, a thyroid scan can be done in lactating females with a stoppage of breastfeeding for 4 hours.
- Although the radiation exposure is very low, in the case of pregnancy, the procedure would be performed only, if necessary, at that time (benefit vs. risk evaluation).

TABLE 2: Various factors affecting iodine uptake are listed below.

Decrease uptake	Duration of effect
Thyroid hormones	
L: Thyroxine (T$_4$)	4–6 weeks
L: Triiodothyronine (T$_3$)	2 weeks
Excess iodine (expanded iodine pool)	
Potassium iodide, cyanate, and thiocyanate	2–4 weeks
Mineral supplements, cough medicines, vitamins, and iodinated skin ointment	2–4 weeks
Iodine food supplements, cabbage, turnips, and goitrogenic foods	2–4 weeks
Iodinated drugs (e.g., amiodarone)	Months
Radiographic contrast media	
Water-soluble intravascular media	3–4 weeks
Fat-soluble media (lymphography)	Months to years
Pathological condition	
Renal failure	
Congestive heart failure	
Noniodine-containing drugs	
Adrenocorticotropic hormone and adrenal steroids	Variable
Monovalent anions (perchlorate)	Variable
Penicillin	Variable
Antithyroid drugs	
Propylthiouracil	3–5 days
Methimazole	5–7 days
Prior radiation to the neck	
Increased uptake	
Iodine deficiency	
Pregnancy	
Rebound after therapy withdrawal	
Recombinant thyrotropin (rhTSH and genotropin)	

Principles of Thyroid Scan Interpretation

Scintigraphy of the thyroid provides a visualization of the radiotracer distribution in the thyroid parenchyma. It helps to detect thyroid disorders based on the level of radiotracer uptake relative to surrounding structures, radiotracer distribution in the thyroid, and any extrathyroidal uptake. It provides information on thyroid location, morphology, size, shape, and overall thyroid function qualitatively and quantitatively. Thyroid scintigraphy scans are used to calculate the thyroid uptake ratio. Percentage uptake value of more than 3 indicated increased thyroid uptake (normal value 0.3–3%).

Normal Thyroid Imaging

Typically, the gland is symmetrical, and the lobes have straight to convex lateral margins. Tracer is typically detected in salivary glands, and the capillary network of the neck tissue referred to as the "blood pool." This appears as a light background along the curvature of the neck (**Fig. 3**).

Graves' Disease

The workup of these patients would be completed by combining typical clinical features of Graves' disease with biochemical parameters and a thyroid scan. Radioiodine therapy is the preferred treatment for uncomplicated, small to medium-sized goiters. Thyroid scintigraphy typically demonstrates uniform diffuse enlargement (**Fig. 4A**). The tracer is evenly distributed throughout the thyroid. A previously unseen pyramidal lobe (a remnant of the thyroglossal duct) can be seen in a hypertrophied gland. The tracer is barely trapped in salivary glands because there is less tracer available for extraction due to higher trapping by the thyroid.

Thyroiditis

Thyroiditis symptoms include features of hyperthyroidism with neck pain and a recent onset of an upper respiratory tract infection. A thyroid scan reveals little or no uptake in the thyroid; however, salivary gland shows normal radiotracer uptake (**Fig. 4B**). This results from the thyrocyte's stupor during the acute phase of inflammation. These patients can be conservatively treated with nonsteroidal anti-inflammatory drugs, low-dose corticosteroids, and β-blockers. After 6–12 weeks, a repeat scan would reveal a resolving thyroid at various phases exhibiting diverse forms of uptake. The scan verifies that recovery has occurred and acts as a benchmark for the future.

Solitary Thyroid Nodule

They are typically palpable nodules that are assessed primarily to rule out malignancy. On thyroid imaging, the following subtypes are distinguished:
- *Warm*: Tracer uptake equal to that of normal tissue, indicating a normal function in that location. Have a low likelihood of being malignant.

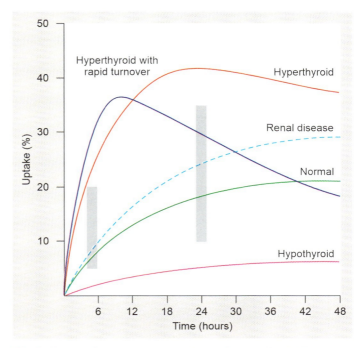

Fig. 3: Thyroidal reference radioactive iodine uptake (RAIU) curves in normal and various pathophysiological conditions. Note the early uptake and rapid turnover in a few hyperthyroid patients. Prolonged uptake in renal disease patients is due to decreased urinary excretion.

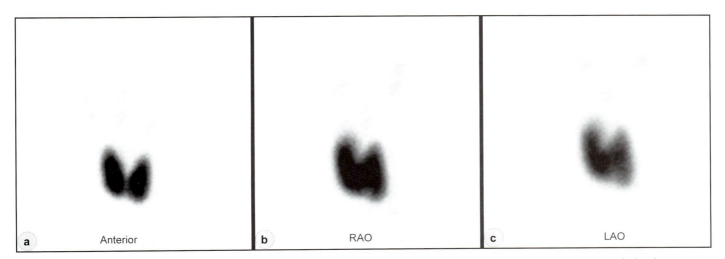

Fig. 4A: Graves' disease—^{99m}TC thyroid scintigraphy in a case reveals increased uptake in the bilaterally enlarged thyroid gland in anterior (a) left anterior oblique (LAO) view (b), and right anterior oblique (RAO) view (c). Note that the uptake in the salivary gland and background is suppressed.

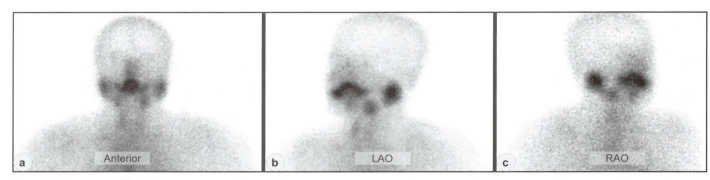

Fig. 4B: Thyroiditis—^{99m}TC thyroid scintigraphy reveals absent uptake in the thyroid gland in anterior (a), left anterior oblique (LAO) view (b), and right anterior oblique (RAO) view (c). Note that the salivary gland and background uptake appears to be increased.

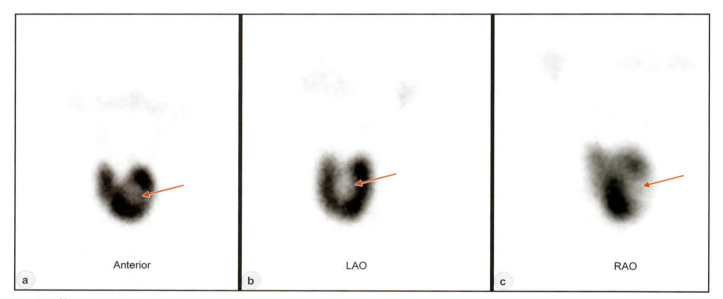

Fig. 4C: ^{99m}TC thyroid scintigraphy reveals increased uptake in both lobes of the thyroid gland in the anterior (a), left anterior oblique (LAO) view (b), and right anterior oblique (RAO) view (c). The left lobe of the thyroid is enlarged than the right lobe, and an area of decreased uptake is noted in the midpolar region of the left thyroid lobe, suggestive of the cold nodule (red arrow).

- *Cold*: Absent tracer uptake or less than normal tissue indicates a nonfunctioning nodule. These nodules may be caused by cystic alterations, fibrosis, hemorrhage, adenoma, cancer, etc., and are likely malignant **(Fig. 4C)**.
- *Hot*: Tracer uptake greater than normal tissue, indicating greater than normal function. They can be thyroid nodules that function independently (AFTN). Have a low likelihood of being malignant.

Multinodular Goiter

It typically occurs in populations residing in iodine-deficient regions due to periods of nutritional iodine shortage interspersed with iodine sufficiency, resulting in compensatory thyroid hypertrophy and regression to normalcy, respectively. This results in glandular nodularity, localized hemorrhages, calcifications, cyst development, and scarring. Typically, the thyroid is substantially enlarged with nonuniform growth. In a nodular pathology, the tracer distribution may be heterogeneous because different areas/nodules may have varying levels of function **(Fig. 4D)**. Therefore, the tracer trapping on scintigraphy is varied, higher/lower than typical in some locations. Some nodules may become autonomous, i.e., independent of TSH regulation, and may exhibit hyperfunction resulting in the production of toxic multinodular goiter (MNG). In such instances, regions of enhanced radiotracer absorption, often known as hot nodules, are visible. The toxic multinodular goiter must be treated to prevent long-term TSH suppression-related problems. High dosages of radioiodine (15–25 mCi) are typically effective for subclinical toxicosis management. However, if compression symptoms are present, surgical treatment is more advantageous.

Toxic Autonomous Nodule

It is also known as an AFTN, which means it functions independently of TSH. The image depicts enhanced tracer

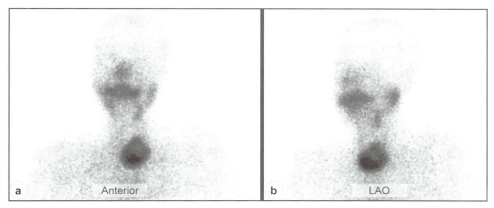

Fig. 4D: ^{99m}TC thyroid scintigraphy in a case of autonomously functioning thyroid nodules (AFTN) reveals a large area of increased uptake in the left thyroid lobe of the thyroid gland in the anterior (a), left anterior oblique (LAO) view (b). The right thyroid lobe is not visualized. Physiological tracer uptake is noted in the background and salivary glands.

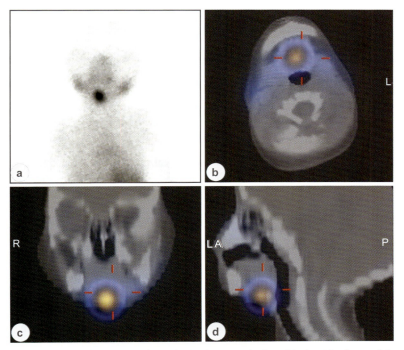

Fig. 4E: ^{99m}TC thyroid planar scintigraphy reveals increased uptake in the ectopic thyroid gland in the neck in anterior view (a). Fused single-photon emission computerized tomography (SPECT)/computed tomography (CT) in axial (b), coronal (c), and sagittal section (d) revealed increased uptake in the thyroid gland in the neck region near the base of the tongue, suggestive of ectopic lingual thyroid.

uptake localized to a nodule that occupies most of the entire thyroid lobe. The remaining gland cannot be seen due to the complete suppression of TSH activation. These patients may be successfully treated with radioiodine therapy and/or surgery.

Thyroid Dysgenesis, Agenesis, and Ectopic Development

The gold standard for imaging functioning thyroid tissue in the body is thyroid scanning with I-123/I-131. If indicated, a screening with Tc-^{99}m imaging **(Fig. 4E)** can be followed with I-123/I-131 imaging. The scan reveals thyroid tissue in ectopic locations, more commonly near the root of the tongue, i.e., lingual thyroid.

Suppression Thyroid Scintigraphy

Suppression scans are performed to visualize thyroid tissue capable of functioning independently of the hypothalamic–pituitary–thyroid axis. Respectively before and after the administration of a thyroxine preparation or triiodothyronine for 7–14 days, thyroid scintigraphy with radioiodine uptake measurement is performed. The recommended daily

L-triiodothyronine or levothyroxine is 80 μg or 150 μg, respectively. In a healthy gland, the thyroid hormone reduces the accumulation of radioactive iodine by at least 50%. A decrease in iodine absorption of <30% indicates an autoimmune process. In place of iodine, this test can also be conducted by measuring ^{99m}Tc uptake. An autonomous nodule that is warm on the initial image becomes hot as the surrounding normal tissue is suppressed. Therefore, in some centers, the suppression test is also used to prepare for radioiodine treatment of a nontoxic nodular goiter.

■ Potassium Perchlorate Test

Iodine organification abnormalities are diagnosed using the potassium perchlorate test. Under normal circumstances, iodide ions are oxidized by thyroid peroxidase and integrated into thyroglobulin tyrosyl residues. After entering the cell via NIS. This procedure takes between 2 and 3 hours. In the case of an organification deficiency (peroxidase deficiency in Pendred syndrome), unorganized iodine is washed out of the cell. The NIS is inhibited by potassium perchlorate, which reduces the influx of iodide into the cell. Thus, in the absence of peroxidase, perchlorate administration reduces the iodine concentration in the thyroid gland due to iodine washout. The test measures iodine uptake 2–3 hours after intravenous administration of ^{123}I or oral administration of ^{131}I, followed by a measurement 2 hours after oral administration of potassium or sodium perchlorate (0.5–1.0 g). A minimum 20% decrease in iodine absorption confirms the organification defect. Iodine uptake after perchlorate administration should not be declined in healthy subjects.

IMAGING IN THYROID MALIGNANCY

■ ^{99m}Tc-Methoxyisobutylisonitrile Scintigraphy

In the past few decades, there have been reports of the usefulness of thyroid imaging employing methoxyisobutylisonitrile (^{99m}Tc-MIBI). This tracer's uptake in the mitochondria of cancer cells correlates with an increase in the quantity and activity of mitochondria and an increase in the lesion's perfusion. The ^{99m}Tc-MIBI scan has been suggested for usage in cases with inconclusive biopsy and/or cold nodules. Due to the lack of conclusive outcomes from clinical trials, this approach was not included in the guidelines for managing nodular thyroid disease. There are—however, data indicating that negative ^{99m}Tc-MIBI scintigraphy effectively rules out malignancy.

■ The Radioiodine Whole-body Scan

Traditionally, planar imaging in nuclear medicine has played a pivotal role in treating patients with differentiated thyroid cancer following a total or near-total thyroidectomy.

Typically, diagnostic radioiodine whole-body scan (WBS) is performed (**Figs. 5 to 7**). Because radioiodine is concentrated in functional thyroid tissue, the WBS has multiple functions—(i) to determine the quantity of residue thyroid

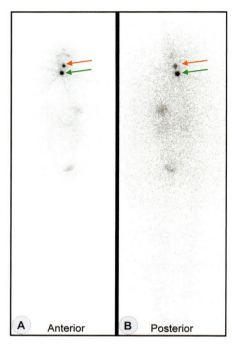

Figs. 5A and B: Whole body radioiodine (WBRI) images in anterior (A) and posterior (B) projection of a patient post total thyroidectomy reveal remnant uptake in the thyroid bed (green arrows) and thyroglossal duct (red arrows).

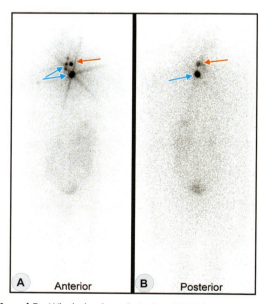

Figs. 6A and B: Whole body radioiodine (WBRI) images in anterior (A) and posterior (B) projection of a patient post total thyroidectomy reveal remnant uptake in thyroid bed (red arrows) and multiple metastatic cervical lymph nodes (blue arrows).

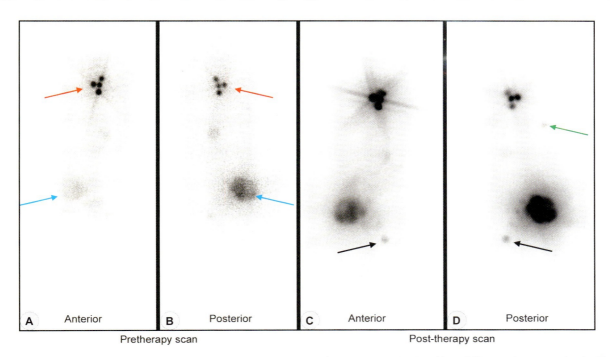

Figs. 7A to D: WBRI of patient; pretherapy planar images in anterior and posterior projection (A and B) reveal remnant bed with multiple metastatic nodes (red arrows) in the neck with the metastatic lesion in the pelvis (blue arrow) with soft tissue (confirmed on SPECT/CT, not shown here). The patient was given 150 mCi I-131 as an ablative dose, and a post-therapy scan in anterior and posterior projection (C and D) revealed a new metastatic lesion in the right rib (green arrow) and left ischium (black arrows).
(SPECT/CT: single-photon emission computerized tomography/computed tomography; WBRI: whole body radioiodine scan)

tissue obtained after a thyroidectomy; (ii) to evaluate metastatic disease; (iii) to guide treatment selection I-131 dose, and (iv) to demonstrate a change in biodistribution. Typically, the results of a WBS are utilized to modify the therapeutic dose of I-131 in combination with clinical, surgical, and diagnostic procedures and pathologic background. The time between the WBS and the timing of I-131 therapy can vary from the same day to several days later, assuming the patient stays hypothyroid until treatment. To optimize the thyroid tissue's avidity for radioiodine in preparation for a WBS, the patient's TSH is permitted to rise over 30 mIU/L following thyroidectomy.

Follow-up testing for identifying recurrent/residual thyroid cancer also requires an elevated TSH. Either withdrawal of thyroid hormone or delivery of recombinant human TSH [recombinant human thyroid-stimulating hormone (rhTSH), thyrogen, and genzyme] can elevate TSH. This latter method entails intramuscular injections of 0.9 mg of rhTSH every day for two days. On the third day, the patient receives a diagnostic dosage of I-131 or I-123. Imaging is conducted on the fourth day with I-123 and the fifth day with I-131. On day 5, a quantitative blood thyroglobulin (Tg) level and anti-Tg antibodies (TgAbs) are obtained to quantify "stimulated" Tg. The diagnostic accuracy of WBS conducted with rhTSH is comparable to hormone withdrawal. To enhance the sensitivity of the WBS, patients can be counseled to have a low-iodine diet for 7–21 days before the test if possible. Avoid exposure to iodinated contrast for 7 days, and if possible, suspend known iodine-rich drugs such as amiodarone. Historically, a WBS was obtained by administering a 3–5 mCi activity of I-131 orally at least 4 weeks following a thyroidectomy.

However, I-123 has gained popularity recently as its availability has increased. Due to the I-123 short half-life, imaging is done at 24 hours. However, the target-to-background ratio may be high. With I-123's short half-life, metastatic thyroid cancer with a sluggish radioiodine metabolism may not be able to concentrate enough radioiodine to be detected. Some publications have recommended employing higher dosages of I-123 (111–185 mBq; 3–5 mCi), allowing for delayed imaging at 48 hours, which could increase the detection rate of mildly avid metastatic thyroid remnants.

The selection of I-123 or I-131 for the WBS is also related to the contentious concept of thyroid stunning. Stunning refers to the diminished uptake of a therapeutic dose of I-131 due to the thyroid cell damage caused by β-emission from a WBS with I-131. Because I-123 is a pure γ-emitter, this isotope should theoretically not be capable of stunning. Silberstein demonstrated that nonmetastatic thyroid cancer patients who had WBS with either 14.8 MBq (0.4 mCi) of I-123 or 74 MBq (2 mCi) of I-131 before ablation with 3.7 GBq (100 mCi) of I-131 did not have significantly different outcomes. Even if stunning occurs with I-131, his findings indicate that it has little effect on ablation rates.

With the greater availability of I-123, stunning concerns are one reason why many universities no longer utilize I-131 for WBS. Because many practitioners know the danger of stunning, they virtually universally utilize significantly lower doses. Overall, the amount of I-131 utilized to treat WBS has decreased with time. Current standards indicate the administration of 37–185 MBq (1–5 mCi) of I-131, followed by a scan 2–3 days later.

Post-therapy Scan

After I-131 ablation, a post-therapy scan (PTS) is frequently performed to confirm localization in the remaining thyroid tissue. American and European recommendations both require routine PTS testing. Post-therapy scan can be obtained anywhere between 3 and 8 days after I-131 therapy, with later imaging yielding a higher ratio of target-to-background. Although the best time to do the PTS remains debatable, recent data suggests that imaging performed 72–96 hours earlier may be superior for detecting metastatic foci. Because the therapeutic dose of I-131 is significantly higher than the minimal dose used for the WBS, the PTS can reveal additional unexpected locations of uptake, such as lung or skeletal lesions, which may affect the staging and prognosis of some patients **(Fig. 7)**.

Consequently, the PTS can influence patient management by requiring rapid further imaging examinations, demanding an earlier follow-up period, or modifying plans for subsequent WBS and extra I-131 therapy. PTS may be more sensitive than WBS for detecting thyroid remnant and metastatic disease since it is frequently acquired several days after therapy, as opposed to 48–72 hours for I-131 WBS. This distinction increases the target-to-background ratio on the PTS. In contrast, significant thyroid bed activity on a PTS can conceal smaller, less iodine-avid regional metastases. Patients with normal WBS and elevated stimulated Tg levels may potentially benefit from the PTS. Raised thyroglobulin (Tg) with negative WBS is an indication for positron emission tomography (PET) scanning using 18F-fluorodeoxyglucose. Empirical I-131 therapy can be given, followed by a PTS to locate the source of the elevated Tg level in the case of a normal PET scan. Either localized uptake on the PTS or low-level hepatic uptake from the metabolism of radioactive Tg indicates that thyroid tissue has been successfully targeted. In addition to a repeat measurement of the stimulated Tg level, a follow-up WBS conducted 6–12 months after I-131 therapy is essential for determining the treatment's efficacy.

Positron Emission Tomography

In oncology, PET/CT using 18F-FDG is used to distinguish benign from malignant lesions, such as in a lung nodule, and for metastatic workup. PET is not indicated for the diagnosis of benign thyroid disease, but there are clinical scenarios in which a thyroid incidentaloma is found inadvertently during a PET/CT scan. In thyroid management, determining the indications for surgery in the event of an ambiguous biopsy or a follicular neoplasm is a common challenge. In such circumstances, the role of PET remains unclear. The specifics are beyond the scope of this text, but here are some common areas in thyroid disorders where PET (with F-18 FDG) is indicated:

- Thyroid incidentalomas are found in about 4% of patients with a PET scan for another reason. These can lead to the detection of several occult/asymptomatic thyroid cancers.
- Preoperative assessment of cytologically indeterminate equivocal thyroid nodules.
- Thyroid carcinoma management (TENIS syndrome—thyroglobulin elevated negative iodine scintigraphy syndrome) **(Figs. 8 and 9)**.
- Anaplastic carcinoma thyroid.
- Response assessment following TKI therapy in thyroid cancer **(Figs. 10 and 11)**.
- Management and follow-up of Hürthle cell **(Fig. 12)**, a tall cell variant of thyroid carcinoma.
- In cases of carcinoma unknown primary (sometimes Ca thyroid present as carcinoma of unknown primary).
- Medullary carcinoma thyroid in poorly differentiated medullary carcinoma thyroid, fluorodeoxyglucose (FDG) PET/CT is recommended; however, well-differentiated MCT ^{68}Ga DoTANOC scan is more sensitive.

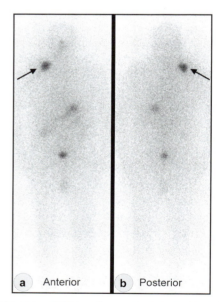

Fig. 8A: In the case of FCT with a metastatic skeletal lesion on the right shoulder, the patient received EBRT for the skeletal lesion; following radiotherapy, WBRI revealed (a and b) persistent iodine uptake in the right shoulder region. However, given very high thyroglobulin (Tg), TENIS was suspected, and FDG PET/CT was done **(Fig. 8B)**.
(EBRT: external beam radiation therapy; FCT: follicular carcinoma of thyroid; FDG: fluorodeoxyglucose; PET/CT: positron emission tomography/computed tomography; TENIS: thyroglobulin-elevated negative iodine scintigraphy; WBRI: whole body radioiodine scan)

CHAPTER 7

Nuclear Imaging in Thyroid Disorders 53

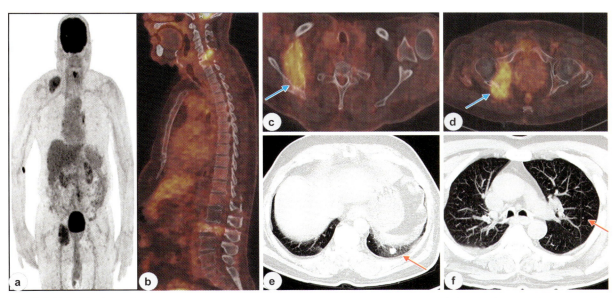

Fig. 8B: 18F-FDG PET/CT of the above patient reveals the normal physiological distribution of FDG in the body with abnormally increased uptake in the right shoulder, neck, and lumbar region in MIP image (a), fused SPECT/CT sagittal section (b) revealed nonmetabolically active multiple sclerotic vertebrae with few metabolically active sclerotic skeletal lesions. Fused PET/CT axial sections (c and d) revealed a skeletal lesion with soft tissue component in the left humerus and scapular region, and in the left acetabular region (blue arrows), CT axial view (e and f) revealed multiple lung nodules in the left lobe of the lung.
(18F-FDG: 18-F fluorodeoxyglucose; MIP: maximum intensity projection; PET/CT: positron emission tomography/computed tomography; SPECT/CT: single-photon emission computerized tomography)

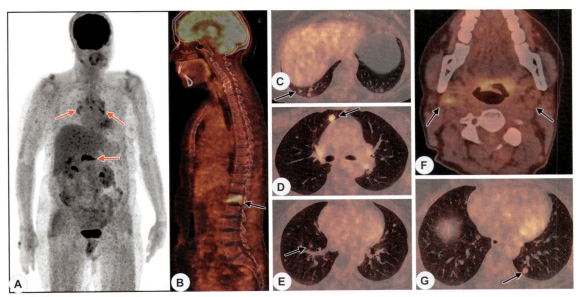

Figs. 9A to G: 18F-FDG PET/CT of a papillary thyroid carcinoma patient (TENIS); thyroglobulin of the patient was raised (>300 ng/mL) despite of negative WBRI scan (not shown), so TENIS was suspected. MIP image (A) of the patient revealed physiological tracer uptake of FDG in the patient with increased tracer uptake in the mediastinal and vertebral region (red arrow); sagittal fused PET/CT (B) revealed a metastatic lesion in L1 vertebrae (black arrow). Fused PET/CT axial view (C to G) revealed FDG avid to non-avid multiple cervical nodes and multiple lung nodules (black arrow).
(18F-FDG: 18-F fluorodeoxyglucose; MIP: maximum intensity projection; PET/CT: positron emission tomography/computed tomography; TENIS: thyroglobulin elevated negative iodine scintigraphy; WBRI: whole body radioiodine scan)

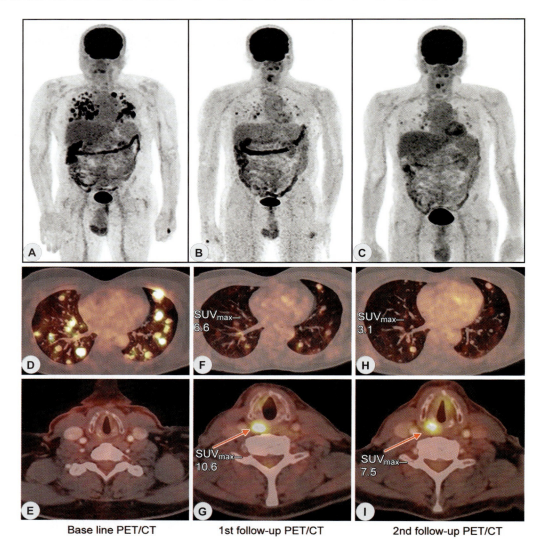

Figs. 10A to I: 18F-FDG PET/CT of a poorly differentiated thyroid carcinoma patient (TENIS), whole body baseline FDG PET/CT MIP image (A) reveals multiple focal uptakes in the lung, fused baseline axial PET/CT (D and E) reveal metabolically active multiple lung nodules in the bilateral lung (D), however, no uptake in noted near postoperative thyroid bed. The patient started on lenvatinib therapy three months after PET/CT was repeated to evaluate therapy response. MIP image (B) revealed decreased focal uptake in the lungs; however, new focal uptake was noted in the neck. First follow-up fused axial PET/CT (F and G) revealed reduced number of lung nodules and decreased uptake (SUV_{max}—6.6) in lung nodules with a new soft tissue lesion (SUV_{max}—10.6) near right cricoid cartilage suggestive of disease progression. The patient was continued on lenvatinib therapy. PET/CT was repeated three months later; second follow up MIP image (C) revealed decreased uptake in lung and neck lesions. Fused axial PET/CT (H and I) revealed further decreased uptake (SUV_{max}—3.1) in lung nodules and neck lesion (SUV_{max}—7.5), suggestive of partial response to lenvatinib treatment.

(18F-FDG: 18-F fluorodeoxyglucose; MIP: maximum intensity projection; PET/CT: positron emission tomography/computed tomography; TENIS: thyroglobulin elevated negative iodine scintigraphy; SUV_{max}: maximum standardized uptake value)

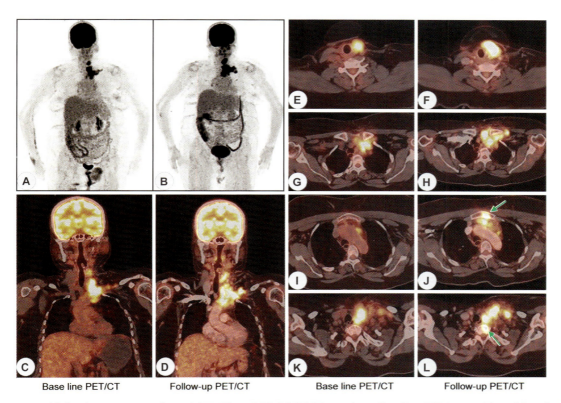

Figs. 11A to L: Case of follicular carcinoma thyroid (TENIS), 18F-FDG PET/CT was done. Baseline MIP image (A) and fused PET/CT coronal image (C) revealed soft tissue lesion in the neck with increased uptake in the left supraclavicular region. Fused axial PET/CT (E and G) revealed a soft tissue lesion in the left thyroid bed with conglomerated lymph nodes in the left supraclavicular (G and K) and mediastinal region (I); however, no metastatic skeletal lesion was noted. The Patient started on TKI, and a follow-up PET/CT was done for response evaluation. Follow-up MIP image (B) and fused coronal PET/CT (D) revealed an increase in size and uptake in previously mentioned neck and supraclavicular lesions. Fused axial PET/CT (F and H) revealed an increase in the size and uptake of neck lesions and supraclavicular and mediastinal lymph nodes. Furthermore, fused axial PET/CT (J and L) revealed metabolically active new lytic lesions in the sternum and vertebrae (green arrow), suggesting disease progression.
(18-F FDG: 18-F fluorodeoxyglucose; MIP: maximum intensity projection; PET/CT: positron emission tomography/computed tomography)

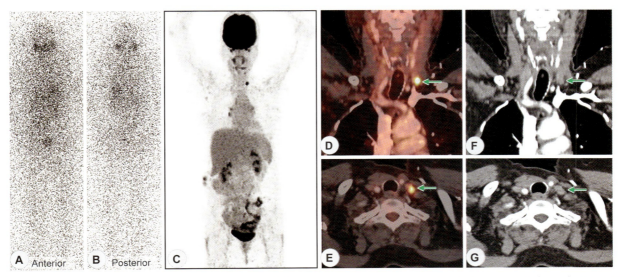

Figs. 12A to G: Case of a Hürthle cell carcinoma thyroid; the patient was treated with radioiodine following total thyroidectomy. However, during follow-up, WBS was found to be negative. No abnormal uptake was noted in the whole body iodine scan (A and B). However, given Hürthle cell carcinoma, 18F-FDG PET/CT was done. MIP image (C) revealed focal increased uptake in the neck. Coronal (D) and axial fused PET/CT (E) revealed increased focal uptake in the right side of the neck with soft tissue lesions (green arrow). Coronal CT (F) and axial CT (G) revealed well-defined soft tissue lesions (green arrow) suggestive of disease recurrence. FNAC from the lesion confirmed it to be a recurrent lesion.
(FNAC: fine needle aspiration cytology; 18F-FDG: 18-F fluorodeoxyglucose; MIP: maximum intensity projection; PET/CT: positron emission tomography/computed tomography; WBS: whole-body scan)

SUGGESTED READINGS

1. Kaminsky SM, Levy O, Salvador C, Dai G, Carrasco N. The Na$^+$/I$^-$ symporter of the thyroid gland. Soc Gen Physiol Ser. 1993;48:251-62.
2. Meller J, Becker W. The continuing importance of thyroid scintigraphy in the era of high-resolution ultrasound. Eur J Nucl Med Mol Imaging. 2002;29 (Suppl 2):S425-38.
3. Czepczyński R. Nuclear medicine in the diagnosis of benign thyroid diseases. Nucl Med Rev Cent East Eur. 2012;15(2):113-9.
4. Gharib H, Papini E, Paschke R, Duick DS, Valcavi R, Hegedüs L, et al. American Association of Clinical Endocrinologists, Associazione Medici Endocrinologi, and European Thyroid Association Medical guidelines for clinical practice for the diagnosis and management of thyroid nodules: executive summary of recommendations. Endocr Pract. 2010;16(3):468-75.
5. Smith JR, Oates E. Radionuclide imaging of the thyroid gland: patterns, pearls, and pitfalls. Clin Nucl Med. 2004;29(3):181-93.
6. Garberoglio S, Testori O. Role of Nuclear Medicine in the Diagnosis of Benign Thyroid Diseases. Front Horm Res. 2016;45:24-36.
7. Durgia H, Nicholas AK, Schoenmakers E, Dickens JA, Halanaik D, Sahoo J, et al. Brief Report: A Novel Sodium/Iodide Symporter Mutation, S356F, Causing Congenital Hypothyroidism. Thyroid. 2022;32(2):215-8.
8. Oh JR, Ahn BC. False-positive uptake on radioiodine whole-body scintigraphy: physiologic and pathologic variants unrelated to thyroid cancer. Am J Nucl Med Mol Imaging. 2012;2(3):362-85.
9. Giovanella L, Avram AM, Iakovou I, Kwak J, Lawson SA, Lulaj E, et al. EANM practice guideline/SNMMI procedure standard for RAIU and thyroid scintigraphy. Eur J Nucl Med Mol Imaging. 2019;46(12):2514-25.
10. Yordanova A, Mahjoob S, Lingohr P, Kalff J, Türler A, Palmedo H, et al. Diagnostic accuracy of [^{99m}Tc]Tc-Sestamibi in the assessment of thyroid nodules. Oncotarget. 2017;8(55):94681-91.
11. Silberstein EB, Alavi A, Balon HR, Becker D, Charkes D, Clarke SEM, et al. Society of Nuclear Medicine Procedure Guideline for Scintigraphy for Differentiated Papillary and Follicular Thyroid Cancer. Reston, VA: Society of Nuclear Medicine; 2006.
12. Pacini F, Schlumberger M, Harmer C, Berg GG, Cohen O, Duntas L, et al. Post-surgical use of radioiodine (^{131}I) in patients with papillary and follicular thyroid cancer and the issue of remnant ablation: a consensus report. Eur J Endocrinol. 2005;153(5):651-9.
13. Robbins RJ, Tuttle RM, Sharaf RN, Larson SM, Robbins HK, Ghossein RA, et al. Preparation by Recombinant Human Thyrotropin or Thyroid Hormone Withdrawal are Comparable for the Detection of Residual Differentiated Thyroid Carcinoma. J Clin Endocrinol Metab. 2001;86(2):619-25.
14. Minambres I, Farran JA, Lopez DA, Estorch M, Perez JI, Moral A, et al. 18F-Fluorocholine PET/CT in patients with primary Hyperparathyroidism and negative or inconclusive ^{99m}Tc-MIBI parathyroid scan: clinicopathological correlations. Endocr Abstr. 2019;63:GP19.
15. Donahue KP, Shah NP, Lee SL, Oates ME. Initial Staging of Differentiated Thyroid Carcinoma: Continued Utility of Posttherapy ^{131}I Whole-body Scintigraphy. Radiology. 2008;246(3):887-94.
16. Ali N, Sebastian C, Foley RR, Murray I, Canizales AL, Jenkins PJ, et al. The management of differentiated thyroid cancer using ^{123}I for imaging to assess the need for ^{131}I therapy. Nucl Med Commun. 2006;27(2):165-9.
17. Park HM, Perkins OW, Edmondson JW, Schnute RB, Manatunga A. Influence of Diagnostic Radioiodines on the Uptake of Ablative Dose of Iodine-131. Thyroid. 1994;4(1):49-54.
18. Silberstein EB. Comparison of Outcomes after (123)I versus (131)I Preablation Imaging before Radioiodine Ablation in Differentiated Thyroid Carcinoma. J Nucl Med. 2007;48(7):1043-6.
19. Mazzaferri EL, Kloos RT. Current Approaches to Primary Therapy for Papillary and Follicular Thyroid Cancer. 2001;86(4):1447-63.
20. Haugen BR, Alexander EK, Bible KC, Doherty GM, Mandel SJ, Nikiforov YE, et al. 2015 American Thyroid Association Management Guidelines for Adult Patients with Thyroid Nodules and Differentiated Thyroid Cancer: The American Thyroid Association Guidelines Task Force on Thyroid Nodules and Differentiated Thyroid Cancer. Thyroid. 2016;26(1):1-133.
21. Hung BT, Huang SH, Huang YE, Wang PW. Appropriate Time for Post-therapeutic I-131 Whole Body Scan. Clin Nucl Med. 2009;34(6):339-42.
22. Schlumberger M, Catargi B, Borget I, Deandreis D, Zerdoud S, Bridji B, et al. Strategies of radioiodine ablation in patients with low-risk thyroid cancer. N Engl J Med. 2012;366(18):1663-73.
23. Dietlein M, Verburg FA, Luster M, Reiners C, Pitoia F, Schicha H. One should not just read what one believes: the nearly irresolvable issue of producing truly objective, evidence-based guidelines for the management of differentiated thyroid cancer. Eur J Nucl Med Mol Imaging. 2011;38(5):793-8.

8 CHAPTER

Clinical and Pathological Aspect of Benign and Malignant Thyroid Nodules

Uma Nahar Saikia, Pranab Dey, Pinaki Dutta, Mayur Parkhi, Ananda Mohan Chakraborty

CLINICAL PERSPECTIVE

INTRODUCTION

The prevalence of thyroid nodule increases with age and more common in women. The prevalence of thyroid nodules is up to 50% in adult population **(Fig. 1)**. It can be either singular, solitary process, or part of a multinodular gland. Multinodularity is defined as having two or more nodules, each being >1 cm in diameter **(Fig. 2)**.

The primary goal of diagnostic assessment of thyroid nodules is to classify them as benign or malignant neoplasm by ultrasound and ultrasound-guided fine needle aspiration (FNA). The risk of thyroid malignancy in a thyroid nodule is approximately 7–15%.

DIAGNOSTIC APPROACH TO THYROID NODULES

Assessment of Clinical and Serological Risk Factors

Assessment of thyroid nodule/s is to prognosticate thyroid cancer via assessment of multiple risk factors including exposure to ionizing radiation or family history. The younger patients (18–50 years) **(Fig. 3)** and men are at a greater risk of thyroid malignancy than older patients (>51 years) and women, respectively **(Fig. 4)**. Additionally, rapid growth of a nodule, persistent hoarseness of voice, dysphagia, persistent and new-onset cervical lymphadenopathy, or worsening, and unexplained neck pain are considered as potentially aggressive nature of thyroid nodule though rare.

High-resolution Ultrasound

The application of high-resolution ultrasound has markedly improved risk stratification of thyroid nodules. Based

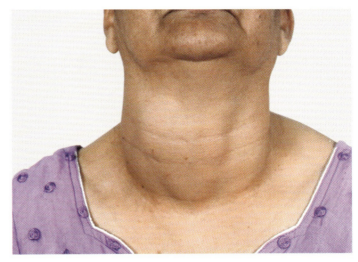

Fig. 1: Diffuse thyroid enlargement in goiter.

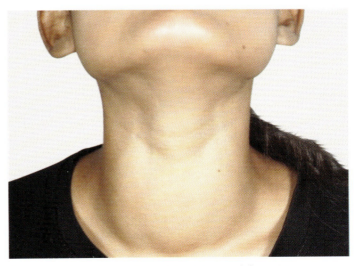

Fig. 2: Multinodular swelling of thyroid in nodular goiter.

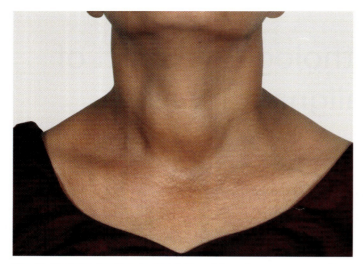

Fig. 3: Nodular swelling in middle-aged female in thyroid papillary carcinoma.

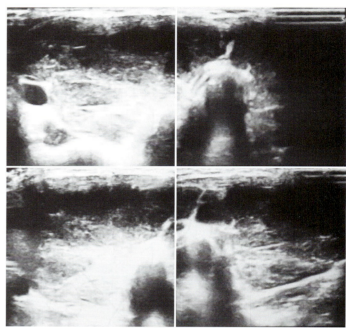

Fig. 5: Irregular borders with hypoechogenicity of the thyroid nodule.

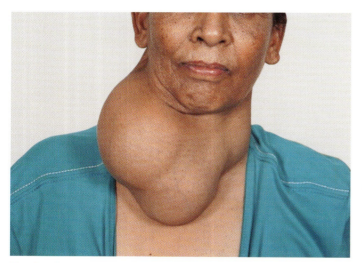

Fig. 4: Huge multinodular swelling of thyroid in follicular thyroid carcinoma.

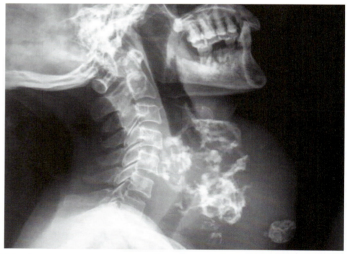

Fig. 6: Micro and macro calcifications in nodular thyroid swelling.

on ultrasonographic findings, the American College of Radiology (ACR) has proposed a thyroid imaging reporting and data system (TI-RADS) for thyroid nodules using a standardized scoring system. It provides recommendations for FNA or ultrasound with follow-up of suspicious nodules, and safely leaves nodules that are benign/not suspicious without surgery.

The TI-RADS scoring is determined from five categories of ultrasound findings. A score of "ONE" is assigned for each of following categories: composition, echogenicity, shape, margin, and echogenic foci. Higher-risk sonographic features, such as microcalcifications, hypoechogenicity, or irregular nodule shape or borders (especially when two or more such features are detected in combination), substantially increases risk of malignancy **(Figs. 5 and 6)**. The individual scores are summed up to determine a TR (TI-RADS) level. Higher the cumulative score, higher is the TR level and likelihood of thyroid malignancy is high. Accordingly, TR1 (0 points) is suggestive of benign disease while TR5 (≥ 7 points) is highly suspicious of malignancy with malignancy rates ranging from 0.3% in TR1 thyroid nodules to 35% in TR5 nodules.

The TI-RADS scoring is an essential guiding tool for selecting next line of action; FNA is not recommended in TR1 and TR2 nodules while suspicious lesions (TR3-TR5) are usually advised to undergo FNA. However, possibility of significant inter-observer variability in interpreting sonographic and FNA findings urges the need of biopsy or early surgery in such nodules.

Hence, a holistic approach including clinical, serological, USG, FNA, and biopsy is required to achieve an accurate and early diagnosis thyroid nodule.

CYTOLOGY AND HISTOPATHOLOGY

ANATOMY

- It normally weighs 20–30 g; two lobes, joined by isthmus; lies across the trachea anteriorly, below the level of cricoid cartilage.
- Rich lymphatic network.

NORMAL HISTOLOGY

Varying sized follicles, single layer of follicular cells, pale acidophilic or amphophilic cytoplasm **(Fig. 7)**.

IMMUNOHISTOCHEMISTRY

- Reactivity for TG, thyroid peroxidase (TPO), triiodothyronine (T3), and thyroxine (T4) both in colloid and cytoplasm of the follicular cells.
- Thyroid transcription factor-1 (TTF-1)—normal follicular cells **(Fig. 8)**.
- Low molecular weight keratin (CK7, CK18, CK8, CK19), EMA, Vimentin, ER, PR—positive.

CYTOPATHOLOGY GUIDELINES

Fine needle aspiration cytology (FNAC) of thyroid lesions is the first line of investigation for rapid diagnosis of thyroid swelling and nodules.

The common indications of FNAC include:
- Visible and palpable thyroid swelling
- Solid nodule on USG
- Dominant nodule

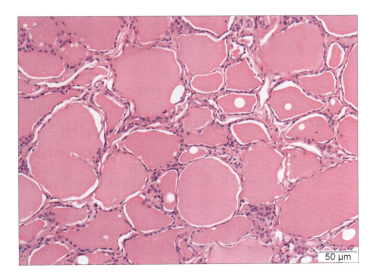

Fig. 7: Normal histology—variable size follicles lined by flattened to low cuboidal epithelium containing abundant colloid (H&E, ×200).

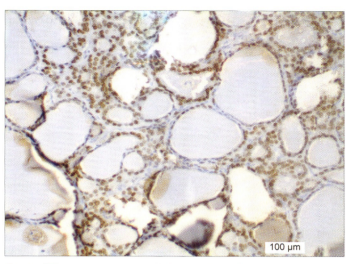

Fig. 8: TTF-1 immunostain highlighting follicular and para-follicular cells (Peroxidase, ×200).

USG or CT guided FNAC is done for:
- Nonvisible or palpable lesions
- Failed first FNAC
- Solid area in a cystic swelling

■ Complications of FNAC

- Minor hemorrhage
- Needle tract seedling rarely

Clinically: The age, sex, duration, size of lesion, and USG findings (if available) are important; thyroid scan report (optional) and history of bleeding diathesis to be noted.

■ Gross Examination of Material

- *Brown color*: Colloid goiter with cystic degeneration
- *Necrotic material*: Anaplastic carcinoma, suppurative inflammation
- *Thick chewing gum like colloid*: Papillary carcinoma

■ Microscopic Examination

- *Colloid* **(Fig. 9)**: Light to deep blue
- *Thyroid follicular cells* **(Fig. 10)**: Follicular arrangement or loose clusters, round cells with scanty cytoplasm having round monomorphic nuclei.
- *Hürthle cells* **(Fig. 11)**: Large cells with abundant cytoplasm, central to eccentric monomorphic nuclei. Abundant mitochondria on electron microscopy.
- *Foamy macrophages* **(Fig. 12)**: Large cells with abundant vacuolated cytoplasm.

■ Adequacy of FNAC

- At least six clusters of cells having at least 10 thyroid follicular cells in each cluster.
- Abundant colloid in colloid goiter with few thyroid follicular cells is adequate.

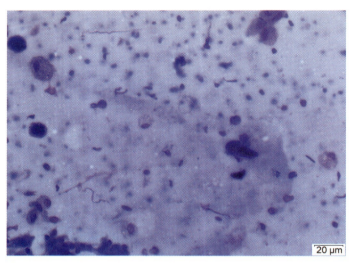

Fig. 9: Abundant bluish thin colloid in a colloid goiter (MGG, ×400).

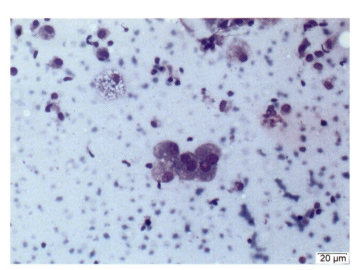

Fig. 12: Foamy macrophages—the cells with abundant vacuolated cytoplasm (MGG, ×400).

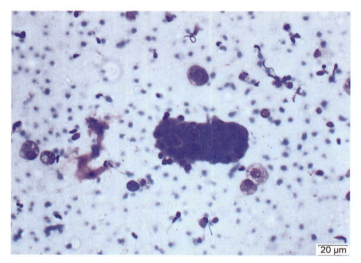

Fig. 10: Thyroid follicular cells—the cells with scanty cytoplasm and monomorphic round nuclei (MGG, ×400).

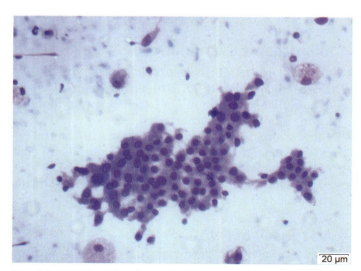

Fig. 11: Hürthle cells—the cells with abundant cytoplasm having central to eccentric monomorphic nuclei (MGG, ×400).

■ The Bethesda Terminology of Reporting Thyroid FNAC

The Bethesda terminology of reporting thyroid FNAC is mentioned in **Table 1**.

■ Thyroglossal Duct Cyst

- *Gross*: Smooth-walled cyst (2–85 mm) containing clear, mucinous fluid to purulent material when secondarily infected.
- *Microscopy*: Cyst lined by respiratory or squamous or both and contains thyroid follicular epithelium in the wall. On rupture, fibrosis, collection of histiocytes, cholesterol cleft, and foreign body giant cell reaction seen **(Fig. 13)**.
- *Differential diagnosis (D/Ds)*: Epidermal inclusion cyst, dermoid cyst, branchial cleft cyst, bronchogenic cyst, cervical thymic cyst, and metastatic papillary thyroid carcinoma (PTC).

■ Thyroglossal Duct Carcinoma

Malignancy seen in about 3% of thyroglossal duct cyst (TGDC), PTC accounting for >95% **(Fig. 14)**.

THYROID ENDOCRINE ABNORMALITIES

- *Hyperthyroidism*: Papillary hyperplasia lacking fibrovascular cores, stromal lymphocytic rich infiltrate, small or occluded lumens containing pale or little colloid with scalloping.
- *Hypothyroidism*: Primary hypothyroidism (hyperplastic follicles, occasional papillary folding, follicle cells from cuboidal to columnar with clear cytoplasm, scant colloid material, lymphocytic infiltrate).

Clinical and Pathological Aspect of Benign and Malignant Thyroid Nodules

TABLE 1: Bethesda terminology of reporting thyroid FNAC.			
Category	Different diagnostic entities	Risk of malignancy	Management
I: Inadequate for opinion	• Low cellularity • Mainly blood • Poor quality	1.4%	Repeat aspiration
II: Benign	Consistent with: • Colloid goiter • Lymphocytic thyroiditis • Hyperplastic nodule	0–3%	Clinical follow-up
III: Follicular lesions of undetermined significance (FLUS)/atypia of undetermined significance (AUS)	Subdivision: • *Cytological atypia*: Nuclear atypia • *Architectural atypia*: Many micro-follicles • Both cytologic and architectural atypia • Atypia, not otherwise specified	6–30%	• Repeat FNAC • Molecular test, if possible • Surgical removal rarely
IV: Follicular neoplasm (FN)/ suspicious of follicular neoplasm (SFN)	Noninvasive follicular thyroid neoplasm with papillary (NIFTP) such as nuclear features	15–30%	• lobectomy • Molecular testing
V: Suspicious for malignancy	• Suspicious for follicular variant of papillary carcinoma, medullary, or other carcinomas • Suspicious for lymphoma	50–75%	Near-total thyroidectomy
VI: Malignant	Confirmed specify the type of malignancy	97–99%	Thyroidectomy

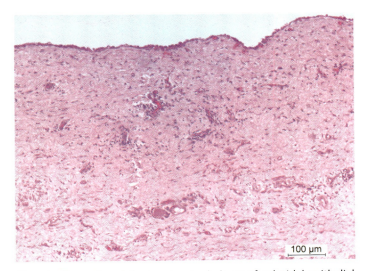

Fig. 13: Thyroglossal duct cyst—single layer of cuboidal epithelial cells with fibrosis, mild chronic inflammation and few benign thyroid follicles (H&E, ×100).

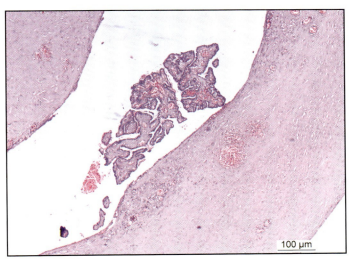

Fig. 14: Thyroglossal duct carcinoma—PTC in a background of thyroglossal cyst (H&E, ×100).

Thyroiditis

Clinically, it includes painless (silent or subacute) thyroiditis that can be sporadic or postpartum, juvenile or hashitoxicosis (initial phase). Usually presents with clinical symptoms of hypothyroidism with diffuse swelling of thyroid gland.

- *Acute/infectious thyroiditis*:
  - Very rare, usually due to extension from surrounding inflammation or disseminated infection showing neutrophilic infiltrate and tissue necrosis.
  - FNAC usually avoided
    - Large number of neutrophils with necrosis
    - Degenerated thyroid follicular cells
- *Autoimmune thyroiditis*:
  - *Lymphocytic thyroiditis*
    - Cytology: **(Figs. 15 to 18)**
      - Lymphocytes infiltrating follicular cells causing destruction of follicles
      - Occasional histiocytic collection and multi-nucleated giant cells

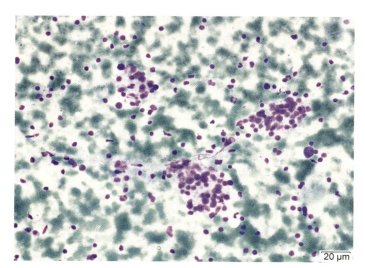

Fig. 15: Lymphocytic thyroiditis—multiple thyroid follicle in the background of lymphocytes (MGG, ×200).

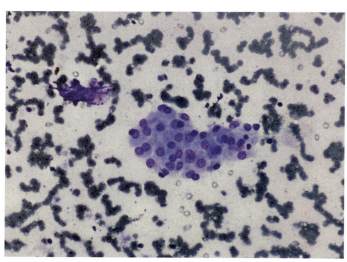

Fig. 18A: Lymphocytic thyroiditis— Hürthle cells (MGG, ×400).

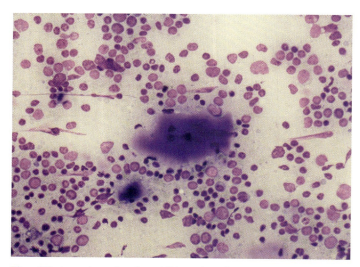

Fig. 16: Lymphocytic thyroiditis—abundant reactive lymphoid cells and colloid (MGG, ×400).

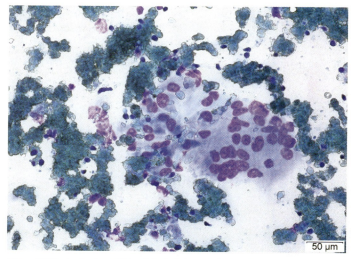

Fig. 18B: Lymphocytic thyroiditis—multinucleated giant cells (MGG, ×400).

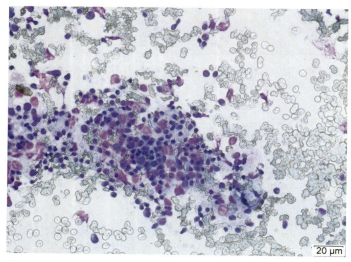

Fig. 17: Lymphocytic thyroiditis—thyroid follicles are infiltrated with lymphocytes (MGG, ×400).

- D/Ds (cytology):
    - Non-Hodgkin's lymphoma (NHL)
    - Hürthle cell neoplasm: Hürthle cells (>75%) without background lymphoid cells.
    - PTC: Presence of papillae and nuclear features absent
- Histopathology: Lymphocytic infiltration with few lymphoid follicles, focal oncocytic change. **(Fig. 19)**
  - *Drug-induced thyroiditis*: Amiodarone, lithium, immunomodulatory drugs, cancer immunotherapy, and cancer vaccines.
  - *Focal lymphocytic thyroiditis (nonspecific or focal autoimmune thyroiditis)* **(Fig. 20)**
  - *Hashimoto's thyroiditis*: Similar to lymphocytic thyroiditis with extensive destruction and oncocytic change **(Fig. 21)**.

Clinical and Pathological Aspect of Benign and Malignant Thyroid Nodules

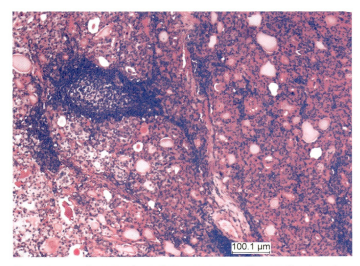

Fig. 19: Lymphocytic thyroiditis—presence of extensive lymphocytic infiltrate forming aggregates and follicles causing destruction of native thyroid follicles (H&E, ×100).

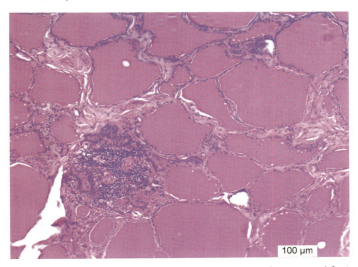

Fig. 20: Focal lymphocytic thyroiditis—presence of occasional foci of lymphocytic aggregate with mild destruction of native thyroid follicles (H&E, ×100).

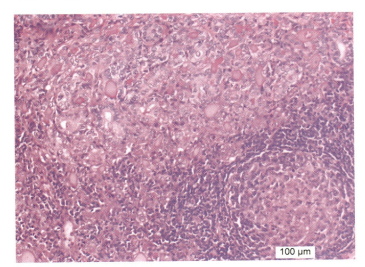

Fig. 21: Hashimoto's thyroiditis—reactive lymphoid follicles with germinal centres causing destruction and Hürthle cell change in follicular cells (H&E, ×100).

- *Hashimoto-fibrous*:
    - Similar to Hashimoto thyroiditis with extensive fibrosis (dense hyaline type).
    - D/D: Malignant neoplasm with extensive fibrosis, immunoglobulin G4 (IgG4) related disease.
- *Palpation thyroiditis (multifocal granulomatous folliculitis)*: It occurs secondarily to vigorous palpation usually in younger population.
- *Radiation thyroiditis*: Histologic changes vary with dose and type of radioactive isotope. Nodular hyperplasia, follicular disruption and atrophy, focal hemorrhagic necrosis, inflammatory cell infiltration (acute, chronic, or mixed), marked cellular atypia with oncocytic metaplasia, and fibrosis.
- *Riedel's thyroiditis (Riedel struma/fibrous thyroiditis/ invasive thyroiditis/IgG4 related disease)*:
    - *Gross*: Thyroid gland enlargement with extra-thyroidal extension. Stony hard and cuts with great resistance.
    - *Microscopy*: Presence of extensive fibrosis replacing thyroid follicles with extrathyroidal extension (absent in fibrous Hashimoto's thyroiditis).
- *Subacute granulomatous thyroiditis* **(Figs. 22 to 24)**:
    - Reactive lymphoid cells infiltrating follicular cells
    - Epithelioid cell granulomas and multinucleated giant cells

Hyperplasia/Goiter

- *Amyloid goiter*:
    - *Gross*: Enlarged gland with bosselated surface, salmon cut surface.
    - *Microscopy*: Deposition of amorphous eosinophilic material in perifollicular and perivascular regions **(Fig. 25A)**.
    - Congophilic **(Fig. 25B)** and apple-green birefringence under-polarized microscope **(Fig. 25C)**.

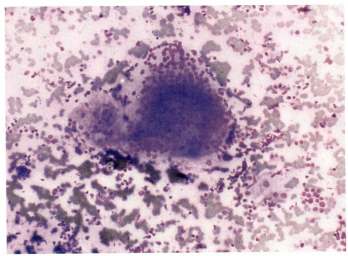

Fig. 22: Subacute granulomatous thyroiditis—epithelioid cell granulomas and multinucleated giant cells (MGG, ×200).

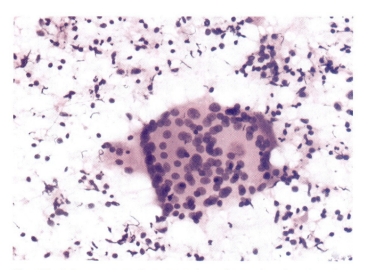

Fig. 23: Subacute granulomatous thyroiditis—abundant lymphocytes and multinucleated giant cells (MGG, ×400).

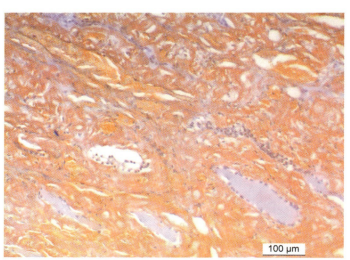

Fig. 25B: Amyloidosis—amorphous, homogenous, eosinophilic material is congophilic on Congo red stain (Congo red stain, ×200).

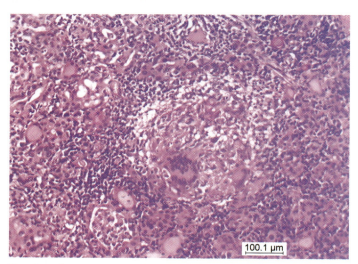

Fig. 24: Subacute granulomatous thyroiditis—presence of non-necrotizing epithelioid cell granulomas with occasional multi-nucleated giant cells (H&E, ×200).

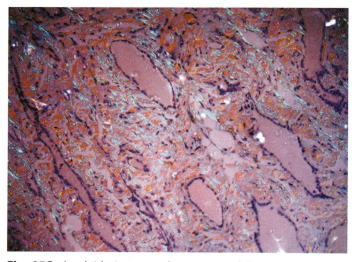

Fig. 25C: Amyloidosis—amorphous eosinophilic material reflects apple-green birefringence on polarizer microscope (×200).

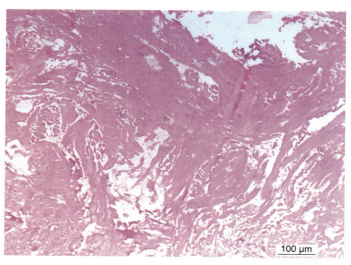

Fig. 25A: Amyloidosis—thyroid parenchyma is replaced by deposition of amorphous, acellular, eosinophilic, and fibrillary material (H&E, ×100).

- *C-cell hyperplasia*:
  - Diffuse or nodular, interfollicular, or intrafollicular.
  - Approximately >6 cells per thyroid follicle and/or >50 intrafollicular calcitonin positive cells (at least one low power field).
- *Dyshormonogenetic goiter*:
  - Enlargement of gland due to defect in synthesis of thyroid hormones.
  - Follicles hyperplastic, lined by follicular cells with marked nuclear pleomorphism.
- *Endemic goiter*:
  - Due to low iodine content in water and soil
  - Hyperactive thyroid with tall follicular epithelium and scanty colloid (parenchymatous goiter). Later follicular atrophy with massive colloid **(Fig. 26)**
  - *Cytology*: **(Figs. 27 to 29)**
    – Abundant colloid with scanty thyroid follicular cells
    – Macrophages in case of cystic degeneration.

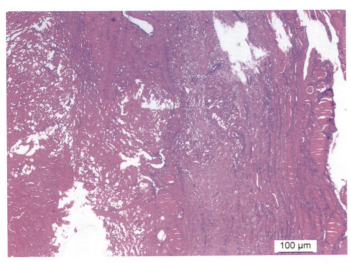

Fig. 26: Colloid goiter—large cyst containing abundant colloid (left) with rupture causing histiocytic and giant cell collection (H&E, ×100).

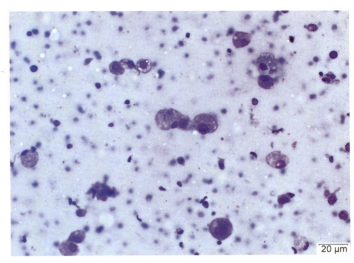

Fig. 29: Colloid goiter—abundant foamy macrophages and colloid (MGG, ×400).

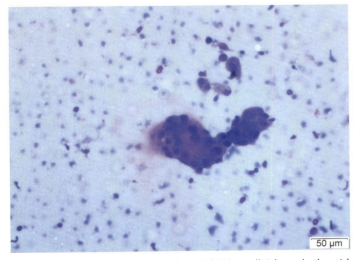

Fig. 27: Colloid goiter—abundant bluish colloid and thyroid follicular cells (MGG, ×400).

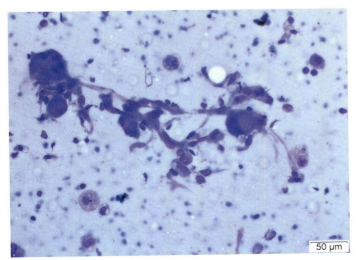

Fig. 28: Colloid goiter—metaplastic cells in a background of colloid (MGG, ×400).

- *D/Ds (cytology)*:
  - Follicular neoplasm: High cellularity with follicular arrangement
  - Lymphocytic thyroiditis: Lymphocytic infiltration of follicles
- *Graves' disease (diffuse toxic goiter)*:
  - Hyperplastic papillae protruding into dilated follicles in diffuse hyperplasia.
  - *Cytology*:
    - Scanty thin colloid with follicular cells in loose clusters
    - Fire flare around follicles
- *Multinodular goiter*:
  - Most common cause for thyroid enlargement with nodule formation.
  - Clinically euthyroid; sometimes can have compression symptoms.
  - *Microscopy*: Nonencapsulated nodular hyperplasia with variable-sized follicles **(Fig. 30)**.

WORLD HEALTH ORGANIZATION CLASSIFICATION OF THYROID NEOPLASMS

Developmental Abnormalities

- Thyroglossal duct cyst (TGDC)
- Other congenital thyroid abnormalities

Follicular Cell-derived Neoplasms

- *Benign tumors*:
  - Thyroid follicular nodular disease (FND)
  - Follicular adenoma (FA)
  - FA with papillary architecture
  - Oncocytic adenoma of the thyroid

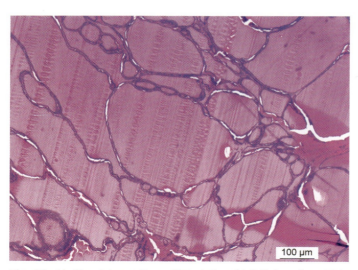

Fig. 30: Multinodular goiter—dilated thyroid follicles of variable size with abundant colloid and single layer of benign cuboidal cells (H&E, ×100).

- *Low-risk neoplasms*:
  o Noninvasive follicular thyroid neoplasm with papillary-like nuclear features
  o Thyroid tumors of uncertain malignant potential
  o Hyalinizing trabecular tumor (HTT)
- *Malignant neoplasms*:
  o Follicular thyroid carcinoma
  o Invasive encapsulated follicular variant papillary carcinoma
  o Papillary thyroid carcinoma
  o Oncocytic carcinoma of the thyroid
  o *Follicular-derived carcinomas, high-grade*:
    – Differentiated high-grade thyroid carcinoma (DHGTC)
    – Poorly differentiated thyroid carcinoma (PDTC)
  o Anaplastic follicular cell-derived thyroid carcinoma

Thyroid C-cell–derived Carcinoma

Medullary thyroid carcinoma (MTC).

Mixed Medullary and Follicular Cell-derived Carcinomas

- Quite rare and difficult to diagnose
- Detailed gross and histological examination with IHC is required to confirm the diagnosis

Salivary Gland-type Carcinomas of the Thyroid

- Mucoepidermoid carcinoma of the thyroid
- Secretory carcinoma of salivary gland type

Thyroid Tumors of Uncertain Histogenesis

- Sclerosing mucoepidermoid carcinoma with eosinophilia (SMECE)
- Cribriform morular thyroid carcinoma

Thymic Tumors within the Thyroid

- Thymoma family
- Spindle epithelial tumor with thymus-like elements
- Thymic carcinoma family

Embryonal Thyroid Neoplasms

Thyroblastoma.

FOLLICULAR CELL–DERIVED NEOPLASMS

- *Benign tumors*:
  o *Thyroid FND*:
    – Gross: Unilateral or bilateral. Nodules of variable size and shapes with degeneration.
    – Microscopy:
      ▪ Nodular hyperplasia with follicular or papillary growth patterns.
      ▪ Low cuboidal to tall columnar epithelium with absent PTC nuclear features.
    – Hemorrhage, fibrosis, and calcification may be present
    – Clinical application: Recurrence ~30%; subtotal thyroidectomy required.
  o *Follicular adenoma*:
    – Cytology: **(Figs. 31A and B)**
      ▪ Abundant microfollicles consisting of 10–18 follicular cells
      ▪ Scanty thin colloid
      ▪ On FNAC "follicular neoplasm" is suggested.
      ▪ Follicular carcinoma: Coarsely clumped chromatin, increased mitotic figures
    – D/Ds (cytology):
      ▪ Follicular hyperplasia: More colloid and fire-flare
      ▪ Follicular carcinoma
      ▪ Follicular variant of PTC (FVPTC)
      ▪ Parathyroid neoplasm: Extremely difficult to diagnose on FNAC. Clinical history and relevant investigations required. Absent colloid, follicles with vascularity, and discrete naked cells are suggestive of parathyroid neoplasm **(Figs. 32A and B)**. Cells are positive for parathormone.
    – Gross: Solitary, round to oval encapsulated nodules (20–30 mm). Cut surface usually homogeneous, greyish-white, tan, or brown.
    – Microscopy:
      ▪ Encapsulated, follicular-pattern (microfollicular, normofollicular, or macrofollicular) tumor, lack capsular, or vascular invasion **(Fig. 33A)**.
      ▪ Absence of PTC nuclear features **(Fig. 33B)**.
      ▪ Mitoses rare (<3 mitoses/2 mm^2)
    – Histological patterns: FA with papillary hyperplasia, clear cell FA, signet-ring-cell pattern, FA with bizarre nuclei, spindle cell variant OR Black FA.

Clinical and Pathological Aspect of Benign and Malignant Thyroid Nodules

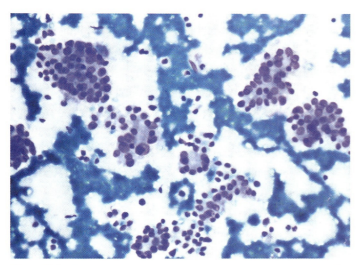

Fig. 31A: Follicular neoplasm—abundant microfollicles (MGG, ×200).

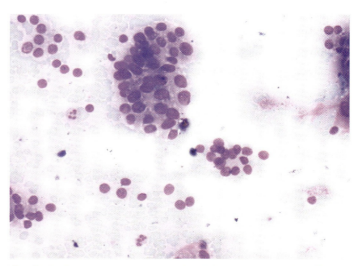

Fig. 31B: Follicular neoplasm—microfollicles consist of 10–15 cells (MGG, ×400).

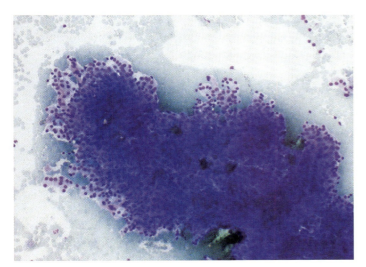

Fig. 32A: Parathyroid neoplasm—cohesive cluster of tumor cells (MGG, ×200).

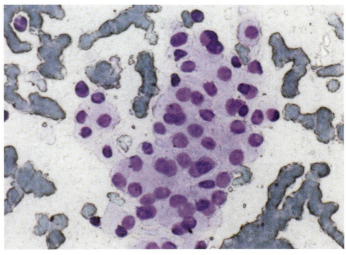

Fig. 32B: Parathyroid neoplasm—the cells show abundant clear cytoplasm and central monomorphic round nuclei (MGG, ×400).

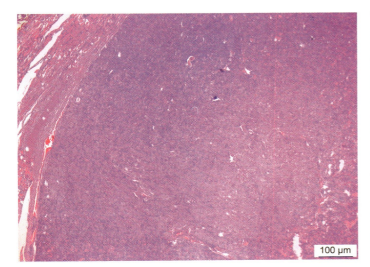

Fig. 33A: Follicular adenoma—well-encapsulated tumor showing dominantly microfollicular arrangement without capsular or vascular invasion (H&E, ×40).

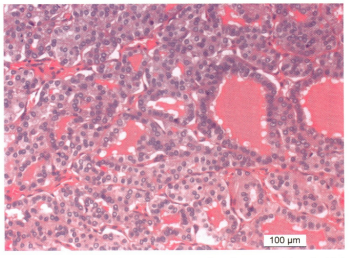

Fig. 33B: Follicular adenoma—encapsulated tumor with cuboidal tumor cells having moderate eosinophilic cytoplasm, round nuclei, and coarse chromatin (H&E, ×400).

- IHC:
  - Positive: CAM5.2, EMA, CK7, PAX8, and TTF-1
  - Negative: CK20, calcitonin, Galectin-3, HBME1, and CITED1
  - Ki-67 proliferation index <5%
- D/Ds: Follicular thyroid carcinoma, multifocal nodular hyperplasia.
- Clinical implication: Good with partial thyroidectomy

o *Follicular adenoma with papillary architecture*:
  - Gross: Distinct capsule with beefy red cut surface.
  - Microscopy:
    - Mixed follicular and papillary architecture
    - One large follicle with complex papillary infoldings having broad papillae with an organized centripetal orientation, edematous cores embedded within follicles.
    - Sanderson's pollsters (subfollicles within follicles).
    - Bubbly colloid with peripheral scalloping.
    - Crowded columnar cells, basally located, uniformly lack PTC nuclear features.
  - Clinical implication: Good with partial thyroidectomy.

o *Oncocytic adenoma of the thyroid (OA)*:
  - Cytology: **(Figs. 34 to 36)**
    - Large number of Hürthle cells (>75%) in follicles or sheets.
    - Large cells with abundant granular cytoplasm with central prominent nuclei
    - Electron microscopy: Abundant mitochondria
    - ICC: Positive for GLUT-4, CK 14, CEA, and thyroglobulin.
  - Gross: Solitary, encapsulated nodules, and homogenous (20–30 mm).
  - Microscopy:
    - Encapsulated, follicular-pattern (microfollicular, normofollicular, few macrofollicular) tumor, lack capsular, or vascular invasion **(Fig. 37A)**.
    - Solid or trabecular growth (more frequent in oncocytic carcinoma).
    - >75% oncocytic cells **(Fig. 37B)**
    - Punctuated nuclei with "endocrine atypia" **(Fig. 37C)**
    - Mitoses infrequent.
  - D/Ds: Oncocytic carcinoma, oncocytic hyperplastic nodule.
  - Note: Noninvasive, encapsulated, follicular-cell-derived neoplasms composed of <75% oncocytic cells, considered FAs with oncocytic features.
  - Clinical implication: Good prognosis following partial thyroidectomy.

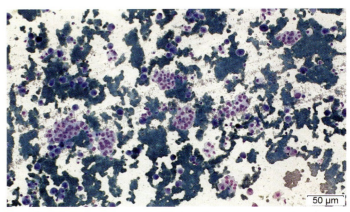

Fig. 34: Oncocytic adenoma—abundant. Hürthle cells in small clusters and discretely arranged (MGG, ×200).

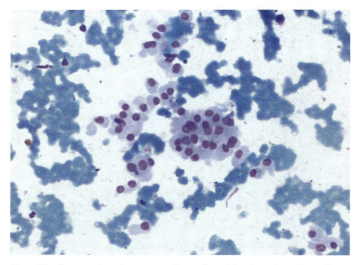

Fig. 35: Oncocytic adenoma—the cells with abundant cytoplasm and centrally placed monomorphic nuclei (MGG, ×400).

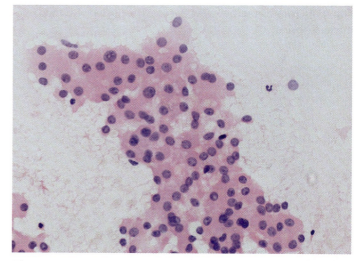

Fig. 36: Oncocytic adenoma—the cells with abundant cytoplasm having indistinct margin (Papanicolaou stain, ×400).

Clinical and Pathological Aspect of Benign and Malignant Thyroid Nodules

- *Low-risk neoplasms*:
  - *Noninvasive follicular thyroid neoplasm with papillary-like nuclear features (NIFTP)*:
    – Subtypes:
      - Subcentimeter: <10 mm in size
      - Oncocytic: NIFTP with at least 75% oncocytic cells
    – Gross: Well delineated or encapsulated solid nodule with white/tan to brown color.
    – Microscopy:
      - Encapsulated or circumscribed (**Fig. 38A**).
      - Follicular growth pattern with following criteria: <1% true papillae; no psammoma bodies; <30% solid/trabecular/insular growth pattern.
      - Nuclear features of papillary carcinoma (nuclear score of 2–3) (**Fig. 38B**).
      - No vascular or capsular invasion
      - Low mitotic count (<3 mitosis/2 mm^2)

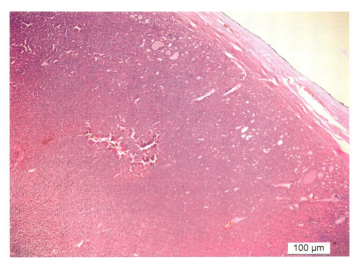

Fig. 37A: Oncocytic adenoma—well encapsulated tumor with micro follicular growth pattern without capsular or vascular invasion (H&E, ×40).

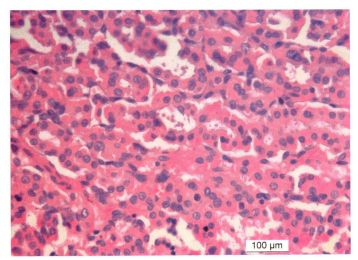

Fig. 37B: Oncocytic adenoma—tumor cells containing abundant granular eosinophilic cytoplasm, sharp cytoplasmic borders, round-to-oval nuclei and prominent nucleoli (H&E, ×200).

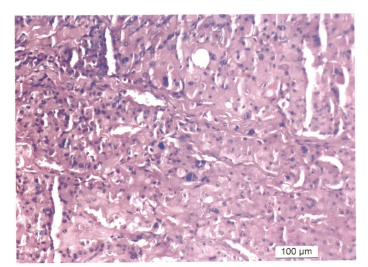

Fig. 37C: Oncocytic adenoma—tumor cells showing sudden nuclear (endocrine) atypia (H&E, ×200).

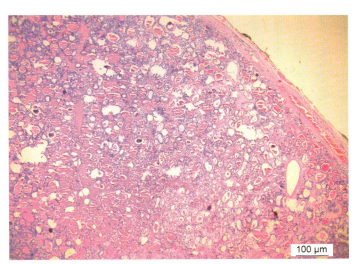

Fig. 38A: Noninvasive follicular thyroid neoplasm with papillary-like nuclear features (NIFTP)—encapsulated tumor with follicular pattern without capsular or vascular invasion seen (H&E, ×40).

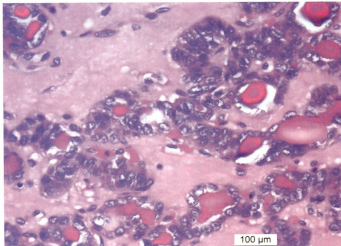

Fig. 38B: Noninvasive follicular thyroid neoplasm with papillary-like nuclear features (NIFTP)—tumor displaying nuclear features of PTC (score 2 or 3) (H&E, ×400).

- IHC: BRAF and NRAS
- D/Ds: FVPTC, classic follicular predominant PTC, FA
- Clinical implication: Recurrence due to inadequate resection hence total thyroidectomy may be needed.

o *Thyroid tumors of uncertain malignant potential*:
  - Subtype(s):
    - Follicular tumor of uncertain malignant potential (FT-UMP)
    - Well-differentiated tumor (WDT) of UMP
  - Gross: Nodular thyroid enlargement
  - Microscopy:
    - Similar to encapsulated well-differentiated follicular-patterned neoplasms, i.e., FA, follicular carcinoma, or encapsulated follicular variant PTC.
    - FT-UMP: Tumor cells are regular with round nuclei and lack nuclear features of PTC.
    - WDT-UMP: Tumor cells have PTC-type nuclear alterations (nuclear score of 2–3); if invasion is thoroughly excluded, term NIFTP should be used.
  - Clinical implication: Good prognosis in absence of vascular or capsular invasion.

o *Hyalinizing trabecular tumor*:
  - Cytology:
    - Papillae like clusters, absent true papillae
    - Hyalinized pinkish globules surrounded by follicular cells
    - Cells have moderate cytoplasm with longitudinal nuclear groove and often intranuclear inclusions
    - D/D: PTC (monomorphic nuclei and lack of papillae in HTT)
  - Gross: Well-circumscribed, solid (5–75 mm), firm with lobulated appearance
  - Microscopy:
    - Well-circumscribed or encapsulated, wide trabeculae delimited by stromal bundles.
    - Variably abundant eosinophilic hyaline amorphous basal membrane material within trabeculae (congo red–negative; periodic acid–Schiff (PAS) positive diastase resistant).
    - Nuclei are large, elongated, and convoluted with prominent grooves.
    - Frequent intratrabecular and stromal calcifications.
  - IHC:
    - Positive: TG, TTF-1, Galectin 3, MIB1 (membranous; characteristic), GLIS3
    - D/Ds: Follicular cell-derived neoplasms with trabecular growth (FA, papillary and poorly differentiated carcinomas), MTC, and paraganglioma.
  - Clinical implication: Clinically benign, rare lymph node or distant metastasis

- *Malignant neoplasms*:
  o *Follicular thyroid carcinoma*:
    - Gross: Majority capsulated (>20 mm). The capsule is thicker (compared to FA). Extrathyroidal extension is evident in widely invasive FTC.
    - Microscopy:
      - Follicular pattern
      - Capsular and/or vascular invasion is must for diagnosis.
      - Minimally invasive FC (MIFC): Capsular penetration with mushroom-shaped growth with 2–4 small to medium-sized vascular invasion (**Fig. 39A**).
      - Encapsulated angioinvasive FTC: Limited invasion of vessels (<4 foci) and invasion within tumor capsule or beyond (**Fig. 39B**).
      - Widely invasive FTC: Thick capsule, extensive invasion of thyroid and extrathyroidal soft tissues, extensive vascular invasion (four or more foci of invasion) (**Fig. 39C**).
      - Solid or trabecular growth: Exclude PDTC.
      - Mitotic count: <3/mm^2 (solid or trabecular growth) and <5/mm^2
    - Histological patterns: Clear cell (most frequent; >50% clear cells), signet-ring-cell, glomeruloid pattern, spindle cell.
    - IHC: It does not distinguish FTC from FA. Ki-67 proliferative index: <5%.
    - Clinical implication:
      - A total of 40-month disease-free survival of 97%, 81%, and 45% for minimally invasive, encapsulated angioinvasive, and widely invasive FTC, respectively.

  o *Invasive encapsulated follicular variant papillary carcinoma (IEFVPTC)*:
    - Gross: 20–30 mm, thick capsule
    - Microscopy:
      - Follicular pattern
      - Capsular and/or vascular invasion is must for diagnosis
      - PTC nuclear features are often variable and pronounced at periphery.
      - True papillae with PTC nuclear features (<1%).
    - IHC: Ki-67 index <5%.
    - D/Ds: NIFTP, follicular thyroid carcinoma.
    - Clinical implication: Similar to FTC

  o *Papillary thyroid carcinoma*:
    - Cytology: (**Figs. 40 to 44**)
      - Multiple papillae
      - Nuclear overcrowding with longitudinal nuclear groove and intranuclear pseudo-inclusions(>90%), prominent in Papanicolaou's (PAP) stain.

CHAPTER 8

Clinical and Pathological Aspect of Benign and Malignant Thyroid Nodules | 71

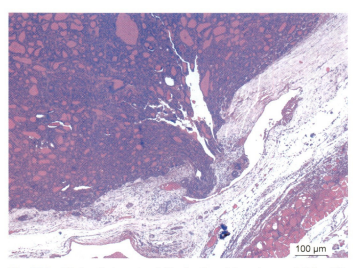

Fig. 39A: Minimally invasive follicular thyroid carcinoma (H&E, ×40).

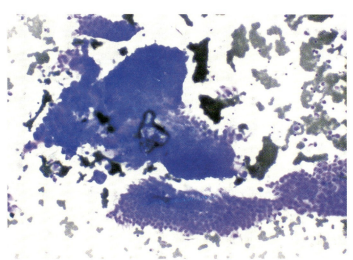

Fig. 40A: Papillary carcinoma of thyroid—multiple papillae and calcified material (MGG, ×200).

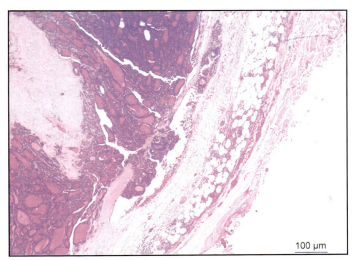

Fig. 39B: Encapsulated angioinvasive follicular thyroid carcinoma (H&E, ×40).

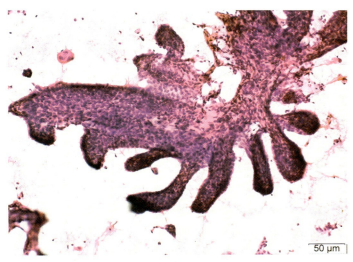

Fig. 40B: Papillary carcinoma of thyroid—multiple papillae with fibrovascular core (H&E, ×200).

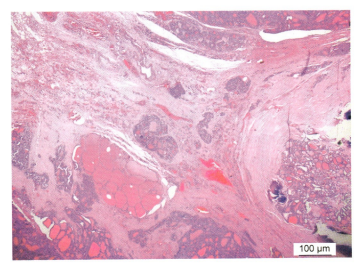

Fig. 39C: Widely invasive follicular thyroid carcinoma (H&E, ×40).

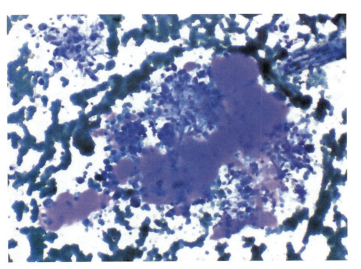

Fig. 41: Papillary carcinoma of thyroid—thyroid follicular cells along with inspissated colloid (MGG, ×200).

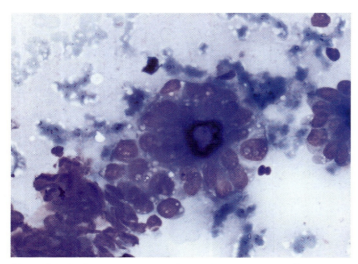

Fig. 42A: Papillary carcinoma of thyroid—psammoma body with concentric layers of calcification (MGG, ×400).

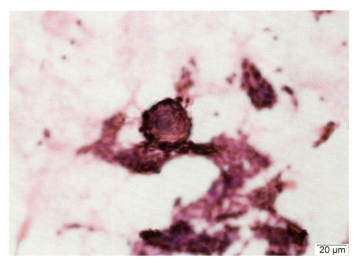

Fig. 42B: Papillary carcinoma of thyroid—psammoma body with concentric layers of calcification is better seen in hematoxylin and eosin stain (H&E, ×400).

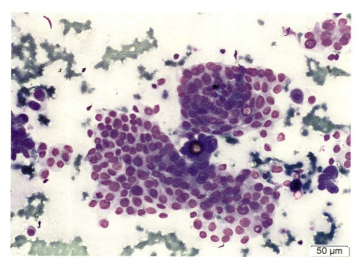

Fig. 43: Papillary carcinoma of thyroid—cells showing longitudinal nuclear grooves, intranuclear inclusions, and calcification (MGG, ×440).

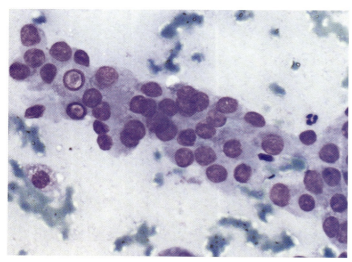

Fig. 44: Papillary carcinoma of thyroid—many intranuclear inclusions (MGG, ×400).

- Optically clear nucleus: Known as "Orphan Annie eye"
- Psammoma bodies: Characteristic of PTC seen in 10–35% cases.
- D/Ds: lymphocytic thyroiditis, hyalinizing trabecular adenoma
- Gross:
    - Average 20–30 mm, firm, and white with focal intratumoral calcification
    - Necrosis absent, if present suggests transformation to poorly differentiated or undifferentiated carcinoma.
- Microscopy:
    - Conventional PTC: Papillae with fibrovascular cores **(Fig. 45A)**.
    - Nuclei: Elongated or oval, overlapping and crowded. Nuclear pseudoinclusions, prominent intranuclear grooves, and optically clear nucleoplasm **(Fig. 45B)**.
    - Psammoma bodies and calcific concretions **(Fig. 45C)**.
    - Regional lymph node metastases ≥80% at initial presentation **(Fig. 45D)**.
    - PTC with poorly differentiated areas **(Fig. 45E)**.
- IHC:
    - Positive: TTF-1, PAX8, TG, and cytokeratins (pan-cytokeratin, AE1/AE3, CK7, and CAM5.2).
    - Negative: CK20, calcitonin and neuroendocrine markers.
    - HBME1, Galectin-3, CK19, and CD56: For differentiating PTC and benign lesions with papillary architecture and/or atypical nuclei.
    - BRAF p.V600E (VE1 clone): Highly sensitive and cytoplasmic and diffuse (≥90% staining in 40–60% cases).

CHAPTER 8

Clinical and Pathological Aspect of Benign and Malignant Thyroid Nodules 73

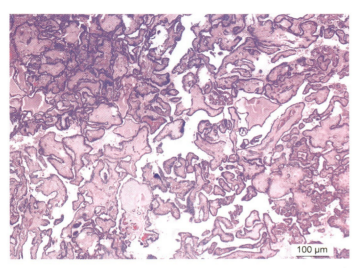

Fig. 45A: Papillary thyroid carcinoma (conventional)—tumor with papillary arrangement having fibrovascular core (H&E, ×100).

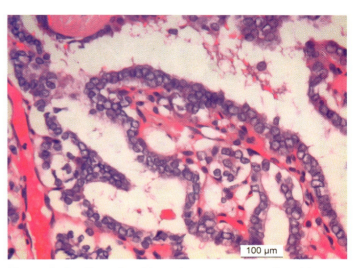

Fig. 45B: Papillary thyroid carcinoma—tumor cells with overcrowding and overlapping. Nuclei with chromatin clearing and nuclear grooving (H&E, ×400).

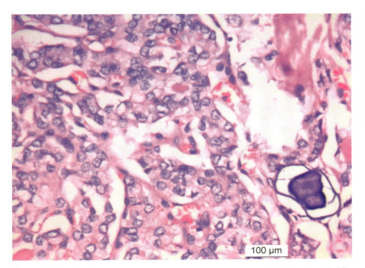

Fig. 45C: Papillary thyroid carcinoma—psammomatous calcification (H&E, ×400).

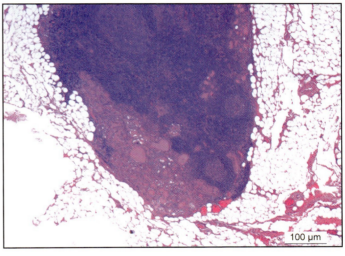

Fig. 45D: Papillary thyroid carcinoma—lymph node metastasis (H&E, ×100).

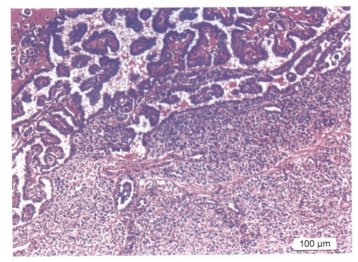

Fig. 45E: Papillary thyroid carcinoma—classic PTC with poorly differentiated component (solid, trabecular, and insular growth pattern; <30%) (H&E, ×100).

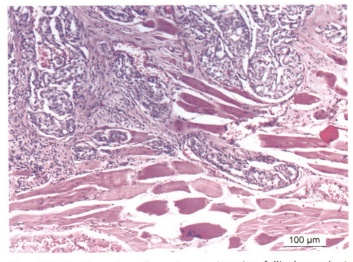

Fig. 45F: Papillary thyroid carcinoma, invasive follicular variant (H&E, ×100).

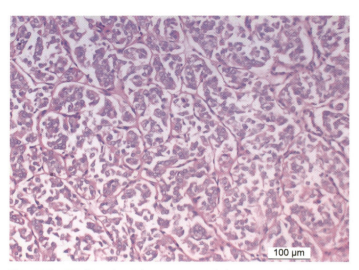

Fig. 45G: Papillary thyroid carcinoma, oncocytic variant (H&E, ×200). Fig. 45H: Papillary thyroid carcinoma, solid variant (H&E, ×200).

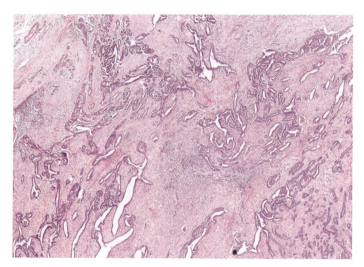

Fig. 45I: Papillary thyroid carcinoma with fibromatosis/fasciitis-like/desmoid-type-stroma-nonencapsulated, well circumscribed tumor with biphasic growth pattern. The epithelial component showing an arrangement of tubulo-papillary and leaf-like or animal-like patterns (H&E, ×40).

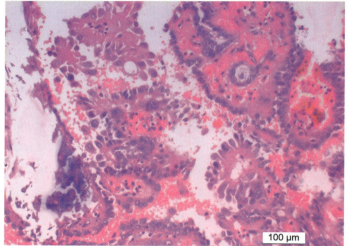

Fig. 45J: Papillary thyroid carcinoma, hobnail variant (H&E, ×400).

- Histologic subtypes:
    - Encapsulated
    - Infiltrative follicular variant (**Figs. 45F and 46**)
    - Oncocytic (**Figs. 45G, 47 and 48**)
    - Warthin-like
    - Clear cell subtype
    - Diffuse sclerosing
    - Solid/trabecular (**Fig. 45H**)
    - PTC with fibromatosis/fasciitis-like/desmoid-type stroma (**Fig. 45I**)
    - Spindle cell
    - Tall cell
    - Hobnail (**Fig. 45J**)
    - Columnar cell

– Clinical implication: Conventional PTC—long-term survival with subtotal or total thyroidectomy >90%. Tall cell, hobnail, and columnar subtypes—poor prognosis
○ *Oncocytic carcinoma of thyroid (OCA)*:
– Cytology:
  ■ Nuclear crowding with significant nuclear atypia
  ■ Irregular nuclear contour and prominent nucleoli
– D/Ds: Medullary thyroid carcinoma
– Gross: Solitary nodule (30–40 mm), encapsulated, thicker capsule (compared to OA), often partly calcified; solid and tan to mahogany color.
– Microscopy:
  ■ Thick capsule with capsular and/or vascular invasion classified as minimally invasive, encapsulated with vascular invasion and widely invasive (**Fig. 49**).

Clinical and Pathological Aspect of Benign and Malignant Thyroid Nodules

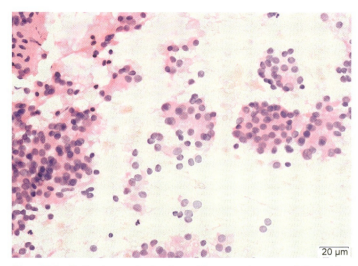

Fig. 46A: Follicular variant of papillary carcinoma of thyroid—multiple follicles and loose clusters of tumor cells (H&E, ×240).

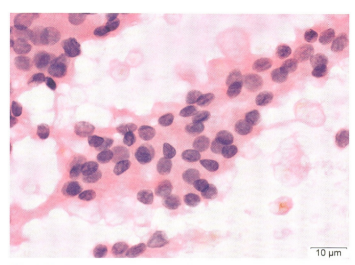

Fig. 46B: Follicular variant of papillary carcinoma of thyroid—cells showing longitudinal nuclear grooves (H&E, ×1,000).

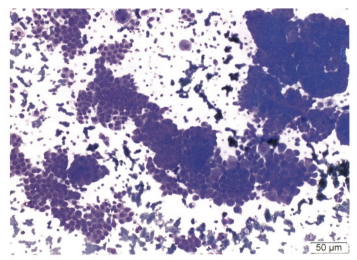

Fig. 47: Oncocytic variant of papillary carcinoma of thyroid—papillae, sheets, and discrete cells present (MGG, ×200).

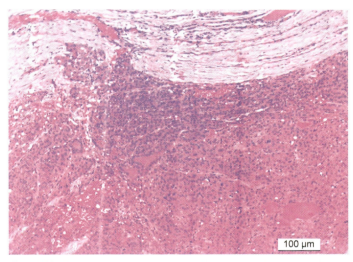

Fig. 49: Oncocytic carcinoma of thyroid—similar to follicular adenoma with oncocytic change with capsular invasion (H&E, ×40).

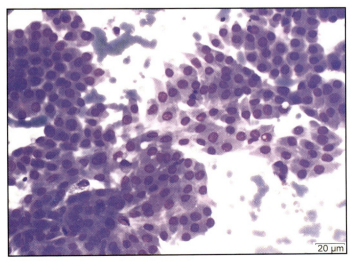

Fig. 48: Oncocytic variant of papillary carcinoma of thyroid—predominantly Hürthle cell with nuclear features of papillary carcinoma (MGG, ×400).

- Electron microscopy: Numerous mitochondria.
- IHC: Cannot distinguish OCA from oncocytic adenoma.
- Clinical implication: Survival near 100% in minimally invasive (capsular invasion only) to 10% for widely invasive.
  o *Follicular-derived carcinomas, high-grade*:
    - Cytology: **(Figs. 50 to 52)**
      ▪ Hypercellular smear with microfollicles and papillae with scanty to nil colloid
      ▪ Cells are round, mild nuclear pleomorphism with hyperchromatic nuclei.
      ▪ ICC: Positive for thyroglobulin, TTF-1, and PAX-8. Negative for calcitonin.
      ▪ D/Ds: PTC, follicular neoplasm
    - Gross: 40–60 mm, mostly invasive, solid, light brown to grey with necrosis.

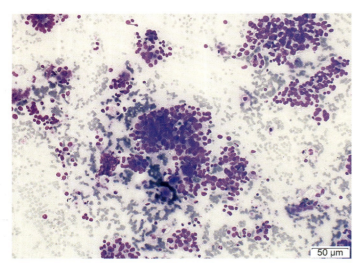

Fig. 50A: Poorly differentiated thyroid carcinoma—multiple clusters of cells (MGG, ×120).

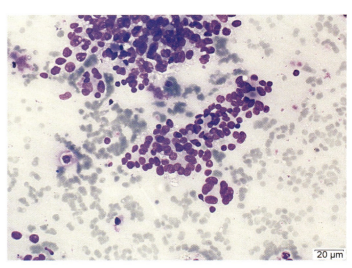

Fig. 50B: Poorly differentiated thyroid carcinoma—the cells with overlapping nuclei (MGG, ×200).

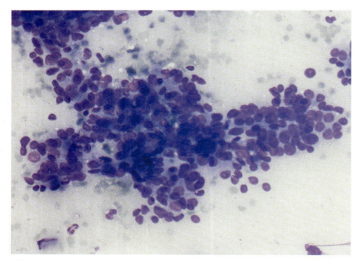

Fig. 51: Poorly differentiated thyroid carcinoma—occasional follicle like arrangement is seen (MGG, ×200).

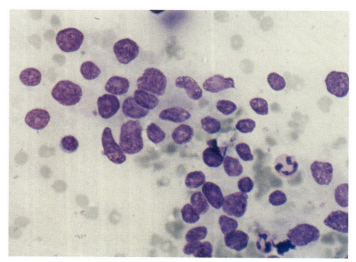

Fig. 52: Poorly differentiated thyroid carcinoma—higher magnification of the cells showing round mildly pleomorphic nuclei and scanty cytoplasm (MGG, ×400).

- Microscopy:
    - Poorly differentiated thyroid carcinoma
        - Solid/trabecular/insular pattern **(Fig. 53A)**.
        - Absence of PTC nuclear features **(Fig. 53B)**.
        - Mitotic count ≥ 3/mm^2, tumor necrosis required for diagnosis **(Fig. 53C)**.
        - Poorly differentiated though lack anaplastic cellular morphology
    - Differentiated high-grade thyroid carcinoma
        - Presence of ≥5 mitoses mm^2 and/or tumor necrosis, with invasion **(Figs. 53D and E)**.
- Clinical implication: Intermediate between well-differentiated carcinomas and anaplastic carcinoma

  o *Anaplastic follicular cell–derived thyroid carcinoma (ATC)*:
    - Cytology: **(Figs. 54 to 56)**
        - Background necrosis with polymorphs
        - Large cells with enlarged bizarre nuclei and large nucleoli.
        - Spindle cells, squamoid cells, and multinucleated giant cells may be seen.
        - ICC: Positive for Vimentin, CK, and EMA. Negative for TG and TTF 1.
        - D/Ds: Spindle cell variant of medullary carcinoma, sarcomas.
    - Gross: Up to 150 mm, bulky tumor, involve both lobes with extrathyroidal growth.
    - Microscopy:
        - Infiltrative tumor with frequent extrathyroidal growth, necrosis, prominent mitotic activity, atypical mitoses, significant nuclear pleomorphism, and angiolymphatic invasion **(Fig. 57)**.

Clinical and Pathological Aspect of Benign and Malignant Thyroid Nodules

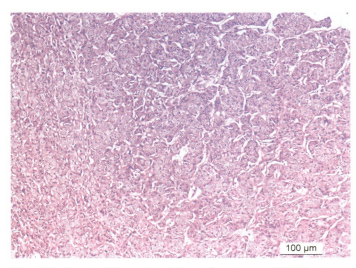

Fig. 53A: Poorly differentiated thyroid carcinoma (PDTC)—tumor with solid, trabecular and insular growth pattern (H&E, ×100).

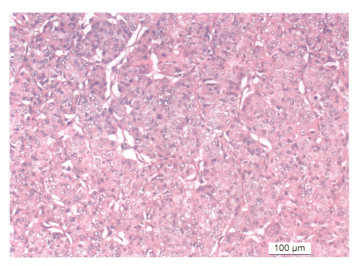

Fig. 53B: Poorly differentiated thyroid carcinoma (PDTC)—absence of PTC nuclear features (H&E, ×200).

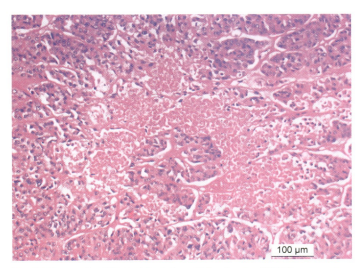

Fig. 53C: Poorly differentiated thyroid carcinoma (PDTC)—presence of microscopic foci of tumor necrosis (H&E, ×200).

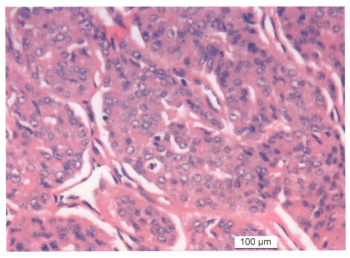

Fig. 53D: Differentiated high-grade thyroid carcinoma (DHGTC)—tumor showing brisk mitotic activity with follicular differentiation (H&E, ×400).

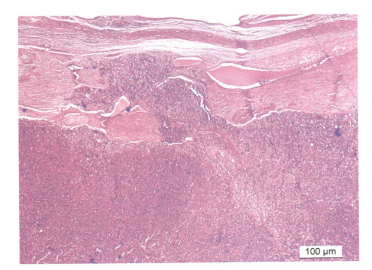

Fig. 53E: Differentiated high-grade thyroid carcinoma (DHGTC)—tumor showing capsular invasion (H&E, ×40).

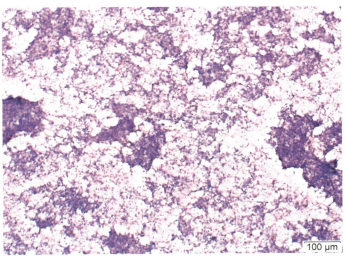

Fig. 54: Anaplastic carcinoma—abundant discrete cells in a background of necrosis (MGG, ×120).

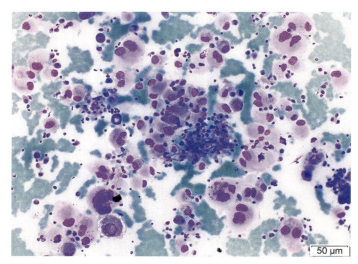

Fig. 55: Anaplastic carcinoma—large pleomorphic cells with severe nuclear pleomorphism (MGG, ×200).

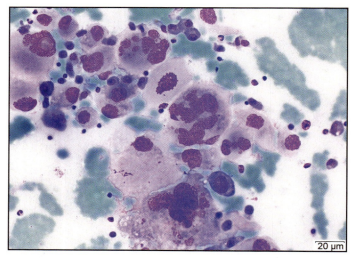

Fig. 56: Anaplastic carcinoma—many cells with bizarre nuclei (MGG, ×400).

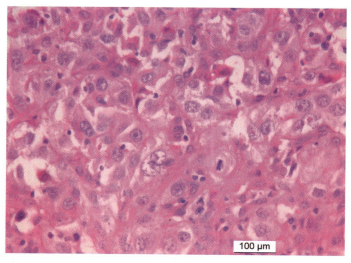

Fig. 57: Anaplastic follicular-cell derived thyroid carcinoma—tumor cells showing marked nuclear pleomorphism with prominent nucleoli and brisk mitotic activity. No nuclear features of PTC seen (H&E, ×400).

- IHC:
    - Positive: Cytokeratin, TTF1, TG, PAX8, p53, and high Ki-67.
    - ATC with squamous cell carcinoma: Positive for high molecular weight keratins, 34BE12 and keratin 5/6, p63, p40, and occasionally for TTF1.
    - ATC with pure squamous cell carcinoma: PAX8 and p53 positivity.
- D/Ds: Primary thyroid sarcoma (synovial sarcoma, malignant peripheral nerve sheath tumor, angiosarcoma, leiomyosarcoma, and rhabdomyosarcoma); melanoma; MTC; mucoepidermoid carcinoma; SMECE; Riedel thyroiditis; NUT carcinoma.
- Clinical implication: Highly aggressive, almost always lethal.

Thyroid C-cell–derived Carcinoma

- *Medullary thyroid carcinoma*:
    - *Cytology*: **(Figs. 58 to 61)**
        - Three types of cells: Round cells with eccentric nuclei (plasmacytoid cells), spindle cells with elongated nuclei, and polygonal cells
        - Cytoplasmic reddish granules with "salt and pepper" nuclear chromatin.
        - Almost 60–80% MTC shows amyloid material.
        - ICC: Positive for calcitonin, chromogranin, neuron-specific enolase (NSE), synaptophysin, and carcinoembryonic antigen (CEA). negative for thyroglobulin
    - *D/Ds*: Hürthle cell neoplasm, follicular neoplasm, papillary carcinoma rarely, thyroid spindle epithelial tumor with thymus-like differentiation (SETTLE)
    - *Gross*:
        - Unilateral (sporadic), bilateral, and multicentric (familial)
        - Medullary microcarcinoma: Size <10 mm.
    - *Microscopy*:
        - Solid, nested, insular, or trabecular growth patterns with fibrovascular stroma **(Fig. 62A)**.
        - Polygonal cells with granular amphophilic cytoplasm and fine nuclear chromatin **(Fig. 62B)**.
        - Plasmacytoid to spindle shaped, with frequent admixtures **(Fig. 62C)**.
        - Low-to-moderate nuclear atypia, focal bizarre nuclei, and multinucleation **(Fig. 62D)**.
        - Variable mitotic activity; focal tumor necrosis **(Fig. 62E)**.
        - Stromal amyloid deposition (50–90%) **(Fig. 62F)**.
    - *Histological patterns*: Papillary, pseudopapillary, follicular (tubular/glandular), spindle cell, plasmacytoid cells, clear cells, oncocytic cells, and melanotic

CHAPTER 8

Clinical and Pathological Aspect of Benign and Malignant Thyroid Nodules 79

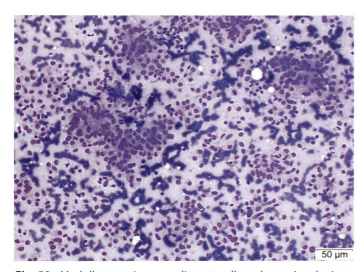

Fig. 58: Medullary carcinoma—discrete cells and occasional microfollicles (MGG, ×200).

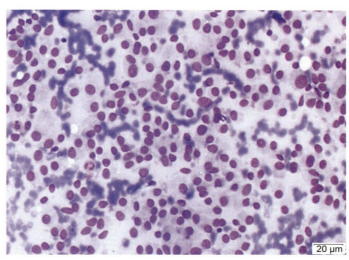

Fig. 59: Medullary carcinoma—abundant discrete tumor cells with round to oval nuclei (MGG, ×200).

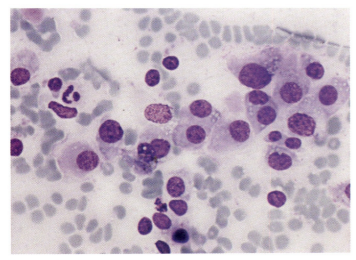

Fig. 60: Medullary carcinoma—the cells show moderate amount of cytoplasm and eccentric nuclei. Chromatin shows salt and pepper like appearance (MGG, ×400).

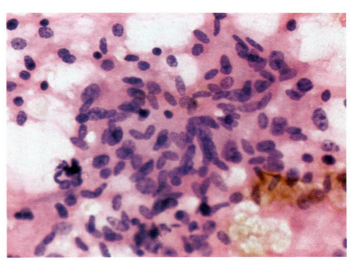

Fig. 61: Medullary carcinoma—many spindle cells may be noted (MGG, ×200).

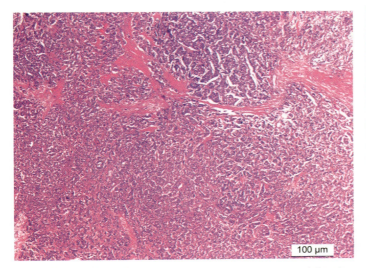

Fig. 62A: Medullary thyroid carcinoma—tumor showing solid, trabecular, nesting, insular, and microfollicular growth patterns (H&E, ×40).

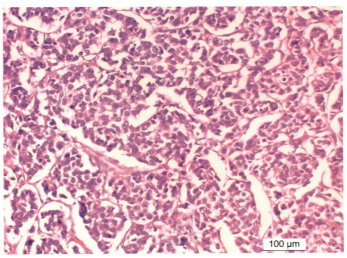

Fig. 62B: Medullary thyroid carcinoma—tumor cells displaying plasmacytoid cell morphology with eccentric round nuclei showing dispersed chromatin (H&E, ×400).

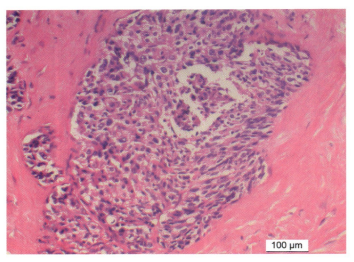

Fig. 62C: Medullary thyroid carcinoma—polygonal tumor cells with central round nuclei, fine chromatin and granular amphophilic cytoplasm. Spindle cell morphology also evident (H&E, ×200).

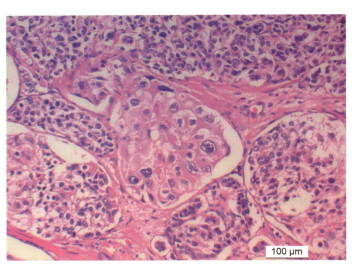

Fig. 62D: Medullary thyroid carcinoma—tumor showing low to moderate nuclear atypia with bizarre nuclei (H&E, ×200).

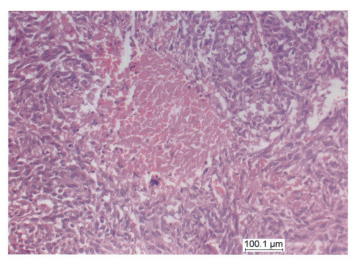

Fig. 62E: Medullary thyroid carcinoma—tumor necrosis (H&E, ×200).

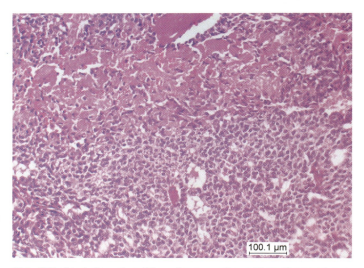

Fig. 62F: Medullary thyroid carcinoma—deposition of amorphous, eosinophilic, and fibrillary material (H&E, ×200).

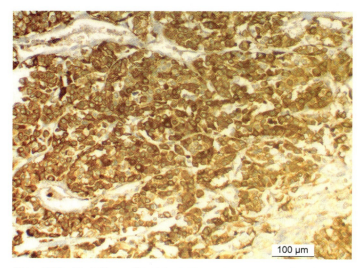

Fig. 62G: Medullary thyroid carcinoma—tumor cells showing diffuse cytoplasmic positivity for calcitonin (Peroxidase, ×200).

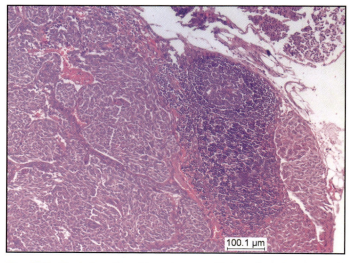

Fig. 62H: Medullary thyroid carcinoma with lymph node metastasis (H&E, ×100).

- IHC:
    - Positive: Calcitonin (95%) **(Fig. 62G)**, neuroendocrine markers, calcitonin gene-related peptide (CGRP), CEA, TTF-1, polyclonal PAX8 (variable and weak), SSTR-2a, and SSTR-5.
    - Negative: TG, monoclonal PAX8.
- *Clinical implication*: Lymph node involvement (75%) **(Fig. 62H)**, distant metastasis (10%), total thyroidectomy required.

Mixed Medullary and Follicular Cell-derived Carcinomas

Mixed medullary with follicular carcinoma OR with papillary carcinoma **(Figs. 63A to C)**, oncocytic carcinoma, poorly differentiated carcinoma OR anaplastic carcinoma

Thyroid Tumors of Uncertain Histogenesis

- Sclerosing mucoepidermoid carcinoma with eosinophilia
- Cribriform-morular thyroid carcinoma (CMTC)

Thymic Tumors within the Thyroid

- *Thymoma family (ectopic thymoma)*: An organotypic thymic epithelial tumor occurring within or attached to thyroid gland.
- *Spindle epithelial tumor with thymus-like elements*: **(Figs. 64A and B)**
- Thymic carcinoma family

Embryonal Thyroid Neoplasms

Thyroblastoma: An embryonal high-grade neoplasm composed of primitive thyroid-like follicular cells surrounded by a primitive small cell component and mesenchymal stroma.

Ancillary Tests in Thyroid

- Immunocytochemistry
- *Flow cytometry*: Useful in differentiating non-Hodgkin's lymphomas.
- Molecular tests for genetic abnormalities

Immunohistochemistry (Table 2)

Molecular markers: The clinicians need to be aware of the molecular markers for targeted therapy and need to ask the pathologists to provide this relevant information for prognostication of the various thyroid tumors.

Papillary thyroid carcinoma:
- *RET/PTC translocation* in 20% cases
- *BRAF mutation*: 50% cases
- *RAS mutation*: 15% cases

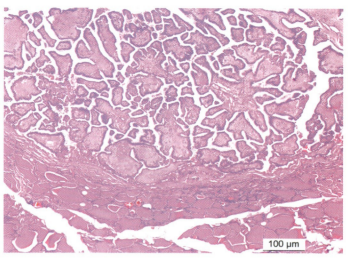

Fig. 63A: Mixed medullary-papillary carcinoma—presence of separate distinct foci of classic PTC (H&E, ×100).

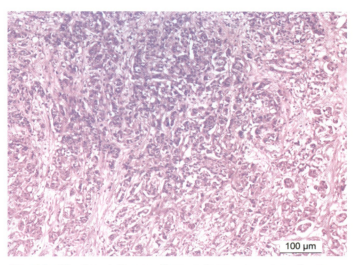

Fig. 63B: Mixed medullary-papillary carcinoma—presence of separate distinct component of medullary thyroid carcinoma (H&E, ×100).

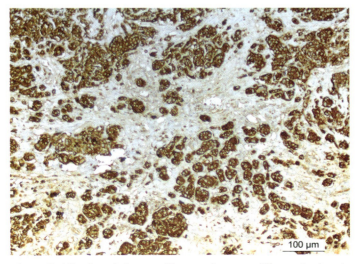

Fig. 63C: Mixed medullary-papillary carcinoma—diffuse cytoplasmic positivity on Calcitonin in medullary thyroid carcinoma (Peroxidase, ×100).

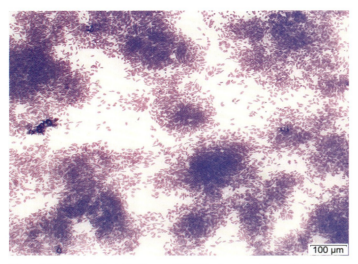

Fig. 64A: Thyroid spindle epithelial tumor with thymus-like differentiation—abundant cells in clusters and discrete (MGG, ×200).

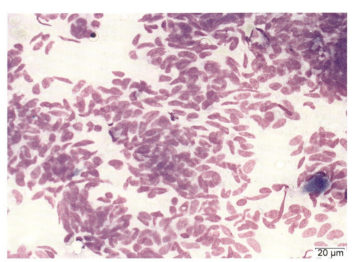

Fig. 64B: Thyroid spindle epithelial tumor with thymus-like differentiation—the cells have scanty cytoplasm with elongated spindle cells (MGG, ×400).

TABLE 2: The expression of different markers in the thyroid tumors.

Tumors	HBME-1	Galectin-3	Ck19	TG	TTF-1	Calcitonin
PTC	+	+	+	+	+	–
FC	+/–	+/–	+/–	+	+	–
FA	–	–	–	+	+	–
MC	+	–	–	–	–	+
PDTC	+/–	–	+/–	–/+	–/+	–
AC	–	+	+/–	–	–	–

[AC: anaplastic carcinoma; FA: follicular adenoma; FC: follicular carcinoma; MC: medullary carcinoma; PDTC: poorly differentiated thyroid carcinoma; PTC: papillary thyroid carcinoma; TG: thyroglobulin; (+): positive; (-): negative].

Follicular carcinoma:
- *RAS mutation*: 35% cases
- FC does not show any *BRAF* mutation.

MANAGEMENT

On the basis of clinical, biochemical, and FNAC diagnosis, thyroid lesions are managed accordingly **(Flowchart 1)**. Management of most commonly encountered thyroid lesion will be discussed one by one.

MANAGEMENT OF GRAVES' DISEASE

Graves' disease is a pathological sequela of TSH-R antibody. Most of the time these antibodies are stimulating antibodies, thus primary hyperthyroidism is the most common manifestation. Rarely this antibody may act like an inhibitory antibody and it may produce hypothyroidism. On rarest occassion periodic activating and inactivating antibody may appear in the serum and consequently periodic hyper and hypothyroidism could be encountered.

Graves' disease often associated with other manifestations, such as orbitopathy, dermopathy, and acropachy. The management of Graves' disease consists of three main modalities of treatment
- Anti-thyroid drugs (propaylthiouracil/carbimazole/methimazole)
- Radioactive Iodine usual dose 5–15 mCi.
- Surgery

ANTITHYROID DRUGS

Most commonly used drug is carbimazole, which is a prodrug that is converted to methimazole is the body. Propylthiouracil is recommended to use in first trimester of pregnancy and in thyrotoxic crisis. Antithyroid drug should be continued for atleast 1–2 years for optimum outcome. Dose titration is based on thyroid hormone level. A commonly employed strategy is shown in the **Table 3**.

For radioactive iodine therapy ideally thyroid gland weight and volume should be measured. Since it is cumbersome and practically not feasible, dose of millicurie (mCi) for per gram of thyroid tissue determined empirically. Higher doses required in case of toxic multinodular goiter, low 24 hours radio-iodine uptake, large goiter, and those with severe thyrotoxicosis.

Surgery is recommended for large goiter with compressive symptoms, intolerance to antithyroid drugs, and contraindication to radioactive iodine.

Each modality has got its own advantages and disadvantages. Radioactive iodine may exacerbate Graves' orbitopathy and it is teratogenic. Surgery can be disfiguring and can render patient hypoparathyroid and there may be injury to recurrent laryngeal nerve. Antithyroid drugs are not out of complications. Common side effects are hepatitis, skin rash, gastrointestinal intolerance, granulocytopenia. Rarely agranulocytosis and vasculitis may be encountered.

Outcome of treatment of Graves' disease with antithyroid drugs can be predicted by a scoring system, known as the 'GREAT' scoring system or a more precise from of that 'GREAT PLUS' scoring system **(Table 4)**.

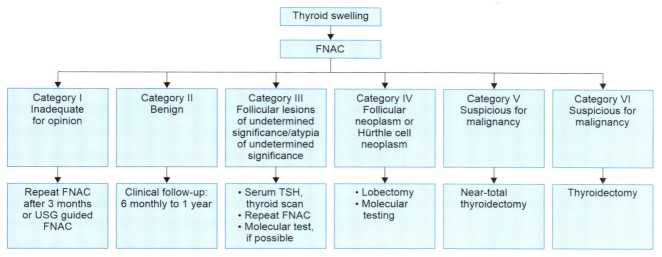

Flowchart 1: Showing approach to thyroid swelling as per Bethesda category following FNAC.
(FNAC: fine needle aspiration cytology; TSH: thyroid stimulating hormone; USG: ultrasonography)

TABLE 3: Dosing of antithyroid drug (methimazole) based on free thyroxine elevation above the upper limit of normal.	
Free T4 (fold above the ULN)	**Methimazole dose (mg/day)**
1–1.5 times	5–10
1.5–2 times	10–20
2–3 times	30–40

TABLE 4: Predictive scores for the risk of recurrent Graves' hyperthyroidism after 1-year treatment with antithyroid drugs.				
			GREAT score	
Items (assessed before starting therapy)		**GREAT score range 0–6**	**Risk class**	**Recurrences**
Age (year)	≥40	0	Class I (score 0–1)	16%
	<40	+1	Class II (score 2–3)	44%
FT4 (pmol/L)	<40	0	Class III (score 4–6)	68%
	≥40	+1		
TBII (U/L)	<6	0		
	6–19.9	+1		
	≥20	+2		
Goiter size[a]	Grade 0–1	0		
	Grade II–III	+2		

Continued

Continued

Items added		GREAT+ score range 0–10	GREAT+ score	
			Risk class	Recurrences
PTPN22 C/C Wild type		0	Class I + (score 0–2)	4%
C/T		+1	Class II + (score 3–4)	21%
HLA number[b] 0		0		
1–2		+2	Class III + (score 5–6)	49%
3 (LD)		+3	Class IV+ (score 7–10)	84%

[a] Goiter size: grade 0, thyroid not or distinctly palpable but usually not visible; grade I, thyroid easily palpable and visible with head in normal or raised position; grade II, thyroid easily visible with the head in a normal position; grade III, goiter visible at a distance.
[b] Number of HLA subtypes (DQB1-02, DQA1-05, DRB1-03) present.

(FT4: free thyroxine; GREAT: Graves' Recurrent Events After Therapy; HLA: human leukocyte antigen; LD: linkage disequilibrium; TBII: thyroid-stimulating hormone-binding inhibitory immunoglobulins)

Source: Tallini G, Mete O, Baloch ZW, et al., editors. Chapter 3: Thyroid gland. In: WHO Classification of Tumours Editorial Board. Endocrine and Neuroendocrine tumours. (WHO classification of tumours series) 5th edition; vol. 8. Lyon (France): International Agency for Research on Cancer; 2022.

MANAGEMENT OF MULTINODULAR GOITER

Multinodular goiter patients are often older and they often have multiple comorbidities. They require higher doses of radioactive iodine usually 8–15 mCi. Initial therapy always consists of antithyroid drugs. Surgery is often required for large Multinodular goiter with retrosternal extension and in presence of compressive symptoms.

MANAGEMENT OF THYROID NODULE

It depends on clinical, imaging, and cytological characterization of the lesion. The cases of unequivocal malignancy are managed by total thyroidectomy. The Bethesda category III, i.e., follicular lesions of undetermined significance/atypia of undetermined significance, subjected to repeat FNAC with ancillary tests to achieve specific diagnosis. Benign lesion is usually kept under follow-up with reassurance.

MANAGEMENT OF DIFFERENTIATED THYROID CARCINOMA OF EPITHELIAL ORIGIN

Surgery is the mainstay of therapy. Usually, total thyroidectomy is considered unless very early stage of carcinoma like papillary micro-carcinoma is detected. Neck dissection depends on regional lymph node involvement. Postoperatively suppressive dose of levothyroxine is used to suppress TSH and subsequent tumor recurrence. Radioactive iodine ablation of remnants is one of the strategies employed in differentiated thyroid carcinoma. Other modalities such as external beam radiotherapy for metastatic disease and tyrosine kinase inhibitor often use in difficult to treat cases **(Table 5)**.

Medical therapy consists of levothyroxine therapy to suppress TSH and biologically targeted therapy.

Initial TSH goals depend on comorbidity and risk-stratification. High risk patients should have TSH <0.1 mU/L, intermediate risk patients should have TSH 0.1–0.5 mU/L, and low risk patient should have TSH 0.5–2 mU/L.

Drugs such as lenvatinib, sorafinib, vandetanib, and cabozantinib can be used. Dedifferentiated tumor can be tried with selumetinib and selpercatinib, debrafinib for redifferentiation and subsequent RAI responsive.

MANAGEMENT OF MEDULLARY CARCINOMA OF THYROID

Surgery is the mainstay of therapy. Alternative add on therapies are TKIs, external beam radiotherapy, protein receptor radiotherapy, and chemotherapy. Among the TKIs, sorafinib, lenvatinib, cabozantinib and mTor inhibitor everolimus can be used as an alternative.

CONCLUSION

In this chapter, we are tried to focus on the commonly encountered pathology of thyroid nodules. Initially we discussed diagnostic approach and then management of specific etiology. Ultrasonography and TI-RADS grading considered as the cornerstone of thyroid swelling diagnosis. FNAC is the key strategy to categorized the lesion as per FNAC grading. Management depends on the specific etiology. For benign disease we prefer drug therapy, for malignant lesion, thyroidectomy is the first option as per as feasible.

TABLE 5: Dynamic risk stratification definitions for differentiated thyroid cancer.

	Total thyroidectomy and RAI ablation	Total thyroidectomy without RAI ablation	Lobectomy
Excellent	Nonstimulated Tg <0.2 ng/mL OR Stimulated Tg<1 ng/mL AND Undetectable TgAb AND Negative imaging	Nonstimulated Tg <0.2 ng/mL OR Stimulated Tg <2 ng/mL AND Undetectable TgAb AND Negative imaging	Stable, nondetectable Tg level <30 ng/mL AND Undetectable TgAb AND Negative imaging
Intermediate	Nonstimulated Tg 0.2–1 ng/mL OR Stimulated Tg 1–10 ng/mL AND TgAb levels stable or declining in absence of structural and functional disease AND Nonspecific findings on imaging study OR faint uptake in thyroid bed on RAI scanning	Nonstimulated Tg 0.2–5 ng/mL OR Stimulated Tg 2–10 ng/mL AND TgAb levels stable or declining in absence of structural and functional disease AND Nonspecific findings on imaging study OR faint uptake in thyroid bed on RAI scanning	Nonspecific findings on imaging study OR TgAb levels stable or declining in the absence of structural and functional disease
Biochemical incomplete	Nonstimulated Tg >1 ng/mL OR Stimulated Tg >10 ng/mL AND Increased TgAb AND Negative imaging	Nonstimulated Tg >5 ng/mL OR Stimulated Tg >10 ng/mL AND Increased TgAb AND Negative imaging	Nonstimulated Tg >5 ng/mL OR Stimulated Tg >10 ng/mL AND Increased TgAb AND Negative imaging
Structural incomplete	Structural and functional evidence of disease regardless Tg and TgAb level	Structural and functional evidence of disease regardless Tg and TgAb level	Structural and functional evidence of disease regardless Tg and TgAb level

SUGGESTED READINGS

1. Alexander EK, Cibas ES. Diagnosis of thyroid nodules. Lancet Diabetes Endocrinol. 2022;10:533-9.
2. Angell TE, Maurer R, Wang Z, Kim MI, Alexander CA, Barletta JA, et al. A Cohort analysis of clinical and ultrasound variables predicting cancer risk in 20,001 consecutive thyroid nodules. J Clin Endocrinol Metab. 2019;104:5665-72.
3. Barroeta JE, Wang H, Shiina N, Gupta PK, LiVolsi VA, Baloch ZW. Is Fine-Needle Aspiration (FNA) of multiple thyroid nodules justified? Endocr Pathol. 2006;17:61-6.
4. Wang CCC, Friedman L, Kennedy GC, Wang H, Kebebew E, Steward DL, et al. A large multicenter correlation study of thyroid nodule cytopathology and histopathology. Thyroid. 2011;21:243-51.
5. Tessler FN, Middleton WD, Grant EG, Hoang JK, Berland LL, Teefey SA, et al. ACR thyroid imaging, reporting and data system (TI-RADS): white paper of the ACR TI-RADS Committee. J Am Coll Radiol. 2017;14:587-95.
6. Middleton WD, Teefey SA, Reading CC, Langer JE, Beland MD, Szabunio MM, et al. Multiinstitutional analysis of thyroid nodule risk stratification using the American college of radiology thyroid imaging reporting and data system. Am J Roentgenol. 2017;208:1331-41.
7. Tallini G, Giordano TJ. Chapter 8: Rosai and Ackerman's Surgical Pathology, 11th edition. Philadelphia, PA: Elsevier; 2018. pp. 278-354.
8. Cibas ES, Ali SZ; NCI Thyroid FNA State of the Science Conference. The Bethesda System For Reporting Thyroid Cytopathology. Am J Clin Pathol. 2009;132(5):658-65.
9. Cibas ES, Ali SZ. The 2017 Bethesda System for Reporting Thyroid Cytopathology. Thyroid. 2017;27(11):1341-6.
10. Dey P. Chapter 7: Thyroid in Fine needle aspiration cytology: Interpretation and diagnostic difficulties. New Delhi: Jaypee Brothers Medical Publishers; 2015. pp. 109-55.
11. Tallini G, Mete O, Baloch ZW, et al., editors. Chapter 3: Thyroid gland. In: WHO Classification of Tumours Editorial Board. Endocrine and Neuroendocrine tumours. (WHO classification of tumours series) 5th edition; vol. 8. Lyon (France): International Agency for Research on Cancer; 2022.
12. Baloch ZW, Asa SL, Barletta JA, Ghossein RA, Juhlin CC, Jung CK, et al. Overview of the 2022 WHO Classification of Thyroid Neoplasms. Endocr Pathol. 2022;33(1):27-63.
13. Sobrinho-Simões M, Eloy C, Magalhães J, Lobo C, Amaro T. Follicular thyroid carcinoma. Mod Pathol. 2011;24 (Suppl 2):S10-8.
14. Mai KT, Landry DC, Thomas J, Burns BF, Commons AS, Yazdi HM, et al. Follicular adenoma with papillary architecture: a lesion mimicking papillary thyroid carcinoma. Histopathology. 2001;39(1):25-32.
15. McFadden DG, Sadow PM. Genetics, Diagnosis, and Management of Hürthle Cell Thyroid Neoplasms. Front Endocrinol (Lausanne). 2021;12:696386.

16. Seethala RR, Baloch ZW, Barletta JA, Khanafshar E, Mete O, Sadow PM, et al. Noninvasive follicular thyroid neoplasm with papillary-like nuclear features: a review for pathologists. Mod Pathol. 2018;31(1):39-55.
17. Hofman V, Lassalle S, Bonnetaud C, Butori C, Loubatier C, Ilie M, et al. Thyroid tumours of uncertain malignant potential: frequency and diagnostic reproducibility. Virchows Arch. 2009;455(1):21-33.
18. Podany P, Gilani SM. Hyalinizing trabecular tumor: Cytologic, histologic and molecular features and diagnostic considerations. Ann Diagn Pathol. 2021;54:151803.
19. Bishop JA, Ali SZ. Hyalinizing trabecular adenoma of the thyroid gland. Diagn Cytopathol. 2011;39(4):306-10.
20. O'Neill CJ, Vaughan L, Learoyd DL, Sidhu SB, Delbridge LW, Sywak MS. Management of follicular thyroid carcinoma should be individualised based on degree of capsular and vascular invasion. Eur J Surg Oncol. 2011;37(2):181-5.
21. Barletta J, Fadda G, Kakudo K. Invasive encapsulated follicular variant papillary carcinoma. In: WHO Classification of Tumours Editorial Board. Endocrine and Neuroendocrine tumours [Internet]. (WHO classification of tumours series) 5th edition; vol. 8. Lyon (France): International Agency for Research on Cancer; 2022.
22. Volante M, Collini P, Nikiforov YE, Sakamoto A, Kakudo K, Katoh R, et al. Poorly differentiated thyroid carcinoma: the Turin proposal for the use of uniform diagnostic criteria and an algorithmic diagnostic approach. Am J Surg Pathol. 2007;31(8):1256-64.
23. Hiltzik D, Carlson DL, Tuttle RM, Chuai S, Ishill N, Shaha A, et al. Poorly differentiated thyroid carcinomas defined on the basis of mitosis and necrosis: a clinicopathologic study of 58 patients. Cancer. 2006;106(6):1286-95.
24. Rindi G, Mete O, Uccella S, Basturk O, La Rosa S, Brosens LAA, et al. Overview of the 2022 WHO Classification of Neuroendocrine Neoplasms. Endocr Pathol. 2022;33(1):115-54.
25. Farhat NA, Faquin WC, Sadow PM. Primary mucoepidermoid carcinoma of the thyroid gland: a report of three cases and review of the literature. Endocr Pathol. 2013;24(4):229-33.
26. Dettloff J, Seethala RR, Stevens TM, Brandwein-Gensler M, Centeno BA, Otto K, et al. Mammary Analog Secretory Carcinoma (MASC) involving the thyroid gland: a report of the first 3 cases. Head Neck Pathol. 2017;11(2):124-30.
27. Hirokawa M, Takada N, Abe H, Suzuki A, Higuchi M, Miya A, et al. Thyroid sclerosing mucoepidermoid carcinoma with eosinophilia distinct from the salivary type. Endocr J. 2018;65(4):427-36.
28. Boyraz B, Sadow PM, Asa SL, Dias-Santagata D, Nosé V, Mete O. et al. Cribriform-morular thyroid carcinoma is a distinct thyroid malignancy of uncertain cytogenesis. Endocr Pathol. 2021;32(3):327-35.
29. Iwasa K, Imai MA, Noguchi M, Tanaka S, Sasaki T, Katsuda S, et al. Spindle epithelial tumor with thymus-like differentiation (SETTLE) of the thyroid. Head Neck. 2002;24(9):888-93.
30. Agaimy A, Witkowski L, Stoehr R, Castillo Cuenca JC, González-Muller CA, Brütting A, et al. Malignant teratoid tumor of the thyroid gland: an aggressive primitive multiphenotypic malignancy showing organotypical elements and frequent DICER1 alterations-is the term "thyroblastoma" more appropriate?. Virchows Arch. 2020;477(6):787-98.
31. Dey P. Chapter 9: Applications of immunocytochemistry in head, neck, salivary gland and thyroid lesions in Immunocytochemistry in diagnostic cytology. New Delhi: Jaypee Brothers Medical Publishers (P) Ltd.; 2021.
32. Braverman LE. Werner and Ingbar's The Thyroid: A Fundamental and Clinical Text, 11th edition. Philadelphia: Wolters Kluwer; 2020.
33. Vos XG, Endert E, Zwinderman AH, Tijssen JG, Wiersinga WM. Predicting the risk of recurrence before the start of antithyroid drug therapy in patients with Graves' hyperthyroidism. J Clin Endocrinol Metab. 2016;101(4):1381-9.
34. Haugen BR, Alexander EK, Bible KC, Doherty GM, Mandel SJ, Nikiforov YE, et al. 2015 American Thyroid Association Management Guidelines for Adult Patients with Thyroid Nodules and Differentiated Thyroid Cancer: The American Thyroid Association Guidelines Task Force on Thyroid Nodules and Differentiated Thyroid Cancer. Thyroid. 2016;26(1):1-133.
35. Anderson RT, Linnehan JE, Tongbram V, Keating K, Wirth LJ. Clinical, safety, and economic evidence in radioactive iodine-refractory differentiated thyroid cancer: a systematic literature review. Thyroid. 2013;23(4):392-407.

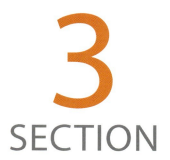

SECTION 3

Hypothyroidism

CHAPTER 9

Hypothyroidism in Adults

Sarita Bajaj

INTRODUCTION

Hypothyroidism is a common endocrine disorder where the thyroid gland does not produce and release thyroid hormone in sufficient quantities leading to thyroid hormone deficiency.

Primary hypothyroidism indicates decreased secretion of thyroid hormone by factors affecting the thyroid gland. A decreased secretion in thyroid hormone may also be due to insufficient stimulation of the thyroid gland by thyroid-stimulating hormone (TSH), because of factors directly interfering with pituitary TSH release (secondary hypothyroidism) or indirectly by decreasing release of hypothalamic thyrotropin-releasing hormone (TRH, tertiary hypothyroidism). Rarely features of thyroid hormone deficiency are caused by the inability of tissues to respond to thyroid hormone by mutations in the nuclear thyroid receptor (thyroid hormone resistance).

Thyroid disorders are among the most common endocrine disorders worldwide and India is no exception to this fact. Prevalence of thyroid disorders in India is about 42 million. Hypothyroidism, specifically, is the most common of thyroid disorders, affecting one in 10 adults. The prevalence of hypothyroidism in India is 11%, compared with only 2% in the UK and 4.6% in the USA. Compared with coastal cities (e.g., Mumbai, Goa, and Chennai), cities located inland (e.g., Kolkata, Delhi, Ahmedabad, Bangalore, and Hyderabad) have a higher prevalence (11.7% vs. 9.5%). Hypothyroidism is easily diagnosed and has a good prognosis but might be potentially fatal in severe cases, if inadequately treated. Some hindrances in the diagnosis and treatment are the facts that there is a large variation in the spectrum of clinical presentation, absence of symptom specificity, and diagnosis is predominantly biochemical.

PATHOPHYSIOLOGY

Tetraiodothyronine or thyroxine (T4) and triiodothyronine (T3) is produced by the thyroid gland utilizing iodide obtained from dietary sources, by metabolism of thyroid hormones and from different iodinated compounds. About, 100 µg of iodide is needed daily to produce sufficient amount of thyroid hormone. The thyroid gland has specialized thyroid epithelial cells which have a Na^+/I^- symporter (NIS) which helps to concentrate iodide 30–40 times the level in plasma to provide sufficient amounts for the production of thyroid hormone. Iodide trapped is subsequently oxidized by thyroid peroxidase (TPO) to iodine. A series of organic reactions ensue within the thyroid gland to produce T4 and T3. T3 is also produced in pituitary, liver, and kidney by the removal of an iodine molecule from T4. T4 is like a prohormone and T3 is the most potent thyroid hormone produced. Thyroglobulin protein of the thyroid stores T4 and T3 while the action of pituitary derived thyrotropin (TSH) releases them into circulation. A normal individual produces approximately 90–100 µg of T4 and 30–35 µg of T3 on a daily basis. About 80% of T3 produced every day in humans is obtained from peripheral metabolism (5′-monodeiodination) of T4, and only about 20% is secreted directly from the thyroid gland. On a weight basis, T3 is about 3–5 times more potent as a thyroid hormone than T4 and is believed to be the biologically active form of the hormone. The circulation of T4 and T3 occurs predominantly in the bound form, both T3 and T4 are bound to carrier proteins. T4 binds with strong affinity to thyroxine-binding globulin (TBG, ~75%) and weakly to thyroxine-binding prealbumin (TBPA, transthyretin, ~20%) and albumin (~5%). T3 binds strongly to TBG and weakly to albumin, with almost negligible binding to TBPA. Approximately, 8 µg/dL is the geometric average for serum T4 in normal individuals, mean for T3 level is approximately 130 ng/dL. In normal conditions, all but 0.03% of serum T4 is protein bound whereas 0.3% of serum T3 is protein bound. A miniscule quantity of unbound (or free) T4 (~2 ng/dL) and T3 (~0.3 ng/dL) circulates in a free state, and it is this that is regarded as responsible for the biological effects of the thyroid hormones **(Flowchart 1)**.

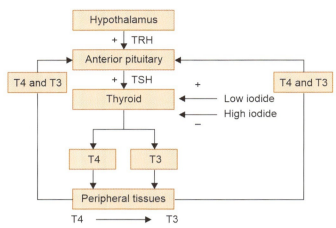

Flowchart 1: Pathway for secretion of thyroid hormones (the hypothalamic–pituitary–thyroid axis governs thyroid hormone secretion. Levels of circulating thyroid hormones are regulated by a complex feedback system involving the hypothalamus and pituitary gland).
(TRH: thyrotropin-releasing hormone; TSH: thyroid-stimulating hormone)

CAUSES

■ Primary Hypothyroidism

- *Congenital*:
  - Thyroid dysgenesis: Ectopy, agenesis, hypoplasia
  - Iodide transport or utilization defect (NIS or pendrin mutations)
  - Iodotyrosine dehalogenase deficiency
  - TSH receptor defects
  - Idiopathic TSH unresponsiveness
  - Organification disorders (TPO dysfunction or deficiency)
- *Acquired hypothyroidism*:
  - Iodine deficiency (endemic goiter)
  - Chronic autoimmune thyroiditis (goitrous or atrophic)
  - Iatrogenic (radioiodine treatment, total or subtotal thyroidectomy, external beam radiation)
  - Thyroid infiltration (hemochromatosis, amyloidosis, sarcoidosis, scleroderma, cystinosis, Riedel's thyroiditis)
  - Drugs: Antithyroid drugs, lithium, iodine, iodinated contrast media, amiodarone, sulfonamide, ethionamide, interferon-α, aminoglutethimide, tyrosine kinase inhibitor sunitinib
  - Hashimoto's thyroiditis
  - Drugs blocking synthesis or release of T4 (e.g., lithium, ethionamide, sulfonamides, iodide)
  - Goitrogens in foodstuffs or as endemic substances of pollutants
  - Cytokines (interferon-γ, interleukin-2)
  - Thyroid infiltration (amyloidosis, hemochromatosis, sarcoidosis, Riedel's struma, cystinosis, scleroderma)
  - Postablative thyroiditis due to ^{131}I surgery or therapeutic irradiation for nonthyroidal malignancy

■ Transient Hypothyroidism
- Following silent, subacute, or postpartum thyroiditis
- After withdrawal of thyroxine in euthyroid patients

■ Consumptive Hypothyroidism
Rapid destruction of thyroid hormone is due to overexpression of type 3 deiodinase by large hemangioma or hemangioendothelioma.

■ Central Hypothyroidism
Central hypothyroidism (secondary or tertiary) results when the hypothalamic-pituitary axis is damaged. The following potential causes should be considered:
- Pituitary adenoma, pituitary or hypothalamic disease, tumors impinging on the hypothalamus
- Severe illness
- Lymphocytic hypophysitis
- Sheehan's syndrome
- History of brain or pituitary irradiation
- Drugs (e.g., dopamine, prednisone, or opioids)
- Congenital nongoitrous hypothyroidism
- Resistance to thyroid hormone
- TRH deficiency

Iodine Deficiency or Excess
Primary hypothyroidism is one of the most common endocrine disorders in clinical practice. It can be endemic in iodine deficient areas, but it is also common in iodine sufficient areas. Excessive iodine, as is present in radiocontrast dyes, amiodarone, health tonics, and seaweed, can temporarily stop iodide organification and thyroid hormone synthesis, this is known as the Wolff–Chaikoff effect. Usually, healthy individuals have a natural physiologic escape from Wolff–Chaikoff effect after 10–14 days, but in patients who have iodine overload, sodium iodide symporter NIS shuts down, allowing intracellular iodine levels to plummet and hormone secretion to resume. Wolff–Chaikoff effect is temporary as NIS has the capacity of quick downregulation. But, exposure to excess iodine can result in serious and prolonged hypothyroidism in individuals with abnormally functioning thyroid glands which may be from autoimmune thyroiditis, subtotal thyroidectomy, or prior radioiodine therapy.

■ Chronic Lymphocytic Thyroiditis
Chronic lymphocytic thyroiditis (CLT, Hashimoto's thyroiditis) is the most common cause of acquired hypothyroidism. The immune system misconstrues the thyroid antigens as foreign, and a chronic immune reaction follows, resulting in lymphocytic infiltration of the gland and progressive destruction of functional thyroid tissue.

Most of the affected individuals will have circulating antibodies to thyroid tissue. Antithyroid peroxidase (anti-TPO) antibodies are characteristic of this disease. Although, antibody levels can change over time, it is possible that they might be absent in the initial disease phase and generally disappear with time. Absence of antibodies however, does not eliminate the diagnosis of chronic lymphocytic (autoimmune) thyroiditis. A study by Bothra et al. reported that, compared with the general population, first-degree relatives of persons with Hashimoto thyroiditis have a ninefold greater risk of developing it. A literature review by Lee et al. indicated that pathologically confirmed Hashimoto thyroiditis has been identified in cases of papillary thyroid carcinoma more frequently than in benign thyroid disorders or other carcinomas, the occurrence rates being 2.8 and 2.4 times greater, respectively.

Postpartum Thyroiditis

Approximately, 10% of postpartum women may develop lymphocytic thyroiditis (postpartum thyroiditis) in the 2–12 months post delivery. The frequency could be up to 25% in women with type 1 diabetes mellitus. Even though a short spell of treatment with levothyroxine (LT4) might be required yet, the condition is frequently transient (2–4 months). After initiation, hypothyroidism arising from postpartum thyroiditis can last for as long as a year before resolving on its own, and patients with postpartum thyroiditis (anti-TPO-positive) are at increased risk for permanent hypothyroidism or recurrence of postpartum thyroiditis with future pregnancies. High titers of anti-TPO antibodies during pregnancy have been reported to be correlated with high sensitivity and specificity for postpartum autoimmune thyroid disease.

Subacute Granulomatous Thyroiditis

Is also called as de Quervain's, or painful thyroiditis. Subacute granulomatous thyroiditis is a relatively uncommon disease that occurs most commonly in women (5:1) and is rare in the elderly. Disease features include low-grade fever, thyroid pain, dysphagia, and elevated erythrocyte sedimentation rate (ESR). The disease is usually self-limiting and does not generally result in long-standing thyroid dysfunction. Inflammatory conditions or viral syndromes may be associated with transient hyperthyroidism followed by transient hypothyroidism (i.e., de Quervain's thyroiditis and subacute thyroiditis). Several studies have shown a correlation between coronavirus disease 2019 (COVID-19) and the development of subacute thyroiditis.

Riedel's Thyroiditis

The hallmark is dense fibrosis of the thyroid gland. It commonly occurs between 30 to 60 years of age and is more frequent in women (3–4:1). It presents with a rock hard, fixed, and painless goiter. Symptoms are mostly related to compressive effects on surrounding structures or hypoparathyroidism due to extension of the fibrosis. The disease has been linked to immunoglobulin G4 (IgG4) and is associated with a systemic fibrotic process. Most patients initially present with euthyroidism but later develop hypothyroidism as normal thyroid tissue is replaced. ESR levels are often normal, but high concentrations of anti-TPO antibodies are frequently present (~67% of patients). Open biopsy confirms the diagnosis, and treatment is usually surgical, although some studies have shown that early treatment with glucocorticoids, methotrexate, or tamoxifen may be beneficial.

Systemic Lupus Erythematosus

Between 15 and 19% of patients with systemic lupus erythematosus (SLE) have primary hypothyroidism. Although all age groups of individuals with SLE have a greater frequency of hypothyroidism, this is especially true in patients under age 20 years, the odds ratio (OR) being 8.38. Proclivity to develop clinical or subclinical hypothyroidism is higher in female patients with SLE as compared to males.

Drug-induced and Iatrogenic Hypothyroidism

The following medications reportedly have the potential to cause hypothyroidism:
- Iodinated contrast
- Amiodarone
- Interferon-α
- Thalidomide
- Lithium
- Stavudine
- Oral tyrosine kinase inhibitors—sunitinib and imatinib
- Bexarotene
- Perchlorate
- Interleukin 2 (IL-2)
- Ethionamide
- Rifampin
- Phenytoin
- Carbamazepine
- Phenobarbital
- Aminoglutethimide
- Sulfisoxazole
- p-aminosalicylic acid
- Immune checkpoint inhibitors—ipilimumab, pembrolizumab, nivolumab

Genetic Causes

Studies have revealed that a single-nucleotide polymorphism near the *FOXE1* gene has the strongest association with hypothyroidism. Individuals who have GG at this locus had an OR of 1.35 for development of hypothyroidism, those who have AG had OR of 1.00, and those having AA had an OR of 0.74. About 10% of cases with congenital hypothyroidism have some kind of an error in thyroid hormone synthesis, mutations in the *TPO* gene seem to be the most common error, resulting in failure to produce sufficient quantities of TPO. Mutations in TSH receptor (*TSHR*) and *PAX8* genes lead to congenital hypothyroidism without goiter.

CLINICAL MANIFESTATIONS

The clinical features of hypothyroidism are diverse and the spectrum ranges from life threatening—as in myxedema coma—to no signs or symptoms in some cases. Myxedema coma which is the result of prolonged untreated, severe hypothyroidism, is now a rare condition, still early diagnosis is extremely important as it has a mortality of 40% in spite of treatment. Myxedema coma causes altered mental status, hypothermia, progressive lethargy, and bradycardia and can eventually result in multiple organ dysfunction syndrome and even, death.

Presentation of hypothyroidism depends upon the age at onset, duration, severity of the disease and presence or absence of other comorbidities. Hypothyroidism can affect all organ systems **(Table 1)**.

TABLE 1: System wise clinical manifestations of hypothyroidism.

System affected	Symptoms/Presentation	Signs	Uncommon presentation
General metabolism	• Increased weight • Cold intolerance • Fatigue	• Increased BMI • Low BMR • Hypertension • Increased waist circumference • Dyslipidemia • Increased total cholesterol • Increased low-density lipoprotein • Increased homocysteine concentration	• Myxedema • Hypothermia
Cardiovascular	• Fatigue on exertion • Shortness of breath	• Dyslipidemia • Bradycardia • Hypertension • Increased vascular resistance • Decreased cardiac output • Decreased left ventricular function • Changes in several other markers of cardiovascular contractility • Myocardial injuries • Pericardial effusion	• Endothelial dysfunction • Increased intima media thickness • Diastolic dysfunction • Hyperhomocysteinemia • Electrocardiogram changes
Neurosensory	• Hoarseness of voice • Decreased taste, vision or hearing	• Neuropathy • Cochlear dysfunction • Decreased olfactory and gustatory sensitivity • Lack of taste in food	
Neurological and psychiatric	• Impaired memory • Paresthesia: Typically tingling or pricking ("pins and needles") • Mood impairment	• Impaired cognitive function delayed relaxation of tendon reflexes • Altered mental status	• Depression • Dementia (reversible dementia) • Ataxia • Carpal tunnel syndrome and other nerve entrapment syndromes • Myxedema coma • Severe primary hypothyroidism can lead to pituitary hyperplasia with concomitant pituitary pathology (e.g., secondary adrenal insufficiency) and symptoms (e.g., amenorrhea)

Continued

Continued

System affected	Symptoms/Presentation	Signs	Uncommon presentation
Gastrointestinal	Constipation	Reduced esophageal motility	• Nonalcoholic fatty liver disease • Ascites (very rare)
Endocrinological	Infertility and subfertility, menstrual disturbance, galactorrhea	• Goiter • Glucose metabolism dysregulation • Infertility • Sexual dysfunction • Increased prolactin	Pituitary hyperplasia
Musculoskeletal	Muscle weakness, muscle cramps, arthralgia	Creatine phosphokinase elevation	Hoffman's syndrome, osteoporotic fracture (most probably caused by overtreatment)
Hematological	Bleeding, fatigue		• Mild anemia • Acquired von Willebrand disease • Decreased protein C and S • Increased red cell distribution width • Increased mean platelet volume
Skin and hair	Dry skin, hair loss	Coarse skin	Loss of lateral eyebrows, yellow palms of the hand, alopecia areata
Electrolytes and nephrological	Deterioration of kidney function	Decreased estimated glomerular filtration rate	Hyponatremia

(BMI: body mass index; BMR: basal metabolic rate)

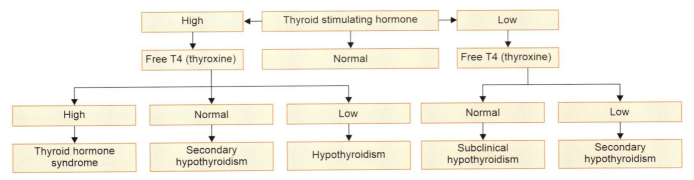

Flowchart 2: Algorithm for the diagnosis of hypothyroidism.

Diagnosis and Treatment

The clinical evaluation of a patient with suspected hypothyroidism should be directed towards confirming the presence and identifying the cause of the hormone deficiency. TSH is the single most sensitive test to diagnose thyroid dysfunction. The combination of FT4 and TSH appears to correctly establish hypothyroidism and its cause in most of the cases. Pituitary dysfunction is uncommon and if present is almost never found in isolation. An elevated TSH in the presence of a low FT4 establishes thyroid dysfunction and primary hypothyroidism. A low TSH in the presence of a low FT4 suggests a pituitary cause and should prompt imaging of the sella. A raised TSH in the presence of a normal FT4 suggests subclinical hypothyroidism **(Flowchart 2)**. If TSH exceeds 10 mIU/L then progression to overt hypothyroidism is likely.

Serum antithyroid antibodies need not be measured routinely in patients with overt hypothyroidism. Anti-TPO antibody testing may be useful to predict the likelihood of progression to permanent hypothyroidism in patients with subclinical hypothyroidism, thyroiditis – whether painless or postpartum **(Boxes 1 & 2, and Table 2)**. In patients taking thyroid hormone without confirmed hypothyroidism, one may stop or reduce dose of T4 by half for 4 weeks, then reassess thyroid function.

Table 2 shows the effect of various drugs on TSH.

> **BOX 1:** Treatment monitoring and follow-up in hypothyroidism.
>
> - One should withdraw blood for testing before LT4 administration in order to maintain TSH within reference range
> - Clinical improvement is gradual, over several weeks and full effect requires about 2–3 months
> - If symptoms persist, then dose adjustment should be done for optimal well-being but TSH suppression should be avoided
> - FT4 should be in middle to upper part of normal range. Serum FT4 rises to normal range by 2 weeks
> - TSH usually requires 6 weeks to normalize. Monitoring of TSH and FT4 should be done every 4–6 weeks after dose adjustment to check the treatment adequacy
> - In long-standing untreated hypothyroidism with very high TSH, it may take 6 months to normalize
> - In such cases, monitoring of TSH should be done every 3 months until stabilized. After obtaining two measurements in the reference range once a year testing is appropriate
> - Excessive LT4 causes subclinical or overt thyrotoxicosis which increases risk of bone loss and arrhythmias
>
> (FT4 : free T4; LT4: levothyroxine; TSH: thyroid-stimulating hormone)

> **BOX 2:** Conditions associated with altered levothyroxine requirement.
>
> - Increased requirement
> - Pregnancy
> - Weight gain
> - *Malabsorption*: Mucosal disease, short bowel syndrome
> - *Drugs*:
>   - Reduce absorption: Sucralfate, aluminum hydroxide, ferrous sulfate, cholestyramine, calcium carbonate, omeprazole, and other proton pump inhibitors
>   - Increased metabolism: Rifampicin, phenytoin, phenobarbitone, carbamazepine, imatinib, sunitinib
>   - Reduced T4 to T3 conversion: Amiodarone, selenium deficiency
>   - Unknown mechanism: Sertraline, lovastatin
> - Decreased requirement
> - Aging
> - Androgen therapy

TABLE 2: Effect of drugs on thyroid-stimulating hormone (TSH).

Decrease secretion of TSH	Increase secretion of TSH
Dopamine	Dopamine antagonist
High-dose glucocorticoids	Amiodarone
Phenytoin	Sodium ipodate
Somatostatin analogs	

Secondary and Tertiary (Central) Hypothyroidism

Secondary and tertiary hypothyroidism should be suspected in the following circumstances:
- In the presence of known hypothalamic or pituitary disease
- A mass lesion in pituitary gland
- Association of signs and symptoms of hypothyroidism with other hormonal deficiencies

DIAGNOSIS AND TREATMENT

Replacement with Thyroxine

Thyroxine is prescribed as LT4 sodium; sodium salt increases the gastrointestinal absorption of LT4. Absorption is greater in the fasting state (80%) than in the fed state.

Orally administered LT4 is well-absorbed, 80% intestinal absorption, predominantly jejunum. Differences in bioavailability have been reported between different brands. Therefore, patient should continue same brand that was initially prescribed. The half-life of serum T4 is approximately 7 days which allows to a single daily dose. **Flowchart 3** gives the approach to management of hypothyroidism. **Box 1** elaborates monitoring and follow-up in hypothyroidism.

There is limited utility of using liothyronine (LT3) for replacement therapy because about 80% is produced in

---

If hypothyroidism is suspected then:
- TSH should be measured
- If TSH is elevated or if there is suspicion of disorders other then primary hypothyroidism then, free thyroxine should be measured
- Diagnosis should be based on two measurements

↓

Indication for treatment:
- Treatment should be started with 1.5–1.8 μg/kg of levothyroxine and initiate with full dose
- Start with 12.5–25 μg/day of levothyroxine in patients with cardiac symptoms and elderly patients with many comorbidities
- One should inform women of childbearing age and women intending pregnancy about the 30% increase in dose which is required once the individual is pregnant
- Repeat TSH measurement after 4–12 weeks and then every 6 months when stable

↓

- If treatment targets have not been reached: Consider reasons for treatment failure
- If treatment targets have been reached: One should advise for annual serum TSH measurement

Flowchart 3: Approach to management of hypothyroidism.
(TSH: thyroid-stimulating hormone)

peripheral tissue by deiodination of T4. Due to the short half-life of approximately 1 day, LT3 has been sometimes recommended for the management of patient with thyroid cancer.

INITIATION OF THERAPY

The initial dose of T4 should be based on the age of the patient severity, duration of hypothyroidism, and the presence of any other associated disorder. Healthy patient under the age of 60 years with no history of cardiac or respiratory disease can be started with the average replacement dose of T4 of 1.6 ug/kg body weight per day. In case of more severe, long-standing hypothyroidism, older age, and presence of ischemic heart disease, it is better to start with a low dose (12.5–25 µg daily). The dose can be increased by 12.5–25 µg every 4 weeks and it takes 3–6 months for euthyroid state. **Box 2** details the conditions associated with altered LT4 requirement.

SCREENING

All patients with symptoms of hypothyroidism should be evaluated for hypothyroidism. Screening of asymptomatic individuals is controversial as there is absence of data showing any benefit of population-based screening. Routine screening is not recommended in asymptomatic nonpregnant adults. Screening is suggested for subjects with laboratory or radiological abnormalities. **Box 3** gives the indications for screening.

High serum TSH concentrations may also occur in TSH-induced hyperthyroidism, primary adrenal insufficiency, and factitiously in patients who have antibodies to the murine immunoglobulins used in the assay. Since errors may be made when only TSH is measured in patients with secondary or central hypothyroidism or TSH-mediated hyperthyroidism, it is recommended that both TSH and FT4 be measured in all patients for screening purposes.

This approach adds cost to screening and is likely to pick up few cases of unsuspected pituitary disease.

Unnecessary laboratory testing may be limited by the following approach:
- *Serum TSH normal*: No further testing performed
- *Serum TSH high*: Free T4 added to determine the degree of hypothyroidism

Screening in hospitalized patients is a more difficult problem and is not recommended unless thyroid disease is strongly suspected since changes in thyroid hormones, binding proteins, and TSH concentrations occur in nonthyroidal illness.

THYROID DEFICIENCY IN THE ELDERLY

Hypothyroidism in elderly patients usually presents with vague symptoms. Clinical manifestations are easy fatigability, lethargy, loss of interest in routine activities, sluggish ankle jerk, dry and coarse skin, hoarseness of voice, and bradycardia. A strong clinical suspicion is warranted to diagnose hypothyroidism in the elderly as a lot of these symptoms mimic aging.

Hypothyroidism in the elderly is correlated with significant morbidity if left untreated. Dyslipidemia is relatively more common in elderly with hypothyroidism when compared to elderly in euthyroid state. Cognitive decline in the elderly is associated with both overt and subclinical hypothyroidism. Other symptoms include reversible dementia, depression, cerebellar dysfunction, neuropathy, and macrocytic anemia. Patients above 60

BOX 3: Indications for screening of hypothyroidism.

Screening for hypothyroidism should be done in cases with laboratory or radiologic abnormalities indicative of hypothyroidism, subjects with risk factors for hypothyroidism, and patients taking drugs that may impair thyroid function. Thyroid function should be measured in:
- Dyslipidemia
- Hyponatremia, often resulting from inappropriate secretion production of antidiuretic hormone
- Increased serum muscle enzymes
- Macrocytic anemia
- Pericardial or pleural effusions
- Previous thyroid injury (e.g., radioiodine therapy, thyroid or neck surgery, external radiation therapy)
- Pituitary or hypothalamic disorders
- History of autoimmune diseases

TSH may not be a useful tool for the diagnosis of hypothyroidism under the following circumstances:
- If pituitary or hypothalamic disease is known or suspected
- In hospitalized patients, since there are many other factors in acutely or chronically ill euthyroid patients that influence TSH secretion
- In patients receiving drugs or with underlying diseases which affect TSH secretion:
  - Drugs that decrease TSH secretion include dopamine, high doses of glucocorticoids, phenytoin, and somatostatin analogs (octreotide).
  - Drugs that increase TSH secretion include dopamine antagonists (metoclopramide or domperidone), amiodarone, and oral cholecystographic dyes (sodium ipodate)

> **BOX 4: Treatment of elderly patients of hypothyroidism.**
>
> - Thyroid dysfunction affects about one-fourth of the geriatric population
> - Subclinical and overt hypothyroidisms are equally common in the elderly. Hypothyroidism occurs in 10% of female elderly patients and 2% of male elderly patients (60 years)
> - An age-related increase is seen for hypothyroidism
> - Younger patients require higher dose than older
> - Low and slow approach in elderly/ischemic heart disease patients because restoration of euthyroidism may increase demands, worsen angina and precipitate arrhythmias
> - Starting doses are 12.5 and 25 µg/day with dose adjustments every 4 weeks by 12.5–25 µg
> - Start full replacement dose of 1.5–1.8 µg/kg ideal body weight of LT4 in adults <60 years with no history of cardiovascular disease
> - Association between cognitive impairment and subclinical and overt hypothyroidism in elderly
> - In patients with coexistent hypocortisolism, glucocorticoid replacement should precede thyroxine replacement
> - Conditions that interfere with absorption or metabolism of LT4 necessitate dose changes
> - Excess of LT4 has adverse impact on cardiac and skeletal system

years should undergo screening for thyroid dysfunction. Since, The elderly have relatively increased sensitivity to LT4, hormone replacement therapy in the elderly should be initiated at low doses and gradually titrated to reach the euthyroid state. Starting doses with or without cardiovascular morbidities are 12.5 and 25 µg/day, respectively in the elderly cohort. Daily dose can subsequently be increased by 12.5–25 µg every 4 weeks until serum TSH levels are normalized. The treatment of subclinical hypothyroidism should be individualized on the basis of TSH levels keeping in mind the potential risk of overtreatment which could result in cardiac arrhythmias and osteoporosis. Adverse drug reactions may be seen in the elderly because of associated comorbidities, polypharmacy, and decreased renal excretion. There is evidence to suggest that treatment of subclinical hypothyroidism with serum TSH of up to 10 mU/L should in all probability be avoided in patients older than 85 years because subclinical hypothyroidism in this population does not result in deleterious effects and is on the contrary, found to be related with extended life span **(Box 4)**.

CONCLUSION

Prevalence of hypothyroidism, is highest in people aged 46–54 years (13·1%), with people aged 18–35 years being least affected (7.5%). Thyroid diseases are relatively easy to diagnose and treatment is within reach of the patient. In spite of this, it often remains undetected, untreated and hampers the work performance and economic productivity. Early diagnosis and treatment therefore remain the cornerstone of management. India is currently iodine replete and this with a possible resultant surge in autoimmune thyroid disorders. This situation is reflected globally with the era of iodization; autoimmune thyroid diseases having become the most common cause of hypothyroidism.

SUGGESTED READINGS

1. Bajaj S, Sachan S, Misra V, Varma A, Saxena P. Cognitive function in subclinical hypothyroidism in elderly. Indian J Endocrinol Metab. 2014;18(6):811-4.
2. Nair A, Jayakumari C, Jabbar PK, Jayakumar RV, Raizada N, Gopi A, et al. Prevalence and Associations of Hypothyroidism in Indian Patients with Type 2 Diabetes Mellitus. J Thyroid Res. 2018;2018:5386129.
3. Bagcchi S. Hypothyroidism in India: more to be done. Lancet Diabetes Endocrinol. 2014;2(10):778.
4. Baloch Z, Carayon P, Conte-Devolx B, Demers LM, Feldt-Rasmussen U, Henry JF, et al. Laboratory medicine practice guidelines. Laboratory support for the diagnosis and monitoring of thyroid disease. Thyroid. 2003;13(1):3-126.
5. Hollowell JG, Staehling NW, Flanders WD, Hannon WH, Gunter EW, Spencer CA, et al. Serum TSH, T(4), and thyroid antibodies in the United States population (1988 to 1994): National Health and Nutrition Examination Survey (NHANES III). J Clin Endocrinol Metab. 2002;87(2):489-99.
6. Larsen PR, Davies TF, Schlumberger MJ, Hay ID. Thyroid physiology and diagnostic evaluation of patients with thyroid disorders. In: Larsen PR, Kronenberg HM, Melmed S, Polonsky K (Eds). Williams' Textbook of Endocrinology, 10th edition. Philadelphia: WB Saunders Company; 2003. pp. 389-516.
7. Jabbar PK, Danish E. Hypothyroidism: introduction, etiology and clinical features. In: Jayakumar RV (Ed). ITS Clinical Manual of Thyroid Disorders, 1st edition. Philadelphia: Elsevier Limited; 2012. pp. 129-30
8. Bothra N, Shah N, Goroshi M, Jadhav S, Padalkar S, Thakkar H, et al. Hashimoto's thyroiditis: Relative recurrence risk ratio and implications for screening of first-degree relatives. Clin Endocrinol. 2017;87(2):201-6.
9. Sabra M. Thyroid cancer: Is there a relationship between thyroid cancer and Hashimoto's thyroiditis? Clin Thyroidol Pub. 2012;6(7):6.
10. Lee JH, Kim Y, Choi JW, Kim YS. The association between papillary thyroid carcinoma and histologically proven Hashimoto's thyroiditis: a meta-analysis. Eur J Endocrinol. 2013;168(3):343-9.

11. Cleveland clinic. Postpartum Thyroiditis. [online]. Available from https://my.clevelandclinic.org/health/diseases/15294-postpartum-thyroiditis [Last accessed December, 2022].
12. Muller I, Cannavaro D, Dazzi D, Covelli D, Mantovani G, Muscatello A, et al. SARS-CoV-2-related atypical thyroiditis. Lancet Diabetes Endocrinol. 2020;8(9):739-41.
13. Pearce EN, Farwell AP, Braverman LE. Thyroiditis. N Engl J Med. 2003;348(26):2646-55.
14. Klionsky Y, Antonelli M. Thyroid Disease in Lupus: An Updated Review. ACR Open Rheumatol. 2020;2(2):74-8.
15. Park SM, Chatterjee VK. Genetics of congenital hypothyroidism. J Med Genet. 2005;42(5):379-89.
16. Chaker L, Bianco AC, Jonklaas J, Peeters RP. Hypothyroidism. Lancet. 2017;390(10101):1550-62.
17. Singh SK, Bajaj S, Patel VH. Hypothyroidism. In: Bajaj S (Ed). ESI Manual of Clinical Endocrinology, 2nd edition. New Delhi: Jaypee Brothers Medical Publishers; 2015.
18. Singh RK, Singh SK. Hypothyroidism. In: Wangnoo SK, Ahmad J, Siddiqui MA (Eds). Principles and Practices of Thyroid Gland Disorders. New Delhi: Jaypee Brothers Medical Publishers; 2018.
19. Kalra S, Das AK, Bajaj S, Saboo B, Khandelwal D, Tiwaskar M, et al. Diagnosis and Management of Hypothyroidism: Addressing the Knowledge–Action Gaps. 2018;35(10):1519-34.
20. Bensenor IM, Olmos RD, Lotufo PA. Hypothyroidism in the elderly: diagnosis and management. Clin Interv Aging. 2012;7:97-111.

CHAPTER 10

Refractory Hypothyroidism

Soumya S, PK Jabbar

INTRODUCTION

There is a proportion of hypothyroid patients whose thyroxine stimulating hormone (TSH) remains elevated refractory to usual thyroxine treatment and requires unusually higher doses. A multicentric study from Brazil described 28% of 2,292 hypothyroid patients on optimal thyroxine therapy had elevated TSH. Refractory hypothyroidism is defined as biochemical (serum level of TSH above the upper target level, following a 6-week interval after the dosage was last increased) or clinical evidence of hypothyroidism (unresolved hypothyroid symptoms), despite increasing dosages of levothyroxine beyond 1.9 µg/kg/day. Supratherapeutic doses of thyroxine can cause deleterious effects on cardiovascular health and bone, especially in the elderly.

CAUSES OF REFRACTORY HYPOTHYROIDISM

The factors causing treatment refractory hypothyroidism can be classified into preluminal, luminal, intramural, increased demand, and those affecting serum TSH **(Table 1)**.

Preluminal factors: Levothyroxine tablet exposure to humidity, light, and high temperature was described as a cause of refractory hypothyroidism by Benvenga, et al. A study from Delhi has shown that 9.6% of hypothyroidism patients were having poor compliance to treatment. Noncompliance and errors in tablet storage and administration is the most common cause of refractory hypothyroidism. The reason being either inconvenience to take the medication in empty stomach and avoiding other medications that may interfere with thyroxine absorption along with it, or waiting for 1 hour for meal or beverage. CONTROL Surveillance Project by McMillan, et al. reported that among 925 patients on levothyroxine therapy >21% patients do not take thyroxine therapy as indicated. Substitution of levothyroxine prescriptions with different pharmaceutical preparations at the pharmacy has also been shown to cause inadequate control of hypothyroidism.

Luminal factors: Levothyroxine has a half-life of about 7 days and 80% oral bioavailability in optimal condition. Levothyroxine preparation is a pentahydrated sodium salt which is insoluble in water and exists in different zwitterionic forms at different pH. Acidic pH causes disintegration and ionization of molecule making it soluble so that it can be absorbed from the jejunum and ileum. Factors which have been shown to affect the absorption of levothyroxine include inadequate spacing between levothyroxine administration and meals or beverages, adsorption to

TABLE 1: Causes of refractory hypothyroidism.	
Preluminal factors	• Improper thyroxine storage • Noncompliance • Poor tolerability • Switching to generic levothyroxine with different bioavailability
Luminal factors	• Food, beverages (coffee) • Achlorhydria • Medications that reduce gastric acid • Medications that bind thyroxine • Medications that alter intestinal motility
Intramural factors	• Celiac disease • Atrophic gastritis • *Helicobacter pylori* infection • Intestinal infections and small intestinal bacterial overgrowth • *Liver diseases*: Cirrhosis and obstructive liver disease • *Pancreatic diseases*: Pancreatic insufficiency • Previous gastrointestinal surgery, jejunostomy, and jejunoileal bypass • Short bowel syndrome • Lactose intolerance (in case of lactose containing thyroxine preparations) • Inflammatory bowel disease • Infiltrative enteropathy • Nephrotic syndrome

Continued

Continued		

Increased demand	• Weight gain
	• Pregnancy
	• *Increased metabolism of thyroxine:*
	  ○ Rifampin, carbamazepine, phenytoin, estrogen (induces CYP3A4 in liver)
	• *Drugs that increase serum thyroxine-binding globulin (TBG) concentration:*
	  ○ Estrogens, tamoxifen, raloxifene, heroin, methadone, mitotane, fluorouracil, capecitabine, clofibrate
	• *Drugs affecting deiodinase activity (blocks conversion of T4 to T3):*
	  ○ Amiodarone, glucocorticoids, beta-blocking drugs
	• Selenium deficiency (cofactor of deiodinase enzyme)	

Factors affecting serum TSH	• Addison's disease • Altered regulation of the hypothalamic–pituitary–thyroid axis • Thyroxine stimulating hormone (TSH) heterophile antibodies • Macro-TSH	
Others	• Type 2 deiodinase polymorphisms, e.g., Thr92Ala polymorphism • Partial thyroid hormone resistance syndrome • Idiopathic	

coadministered medications such as sucralfate, aluminum hydroxide, calcium carbonate, ferrous sulfate, lovastatin or various resins, concomitant use of nutritional supplements or vitamins, medications affecting gastric pH like histamine receptor blockers, proton pump inhibitors, aluminum hydroxide, and drugs modifying gastrointestinal motility.

Intramural factors: Malabsorption of levothyroxine is another cause for refractory hypothyroidism in a significant proportion of hypothyroid patients. There can be concomitant gastrointestinal diseases or autoimmune cause of malabsorption which are more likely to be present in hypothyroid patients with autoimmune hypothyroidism. Gastrointestinal diseases which can cause malabsorption of levothyroxine include atrophic gastritis, *Helicobacter pylori* infection, primary or secondary gastroparesis, inflammatory bowel disease, celiac disease, lactose intolerance, and surgeries such as gastric bypass, biliopancreatic diversion, and Roux-en-Y duodenal diversion. Excipients present in thyroxine preparation can also trigger a disease exacerbation as in case of lactose intolerance or gluten in celiac disease.

Increased demand: The total daily dose of levothyroxine is usually higher in individuals who are obese, the dose per kilogram tends to be lower. Weight change is an important factor contributing to increased demand of levothyroxine. Sudden weight loss associated with serious illnesses such as human immunodeficiency virus (HIV), malignancies, bariatric surgery, and malnutrition has also been shown to affect oral levothyroxine homeostasis. Pregnancy is associated with an increased levothyroxine requirement of up to 50% early in the first trimester, which peaked midway through pregnancy and remained constant until delivery. Drugs such as rifampin, carbamazepine, phenytoin, and estrogen induce CYP3A4 in liver and cause increased metabolism of thyroxine. An obligatory effect of amiodarone is to block conversion of T4 to T3 and cause an increased demand. Selenium being a cofactor for deiodinase enzyme, the deficiency causes decreased activity of deiodinase and increased demand for thyroxine.

Factors affecting serum TSH: Patients with hypocortisolism can have higher TSH levels. Both the pituitary-adrenal as well as the pituitary-thyroid axis follow diurnal rhythms, but are out of phase so that peak TSH levels occur at a time when the serum cortisol levels are at the lowest. Dysfunction in the hypothalamo-pituitary-thyroid axis due to partial pituitary resistance to thyroid hormone or TSH receptor mutations is rarer cause. Heterophile antibodies cause TSH assay interference leading to elevated TSH levels.

Heterophile antibodies are triggered by external antigens but they can cross react with self antigens. Common example is the heterophile human anti-mouse antibody present in the serum of many persons which can cause laboratory assay interference with immunometric assays such as TSH estimation and can cause falsely high or low TSH values.

Another cause of lab assay interference is the presence of macro TSH in serum. Macro TSH is TSH bound to immunoglobulins in the serum. The binding alters the half-life and neutralizes its bioactivity but leaves the epitope open for analytical antibodies of immunoassay to interact. This leads to falsely high values in assay. There are laboratory methods to detect the presence of Macro TSH such as linearity test, polyethylene glycol (PEG) precipitation TSH sequestration test and gel filtration chromatography.

Others: Polymorphisms of genes coding deiodinase enzyme can also cause inadequate TSH normalization with levothyroxine treatment. The most studied deiodinase gene polymorphism that is likely to have a clinical significance is the Thr92 substitution for Ala in deiodinase 2 (Thr92Ala-DIO2). The polymorphism leads to decreased activity of the enzyme and hence decreased conversion of levothyroxine to T3. This leads to decreased feedback inhibition at the pituitary causing inadequate TSH normalization in primary hypothyroidism. One study showed that the DIO2-Thr92Ala polymorphism predicted the need for a higher dose of LT4 in order to achieve near suppression of the serum TSH in thyroid cancer patients. These polymorphisms can diminish thyroid hormone signaling and/or disrupt normal cellular function and can cause localized/systemic hypothyroidism. Around 10–20% of refractory hypothyroidism patients are deemed idiopathic even after meticulous evaluation.

DELETERIOUS EFFECTS OF SUPRATHERAPEUTIC DOSES OF THYROXINE (TABLE 2)

- Osteoporosis and increased risk of fractures. Those with undetectable TSH levels (<0.03 mIU/L) were shown to have a twofold increased risk for fractures as compared to those with TSH levels in the normal range.
- Increase in cardiovascular conditions such as tachycardia, left ventricular hypertrophy, poor diastolic relaxation, and atrial fibrillation.
- Increased use of healthcare resources.

DIAGNOSIS OF ETIOLOGY OF TREATMENT REFRACTORY HYPOTHYROIDISM

When encountered with hypothyroidism refractory to treatment clinician should employ a systematic approach to gathering information and determining an etiology and an effective therapeutic strategy. A stepwise approach is given below here:

- *Step 1—Confirm the diagnosis and laboratory results*: Repeat TSH, T4/Free T4, T3. Markedly elevated TSH levels in the absence of low or at least low-normal thyroid hormones suggest assay interference with heterophile antibodies or macro-TSH (as earlier).
- *Step 2—Ask about compliance*: Enquire in a nonaccusatory and nonjudgmental manner. Patient report or pill check can be done to assess compliance. Supervised levothyroxine absorption test may be useful if poor adherence to oral treatment is suspected **(Box 1)**.
- *Step 3*—Review the thyroxine storage and ingestion history
- *Step 4*—Check the patient's medication bottles and tablets
- *Step 5—Investigate for levothyroxine malabsorption*: A systematic approach for evaluation of malabsorption has been depicted in **Flowchart 1**.
- *Step 6*—Consider increased turnover or excretion.

TABLE 2: Consequences of over- and undertreatment with L-T4.

Potential consequences of overtreatment with L-T4	Potential consequences of undertreatment with L-T4
• Symptoms of hyperthyroidism • Accelerated bone loss • Fractures • Atrial fibrillation • Heart failure • Coronary heart disease (CHD) events	• Symptoms of hypothyroidism • Elevated total cholesterol and LDL-cholesterol • Impaired cognition • Increased diastolic blood pressure (BP) • Increased body weight • Increased risk of CHD events and mortality • Increased risk of heart failure (HF)

BOX 1: Protocol for thyroxine absorption test.

- Test is conducted in a supervised medical setting
- The patient is kept on an overnight fast except for water
- The regular LT4 dose is held
- Patients are weighed on the morning of the examination and weight is recorded in kg
- An oral levothyroxine load with 600–1,000 µg is administered with a glass of water under medical supervision (50 µg or 100 µg tablets are preferred)
- Blood samples are drawn at times—30, 0, 30, 60, 120, 240, 360 minutes
- Impaired bioavailability is suspected if the percent increase from baseline is <50% (*normal values*: approximately 100–200%). With intermediate results (50–100%)
- Percent increase = peak serum fT4–baseline serum fT4 divided by baseline serum fT4 × 100

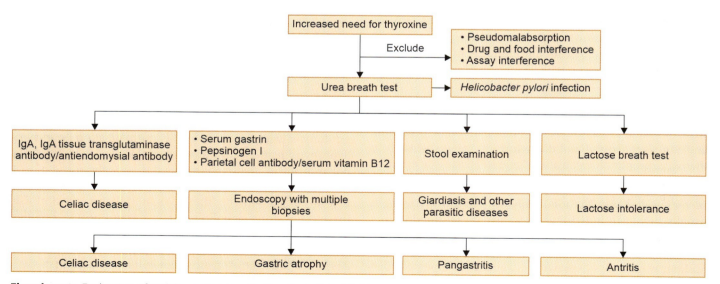

Flowchart 1: Evaluation of malabsorption in refractory hypothyroidism.

MANAGEMENT OF REFRACTORY HYPOTHYROIDISM

The most common approach to refractory hypothyroidism is to increase the dose of levothyroxine further until a target TSH normalization is achieved. Identification of the causative factor and correction of the same is the preferred approach.

Proper patient education regarding storage and administration of thyroxine can improve TSH in most cases. Patient should be advised to store levothyroxine away from heat, light, and humidity. The most efficient way to take levothyroxine is to ingest the tablets on an empty stomach and avoid other medications or food for 30–60 minutes (preferably 60) thereafter. In case of patients who prefer to take at bedtime or in special situations, thyroxine may also be taken 3 hours after a meal. A 4-hour separation is required for interfering medications such as calcium carbonate, ferrous sulfate, and sucralfate.

Once weekly thyroxine oral administration is an option for uncorrectable noncompliance. Owing to its long half-life of approximately 7 days, the weekly dosage requirement can be given together on one day/week. The dose can be calculated as 1.6–1.8 µg per kilogram multiplied by 7 and rounded off to nearest 50 µg. A study from authors institution has demonstrated higher efficacy of once weekly thyroxine over standard daily dose with no adverse effects in patients with refractory hypothyroidism due to poor compliance.

Alternative preparations of levothyroxine like softgel or liquid preparation that are less susceptible to malabsorption or intolerance may also be considered. But these are not available in most parts of the world. A recent retrospective study, the CONTROL Switch, which included 99 hypothyroid patients suggested that switching from levothyroxine tablets to gelcapsules reduce the need for increased dose, while improving the hypothyroidism and TSH normalization.

Role of T3 therapy: The routine use of T3 or combination of T4 and T3 is not recommended by most thyroid association guidelines due to insufficient evidence. However, few selected patients may benefit from combination therapy, e.g., those with type 2 deiodinase polymorphisms.

Thyromimetics: Thyroid hormone analogues are not routinely recommended for treatment of hypothyroidism. Selective thyromimetics are synthetic analogs of thyroid hormones that can selectively stimulate TR-beta present on liver and pituitary thereby action on cholesterol metabolism and obesity, avoiding harmful effects on the heart and bone which are mediated by thyroid hormone receptor (TR) alpha. Examples are:

- *3,5,3-Triiodothyroacetic acid (TRIAC)*: TRIAC is formed by the decarboxylation and deamination of tetraiodothyroxine. It is a naturally occurring metabolite of tetraiodothyroxine with thyromimetic activity. It has 10–20 times affinity for thyroid hormone receptors, as compared to triiodothyroxine (T3). It also has selectivity for TR-beta1 without affecting TR-alpha1, hence having potential for utility in the treatment of symptomatic patients with selective pituitary resistance to thyroid hormone.
- *Sobetirome*: Sobetirome, or GC-1 (3,5-dimethyl-4–4-hydroxy-3-isopropylbenzyl phenoxyacetic acid), is a selective thyromimetic with 10-fold preferential action on TR-beta 1.
- *KB141*: Another agent with TR-beta agonism. It has about 15 times more selectivity for TR-beta than for TR-alpha in vitro and hence it has the potential to induce weight loss and decrease cholesterol and lipoprotein (a) without increasing heart rate.
- *Eprotirome (KB2115):* It is also a TR-beta-selective ligand that is preferentially taken up by the liver.

CONCLUSION

Treatment refractory hypothyroidism is not an uncommon clinical scenario. The etiology could range right from common factors such as noncompliance or erratic administration or timing from meals to less common ones like malabsorption to rare entities like deiodinase gene polymorphisms. A thorough and systematic look into the causative factors with a detailed history and clinical examination and judicious laboratory evaluation will help to delineate the cause. Thyroxine absorption test may be performed to differentiate noncompliance from other pathological causes. Proper patient education, treatment of the cause, and careful titration of levothyroxine dosage are the management principles.

SUGGESTED READINGS

1. Vaisman F, Coeli CM, Ward LS, Graf H, Carvalho G, Montenegro R Jr, et al. How good is the levothyroxine replacement in primary hypothyroidism patients in Brazil? Data of a multicentre study. J Endocrinol Invest. 2013;36(7):485-8.
2. Lips DJ, van Reisen MT, Voigt V, Venekamp W. Diagnosis and treatment of levothyroxine pseudomalabsorption. Neth J Med. 2004;62(4):114-8.
3. Benvenga S, Papi G, Antonelli A. Refractory Hypothyroidism due to Improper Storage of Levothyroxine Tablets. Front Endocrinol. 2017;8:155.
4. Kumar P, Khandelwal D, Mittal S, Dutta D, Kalra S, Katiyar P, et al. Knowledge, awareness, practices and adherence to treatment of patients with primary hypothyroidism in Delhi. Indian J Endocr Metab. 2017;21:429-33.

5. Vermeire E, Hearnshaw H, Van Royen P, Denekens J. Patient adherence to treatment: three decades of research. A comprehensive review. J Clin Pharm Ther. 2001;26(5):331-42.
6. McMillan M, Rotenberg KS, Vora K, Sterman AB, Thevathasan L, Ryan MF, et al. Comorbidities, concomitant medications, and diet as factors afecting levothyroxine therapy: results of the CONTROL Surveillance Project. Drugs RD. 2016;16(1):53-68.
7. Hennessey JV, Malabanan AO, Haugen BR, Levy EG. Adverse event reporting in patients treated with levothyroxine: results of the pharmacovigilance task force survey of the American Thyroid Association, American Association of Clinical Endocrinologists, and the Endocrine Society. Endocr Prac. 2010;16:357-70.
8. Eligar V, Taylor P, Okosieme O, Leese G, Dayan C. Thyroxine replacement: a clinical endocrinologist's viewpoint. Ann Clin Biochem. 2016;53(4):421-33.
9. Flynn RW, Bonellie SR, Jung RT, MacDonald TM, Morris AD, Leese GP. Serum thyroid-stimulating hormone concentration and morbidity from cardiovascular disease and fractures in patients on long-term thyroxine therapy. J Clin Endocrinol Metab. 2010;9: 186-93.
10. Centanni M, Benvenga S, Sachmechi I. Diagnosis and management of treatment-refractory hypothyroidism: an expert consensus report. J Endocrinol Invest. 2017;40(12):1289-301.
11. Ramadhan A, Tamilia M. Treatment-refractory hypothyroidism. CMAJ. 2012;184(2):205-9.
12. Jayakumari C, Nair A, Puthiyaveettil Khadar J, Das DV, Prasad N, Jessy SJ, et al. Efficacy and Safety of Once-Weekly Thyroxine for Thyroxine-Resistant Hypothyroidism. J Endocr Soc. 2019;3(12):2184-93.
13. Ernst FR, Sandulli W, Elmor R, Welstead J, Sterman AB, Lavan M. Retrospective study of patients switched from tablet formulations to a gel cap formulation of levothyroxine: results of the CONTROL Switch study. Drugs RD. 2017;17:103-15.
14. Biondi B, Wartofsky L. Treatment with Thyroid Hormone. Endocr Rev. 2014;35(3):433-512.

CHAPTER 11

Hypothyroidism and Associated Comorbidities

Sphoorti P Pai, S Vageesh Ayyar

INTRODUCTION

Hypothyroidism is the deficiency of thyroid hormone action in the peripheral tissues which require thyroid hormones for their normal function. Primary hypothyroidism is the term used when the thyroid gland is diseased. In central hypothyroidism, the pathology lies in the hypothalamus and/or the pituitary. Peripheral hypothyroidism refers to conditions where the thyroid hormone action at the tissue level is impaired. Thyroid hormone deficiency can lead to varied symptoms involving multiple organ systems. Theodor Kocher, a Swiss surgeon and Sir William Horsley, a British surgeon found similar symptoms in patients with cretinism and those who underwent total thyroidectomy. It was then concluded that these symptoms of "myxedema" were due to dysfunction of the thyroid gland. This led to the concept of thyroid hormone replacement. With the advent of therapy, the fatal outcomes of hypothyroidism, frequently due to cardiovascular causes, were reduced. At present, the classical presentation of myxedema is infrequent. Nowadays, due to routine use of thyroid function tests, subclinical hypothyroidism (SCHT) is detected frequently. The prevalence of overt hypothyroidism is 0.3–0.4% and that of SCHT is between 4.3 and 8.5%. Prevalence may vary with age, sex, the cut-offs used, geographical area, and iodine intake. Both overt and SCHT have been associated with multiple comorbidities such as hypertension, dyslipidemia, diabetes, coronary artery disease, depression, and reduced quality of life. In this chapter, the associations between comorbidities and hypothyroidism **(Fig. 1)**, pathophysiology, and outcomes with thyroid hormone replacement therapy have been discussed.

HYPERTENSION AND HYPOTHYROIDISM

Hypertension affects one-fourth of the global population and is a treatable risk factor for cardiovascular mortality. Primary hypertension is the most common cause of hypertension, but approximately 10% can be due to secondary causes. Hypothyroidism is listed as a recognized cause of secondary

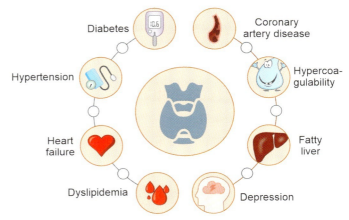

Fig. 1: Hypothyroidism and comorbidities.

hypertension. Patients with hypothyroidism have a threefold higher incidence of diastolic hypertension with frequency of 1–3% among patients with diastolic hypertension. Masked hypertension is defined as normal office blood pressure (BP) measurements despite presence of elevated BP in home or ambulatory BP monitoring. A study by Piantanida et al., found that the prevalence of masked hypertension was significantly higher in patients with both overt and SCHT compared to euthyroid controls. A study done in children and adolescents has shown positive correlation between thyroid-stimulating hormone (TSH) levels, systolic blood pressure (SBP), and diastolic blood pressure (DBP). In an Indian study, the prevalence of hypothyroidism in hypertensive subjects was 31.2%.

The mechanisms postulated for hypertension in hypothyroidism are increased peripheral vascular resistance, reduced endothelial-dependent vasodilation and proinflammatory milieu. Genetic polymorphisms in genes involving the hypothalamus–pituitary–thyroid pathway and deiodinases are found to have associations with hypertension. These studies are controversial with conflicting reports in different studies. Further research in genetics is needed to elucidate the relationship between hypothyroidism and hypertension.

Overt hypothyroidism undoubtedly requires therapy. The dilemma arises in the treatment of SCHT where data regarding benefits are variable. Studies have shown that pulse wave velocity, a surrogate marker for arterial stiffness is higher and it improves with levothyroxine (LT4) therapy in both overt and SCHT. Levothyroxine therapy in SCHT has also been noted to reduce SBP in a meta-analysis which included 10 randomized-controlled trials (RCTs). On analysis of 19 prospective studies, it was noted that both SBP and DBP were reduced by LT4 treatment in SCHT. The limitation in the existing studies is the lack of uniformity in cut offs used for TSH and therapy. Some studies used liothyronine (LT3) therapy or a combination of LT4 and LT3. Available data suggests that treatment of SCHT with LT4 may be beneficial in reducing blood pressure. However, caution must be exercised in older population, especially oldest of the old (>70 years of age), where data suggests increased mortality with LT4 treatment of SCHT. Current guidelines do not recommend use of LT3 in routine practice for therapy of hypothyroidism except for few uncommon conditions.

DIABETES MELLITUS AND HYPOTHYROIDISM

Diabetes mellitus (DM) and hypothyroidism are two of the most commonly encountered conditions in endocrinology. Type1 diabetes mellitus (T1DM) and autoimmune thyroid disorder (AITD) are known to be associated in autoimmune polyglandular syndrome (APS)-3 and also rarely in APS-1 where primary hypoparathyroidism and Addison's disease are the major endocrine components. The prevalence of AITD in T1DM is 17–30%. There is also higher prevalence of hypothyroidism around 6–20% noted among patients with type 2 diabetes mellitus (T2DM). An Indian study done in 2019 by Talwalkar et al., that prevalence of hypothyroidism was 24.8% in T2DM. Age >65 years, female gender, obesity, and presence of thyroid autoantibodies are additional risk factors for hypothyroidism in T2DM.

Joint susceptibility genes are associated with the polyglandular autoimmunity which causes AITD and T1DM. Both AITD and T1DM are organ-specific T-cell mediated diseases and genes involved in immune regulation are implicated. *HLA class II* genes, *PTPN22*, *CTLA-4*, and *FOXP3* are the genes which have a confirmed association with AITD and T1DM. Various other candidate susceptibility genes are also under study which need further evaluation such as interleukin-1 receptor antagonist (IL-1 RA), interleukin 4 (IL-4), *major histocompatibility complex class I chain-related gene A (MICA)*, tumor necrosis factor alpha (TNF-α), Tg, *IL2RA/CD25*, *VNTR (insulin)*, *ERBB3*, *CLEC16A*, and *CD40*. An Indian study showed that positivity for anti-GAD antibodies were significantly higher in subjects with anti-TPO positivity compared to healthy controls that were negative for anti-TPO antibodies.

Hypothyroidism can affect glucose metabolism in multiple ways. HbA1c levels correlate with TSH levels. Increase in TSH levels has been associated with increase in the incidence of T2DM. Higher TSH levels can lead to increased progression from prediabetes to diabetes. Thyroid-stimulating hormone has been positively correlated with insulin resistance even in euthyroid state. It is observed in multiple studies that there is increased risk of diabetic nephropathy and diabetic retinopathy among diabetic patients with overt and SCHT. Treatment of hypothyroidism can improve the renal function in diabetic patients.

It affects multiple pathways in glucose metabolism. Both hyperglycemia and hypoglycemia can be caused by hypothyroidism. T3 modulates the expression of GLUT4, AMP-kinase in skeletal muscle and thus increases peripheral glucose uptake and insulin sensitivity. In patients with diabetes, leptin levels are elevated. Leptin can increase the *TRH* and TSH levels via Janus kinase (JAK)/signal transducers and activators of transcription (STAT) pathway. Mitochondrial dysfunction caused by hypothyroidism is also postulated as one of the mechanisms for increased risk of dysglycemia.

In overt hypothyroidism, tendency for hypoglycemia increases due to reduced absorption in glucose, reduced hepatic gluconeogenesis, hepatic glycogenolysis, reduced renal clearance of insulin. In insulin treated diabetic patients, the exogenous insulin requirement is reduced and doses increase with LT4 therapy. Excess LT4 therapy can suppress TSH and cause worsening of hyperglycemia and HbA1c.

Some antidiabetic medications have been found to alter the hypothalamus–pituitary–thyroid axis. Metformin can suppress the TSH levels in euthyroid and patients with hypothyroidism on LT4 therapy. This is postulated to be due to action of metformin at the level of thyroid receptors in hypothalamic–pituitary level as free thyroid hormones levels remain unaltered. Insulin suppresses the hepatic conversion of T4 to T3, thus increases the free T4 levels and reduces T3 levels. Low T3 state is also caused by uncontrolled hyperglycemia. The clinical implications of these findings need more studies.

In T1DM who are euthyroid, most international guidelines recommend routine screening for thyroid dysfunction. International Society for Pediatric and Adolescent Diabetes (ISPAD) recommends testing of TSH and anti-TPO antibodies at diagnosis of T1DM; then TSH every 2 years, if anti-TPO antibodies are negative and more frequently, if anti-TPO antibodies are positive. With the current data available, it seems beneficial to screen and treat SCHT in diabetes in order to minimize the negative impact of thyroid dysfunction in diabetes. However, currently universal screening is not advised by guidelines in T2DM. Overtreatment with levothyroxine can also have worsening of diabetes. Individualized approach is necessary for better patient outcomes.

DYSLIPIDEMIA AND HYPOTHYROIDISM

Hypothyroidism is a known cause of dyslipidemia. Dr William Greenfield, in 1878, found extensive atherosclerosis in autopsy of a woman who was diagnosed with myxedema. The link between hypercholesterolemia and hypothyroidism was confirmed by Mason et al. in 1930 where they described the significance of thyroid hormones and cholesterol metabolism.

The prevalence of hypothyroidism in patients with dyslipidemia ranges from 1.4 to 13%. Most often subclinical thyroid dysfunction goes undetected which may underestimate the prevalence. Hyperlipidemia is found in 90% of overtly hypothyroid patients. Approximately, a 30% increase in total cholesterol and low-density lipoprotein-cholesterol (LDL-C) is noted in overt hypothyroidism. High-density lipoprotein-cholesterol (HDL-C) and triglycerides may be normal or slightly increased. The data from Indian studies suggest that HDL is reduced in hypothyroidism. A study done in Bastar region of India, found that HDL was reduced in hypothyroid individuals. Another study from Tamil Nadu, also found that HDL-C levels were reduced in hypothyroid subjects compared to controls. These studies represent regional data and included a small number of subjects. The multicentric Indian Council of Medical Research–India Diabetes (ICMR-INDIAB) study also noted that in Indian population the prevalence of low HDL-C levels is as high as 72.3%. Further studies are required in India to find out whether the low HDL-C levels seen widely in Indian population are independently associated with hypothyroidism or not. A sevenfold increased risk for postprandial hypertriglyceridemia was observed in a study. Postprandial hypertriglyceridemia was defined as 80% increase in serum triglycerides after 4–6 hours of meal. Lipoprotein(a) and oxidized LDL-C are also found to be increased. These adverse lipid parameters contribute to atherosclerotic cardiovascular disease (ASCVD). The changes in SCHT are more subtle and variable. A study by Marwaha et al. in 2011, found that significant changes in lipid profile were seen in patients with SCHT and TSH >10 mU/L, but not in patients with TSH <10 mU/L.

Thyroid hormone is required for expression of hepatic hydroxymethylglutaryl coenzyme A (HMG-CoA) reductase and LDL-C receptors in liver. Sterol regulatory element-binding protein-2 (*SREBP-2*) gene mediates the negative feedback of LDL-C receptor expression when the cholesterol synthesis is increased. *SREBP-2* is also regulated by T3. In overt hypothyroidism, there is reduced synthesis of cholesterol and clearance of LDL-C from blood which leads to high total and LDL cholesterol levels. Newer mechanisms involving fibroblast growth factor (FGF)-21 and FGF-19 have been discovered. Thyroid hormones increase FGF21 which in turn stimulates β-oxidation of fatty acids. Cholesterol ester transfer protein, which transfers cholesterol from HDL-C to LDL-C and very low-density lipoprotein cholesterol (VLDL-C), is reduced in overt hypothyroidism which leads to a mild increase in HDL-C levels. Lipoprotein lipase which hydrolyses triglycerides is stimulated by T3. Thyroid hormones inhibit angiopoetin like-3 (ANGPTL3) which cleaves LPL. In hypothyroidism LPL activity is reduced in hypothyroidism contributing to the increased serum triglycerides.

Levothyroxine therapy partially reverses the changes in lipid parameters. Larger improvements in lipid parameters are seen in patients with overt hypothyroidism. The effect of LT4 therapy in SCHT is inconsistent. A Cochrane review in 2007, analyzing effect of LT4 therapy in SCHT concluded that there was a trend toward reduction of total cholesterol levels but no significant effect of treatment on HDL-C, LDL-C, triglycerides or Lp(a) levels. A recent meta-analysis also has concluded that there were significant reductions in total cholesterol, LDL-C, triglycerides, ApoB and Lp(a) after treatment with LT4 in overt hypothyroidism. The mean total cholesterol reduced by 58.4 mg/dL and LDL-C reduced by 41.1 mg/dL after treatment in overt hypothyroidism. In SCHT, the mean total cholesterol reduced by 12.04 mg/dL and LDL-C reduced by 11.05 mg/dL which was also significant though the magnitude of change was lesser. The American Thyroid Association (ATA) and American Association of Clinical Endocrinologists AACE) issued a joint guidelines in 2012, which said treatment with LT4 may be considered for patients with SCHT having symptoms, anti-TPO positivity, ASCVD, those with ASCVD risk factors and heart failure. A 2019 clinical practice guideline published in British Medical Journal (BMJ) recommended that routine treatment of SCHT was not warranted, but this guideline has been somewhat controversial. Further studies are needed for LT4 and LT3 combination therapy. Current data does not support combination therapy.

CORONARY ARTERY DISEASE AND HYPOTHYROIDISM

The cardiovascular system can be affected in multiple ways due to changes in thyroid hormone levels (**Fig. 2**). Hypothyroidism can cause alterations in known cardiovascular (CV) risk factors such as glycemia, lipid profile, and blood pressure. There can be endothelial dysfunction and procoagulant state which can lead to thrombogenesis.

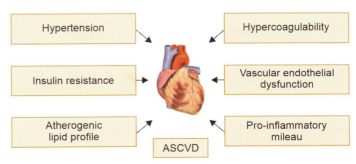

Fig. 2: Risk factors for atherosclerotic cardiovascular disease (ASCVD) in hypothyroidism.

The coagulation abnormalities depend on the severity of the hypothyroidism. *Moderate hypothyroidism* causes increased coagulability and *severe hypothyroidism* leads to increased fibrinolysis.

Subclinical hypothyroidism also has been consistently associated with increased cardiovascular mortality in multiple studies except in the older individuals (>70 years), where it can have a protective effect. One of the important studies with a 20-year follow-up was the Wickham Survey conducted in England. The initial analysis of Wickham Survey had not shown any increase in incident ischemic heart disease (IHD) in SCHT; however, this was due to misclassification at baseline, where some euthyroid individuals had been included in the thyroid disease group because of prevalence of antithyroid autoantibodies. Reclassification and reanalysis of the survey showed an increase in incidence of IHD in SCHT, as well as beneficial effect of LT4 therapy. Surrogate markers of ASCVD such as atherogenic lipid particles, arterial stiffness, and left ventricular function have been studied in SCHT and some studies have shown improvement in these parameters with LT4 therapy. The data supporting therapy for SCHT has, however, been inconsistent for TSH levels <10 mU/L, whereas higher TSH >10 mU/L has shown benefit with therapy in most studies. Most of the data is currently derived from observational studies and small interventional trials. Most international guidelines advise personalized approach according to patient factors such as age, TSH levels, ASCVD risk, and other comorbidities. Large scale RCTs are needed to assess effect of LT4 therapy in SCHT in terms of CV outcomes.

HEART FAILURE AND HYPOTHYROIDISM

Thyroid hormones have chronotropic and inotropic effect on the heart. Hypothyroidism can contribute to heart failure in multiple ways **(Fig. 3)**. In overt hypothyroidism, the cardiac output is reduced due to decreased heart rate and stroke volume. In the absence of heart disease, heart failure (HF) is uncommon despite reduced cardiac output because of the concurrent reduction in peripheral metabolic demand. Diastolic dysfunction is seen in hypothyroidism. This can have adverse consequences in the older population where cardia is already affected by degenerative processes due to aging. Hypothyroidism has shown to cause adverse outcomes in patients with HF. A meta-analysis by Ning et al. which included subjects with HF showed that overt hypothyroidism, SCHT and low T3 syndrome were associated with increased all-cause mortality and increased risk of hospitalization in HF.

Multiple myocyte genes involved in cardiac contractility are regulated by T3. Sarcoplasmic reticulum (SR) calcium ATPase (SERCA2), alpha-myosin heavy chain (α-MHC), Na^+/K^+-ATPase, β-1-adrenergic receptor, voltage gated K^+ channels Kv1.5, Kv4.2, and adenine nucleotide translocase 1 are positively regulated, whereas beta-myosin heavy chain (β-MHC), phospholamban (PLB), Na^+/Ca^{2+} exchanger (NCX1), and adenyl cyclase type V, VI are negatively regulated by thyroid hormone. The cardiac contractility is determined by intracellular calcium (Ca^{2+}) levels, which is released from the SR via ryanodine receptors. Reuptake of Ca^{2+} is via SERCA2. PLB downregulates the SERCA2 activity. T3 increases SERCA2 expression and downregulates PLB expression, thus increasing the intracellular Ca^{2+} levels and cardiac contractility. Cardiac tissue is extremely sensitive to the changes in T3 levels.

The Cardiovascular Health Study noted that therapy with LT4 in SCHT with TSH >10 mU/L may reduce the risk of HF. T3 has been shown to cause an increase in 3–5% of the left ventricular ejection fraction (LVEF), however the results are not consistent in different studies and vary with the severity in baseline LVEF. The American College of Cardiology guidelines recommends screening of all newly diagnosed HF patients for thyroid dysfunction. Though treating SCHT may be beneficial, caution is advised as atrial fibrillation can be precipitated in overtreated older individuals who can worsen the heart failure. Further studies are necessary to determine the role of T3 therapy in heart failure.

NONALCOHOLIC (METABOLIC DYSFUNCTION ASSOCIATED) FATTY LIVER DISEASE AND HYPOTHYROIDISM

Prevalence of nonalcoholic fatty liver disease (NAFLD) has markedly increased in the past few decades due to the substantial increase in the prevalence of obesity. Insulin resistance (IR) is the key contributing factor to NAFLD. NAFLD has been a matter of concern as it may progress to nonalcoholic steatohepatitis (NASH) and cirrhosis. In 2–3% cirrhosis can progress to hepatocellular carcinoma (HCC). NAFLD also has been associated with cardiovascular mortality and morbidity. Numerous observational studies have suggested a relationship between hypothyroidism and NAFLD. Some studies reported prevalence of hypothyroidism in NAFLD, as high as 15.2–36.3%. A meta-analysis which included 13 studies concluded that overt hypothyroidism and SCHT are independently associated with NAFLD.

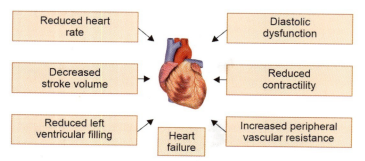

Fig. 3: Pathogenesis of heart failure in hypothyroidism.

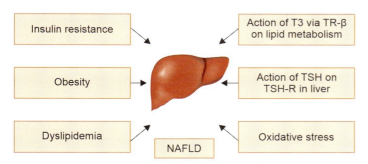

Fig. 4: Pathogenesis of NAFLD in hypothyroidism.
(NAFLD: nonalcoholic fatty liver disease; T3: triiodothyronine; TR-β: thyroid hormone receptor beta; TSH: thyroid-stimulating hormone; TSH-R: thyroid stimulating hormone receptor)

Insulin resistance (IR), obesity, and dyslipidemia especially triglycerides contribute to pathogenesis of NAFLD (**Fig. 4**). As elaborated above, hypothyroidism can lead to occurrence and worsening of the above conditions. Thyroid hormones can directly affect hepatic lipid metabolism via the thyroid hormone beta (TR-β) receptors. Activation of TR-β can lead to reduction in cholesterol and triglyceride levels. Oxidative stress, which is increased in hypothyroidism, can worsen the liver injury.

A study done in 2017 showed that the prevalence of NAFLD significantly reduced with LT4 therapy in SCHT with TSH >10 mU/L. The reduction in NAFLD prevalence after LT4 therapy was not statistically significant the SCHT group with TSH of 4.2–10 mU/L. Thyromimetics, eprotirome, and sobetirome studied in 2015, showed significant reduction of cholesterol level in animal studies. However, these drugs were abandoned due to cartilage toxicity. The latest TR-β agonist resmetirom shows specificity for liver and initial phase 2 studies in NASH have given promising results in terms of liver fat reduction, decrease in liver enzymes, and improvement in lipid profile. A phase 3 study with resmetirom, MAESTRO-NASH trial is expected to be completed by 2024. Other newer TR-β agonists are also under development for NASH. There is no specific treatment for NASH which is USFDA approved, though many drugs have been used off-label for the same. In India, drug controller general of India (DCGI) has given approval for Saroglitazar for the treatment of NASH. Data on CV outcomes and usage of this drug in patients with NAFLD and hypothyroidism are lacking.

PSYCHIATRIC AND COGNITIVE MANIFESTATIONS IN HYPOTHYROIDISM

The thyroid hormones are essential for neurodevelopment and cognitive functions. Mental disturbances in patients with myxedema had been described in the 19th century ranging from mild irritability to severe melancholy and "myxedema madness." Nowadays, patients rarely present with severe psychiatric symptoms due to hypothyroidism but still a vast number of behavioral and cognitive complaints are seen in hypothyroidism. Commonly occurring symptoms in overt hypothyroidism such as slow thought and speech, poor concentration, decreased memory, and decreased attentiveness can be confused with depression. Subtle alterations in mood due to hypothyroidism can go unnoticed for a longtime. Anxiety and frank psychotic symptoms such as visual or auditory hallucinations, paranoia, anger outbursts, and agitation have also been reported in hypothyroidism.

Cognitive decline has been consistently reported in multiple studies with overt hypothyroidism but the data is less convincing in subjects with SCHT. The degree of cognitive dysfunction also varies; most commonly affected domain is memory. Changes in language, attention/concentration, and executive function have also seen in many studies.

Since hypothyroidism is known to cause multiple cognitive and behavioral changes, it is advisable to check TSH levels in all patients with psychiatric and cognitive ailments. A recent meta-analysis which included 348,104 participants found association of hypothyroidism and clinical depression especially in females more than males. There was no significant association of anti-TPO antibodies with depression. Objective evidence for treatment with LT4 in SCHT has not been promising, as RCTs have not demonstrated consistency in improvement of psychological distress scores. Studies focusing on older individuals with SCHT and cognitive decline also have inconsistent results in cognitive effects. If a patient has hypothyroidism and an independent psychiatric diagnosis, both should be treated separately, as treating only hypothyroidism may not completely reverse psychiatric or behavioral changes. More objective data is required before levothyroxine can be recommended for nonspecific behavioral issues in SCHT.

OBESITY AND HYPOTHYROIDISM

The relationship between hypothyroidism and obesity is complex. Overt hypothyroidism has been known to cause weight gain, however the extent of weight gain and the effect of SCHT on weight is still unclear. In 1900s, thyroid extracts were used for inducing weight loss. In 1940s, "rainbow pills" (containing T3 and a combination of other weight loss inducing medications) were used rampantly for achieving weight loss. Severe adverse effects led to the banning of such pills in 1967.

Hypothyroidism has been associated with obesity in many studies. The DanThyr study found that there was a positive correlation between TSH levels and weight gain even within the normal range. There was a negative association between free T4 and obesity. A study conducted in India with 625 subjects, concluded that more subjects were overweight in overt hypothyroidism compared to the SCHT. Among patients who were obese, 33% had overt hypothyroidism and 11% had SCHT.

Thyroid hormones are involved in pathways involving energy expenditure. T3 levels have been associated with resting energy expenditure (REE). It is also noted that small changes in LT4 supplementation can lead to a significant change in REE, in subjects with hypothyroidism on treatment. In brown adipose tissue (BAT), the increased local production of T3 by upregulation of deiodinase type 2 has been implicated in adaptive thermogenesis during cold exposure. These studies imply that, a causal relationship probably exists between hypothyroidism and obesity, though more research is needed to elucidate which pathways play a greater role in SCHT and obesity.

Obesity itself can also increase the TSH levels, which is found to normalize after weight loss. Leptin is an indicator of fat-mass in the body. Leptin regulates the *TRH* gene expression in hypothalamus and an increase in *TRH* leads to increased TSH levels. TSH further stimulates leptin release from adipocytes directly. It is also postulated that TSH secreted in obesity is partially bioinactive, leading to an alteration in negative feedback loop and higher TSH levels. This hypothesis needs proof from studies which is currently lacking. Current guidelines do not recommend starting LT4 or LT3 for obesity as evidence is not very clear. Weight loss may lead to an improvement in TSH levels in some individuals with SCHT, however it is not universal.

CONCLUSION

Hypothyroidism can have implications in management of associated comorbidities and vice-versa. Screening should be routinely utilized for thyroid dysfunction in patients with diabetes, hypertension, dyslipidemia, coronary artery disease (CAD), HF, NAFLD, and depression. Overt hypothyroidism has shown stronger associations with comorbidities such as dyslipidemia, CAD, heart failure, and depression. Therapy for overt hypothyroidism is warranted as benefits are consistent. SCHT has also shown associations with comorbidities, but the results are less convincing. Consistent benefits with LT4 therapy for SCHT are found in those with TSH >10 mU/L and younger age group in most studies. In older population risks versus benefits should be assessed before therapy is initiated. Smaller doses of LT4 should be initiated in older patients requiring therapy. Therapy with LT3 has been shown to be beneficial for some comorbidities such as heart failure and NAFLD, however, some studies have shown harmful effects of T3. Current guidelines do not favor T3 therapy routinely. Thyromimetics or thyroid hormone receptor agonists are newer modalities under study for therapy in comorbidities like NAFLD even for those without hypothyroidism. This is a new area of research which may change the therapeutic approach in future.

SUGGESTED READINGS

1. Young Jr WF, Calhoun DA, Lenders JW, Stowasser M, Textor SC. Screening for endocrine hypertension: an endocrine society scientific statement. Endocrine Reviews. 2017;38(2):103-22.
2. Saito I, Ito K, Saruta T. Hypothyroidism as a cause of hypertension. Hypertension. 1983;5:112-5.
3. Piantanida E, Gallo D, Veronesi G, Pariani N, Masiello E, Premoli P, et al. Masked hypertension in newly diagnosed hypothyroidism: a pilot study. J Endocrinol Invest. 2016;39(10):1131-8.
4. Ittermann T, Thamm M, Wallaschofski H, Rettig R, Völzke H. Serum thyroid-stimulating hormone levels are associated with blood pressure in children and adolescents. J Clin Endocrinol Metab. 2012;97(3):828-34.
5. Talwalkar P, Deshmukh V, Bhole M. Prevalence of hypothyroidism in patients with type 2 diabetes mellitus and hypertension in India: a cross-sectional observational study. Diabetes Metab Syndr Obes. 2019;12:369-76.
6. Gumieniak O, Perlstein TS, Williams JS, Hopkins PN, Brown NJ, Raby BA, et al. Ala92 type 2 deiodinase allele increases risk for the development of hypertension. Hypertension. 2007;49(3):461-6.
7. Fox CS, Maia AL, Hwang SJ, Levy D, Larson MG, Larsen PR. Lack of Association between the Type 2 Deiodinase Thr92Ala Polymorphism and Hypertensive Traits: the Framingham Heart Study. Hypertension. 2008;51(4):e22-3.
8. He W, Li S, Zhang JA, Zhang J, Mu K, Li XM. Effect of levothyroxine on blood pressure in patients with subclinical hypothyroidism: a systematic review and meta-analysis. Front Endocrinol (Lausanne). 2018;9:454.
9. Biondi B, Kahaly GJ, Robertson RP. Thyroid dysfunction and diabetes mellitus: two closely associated disorders. Endocr Rev. 2019;40(3):789-824.
10. Chubb SA, Davis WA, Inman Z, Davis TM. Prevalence and progression of subclinical hypothyroidism in women with type 2 diabetes: the Fremantle Diabetes Study. Clin Endocrinol (Oxf). 2005;62(4):480-6.
11. Marwaha RK, Garg MK, Tandon N, Kanwar R, Narang A, Sastry A, et al. Glutamic acid decarboxylase (anti-GAD) & tissue transglutaminase (anti-TTG) antibodies in patients with thyroid autoimmunity. Indian J Med Res. 2013;137(1):82-6.
12. Gronich N, Deftereos SN, Lavi I, Persidis AS, Abernethy DR, Rennert G. Hypothyroidism is a risk factor for new-onset diabetes: a cohort study. Diabetes Care. 2015;38(9):1657-64.
13. Asvold BO, Bjøro T, Vatten LJ. Association of thyroid function with estimated glomerular filtration rate in a population-based study: the HUNT study. Eur J Endocrinol. 2010;164(1):101-5.
14. Wu J, Yue S, Geng J, Liu L, Teng W, Liu L, Chen L. Relationship between diabetic retinopathy and subclinical hypothyroidism: a meta-analysis. Sci Rep. 2015;5(1):12212.
15. Vigersky RA, Filmore-Nassar A, Glass AR. Thyrotropin suppression by metformin. The J Clin Endocrinol Metab. 2006;91(1):225-7.
16. Mason RL, Hunt HM, Hurxthal L. Blood cholesterol values in hyperthyroidism and hypothyroidism—their significance. N Engl J Med. 1930;203(26):1273-8.
17. Pearce EN. Hypothyroidism and dyslipidemia: modern concepts and approaches. Curr Cardiol Rep. 2004;6(6):451-6.
18. Khan FA, Patil SK, Thakur AS, Khan MF, Murugan K. Lipid Profile in Thyroid Dysfunction: A Study on Patients of Bastar. J Clin Anal Med. 2014;5(1):12-4.
19. Kaliaperumal R, William E, Selvam T, Krishnan SM. Relationship between lipoprotein(a) and thyroid hormones in hypothyroid patients. J Clin Diagn Res. 2014;8(2):37-9.

20. Joshi SR, Anjana RM, Deepa M, Pradeepa R, Bhansali A, Dhandania VK, et al. Prevalence of dyslipidemia in urban and rural India: the ICMR–INDIAB study. PloS One. 2014;9(5):e96808.
21. Tanaci N, Ertugrul DT, Sahin M, Yucel M, Olcay I, Demirag NG, et al. Postprandial lipemia as a risk factor for cardiovascular disease in patients with hypothyroidism. Endocrine. 2006;29(3):451-6.
22. Marwaha RK, Tandon N, Garg MK, Kanwar R, Sastry A, Narang A, et al. Dyslipidemia in subclinical hypothyroidism in an Indian population. Clin Biochem. 2011;44(14-15):1214-7.
23. Liu H, Peng D. Update on dyslipidemia in hypothyroidism: the mechanism of dyslipidemia in hypothyroidism. Endocr Connect. 2022;11(2):e210002.
24. Villar HC, Saconato H, Valente O, Atallah ÁN. Thyroid hormone replacement for subclinical hypothyroidism. Cochrane Database Syst Rev. 2007(3):CD003419.
25. Kotwal A, Cortes T, Genere N, Hamidi O, Jasim S, Newman CB, et al. Treatment of thyroid dysfunction and serum lipids: a systematic review and meta-analysis. J Clin Endocrinol Metab. 2020;105(12):dgaa672.
26. Garber JR, Cobin RH, Gharib H, Hennessey JV, Klein I, Mechanick JI, et al. Clinical practice guidelines for hypothyroidism in adults: cosponsored by the American Association of Clinical Endocrinologists and the American Thyroid Association. Thyroid. 2012;22(12):1200-35.
27. Bekkering GE, Agoritsas T, Lytvyn L, Heen AF, Feller M, Moutzouri E, et al. Thyroid hormones treatment for subclinical hypothyroidism: a clinical practice guideline. BMJ. 2019;365:l2006.
28. Sue LY, Leung AM. Levothyroxine for the treatment of subclinical hypothyroidism and cardiovascular disease. Front Endocrinol. 2020;11:591588.
29. Ning N, Gao D, Triggiani V, Iacoviello M, Mitchell JE, Ma R, et al. Prognostic role of hypothyroidism in heart failure: a meta-analysis. Medicine (Baltimore). 2015;94(30):e1159.
30. Yancy CW, Jessup M, Bozkurt B, Butler J, Casey DE, Colvin MM, et al. 2016 ACC/AHA/HFSA focused update on new pharmacological therapy for heart failure: an update of the 2013 ACCF/AHA guideline for the management of heart failure: a report of the American College of Cardiology/American Heart Association Task Force on Clinical Practice Guidelines and the Heart Failure Society of America. J Am Coll Cardiol. 2016;68(13):1476-88.
31. He W, An X, Li L, Shao X, Li Q, Yao Q, et al. Relationship between hypothyroidism and non-alcoholic fatty liver disease: a systematic review and meta-analysis. Front Endocrinol. 2017;8:335.
32. Liu L, Yu Y, Zhao M, Zheng D, Zhang X, Guan Q, et al. Benefits of levothyroxine replacement therapy on nonalcoholic fatty liver disease in subclinical hypothyroidism patients. Int J Endocrinol. 2017;2017:5753039.
33. Bode H, Ivens B, Bschor T, Schwarzer G, Henssler J, Baethge C. Association of hypothyroidism and clinical depression: A systematic review and meta-analysis. JAMA Psychiatry. 2021;78(12):1375-83.
34. Müller TD, Clemmensen C, Finan B, DiMarchi RD, Tschöp MH. Anti-obesity therapy: from rainbow pills to polyagonists. Pharmacol Rev. 2018;70(4):712-46.
35. Knudsen N, Laurberg P, Rasmussen LB, Bülow I, Perrild H, Ovesen L, et al. Small differences in thyroid function may be important for body mass index and the occurrence of obesity in the population. J Clin Endocrinol Metab. 2005;90(7):4019-24.
36. Verma A, Jayaraman M, Kumar HK, Modi KD. Hypothyroidism and obesity. Cause or Effect? Saudi Med J. 2008;29(8):1135-8.
37. Rosenbaum M, Hirsch J, Murphy E, Leibel RL. Effects of changes in body weight on carbohydrate metabolism, catecholamine excretion, and thyroid function. Am J Clin Nutr. 2000;71(6):1421-32.
38. Al-Adsani H, Hoffer LJ, Silva JE. Resting energy expenditure is sensitive to small dose changes in patients on chronic thyroid hormone replacement. J Clin Endocrinol Metab. 1997;82(4):1118-25.
39. Bianco AC, Maia AL, Da Silva WS, Christoffolete MA. Adaptive activation of thyroid hormone and energy expenditure. Biosci Rep. 2005;25(3-4):191-208.
40. Reinehr T, de Sousa G, Andler W. Hyperthyrotropinemia in obese children is reversible after weight loss and is not related to lipids. J Clin Endocrinol Metab. 2006;91(8):3088-91.
41. Menendez C, Baldelli R, Camina JP, Escudero B, Peino R, Dieguez C, et al. TSH stimulates leptin secretion by a direct effect on adipocytes. J Endocrinol. 2003;176(1):7-12.
42. Reinehr T. Obesity and thyroid function. Mol Cell Endocrinol. 2010;316(2):165-71.

SECTION 4

Disorders of Thyroid Hormone Excess

CHAPTER 12

Clinical Evaluation and Manifestations of Thyroid Hormone Excess

Mini G Pillai, Abilash Nair, Ashwin Valliyot

INTRODUCTION

Thyroid disorders form a major chunk of disease burden worldwide, including India. The prevalence of overt hyperthyroidism ranges from 0.2 to 1.3% in iodine-sufficient parts of the world.

In a community-based epidemiological investigation done in Kochi, the prevalence of subclinical and overt hyperthyroidism was 1.6% and 1.3% respectively.

Subclinical and overt hyperthyroidism were found in 1.6% and 1.2% of participants in a hospital-based study of women in Pondicherry; among these patients antithyroid peroxidase (anti-TPO) antibodies were positive in 33% and goiter was present in 39%.

DISEASES CAUSING THYROID HORMONE EXCESS

Thyrotoxicosis is a clinical state characterized by excess serum and tissue concentrations of thyroxine (T4), triiodothyronine (T3), or both. Hyperthyroidism refers specifically to thyrotoxicosis resulting from hyperactivity of the thyroid gland. Thyrotoxicosis is considered "overt" when the serum thyroid-stimulating hormone (TSH) level is low or undetectable and serum T4 (free or total T4) level, T3, or both are above the reference range, and "subclinical" when the TSH level is low or undetectable but levels of both T4 (free or total T4) and T3 are within the reference range.

GRAVES' DISEASE

Graves' disease (GD) is the most common cause for hyperthyroidism in Iodine replete populations. The disease is caused by TSH receptor autoantibodies (TR-Abs). Stimulating TR-Ab cause hyperthyroidism. Blocking and neutral TR-Ab may also be present in affected individuals. Antithyroid peroxidase antibodies and antithyroglobulin antibodies are also often found elevated though only TR-Ab is causative. The incidence of GD is about 40/100,000 per year. GD is more common in women than in men and is most common in patients aged 30–50 years. In addition to hyperthyroidism, extrathyroid symptoms may be present, including Graves' ophthalmopathy, thyroid dermopathy, and acropachy. Apart from a strong genetic component, various environmental factors such as smoking, excess iodine, ionizing radiation, excessive emotional or physical stress, selenium or vitamin D deficiency and certain infectious agents such as *Yersinia enterocolitica* and hepatitis C virus also predispose to GD. The postpartum period is associated with an increased risk of flare up of autoimmune diseases including GD with maximum risk at 6–12 months postpartum.

Graves' disease is characterized by a soft diffuse goiter with signs of increased thyroid perfusion like bruit or thrill over the thyroid. However, the gland may be nonpalpable in many patients, especially the elderly. Whereas ocular signs of adrenergic hyperactivity such as retracted eyelids and lid lag may be present in thyroid hormone excess of any etiology, signs such as periorbital puffiness, conjunctival congestion, chemosis, restricted eye movements, and exophthalmos are specific markers of Graves' ophthalmic involvement **(Fig. 1)**.

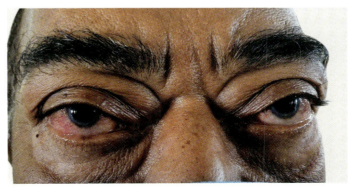

Fig. 1: Graves orbitopathy: Patient with eyelid swelling and erythema, conjunctival redness, and chemosis.

Thyroid dermopathy or pretibial myxedema is an infrequent manifestation of GD forming the third component of the classic triad of Graves' disease (goiter, ophthalmopathy, and dermopathy) present in 0.5–5% of patients. It is usually seen in patients with high titer of TR-Ab and is invariably associated with ophthalmopathy. The incidence of pretibial myxedema has declined probably because of early detection and treatment of GD. The propensity for pretibial site is thought to be due to its dependent position and mechanical factors. Apart from pretibial area, thyroid dermopathy can involve ankle, dorsum of foot, elbows, knees, upper back and neck, and the lesions are characterized by skin thickening, pigmentation, and hyperhidrosis, giving an indurated waxy appearance with prominent hair follicles. They are usually bilaterally symmetrical **(Fig. 2)**, occasionally painful or pruritic, and are more common in females and after middle age. About 20% of patients with dermopathy have thyroid acropachy making it the least common extrathyroidal manifestation of GD. Acropachy is characterized by clubbing of fingers and toes and less commonly there is fusiform soft tissue swelling of digits and toes with periosteal reaction seen radiologically. Metacarpals and metatarsals also may be involved causing diffuse soft tissue swelling of hands and feet.

Graves' disease may also be associated with other autoimmune conditions such as pernicious anemia, vitiligo, type 1 diabetes mellitus (T1DM), autoimmune adrenal insufficiency, systemic sclerosis, myasthenia gravis, Sjögren syndrome, rheumatoid arthritis, and systemic lupus erythematosus which may have their own set of clinical manifestations.

Hashitoxicosis is the rare initial thyrotoxic phase of Hashimoto's thyroiditis. Diffuse goiter may be present, but the signs of increased vascularity are absent clinically as well as sonologically as opposed to Graves' disease. The thyrotoxic phase may last for a few weeks to months and may recur after a period of hypothyroidism. This rare entity may be confused with Graves' disease because of the overlap in antibody profile. Hashitoxicosis is the second most common of thyroid hormone excess in childhood and adolescence.

TOXIC ADENOMA AND MULTINODULAR GOITER

These constitute true thyroid autonomy where thyrocytes hyperfunction independent of TSH receptor stimulation by TSH or TR-Ab. Activating somatic mutations of genes for TSH receptor have been identified in many toxic adenomas as well as nodules of toxic multinodular goiter (MNG). Toxic MNG is the most frequent form of thyroid autonomy and is more common in regions of the world that are relatively iodine deficient. The natural course of goiter is from diffuse thyroid hypertrophy to the development of one or more nodules and ultimately autonomic function of one or more of these nodules with resultant thyrotoxicosis. Because this natural history is generally long, patients with thyrotoxicosis often describe the presence of goiter for years. While GD is the more common etiology in young people with hyperthyroidism, toxic MNG tends to occur more in older age groups. Like most thyroid diseases, toxic adenomas and toxic MNG are also more common in females **(Fig. 3)**.

Solitary toxic thyroid adenomas are generally benign lesions of the thyroid gland. Most guidelines do not recommend fine needle aspiration cytology (FNAC) if scintigraphy shows a toxic nodule. However, malignancy has been reported in many toxic nodules and a recent meta-analysis found that the odds of the nodule harboring malignancy was reduced by 55% in a hot nodule, but was still clinically relevant.

SUBACUTE THYROIDITIS

Subacute thyroiditis (SAT) (also called subacute granulomatous thyroiditis, subacute nonsuppurative thyroiditis, giant cell thyroiditis, painful thyroiditis, or de Quervain's thyroiditis) is a thyroid inflammatory disease, characterized by neck pain or discomfort, a tender diffuse goiter, and a

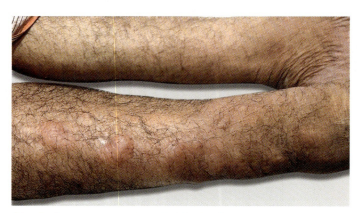

Fig. 2: Graves dermopathy: Multiple plaques and orange peel appearance on the anterior surface of leg.

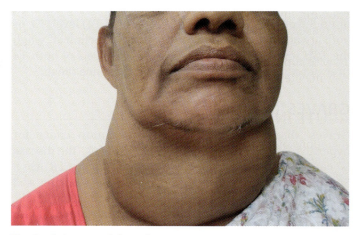

Fig. 3: Goiter—nodular goiter.

predictable course of self-limited thyroid hormone excess. Viral infection is considered the usual SAT triggering factor. Viruses associated with the occurrence of SAT include coxsackieviruses, echoviruses, adenoviruses, influenza viruses, mumps and rubella viruses, parvovirus B19, orthomyxovirus, human immunodeficiency virus (HIV), Epstein–Barr virus, hepatitis E, dengue, and measles virus. Severe acute respiratory syndrome coronavirus 2 (SARS-CoV-2) also frequently causes SAT.

The typical clinical picture of SAT is characterized by history of concomitant or preceding viral infection, presence of anterior neck pain often radiating to the jaw, ear, occiput and upper mediastinum, fever especially at night, marked thyroid tenderness, and a diffuse goiter. This first phase is occasionally also associated with symptoms and signs of thyroid hormone excess such as palpitations and tremors. The fever and pain resolves in the second phase and the thyroid hormone excess gradually comes down. The third phase is a phase of transient hypothyroidism. Each of these phases can last for 2–8 weeks.

Subacute thyroiditis can occur in childhood though rarer compared to adults. A 5-year-old presenting with painful neck swelling, dysphagia, hoarseness of voice, and respiratory distress due to the goiter has been reported from Mangalore recently.

Painless presentation of SAT is frequently recognized off late. This is especially so after the onset of SARS-CoV-2 pandemic where painless thyroiditis has been reported frequently. In a large single center cohort of Post-COVID-19 patients from Eastern India, the incidence of painful and painless SAT was almost equal.

In view of the delay in diagnosis of SAT, often missed by the primary care physicians in addition to the danger of making a false positive diagnosis of SAT in patients with destruction of thyroid and pain caused by capsule invasion due to advanced local malignancies such as anaplastic carcinoma or metastatic disease, a set of diagnostic criteria has recently been proposed. There are two essential major criteria—elevated erythrocyte sedimentation rate (ESR) or C-reactive protein (CRP) and ultrasound scan thyroid showing hypoechoic areas with blurred margin and decreased vascularity along with one of five additional criteria namely thyroid swelling, painful tender gland, elevated Free T4 with suppressed TSH, decreased radioiodine uptake and fine-needle aspiration biopsy (FNAB) result typical of SAT.

ACUTE INFECTIOUS THYROIDITIS

Infections of the thyroid gland are rare. Its innate resistance to infections can be attributed to the rich blood supply, good lymphatic drainage, high iodine content, and presence of capsule. High clinical suspicion is required as a delay in diagnosis can lead to significant morbidity and mortality. Major pathogens include the gram-positive *Staphylococcus aureus* and *Streptococcus* species; however, gram-negative organisms have been found especially in immunocompromised hosts. As in SAT, thyroid hormone excess in this entity also occurs due to release of preformed hormones.

HYPERTHYROIDISM IN PREGNANCY

In women, hyperthyroidism is related to menstrual cycle disorders (oligomenorrhea, amenorrhea) and infertility. As a result, pregnancy in a woman with hyperthyroidism is relatively uncommon. Most of hyperthyroidism in pregnancy is due to Graves' disease though toxic nodular goiters and toxic adenomas are also seen less frequently.

When the diagnosis of hyperthyroidism is made during the first trimester of pregnancy, the human chorionic gonadotropin (HCG)-mediated hyperthyroidism, namely gestational transient thyrotoxicosis (GTT), must be taken into account (prevalence 1–11% of pregnancies). In most cases, this is a subclinical hyperthyroidism, which appears after the 6th week of pregnancy due to the physiological rise in HCG secretion; HCG shares structural homology with TSH and stimulates maternal thyroid function, resulting in decreased TSH levels. GTT has a spontaneous resolution by 14–18 weeks of gestation as HCG values decrease. GTT is more common in conditions with more trophoblastic tissue as in multiple gestations, hyperemesis gravidarum, hydatidiform mole, and choriocarcinoma. Many of the clinical features associated with hyperthyroidism such as anxiety, palpitation, heat intolerance, increased sweating, weight loss in spite of increased appetite, tremors, and goiter may be present in a euthyroid pregnancy. Presence of a markedly enlarged or nodular gland, characteristic eye disease, or dermopathy of GD and markers of thyroid autoimmunity like TR-Ab can help in differentiating hyperthyroidism complicating pregnancy from GTT.

POSTPARTUM THYROIDITIS

The characteristic sequence of postpartum thyroiditis is transient thyrotoxic phase which usually begins 1–4 months after delivery and lasts 2–8 weeks, followed by hypothyroidism which lasts 2 weeks to 6 months followed by recovery. Symptoms and signs are mostly mild and consist mainly of fatigue, weight loss, irritability, etc. The prevalence has been reported as 7% in a study from Urban Kashmir.

DRUG-INDUCED THYROID HORMONE EXCESS

Drug-induced thyroid hormone excess may be due to increased thyroid hormone synthesis due to increased iodine supply, precipitation of thyroid autoimmunity causing Graves' disease, or destructive thyroiditis.
- Amiodarone is a class III antiarrhythmic drug widely used in treating atrial and ventricular arrhythmias; 100 mg amiodarone releases about 3 mg inorganic iodine

into the circulation. It is a lipophilic drug concentrated in adipose tissue, cardiac and skeletal muscle, and the thyroid. Elimination half-life is approximately 100 days and hence toxicity can occur well after stopping the drug. Amiodarone treatment is associated with thyroid dysfunction in up to 30%. Two types of thyroid hormone excess can occur with amiodarone therapy. Type 1 amiodarone-induced thyrotoxicosis (AIT) is seen in people with preexisting MNG or latent GD. Large amounts of iodine contained in amiodarone provides increased substrate for thyroid hormone synthesis and hyperthyroidism results. Type II AIT is a destructive thyroiditis that results in release of preformed hormones and usually occurs in people without underlying thyroid disease. Both types of AIT increases with higher cumulative doses of amiodarone and can occur years after initiating treatment. Mixed forms of AIT can also occur making the diagnosis and treatment more difficult. AIT can cause decompensation and exacerbation of underlying cardiac abnormalities, leading to increased morbidity and mortality, especially in patients with poor left ventricular function.

- *Checkpoint inhibitors*: Immune checkpoint inhibitors are agents used mostly for cancer chemotherapy and act by causing an immune attack on the tumor cells. The enhanced immune function seen with these agents can lead to a variety of immune-related adverse events including thyroid dysfunction. Self-limiting thyroiditis causing transient thyrotoxicosis as well as Graves have been reported with CTLA4 inhibitors such as ipilimumab and tremelimumab as well as PD1 inhibitors like nivolumab.
- Tyrosine kinase inhibitors such as sunitinib, sorafenib, imatinib, and axitinib are also associated with self-limiting thyroiditis and more rarely, Graves.
- *Cytokine-based therapy*: Interferon α and interleukin 2 can cause destructive thyroiditis and rarely, GD. Adalimumab, a TNF-α inhibitor has also been associated with SAT.
- Alemtuzumab, a recombinant anti-CD52 monoclonal antibody used as an immunosuppressive agent as well as in chemotherapy of certain leukemias has been associated with GD as well as subacute thyroiditis. Usually, the thyroid dysfunction occurs during the immune reactivation phase after discontinuation of therapy.
- Thalidomide analog lenalidomide used as an immunomodulator in certain hematological malignancies is also associated with transient thyroiditis.

THYROTROPIN-INDUCED HYPERTHYROIDISM

Conditions causing TSH-induced thyroid hormone excess are TSH-secreting pituitary adenomas (TSH-omas) and thyroid hormone resistance at the pituitary level (PRTH). Both conditions are associated with goiter, more often diffuse, but also occasionally nodular, and mild manifestations of thyroid hormone excess. Family history may be present in PRTH. TSH-omas often present with headache or visual field disturbances. Menstrual disturbances in females, galactorrhea, and acromegaly due to cosecretion of prolactin and growth hormone respectively are other presenting features of TSH-omas.

THYROTOXICOSIS OF EXTRATHYROIDAL ORIGIN

The most common cause for this is probably intentional iatrogenic TSH suppression therapy with levothyroxine used to prevent recurrence in differentiated thyroid cancer. More rarely thyrotoxicosis is caused by surreptitious ingestion of thyroid hormones or desiccated thyroid extract. Hamburger thyrotoxicosis is thyroid hormone excess resulting from ingestion of beef contaminated with bovine thyroid gland.

Struma ovarii is an ovarian teratoma composed predominantly of mature thyroid tissue. It accounts for 5% of all ovarian teratomas. Usually, women aged 40–60 years are affected and present with pain, pelvic mass, and less frequently with ascites or features of thyroid hormone excess. Some of these, especially the larger ones, may be malignant; mostly papillary and occasionally follicular carcinoma has been reported.

Functioning metastatic thyroid carcinoma can also cause thyroid hormone excess.

LIFESTYLE FACTORS CAUSING THYROID HORMONE EXCESS

Smoking

Most investigations on the effects of smoking on TSH and thyroid hormone levels have found that smokers had lower TSH levels and higher T3 and T4 levels.

Gruppen et al. and Kim et al. have independently demonstrated that cigarette smoking lowers TSH levels while increasing FT3 and FT4 levels in large cohorts of 5,766 and 4,249 participants, respectively. It was seen that for every 10 ng/mL increase in serum cotinine, TSH levels dropped by 1.4% percent.

Diet

Most healthy people can tolerate high iodine intakes. But in some, too much iodine can cause thyroid autoimmune diseases leading to both hyperthyroidism and hypothyroidism as well as goiter and/or thyroid cancer. Even intake marginally above physiological needs, may make people more susceptible to thyroid diseases, especially if they already have thyroid illness or have previously been exposed to iodine deficiency.

The Jod–Basedow effect, also known as iodine-induced hyperthyroidism, is most frequently noticed after iodine supplementation or fortification in regions with extremely low iodine intake, where the risk of nodular goiter is raised. TSH hyperstimulation may happen when the thyroid gland experiences prolonged iodine deficiency as an adaptive reaction to the scarce iodine supply. One mechanism may be upregulation of thyroidal H_2O_2 production which may in turn promote mutations leading to development of clusters of autonomously functioning follicular cells.

CLINICAL FEATURES OF THYROTOXICOSIS

The clinical signs and symptoms of thyroid hormone excess are mostly unrelated to the underlying etiology but certain manifestations are seen more frequently with specific etiologies. Graves' disease, for instance, may present with eye and skin features that are unrelated to the elevated serum thyroid hormone concentrations **(Table 1)**.

Most common manifestations of thyrotoxicosis include tachycardia, tremor, nervousness, and excitability, fatigue, palpitations, hyperkinesia, increased sweating, goiter, weight loss despite increased appetite, frequent bowel movements, muscle weakness, and heat intolerance. It can also lead to concentration disorders and deterioration of learning outcomes, menstrual disorders in girls, and systolic hypertension with wide pulse pressure. Dermatological manifestations of thyrotoxicosis are generally non-specific. Smooth and shiny skin is the most common dermatological manifestation of thyrotoxicosis. Alopecia, hyperpigmentation, increased nail growth, and soft nails can also be seen. Brisk tendon reflexes and weakness of proximal muscles may be present. If left untreated, hyperthyroidism in GD progresses dynamically in the vast majority of patients; however, spontaneous remission is possible.

In the elderly, often the characteristic mental and physical hyperactivity of thyroid hormone excess is not present; often they present with lethargy and dis-

TABLE 1: Clinical features of thyroid hormone excess.	
CVS	Palpitation, tachycardia, wide pulse pressure, arrhythmias, cardiomegaly, diffuse and forceful apex beat, enhanced heart sounds, Means–Lerman scratch (scratchy systolic sound along left sternal border), cardiac failure (especially in the elderly and in presence of preexisting heart disease), thromboembolic disease, not necessarily related to AF, Takotsubo cardiomyopathy (a reversible condition occurring during periods of emotional or physical distress)
Metabolism	Increased appetite, heat intolerance and increased sweating, rarely increased basal body temperature, exacerbation of diabetes, decreased total and LDL cholesterol and triglycerides
Nervous system	Nervousness, hyperkinesia, tremors of hands, tongue, lightly closed eyelids, rarely trunk and lower limbs, brisk tendon reflexes, apathy, and lethargy in older patients (apathetic thyrotoxicosis), emotional lability, mental disturbance such as manic depressive, paranoid or schizoid reactions, cognitive impairment, inability to focus and other features mimicking attention deficit hyperactivity disorder and deterioration in school performance in children
Muscles	Muscle wasting and easy fatigability especially of the proximal muscles (thyrotoxic myopathy), association with myasthenia gravis, and hypokalemic periodic paralysis for Graves
Eyes	Lid retraction, lid lag, and globe lag in all forms of thyroid hormone excess; signs of infiltrative ophthalmopathy in Graves
Integument	Warm, moist, flushed skin, palmar erythema, hyperpigmentation, alopecia, thin brittle hair, soft friable nails, onycholysis typically of fourth and fifth fingers (Plummer's sign), association with vitiligo
Respiratory system	Breathlessness and worsening of preexisting chronic lung diseases resulting from decreased vital capacity due to weakness of respiratory muscles coupled with increased oxygen consumption of the hypermetabolic state
Skeletal system	Pathologic fractures especially in elderly women due to accelerated bone loss consequent to increased excretion of Ca and P in urine and stool and increase in bone turnover
Fluid and electrolyte balance	Polyuria, nocturia, hypokalemia associated with periodic paralysis, mild hypercalcemia
Alimentary system	Increased appetite with weight loss, increased frequency of bowel movements, rarely diarrhea, mild steatorrhea, nausea, vomiting, hepatic dysfunction, association with celiac disease, and pernicious anemia for Graves
Hematopoietic system	Splenomegaly, hypercoagulability which can cause thromboembolic phenomena, increased clearance of vitamin K-dependent clotting factors causing enhanced sensitivity to warfarin, normocytic normochromic anemia, and relative neutropenia with lymphocytosis in Graves
Other endocrine organs	Increased cortisol clearance, increased risk of breast and thyroid cancer
Reproductive system	Delayed sexual maturation, menstrual disturbances, subfertility in both sexes, increased risk of miscarriages, gynecomastia and erectile dysfunction in men

(AF: atrial fibrillation; CVS: cardiovascular system; LDL: low-density lipoprotein)

interestedness. This is called apathetic or masked thyrotoxicosis. Weight loss without increased appetite, wasting of muscles, cardiac failure, arrhythmias, motional lability, and occasionally osteoporosis may be the presenting features. Children on the other hand, often do not have weight loss and may have weight gain along with increased appetite.

If left untreated, hyperthyroidism in GD progresses dynamically in the vast majority of patients; however, spontaneous remission is possible.

CONCLUSION

Thyroid hormone excess is one of the common thyroid disorders seen worldwide. It may be transient and self-limiting as in subacute thyroiditis or may have a more prolonged course as in Graves' disease. Associated clinical features often help to identify the pathology behind thyroid hormone excess.

SUGGESTED READINGS

1. Garmendia Madariaga A, Santos Palacios S, Guillen-Grima F, Galofre JC. The incidence and prevalence of thyroid dysfunction in Europe: a meta-analysis. J Clin Endocrinol Metab. 2014;99: 923-31.
2. Usha Menon V, Sundaram KR, Unnikrishnan AG, Jayakumar RV, Nair V, Kumar H. High prevalence of undetected thyroid disorders in an iodine sufficient adult south Indian population. J Indian Med Assoc. 2009;107:72-7.
3. Abraham R, Murugan VS, Pukazhvanthen P, Sen SK. Thyroid Disorders in Women of Puducherry. Indian J Clin Biochem. 2009;24:52-9.
4. Devereaux D, Tewelde SZ. Hyperthyroidism and thyrotoxicosis. Emerg Med Clin North Am. 2014;32:277-92.
5. Ehlers M, Schott M, Allelein S. Graves, disease in clinical perspective. Front. Biosci (Landmark Ed). 2019;24(1):33-45.
6. Niedziela M. Hyperthyroidism in adolescents. Endocr Connect. 2021;10(11):R279-R292.
7. Samuels MH. Hyperthyroidism in Aging. In: Feingold KR, Anawalt B, Boyce A, et al. (Eds). Endotext [Internet]. South Dartmouth (MA): MDText.com, Inc; 2000.
8. Lau LW, Ghaznavil S, Frolkis AD, Stephenson A, Robertson HL, Rabi DM, et al. Malignancy risk of hyperfunctioning thyroid nodules compared with non-toxic nodules: systematic review and a meta-analysis. Thyroid Res. 2021;14:3.
9. Desailloud R, Hober D, Virol J. Viruses and thyroiditis: an update. Virol J. 2009;6:57.
10. Stasiak M, Lewiński A. New aspects in the pathogenesis and management of subacute thyroiditis. Rev Endocr Metab Disord. 2021;22(4):1027-39.
11. Ogawa E, Katsushima Y, Fujiwara I, Iinuma K. Subacute thyroiditis in children: patient report and review of the literature. J Pediatr Endocrinol Metab. 2003;16(6):897-900.
12. Ramineni P, Kamath SP, Josji J, Rao S. Subacute thyroiditis with airway compromise in a 5-year-old boy. BMJ Case Rep. 2020;13(11):e236909.
13. Mondal S, Dasgupta R, Lodh M, Ganguly A. Subacute thyroiditis following recovery from COVID-19 infection: novel clinical findings from an Eastern Indian cohort. Postgrad Med J. 2022:postgradmedj-2021-141429.
14. Siddiqui N, Deletic N, Raal F, Mohamed F. Acute Suppurative Thyroiditis Secondary to *Escherichia coli* Infection. Eur J Case Rep Intern Med. 2021;8(11):003009.
15. Zargar AH, Shah IH, Masoodi SR, Laway BA, Salahuddin M, Bhat IA. Postpartum thyroiditis in India: prevalence of postpartum thyroiditis in Kashmir Valley of Indian sub-continent. Exp Clin Endocrinol Diabetes. 2002;110(4):171-5.
16. Bhattacharya S, Goyal A, Kaur P, Singh R, Kalra S. Anticancer Drug-induced Thyroid Dysfunction. Eur Endocrinol. 2020;16(1):32-9.
17. Nakagawa J, Fujikawa K, Akagi M, Nakaji K, Yasui J, Hanatani Y, et al. Subacute thyroiditis in a patient with psoriatic arthritis switched from secukinumab to adalimumab: a case report and literature review. Mod Rheumatol Case Rep. 2021;5:36-9.
18. Gruppen EG, Kootstra-Ros J, Kobold AM, Connelly MA, Touw D, Bos JHJ, et al. Cigarette smoking is associated with higher thyroid hormone and lower TSH levels: The PREVEND study. Endocrine. 2020;67:613-22.
19. Kim SJ, Kim MJ, Yoon SG, Myong JP, Yu HW, Chai YJ, et al. Impact of smoking on thyroid gland: Dose-related effect of urinary cotinine levels on thyroid function and thyroid autoimmunity. Sci Rep. 2019;9(1):4213.
20. Laurberg P, Cerqueira C, Ovesen L, Rasmussen LB, Perrild H, Andersen S, et al. Iodine intake as a determinant of thyroid disorders in populations. Best Pract Res Clin Endocrinol Metab. 2010;24:13-27.

CHAPTER 13

Management of Thyroid Hormone Excess

K Neelaveni, Beatrice Anne

INTRODUCTION

The term "thyrotoxicosis" refers to a clinical condition that results from inappropriate circulating thyroid hormone (TH) excess irrespective of the cause. The term "hyperthyroidism" is a form of thyrotoxicosis and it is used when the TH excess is due to inappropriately increased synthesis and secretion of the TH from the thyroid gland. Hyperthyroidism can be "subclinical" or "overt" depending on the biochemical severity. Subclinical hyperthyroidism is defined as with low to undetectable thyroid-stimulating hormone (TSH) and normal levels of T3/FT3 and T4/FT4, whereas overt hyperthyroidism is defined as with low to undetectable TSH with elevated T3/FT3, T4/FT4. The presentation of thyrotoxicosis may vary with respect to clinical features and their severity, hence, there may be a delay in the diagnosis. In majority of the patients, history and clinical examination alone may be sufficient to diagnose but in atypical and occult presentations, a high index of suspicion is required with appropriate investigations to establish the accurate diagnosis. The management approaches differ depending on the etiology of thyrotoxicosis, so accurate diagnosis is important for appropriate management.

ETIOLOGY

Thyroid hormone excess may be due to endogenous source or exogenous source.

Endogenous Source

Thyroidal Source
- *Overactive thyroid (TH excess synthesis and secretion)*:
  - *TSH receptor stimulation*: Graves' disease (GD), TSH receptor mutation (McCune–Albright syndrome), TSH-secreting pituitary adenoma (thyrotropinoma), resistance to thyroid hormone (RTH)
  - *Pregnancy associated*: Gestational transient thyrotoxicosis, trophoblastic disease, and familial gestational hyperthyroidism (mutant TSH receptor)
  - *Autonomous thyroid hormone synthesis and secretion*: Toxic adenoma (TA), toxic multinodular goiter (TMNG)
- *Inflammation and destruction of thyroid (preformed TH release)*: Subacute thyroiditis, painless thyroiditis, drug associated [amiodarone, interferon α (IFNα), tyrosine kinase inhibitor (TKI)], and acute thyroiditis

Extrathyroidal Source

Struma ovarii, functioning thyroid metastases.

Exogenous Source

Iatrogenic, excessive self-administration of TH, food, and supplements containing excess TH.

EVALUATION OF SUSPECTED CASE OF THYROID HORMONE EXCESS

Comprehensive history and physical examination are paramount in suspected case of thyrotoxicosis.

History

Onset and progression of symptoms of thyrotoxicosis, etiological history, family history, symptoms suggestive of other systemic involvement, and smoking.

Physical Examination

Bodyweight, vital signs, goiter size, symmetry, nodularity, tenderness, eye manifestations **(Figs. 1 to 4)**, pedal edema, and pretibial myxedema should be assessed along with respiratory, cardiac, and neuromuscular assessment.

Biochemical Evaluation

Diagnosis of Thyrotoxicosis (Flowchart 1)
- *TSH*: Serum TSH measurement is more sensitive in the evaluation of suspected case of thyrotoxicosis.

SECTION 4
DISORDERS OF THYROID HORMONE EXCESS

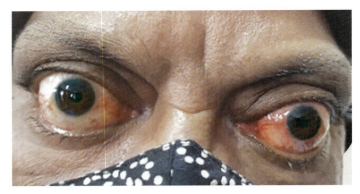

Fig. 1: Patient with active graves ophthalmopathy, conjunctival redness, chemosis left eye.

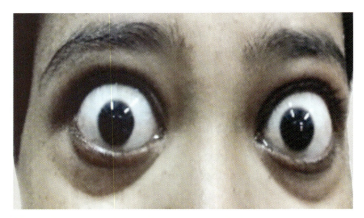

Fig. 2: Patient with bilateral severe exophthalmos.

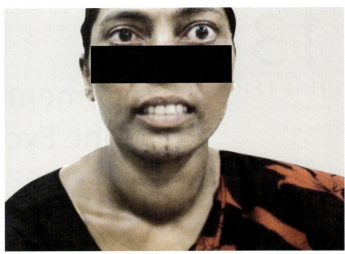

Fig. 3: Patient with diffuse goiter with unilateral exophthalmos.

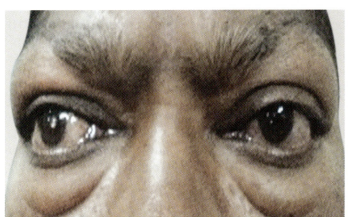

Fig. 4: Graves' ophthalmopathy with periorbital swelling.

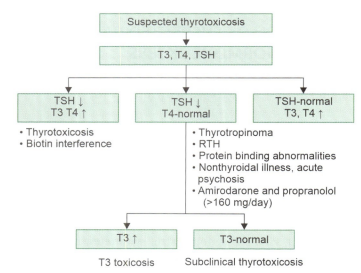

Flowchart 1: Diagnostic scheme for a suspected case of thyrotoxicosis.
(RTH: resistance to thyroid hormone; TSH: thyroid-stimulating hormone)

The relationship between freeT4 and TSH with intact hypothalamic–pituitary–thyroid axis is an inverse log linear one, so small changes in T4 concentrations result in large changes in serum TSH concentrations.

- o *Limitations*:
  - Serum TSH may be normal or elevated in:
    - TSH secreting pituitary adenoma
    - Some phenotypes of RTH
  - Serum TSH is low in:
    - Central hypothyroidism
    - Nonthyroidal illness
    - First trimester of pregnancy

  Hence, low serum TSH alone is not pathognomonic of thyrotoxicosis.

- *Measurement of serum free and total T3, and free and total T4*: Elevated T3 and T4 are useful for detecting and monitoring therapy of thyrotoxicosis
  - o *Limitations*:
    - Euthyroid hyperthyroxinemia
    - Serum T3 and T4 concentrations may be normal in subclinical thyrotoxicosis

  Hence, elevated serum T3 and T4 alone are not pathognomonic of thyrotoxicosis.

Free T4 and T3 measurement: Equilibrium dialysis and ultrafiltration are the most accurate methods for serum FT4 measurement. Assays for measuring FT3 are less robust and not widely validated than those for FT4. Hence, total T3 measurement is frequently preferred over FT3 in clinical practice.

Measurement of serum TSH together with FT3/T3 and FT4/T4 at the initial screening improves the diagnostic accuracy in a suspected case of thyrotoxicosis.

T3/T4 ratio in determining the etiology of thyrotoxicosis: The relative elevations of serum T3 and T4 concentrations may give a clue to the etiology of thyrotoxicosis. Excessive T3 production is common in GD and toxic nodular goiter with T3 (ng/dL):T4 (μg/dL) ratio of >20, T4 predominant thyrotoxicosis with T3:T4 ratio <15 suggests thyroiditis.

Euthyroid Hyperthyroxinemia versus TSH-secreting Adenoma and RTH

Euthyroid hyperthyroxinemia: It refers to elevated T3 and T4 with normal TSH, is due to thyroid-binding protein abnormalities. Most of the T4 (99.97%) in the serum is bound to thyroxine-binding globulin (TBG), transthyretin, prealbumin, or albumin. An increase in the concentrations of any of these proteins especially TBG can cause elevated T3 and T4 levels (hyperthyroxinemia) which can be misinterpreted as thyrotoxicosis.

- Causes:
  - Increased protein binding **(Table 1)**
  - Assay interference (anti-T4 immunoglobulins, biotin)
  - Drugs inhibiting the T4 → T3 conversion (propranolol ≥160 mg/day, amiodarone)
  - Nonthyroidal illness, acute psychosis

Thyroid-stimulating hormone-secreting pituitary adenoma (thyrotropinoma): It should be suspected when T3 and T4 are elevated with normal or elevated TSH levels. In suspected cases, pituitary lesion on magnetic resonance imaging (MRI) and high ratio of serum α-subunit to TSH supports the diagnosis.

Resistance to thyroid hormone: Clinical features with elevated T3 and T4 with normal or elevated TSH.
- Family history
- Genetic testing supports the diagnosis

Biotin effect on thyroid function test (TFT): High doses of biotin ingestion may cause false results in assays that utilize a streptavidin-biotin separation technique. In competitive binding assays, which are used to measure T4, excess biotin competes with biotinylated analog and results in falsely high values. In immunometric assay, which measures TSH, biotin displaces biotinylated antibodies and cause falsely low TSH levels. Biotin supplements should be stopped for at least 2 days then repeat the measurements to get true results.

Determination of Etiology

In majority of the patients, history and clinical examination along with initial biochemical evaluation with T3, T4, and TSH alone are sufficient to make a diagnosis. In a patient with clinical and biochemical thyrotoxicosis with diffuse goiter with thyroid-associated orbitopathy, the diagnosis of GD is clear, no further testing is required in such a scenario. If the diagnosis is not clear based on the initial clinical and biochemical evaluation the following diagnostic testing is indicated depending on the clinical scenario, available expertise, and resources.

Radioactive Iodine Uptake/Tc99 Pertechnetate Thyroid Scan

Radioactive iodine uptake (RAIU) measures the percentage of administered radioactive iodine (RAI), which gets concentrated into the thyroid gland after 24 hours. Technetium-99 pertechnetate is trapped by the thyroid gland but not organified. A technetium uptake measures the percentage of administered technetium that is trapped by the thyroid gland after 20 minutes. This is contraindicated

TABLE 1: Causes of euthyroid hyperthyroxinemia due to increased serum protein binding.

↑TBG concentration	↑Transthyretin concentration	Albumin (mutated form)
Inherited (X-linked trait)	Inherited	Familial dysalbuminemic hyperthyroxinemia
Hyperestrogenic states (pregnancy, exogenous, tumoral production)	• Carcinoma • Pancreas • Hepatoma	
Hepatitis		
HIV		
Drugs: 5-fluorouracil, clofibrate, heroin, methadone		

(HIV: human immunodeficiency virus; TBG: thyroxine-binding globulin)

TABLE 2: Radionuclide imaging in the differential diagnosis of thyrotoxicosis.

Normal or ↑RAIU over the neck	Low RAIU over the neck
• GD • TA/TMNG • TSH-secreting pituitary adenoma • Trophoblastic thyrotoxicosis • RTH (T3 receptor β mutation)	• Painless (silent) thyroiditis • Subacute (granulomatous, de Quervain's thyroiditis) • Acute thyroiditis • Amiodarone induced • Exogenous thyroid hormone excess • Struma ovarii (uptake in ovary) • Thyroid cancer metastases (uptake in tumor metastases)

(GD: Graves' disease; RAIU: radioactive iodine uptake; RTH: resistance to thyroid hormone; TA: toxic adenoma; TMNG: toxic multinodular goiter; TSH: thyroid-stimulating hormone)

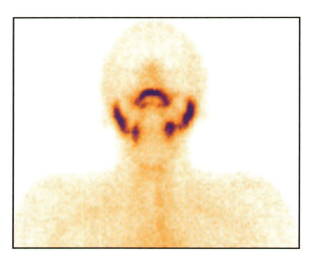

Fig. 5: Technetium-99 scan showing reduced uptake in thyroiditis.

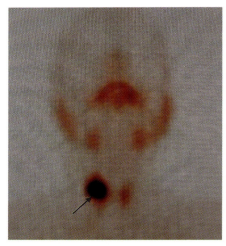

Fig. 7: Technetium-99 scan showing solitary toxic thyroid nodule.

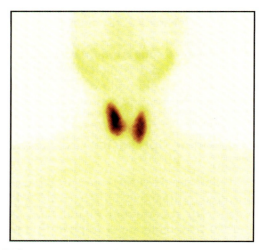

Fig. 6: Technetium-99 scan showing diffuse increased uptake in Graves' disease.

in pregnancy and lactation. Radionuclide imaging of thyroid differentiates the causes of thyrotoxicosis with low radiotracer uptake versus high uptake **(Table 2 and Figs. 5 and 6)** and also the pattern of tracer uptake helps to differentiate Graves **(Fig. 6)** from toxic nodular goiter which have a diffuse tracer uptake and focal regions of tracer uptake respectively **(Figs. 7 and 8)**.

Thyroid-stimulating Hormone Receptor Antibodies

Thyroid-stimulating Hormone Receptor Antibody Assays

TSH-binding inhibitory immunoglobulins (TBIIs): TBIIs are competition assays, which measure inhibition of labeled TSH (or labeled monoclonal anti-TSH-R antibody) binding to recombinant TSH-R by serum antibodies. TBII assays cannot distinguish the TSH-R antibody types.

Bioassays can differentiate the different (stimulating or blocking) antibodies.
- TSI or TS-Ab (thyroid-stimulating immunoglobulins) measure the cyclic adenosine monophosphate (cAMP) production by thyroid cell lines transfected with TSH-R.
- TB-Ab (thyroid blocking antibodies) measure the inhibition of cAMP production by the TSH-R transfected thyroid cell lines.

Clinical utility of TSH receptor antibody (TR-Ab)
- Diagnosis of GD, when the diagnosis is not clinically straightforward, example: euthyroid patient with unilateral proptosis.
- *Treatment*: Predict the likelihood of remission at baseline and during treatment with antithyroid drugs (ATDs) in GD.
- *Pregnancy*: Women with current or previously treated GD, to predict the risk fetal and neonatal thyrotoxicosis.

Ultrasonography with Color Flow Doppler

This test measures peak systolic velocity from inferior thyroid artery and intrathyroidal arteries, and requires expertise to locate the inferior thyroid artery and necessary adjustments to prevent artifacts. This test is particularly useful when radionuclide thyroid scan is contraindicated as in pregnancy and lactation. Doppler flow can distinguish GD from destructive thyroiditis and also useful to differentiate the subtypes of amiodarone-induced thyrotoxicosis (AIT).

Other Tests

Thyroglobulin: Serum thyroglobulin concentrations are increased in patients with hyperactive thyroid gland and thyroiditis but low or undetectable in factitious or iatrogenic thyrotoxicosis. In a suspected case of factitious thyrotoxicosis with positive antithyroglobulin antibodies which interfere with thyroglobulin measurement, an alternative approach is to measure the fecal T4 which is not widely available

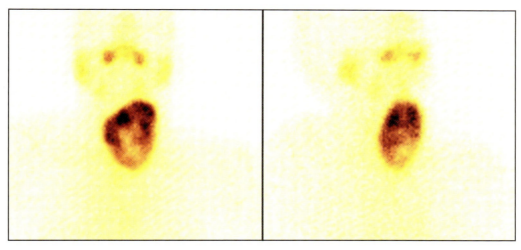

Fig. 8: Technetium-99 scan showing toxic multinodular goiter.

(euthyroid patients–1.03 nmol/g, GD–1.93 nmol/g, factitious thyrotoxicosis–12–24 nmol/g).

Erythrocyte sedimentation rate (ESR) and C-reactive protein (CRP): Most patients with subacute thyroiditis and infective thyroiditis have elevated ESR and CRP, whereas those with painless thyroiditis have normal ESR.

Interleukin 6 (IL-6): IL-6 levels are elevated in type 2 AIT. RAIU scans are not helpful to differentiate between two types of AIT. Measurement of IL-6 along with color flow Doppler ultrasonography thyroid can help to differentiate, so that appropriate treatment can be initiated.

MANAGEMENT OF THYROID HORMONE EXCESS

Management of Graves' Disease

Treatment Modalities
- Antithyroid drugs
- Radioactive iodine therapy (RAI131)
- Surgery

Antithyroid Drugs
They are heterocyclic compounds known as thionamides. They are methimazole (MMI), carbimazole, propylthiouracil (PTU). Carbimazole is rapidly metabolized to MMI (10 mg of carbimazole is converted to approximately 6 mg of MMI), hence, these two drugs can be considered as one. The important pharmacological features of these drugs are depicted in **Table 3**.

Antithyroid drugs do not cure but are very effective in controlling hyperthyroidism.

Mechanism of action
Intrathyroidal effects: ATDs inhibit thyroid peroxidase-mediated iodide oxidation, organification and iodotyrosine coupling, thereby decreasing the TH synthesis.

TABLE 3: Pharmacological features of ATD.

	Methimazole	PTU
Serum half-life	6–8 hours	1–2 hours
Serum protein binding	Nil	>75%
Volume of distribution	40 L	20 L
Transplacental passage	++	+
Levels in breast milk	++	+
Metabolism of drug during illness		
Severe liver disease	Decreased	Normal
Severe renal disease	Normal	Normal
Normalization of T3/T4	6 weeks	12 weeks
Agranulocytosis	0.6%	1–1.5%

(ATD: antithyroid drug; PTU: propylthiouracil)

Extrathyroidal effects: PTU (in large doses), but not MMI, decrease the peripheral conversion of T4 → T3 by inhibiting the activity of type 1 deiodinase.

Immunosuppressive effects of ATD: ATDs may have a beneficial immunomodulatory effect either primarily due to effect on thyroid-specific autoimmunity or secondarily by controlling the hyperthyroidism.

Initiation of ATD therapy: Before initiating ATD, patient should be informed preferably in writing about the side effects (pruritus, jaundice, fever, sore throat) **(Table 4)** and discontinuation of the drug immediately and informing the healthcare provider promptly. Patient should have a baseline complete blood count with differential white blood cell (WBC) count and liver function test (LFT).

Drug choice: MMI is preferred, except in first trimester of pregnancy and thyrotoxic storm where PTU is preferred.

TABLE 4: Adverse effects (AEs).

Minor AEs	Major AEs
Common (1–5%)	*Rare (0.2–0.5%)*
Urticaria, pruritus	Agranulocytosis (granulocyte count <500 neutrophils/mm^3)
Arthralgia	*Very rare (<1%)*
Fever	Aplastic anemia
Transient granulocytopenia	Cholestatic hepatitis (MMI)
Uncommon (<1%)	Toxic hepatitis (PTU)
GI upset	ANCA +ve vasculitis, SLE-like syndrome
Abnormalities of taste	Hypoglycemia (immune mediated, MMI)
Arthritis	↓prothrombin

(ANCA: antineutrophil cytoplasmic antibody; GI: gastrointestinal; MMI: methimazole; PTU: propylthiouracil; SLE: systemic lupus erythematosus)

TABLE 5: Starting methimazole dose based on FT4 levels.

Free T4	Methimazole dose (mg/day)
1–1.5 times above normal	5–10
1.5–2 times above normal	10–20
2–3 times above normal	30–40

TABLE 6: GREAT score.

Parameter (assessed before starting ATD)		GREAT score
Age (years)	≥40	0
	<40	1
FT4 (pmol/L)	<40	0
	≥40	1
TBII (U/L)	<6	0
	6–19.9	1
	≥20	2
Goiter size	Gr 0-1	0
	Gr II-III	2
Total score		6
Risk class (based on GREAT score)		*Recurrence*
Class I (score 0–1)		16%
Class II (score 2–3)		44%
Class III (score 4–6)		68%

(ATD: antithyroid drug; GREAT: Graves' Recurrent Events After Therapy)

TABLE 7: Beta-blockers used in the management of thyrotoxicosis.

Drug	Dosage	Frequency	Considerations
Propranolol	10–40 mg	3–4 times per day	• Nonselective β-adrenergic receptor blockade • Longest experience • May block T4 to T3 conversion at high doses • Preferred agent for nursing and pregnant mothers
Atenolol	25–100 mg	1–2 times per day	• Relative β-1 selectivity • Increased compliance • Avoid during pregnancy
Metoprolol	25–50 mg	2–3 times per day	Relative β-1 selectivity
Nadolol	40–160 mg	1 time per day	• Nonselective-adrenergic receptor blockade • Once daily • Least experience to date • May block T4 to T3 conversion at high doses

Dose: Carbimazole 0.5-1.0 mg/kg bodyweight, PTU 5-10 mg/kg bodyweight in divided doses, ATA guidelines recommend starting doses of MMI based on baseline FT4 levels **(Table 5)**.

Monitoring of patients on ATDs: Initially periodic assessment of T3, T4, and TSH every 4-6 weeks and adjusting the doses accordingly. T4 levels may normalize early despite persistent elevation of T3 and TSH may remain suppressed for several months after initiating therapy. Restoration of euthyroid status is mostly done by titration method, sometimes by block and replace regimen.

Duration of therapy: Medication should be continued for approximately for 12-18 months. Chances of remission are better if during ATD therapy goiter size decreases and TR-Abs and TSH become normal. After discontinuation of ATD, thyroid function should be monitored at 6-12 months for any recurrence.

Predictive score to assess the risk of recurrence after 1 year treatment with ATD

Graves' Recurrent Events After Therapy (GREAT): This score is useful to predict the risk of recurrence after a course of ATD which is done before the start of ATD, based on readily available clinical parameters **(Table 6)**. Addition of specific genotypes PTPN22 (protein tyrosine phosphatase) and number of human leukocyte antigen (HLA) subtypes (GREAT +score) may predict the risk even better.

Beta blockers: Beta blockers are used as an adjunct in the interval before the response to ATDs to ameliorate the thyrotoxic manifestations and they rapidly improve the symptoms of tremulousness, palpitations, and excessive sweating **(Table 7)**. Beta blockers are generally contraindicated in bronchial asthma, chronic obstructive pulmonary disease (COPD), or symptomatic Raynaud's phenomenon. In such cases β1 selective agents or verapamil and diltiazem can be used to control the heart rate.

Radioactive Iodine

Radioiodine causes cell necrosis and inflammation leading to cell death, thereby causing thyroid hypofunction and decrease in thyroid size. Though I-131 emits both β and γ radiation, it is the β radiation that causes thyroid cell death. ATA recommends "sufficient activity of RAI should be administered in a single application, typically a mean dose of 10–15 mCi to render the GD patient hypothyroid". Thyroid function gradually declines within weeks to months after RAI, so thyroid functions should be monitored every 6–8 weeks initially. Retreatment with RAI can be considered after 6 months in case of persistent hyperthyroidism.

Pretreatment with MMI and β-blockers will minimize the risk due to worsening hyperthyroidism after RAI. ATD should be stopped 3–5 days before and after RAI therapy.

Complications of RAI:
- Worsening of Graves' orbitopathy due to increase in TR-Ab levels after RAI
- Thyroiditis
  Absolutely contraindicated in pregnancy and lactation, and patients can plan for pregnancy at least 6 months after RAI both in males and females.

Surgery

Total thyroidectomy has a High Cure Rate.

Preparation for surgery:
- Patient should be rendered euthyroid with ATD
- *Iodine*: SSKI 2–3 drops (50 g iodide/drop) or Lugol's solution (8 mg iodide/drop)—5–7 drops thrice daily, mixed in water or juice, 7–10 days prior to surgery, iodine use is reported to decrease the thyroid gland vascularity
- Calcium and vitamin D status should be assessed and appropriately managed.

Complications: Permanent hypoparathyroidism <2%, recurrent laryngeal nerve injury <1% in the hands of high volume thyroid surgeon.

Choosing the right treatment modality: Choosing an appropriate treatment modality considering the advantages and disadvantages of treatment options **(Table 8)** in a given clinical scenario **(Table 9)** yield the best results.

Management of Other Forms of Thyroid Hormone Excess

Toxic Multinodular Goiter and Toxic Adenoma

The most effective and relatively safe definitive treatment options for TMNG and TA include RAI therapy and thyroid surgery **(Table 10)**. TMNG and TA with high nodular radioiodine uptake and widely suppressed uptake in the perinodular thyroid tissue are good candidates for RAI therapy. The success rate of RAI (definitive hypothyroidism or euthyroidism) is high: 93.7% in TA and 81.1% in TMNG. In patients with TA undergoing RAI therapy, there is a need for continued surveillance as the nodule is rarely eradicated. For patients with TA, the risk of treatment failure is <1% after surgical resection (thyroid lobectomy or isthmusectomy). Euthyroid state is achieved within days after surgery.

TABLE 8: Advantages and disadvantages of treatment options for Graves' hyperthyroidism.

Treatment option	Advantages	Disadvantages
Antithyroid drugs	Chance of permanent remission (~35%)	• Side effects of ATDs • Long duration (12–18 months) • High recurrence risk
Radioactive iodine	• Simplicity • Low recurrence risk	• Risk of orbitopathy • Lifelong LT4 needed • Possible small increase in cancer risk
Thyroidectomy	• Rapidity • Almost no recurrences	• Low but unavoidable morbidity • Lifelong LT4 needed

(ATDs: antithyroid drugs)

TABLE 9: Clinical situations that favor a particular modality of treatment.

ATD preferred	RAI preferred	Surgery preferred
Patients with high likelihood of remission (mild disease, women, small goiter, low TR-Abs)	Failure of medical therapy/major adverse events with ATD	Failure of medical therapy with active GO
Active GO	Liver disease	Associated thyroid malignancy
Pregnancy or planning pregnancy within 4–6 months	Comorbidities with ↑surgical risk and/or limited life expectancy	Coexistent primary hyperparathyroidism requiring surgery
Elderly with comorbidities	Patients with previously operated or with external neck irradiation	Large goiter with signs of compression
	Patients with periodic paralysis	
	Patients with pulmonary HTN and CHF	

(ATD: antithyroid drugs; CHF: chronic heart failure; HTN: hypertension; RAI: radioactive iodine; TR-Abs: TSH receptor antibodies)

TABLE 10: Factors that favor a particular modality as treatment for TMNG or TA.

Factors	RAI	Surgery	ATD
Pregnancy	Contraindicated	Acceptable	Preferred
Advanced age, comorbidities with limited life expectancy	Preferred		Acceptable
Confirmed or suspected thyroid malignancy		Preferred	
Compressive symptoms	Acceptable	Preferred	
Associated hyperparathyroidism		Preferred	
Goiter or nodule with substernal or retrosternal extension	Acceptable	Preferred	
Large goiter	Acceptable	Preferred	

(ATD: antithyroid drug; RAI: radioactive iodine; TA: toxic adenoma; TMNG: toxic multinodular goiter)

The prevalence of hypothyroidism following lobectomy for TA is 2–3%. In patients with TMNG presenting with compressive symptoms, all patients showed resolution of these symptoms after thyroidectomy whereas only 46% of patients undergoing RAI showed improvement in such symptoms. In patients with TMNG, the risk of treatment failure or need for repeat treatment following thyroidectomy is <1%. In patients with TMNG post RAI therapy, the response is 50–60% by 3 months and 80% by 6 months.

Thyroiditis

The treatment of thyroiditis depends on the subtype **(Table 11)**. Antithyroid drugs do not have any role as these are destructive forms of thyroiditis and the TH excess is not due to hyperfunctioning of the thyroid gland **(Table 11)**.

Gestational Thyrotoxicosis

Antithyroid medications are not required in these cases. Severe vomiting and dehydration may warrant parenteral nutrition and intravenous fluid correction. Beta blockers like labetalol, which are considered safe in pregnancy, can be used to control the thyrotoxic symptoms. Treatment of other causes of human chorionic gonadotropin (HCG) excess like trophoblastic diseases, hydatidiform mole, and choriocarcinoma leads to biochemical and clinical resolution.

Treatment of Thyrotoxicosis of Extrathyroidal Origin

Iatrogenic Thyrotoxicosis

The only therapy that may be required would be discontinuation of the thyroid supplements. Beta blockers are recommended for those with sympathetic overactivity. Although even massive doses of TH are well tolerated, it may sometimes require use of gastric lavage and activated charcoal. Those who do not respond to conservative measures or who are at high risk of developing cardiac or neurologic complications such as seizures, myocardial infarction, thyroid storm, or choreoathetosis, other measures such as use of cholestyramine, iopanoic acid, and ipodate sodium may be considered. Plasmapheresis and exchange transfusions are last resort measures in severe and refractory cases.

Thyrotoxicosis Secondary to Metastatic Functioning Thyroid Carcinoma

Patients should first be rendered euthyroid with ATDs before proceeding for debulking surgery with RAI treatment.

TABLE 11: Overview of treatment of thyroiditis.

Type of thyroiditis	Treatment	Follow-up
Sporadic painless thyroiditis	Thyrotoxic phase—β-blockers	Hypothyroidism phase may require treatment with L-thyroxine which can be withdrawn after 6–9 months to reassess recovery
Subacute thyroiditis	• Thyrotoxic phase—β-blockers • Salicylates and nonsteroidal anti-inflammatory drugs for pain • Severe cases—prednisone 40 mg/day for 1 week followed by slow tapering over 4–6 weeks	• Overt and clinical hypothyroidism to be treated with L-thyroxine which can be withdrawn after 6–9 months to reassess recovery. • *Recurrent exacerbations*: Thyroidectomy and radioactive ablation have both been advocated as treatment modalities for recurrent thyroiditis (*Source*: Werner and Ingbar "The Thyroid")
Acute infectious thyroiditis	• Antibiotics for bacterial cause • Incision and drainage for abscess/airway compromise	Recurrent disease—partial lobectomy
Postpartum thyroiditis	Thyrotoxic phase—β-blockers (propranolol or metoprolol)	• Postpartum hypothyroidism—treat with L-thyroxine for 1 year and taper to re-evaluate thyroid function • Annual screening of thyroid functions for transient hypothyroidism/those planning further pregnancy

Tyrosine kinase inhibitors have been found to be equally effective in thyrotoxic metastatic disease as in metastatic nonfunctional thyroid carcinoma.

Struma Ovarii

Patients are initially treated with ATDs to achieve euthyroidism before planning definitive surgery. Surgical options are unilateral or bilateral oophorectomy and salpingectomy with total abdominal hysterectomy. The extent of surgery depends on presence of capsular invasion or metastasis and fertility preservation. If rapid surgical preparation is required, iodine may be used to restore euthyroidism. In case of malignancy, the ovarian surgery is followed by thyroidectomy to enable RAI ablation. This would also assist in differentiating between a malignant struma ovarii from a metastatic thyroid carcinoma. Serum Tg and RAI scans may be used in follow-up to detect recurrence.

Amiodarone-induced Thyrotoxicosis (Type 1 and Type 2)

In AIT-1, excess iodine released from amiodarone by the action of deiodinase enzyme in the liver causes increased organification of iodine in the thyroid follicular cells and thereby increased synthesis of T4 and T3 (the Jod–Basedow effect). Patients with AIT-1 present with thyrotoxic symptoms, elevated THs, suppressed TSH, and presence of thyroid autoantibodies.

AIT-1 usually presents with a diffuse or nodular goiter, increased tracer uptake on RAI or technetium scanning and increased vascularity on color flow Doppler imaging. AIT-1 is mainly treated using antithyroid medications such as thionamides. Because of the prolonged half-life of amiodarone, even if the drug is stopped, treatment with thionamides may need to be continued for a longer time. As the thyroid gland is usually highly iodinated, very large doses of thionamides are needed to control the thyrotoxicosis in AIT-1. Because of the high iodine exposure of thyroid gland in amiodarone treated patients RAIU is usually low and therefore response to RAI is often inadequate but may be considered in those showing an increased uptake. AIT-2 is a destructive form of thyroiditis that usually occurs in patients with normal thyroid glands prior with negative thyroid autoantibodies. Treatment with steroids may be necessary in severe cases, especially in those with unstable cardiac status. Prednisolone with a dose of 40–60 mg/day is the usual steroid regimen that can be gradually tapered over 2–3 months, once euthyroidism is achieved. Total thyroidectomy is not considered as first-line therapy in both forms of AIT but may be useful in those patients with severe/refractory cardiac arrhythmias wherein amiodarone cannot be discontinued. Other therapies to reduce the TH excess in both forms of AIT are cholestyramine, lithium, iodinated contrast agents, and plasmapheresis. Hyperthyroidism in AIT-1 has a higher recurrence rate compared to AIT-1 and hence needs follow-up every 3–6 months. AIT-2 may result in hypothyroidism in a few patients and needs similar frequency of follow-up.

CONCLUSION

Comprehensive history and thorough clinical examination supported by necessary biochemical investigations are sufficient to make a diagnosis in most of the cases. Additional testing with nuclear imaging, TR-Abs, color flow Doppler and other tests should be based on appropriate clinical scenario to differentiate overactive gland from thyroiditis, which is important for choosing appropriate therapy. Graves' disease is the most common cause of thyrotoxicosis. Among the three modalities of treatments with their advantages and disadvantages, the choice of therapy should be guided by the clinical scenario, associated factors, and comorbidities. Thyroiditis-associated transient thyrotoxicosis requires symptomatic treatment with β-blockers and ATD therapy not required. So accurate diagnosis is important for appropriate management of TH excess.

SUGGESTED READINGS

1. Ross DS, Burch HB, Cooper DS, Greenlee MC, Laurberg P, Maia AL, et al. 2016 American Thyroid Association Guidelines for Diagnosis and Management of Hyperthyroidism and Other Causes of Thyrotoxicosis. Thyroid. 2016;26(10):1343-421.
2. Kahaly GJ, Bartalena L, Hegedüs L, Leenhardt L, Poppe K, Pearce SH. 2018 European Thyroid Association Guideline for the Management of Graves' Hyperthyroidism. Eur Thyroid J. 2018;7(4):167-86.
3. Melmed S, Auchus RJ, Goldfine AB, Koenig RJ, Rosen CJ. Williams Textbook of Endocrinology, 14th edition. Philadelphia, PA: Elsevier; 2019.
4. Braverman LE, Cooper DS, Kopp PA. Werner and Ingbar's the Thyroid: A Fundamental and Clinical Text, 11th edition. Philadelphia, USA: Wolters Kluwer; 2020.
5. Elnaggar MN, Jbeili K, Nik-Hussin N, Kozhippally M, Pappachan JM. Amiodarone-induced Thyroid Dysfunction: A Clinical Update. Exp Clin Endocrinol Diabetes. 2018;126(6):333-41.
6. Epp R, Malcolm J, Jolin-Dahel K, Clermont M, Keely E. Postpartum thyroiditis. BMJ. 2021;372:n495.

CHAPTER 14

Rare Forms of Thyroid Hormone Excess

Subhankar Chowdhury, Partha Pratim Chakraborty

INTRODUCTION

Excess thyroid hormone (TH) in circulation is known as thyrotoxicosis; when thyrotoxicosis results from hyperfunction of the thyroid gland itself, the condition is termed as hyperthyroidism. The common etiologies of thyrotoxicosis are hyperthyroidism due to Graves' disease (GD) and toxic nodular goiter, excess release of preformed TH following thyroid follicular destruction due to painful subacute or sporadic painless thyroiditis and inappropriate dosing of levothyroxine (LT4) during treatment of hypothyroidism. Accidental or surreptitious ingestion of exogenous TH, excess circulatory human chorionic gonadotropin (hCG), struma ovarii (SO), functional metastases from differentiated thyroid carcinoma (DTC), and McCune-Albright syndrome (MAS) are relatively uncommon causes of thyrotoxicosis. In all these situations serum thyroid-stimulating hormone (TSH) is appropriately suppressed. At times, elevated total thyroxine (TT4) is present with normal or elevated TSH, a condition known as "euthyroid hyperthyroxinemia" (EH). This may result from qualitative or quantitative abnormalities of the TH-binding proteins, assay interferences, medication use, or rarely from conditions with disrupted negative feedback mechanism or altered TH metabolism. Patients with EH may or may not have elevated total triiodothyronine (TT3) concentration. Excessive secretion of bioactive TSH and subsequent hyperstimulation of the thyroid gland and the consequent thyrotoxicosis is termed as "central hyperthyroidism" or "inappropriate secretion of TSH".

The free and total THs are measured by competitive immunoassay (IA) while TSH is measured by non-competitive IA. Assay interference giving rise to falsely elevated THs with normal or spuriously suppressed TSH is not uncommon in clinical practice. IA interference should always be suspected if abnormal thyroid function test (TFT) is encountered in an otherwise asymptomatic patient. High biotin intake (100–300 mg/day) may result in an abnormal TFT typically characterized by high THs and suppressed TSH when measured in IA platforms using biotin-streptavidin immobilization system (Roche, Beckman, Siemens). Similar pattern of TFT is also encountered in these platforms due to anti-streptavidin antibody interference. However, alteration in TFT due to biotin or anti-streptavidin antibody also varies in different platforms. Falsely elevated THs may also be found due to circulatory anti-Ru antibodies that bind to the ruthenylated anti-TH antibody in some competitive IA platforms [electrochemiluminescence immunoassay (ECLIA), Roche]. Circulating anti-T4 and/or anti-T3 autoantibodies are not uncommon in patients with plasma cell disorders and various connective tissue diseases. Both total and free THs may be overestimated in the commonly performed "one-step" tracer analog method in presence of these antibodies in the analyte. When such interference is suspected, THs should be measured by "two-step" competitive IA or by equilibrium dialysis (ED). Patients having thyrotoxicosis secondary to GD or thyroiditis or LT4 overdose may demonstrate spurious elevation of TSH due to interference by circulatory heterophile or human anti-animal antibodies acting as anti-TSH antibodies in the noncompetitive IA.

The relatively rare forms of true TH excess have been summarized in **Table 1**.

AUTONOMOUS TSH HYPERSECRETION FROM TSH-SECRETING PITUITARY ADENOMA

Thyroid-stimulating hormone-secreting pituitary adenomas (TSPAs) account for about 0.5–1% of all pituitary adenomas with an overall prevalence of about 0.02% in the general population. Though commonly encountered between third and sixth decades of life, TSPAs have been reported in children <10 years of age and in adults in their late 80s. Familial TSPAs occur in association with multiple endocrine neoplasia type 1 (MEN1) syndrome and as familial isolated pituitary adenoma (FIPA) secondary to aryl hydrocarbon receptor interacting protein (AIP) mutation. Though, almost all such tumors originate from pituitary thyrotropes, TSPAs

TABLE 1: Uncommon etiologies of thyroid hormone (TH) excess.

With normal/elevated thyroid-stimulating hormone (TSH)	With suppressed TSH
Elevated serum-binding proteins	Surreptitious ingestion of LT4, accidental overdose of exogenous TH
Familial dysalbuminemic hyperthyroxinemia (FDH)	Iodine-induced thyrotoxicosis or Jod–Basedow phenomenon
TSH-secreting pituitary tumor	Functional metastasis from thyroid carcinoma
Resistance to thyroid hormone	Painful thyroiditis in anaplastic thyroid carcinoma
Disorders of thyroid hormone transport	Painless thyroiditis with immune checkpoint inhibitors
Disorders of thyroid hormone metabolism	Struma ovarii, Struma cordis
Acute psychosis	Trophoblastic tumors
Drugs (amiodarone, heparin)	McCune–Albright syndrome
Non-compliance with LT4 replacement	Hereditary toxic thyroid hyperplasia

arising from ectopic pituitary tissue, located particularly in the nasopharynx, have also been reported. A vast majority of these TSPAs have a diameter of 10 mm or more (macroadenoma) with significant suprasellar and parasellar extension and invasion to the surrounding structures **(Figs. 1A to D)**. Microadenomas constitute about a quarter of such cases. Two-thirds of TSPAs secrete TSH and free α-subunit, with disproportionately high secretion of the latter. Co-secretion of growth hormone (GH) and/or prolactin is encountered in about 25% of cases as thyrotropes, somatotropes and lactotropes share the common transcription factor, Pit-1. TSH in such patients may have normal, increased, or reduced biologic activity relative to its immunoreactivity; thus, TSH concentration varies significantly in TSPA. In addition, the set point of hypothalamo-pituitary-thyroid (HPT) axis is also altered. Discrepancy between biologic activity and immunoreactivity of TSH, secreted from TSPA, results from alteration in post-translational processing of TSH molecule within the tumor cells that includes glycosylation of TSH, necessary for its bioactivity. The TSH secreting tumor cells, though exhibit partial or total resistance to feedback inhibition of elevated circulatory TH, demonstrate preserved or even increased sensitivity to decreasing circulatory TH concentration. TSH-secreting pituitary carcinoma is exceedingly rare. Patients with TSPA have a long history of thyrotoxicosis, are often misdiagnosed as GD, and frequently treated inappropriately by thyroidectomy or radioiodine ablation. Invasive macroadenomas are more prevalent in patients with previous thyroid ablation or thyroid surgery.

Clinical Features

Patients with TSPAs often present with goiter (diffuse or nodular), signs and symptoms of TH excess with/without local mass effects secondary to pituitary tumor, and pituitary hormone deficiency; typically, they do not have features of ophthalmopathy. Goiter may also be found in patients with previous thyroidectomy, as the residual thyroid tissue regrows under TSH stimulation. TSPAs co-secreting GH and prolactin demonstrate features of acromegaly and

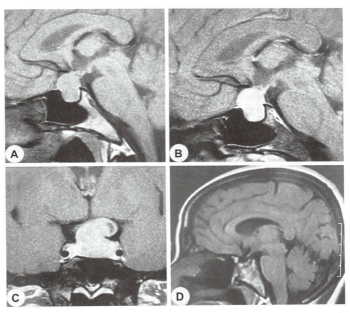

Figs. 1A to D: MRI of hypothalamo-pituitary region in a lady with TSPA. (A) Mid-sagittal non-contrast T1 image; (B and C) Postcontrast T1 images showing contrast enhancement; (D) Following successful transsphenoidal surgery.

galactorrhea, respectively. Unlike primary thyroid diseases, atrial fibrillation and heart failure are rare in TSPAs, possibly due to lesser degree of circulatory TH excess.

Diagnosis

The typical pattern of TFT, encountered in treatment naïve patients with TSPA, is elevated total and free THs (both T4 and T3) and normal or elevated TSH.

The possible differential diagnoses that need to be considered in patients with such a pattern of TFT, particularly in absence of overt signs and symptoms of thyrotoxicosis and/or intracranial mass effects are immunoassay interferences, TH-binding protein alterations, and resistance to thyroid hormone (RTH), pituitary RTH in particular. A suggestive family history often points toward RTH or inherited causes of quantitative/qualitative alterations of TH-binding proteins [thyroxine-binding globulin (TBG), albumin, or transthyretin]. Moreover, high FT4/TT4, normal FT3/TT3, and normal or elevated TSH may also be encountered in LT4-treated patients with poor compliance or following an unusual high dose of LT4 ingested before blood sampling. On rare occasions, LT4-treated patients may have elevated FT4 and normal or elevated TSH levels, despite strict adherence to therapy, possibly due to decreased intrapituitary conversion of T4 to T3 by type 2 deiodinase (D2).

Once such alteration in TFT is encountered, the first step should be to rule out use of medications, known to cause elevation in TBG, and repeat total and free THs and TSH, preferably on a different platform.

The next step particularly in presence of intracranial mass effect(s) is magnetic resonance imaging (MRI) of the hypothalamo-pituitary region. Presence of a pituitary adenoma, microadenoma in particular, may not necessarily clinch the diagnosis of TSPA. Pituitary microincidentalomas are encountered in about 10% of normal population and TSPA has also been reported in rare patients with RTH. The next step is to differentiate between TSPA and RTH. TSH values are more often normal in RTH and elevated in TSPA. TFT of the first-degree relatives should be obtained. Inconclusive MRI and similar pattern of abnormal TFT in first-degree relative(s) suggest underlying *RTH,* and *TRHB* gene should be sequenced.

Determination of α-subunit, though useful both to diagnose TSPA, and differentiate TSPA from RTH in appropriate background, is not widely available. Altered hormone synthesis within the tumor cells results in release of disproportionate quantities of the free α-subunit compared to whole TSH in the circulation, and α-subunit/TSH molar ratio [(α-subunit in μg/L/TSH in mIU/L) ×10] of >1 indicates TSPA. However, it needs to be remembered that hypersecretion of α-subunit is not uncommon in tumors other than TSPA, such as non-functioning pituitary adenomas, gonadotropinomas, and even in rare patients with prolactinomas and somatotropinomas. In addition, postmenopausal women may also have high circulatory α-subunit.

Sex hormone-binding globulin (SHBG), a marker of peripheral TH action is often used to differentiate TSPA and RTH; serum SHBG is high in the former and normal/low in the latter. Rare patients with mixed GH/TSH-secreting adenomas may have normal serum SHBG as GH inhibits SHBG secretion. On the other hand, estrogen treatment in RTH patients may elevate serum SHBG.

Triiodothyronine suppression test and thyrotropin-releasing hormone (TRH) stimulation test, though not performed routinely, may be of use in selected patients with TSPA. TSH and/or α-subunit unresponsiveness following TRH stimulation is seen in about 83% of such patients. Moreover, lack of suppression of TSH after T3 administration (80–100 μg/day for 8–10 days) favors TSPA. T3-suppression test is particularly useful to diagnose TSPA in patients with elevated TSH following previous thyroid ablation with high sensitivity and specificity.

Treatment

Surgical resection either by transsphenoidal or transcranial route remains the first choice of treatment in TSPA. These tumors are often large, invasive with marked fibrosis; hence not amenable to complete resection. Preoperative MRI with diffusion weighted image (DWI) and apparent diffusion coefficient (ADC) maps can be utilized for planning of the appropriate surgical approach. Tumors showing diffusion restriction, i.e., high signal intensity on DWI and corresponding reduced ADC value are soft in nature and easily removed by transsphenoidal route **(Figs. 2A and B)**. Hard tumors should better be operated through transcranial approach. Patients should be made euthyroid with antithyroid drugs (ATDs) or octreotide prior to surgery. The biochemical remission rate following surgery is around 70%. Undetectable TSH 1-week postsurgery likely indicates complete tumor removal, provided presurgical medical

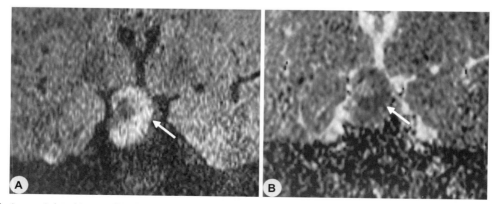

Figs. 2A and B: Diffusion weighted image (DWI) (A) and apparent diffusion coefficient (ADC) maps (B) of a TSPA showing diffusion restriction, i.e., high signal intensity on DWI and corresponding reduced ADC value (white arrows) suggesting soft tumor.

treatments were stopped at least 10 days before surgery. The most sensitive and specific test to document complete surgical resection is T3-suppression test, and complete cessation of both basal and TRH-stimulated TSH secretion following T3 administration denotes cure.

Patient should be evaluated clinically and biochemically two or three times during the first year and then every year following pituitary surgery. Pituitary imaging should be performed every 2 or 3 years, or whenever an increase in serum TSH and/or TH levels is encountered, or clinical symptoms recur. Pituitary radiotherapy, either by conventional fractionated radiotherapy or stereotactic gamma knife surgery should be offered in patients with incomplete tumor resection or in patients, who are poor candidates for surgery.

Long-acting somatostatin receptor ligands (SRL) are the mainstay of medical therapy in TSPA, particularly in highly invasive mixed GH/TSH-producing adenomas. Reduction of TSH is encountered in almost 100% of cases and majority of them achieve euthyroidism. Half of the treated patients experience tumor shrinkage. Resistance to SRL treatment has been documented in <5% of cases. Dopamine agonists are less effective with favorable effects being observed in occasional patients with mixed PRL/TSH secreting adenomas.

RESISTANCE TO THYROID HORMONE

Resistance to thyroid hormone or impaired sensitivity to TH (ISTH) is a group of disorders characterized by reduced responsiveness of various target tissues to circulatory THs. The knowledge of tissue distribution of different TH receptor (TR) isoforms is critical to understand the clinical manifestations and biochemical alterations in different forms of RTH. TRβ1 is widely expressed in various tissues, and is the predominant isoform found in liver and kidneys. TRβ2 expression is found dominantly in hypothalamus, pituitary, inner ear, and retina. TRα1 is a ubiquitously expressed isoform, found in abundance particularly in the central nervous system (CNS), cardiac and skeletal muscles, gastrointestinal tract, and bones. TRα2 also is expressed in a variety of tissues (e.g., brain and testis), but does not seem to bind to the ligand (TH); hence its function is not known.

Clinical Features

Resistance to thyroid hormone can theoretically be classified into RTH-α and RTH-β, of which the latter is much more prevalent than the former. Based on tissue-specific resistance pattern, RTH-β is further subdivided into three groups—pituitary resistance to TH (PRTH), generalized resistance to TH (GRTH), and an extremely rare form, isolated peripheral tissue resistance to TH (PTRTH). The clinical manifestation of RTH-β is a combination of hypothyroidism and hyperthyroidism depending on the relative dominance of GRTH and degree of PRTH. The signs/symptoms of RTH-β in decreasing order of frequency are goiter (66–95%), tachycardia (33–75%), emotional disturbances, attention deficit hyperactivity disorder (ADHD), hyperkinetic behavior (up to 70%), recurrent ear and throat infections (up to 55%), delayed bone age (29–47%), short stature (18–25%), sensorineural hearing loss (10–22%), learning disability, and low IQ. Children with RTH-β, PRTH in particular, may also present with height acceleration and advanced bone age. A proportion of patients with RTH-β is diagnosed on routine thyroid function testing for nonspecific symptoms or during family screening when one of their family members has the disease (**Fig. 3**).

On the other hand, clinical manifestations of RTH-α are typical of hypothyroidism that include poor feeding, coarse cry, umbilical hernia, coarse facies, broad nose, flat nasal bridge, macroglossia, thick lips, delayed eruption of teeth, delayed milestones, delayed closure of fontanelles, patent cranial sutures with wormian bones, short stature, delayed bone age, constipation, bradycardia, and epiphyseal dysgenesis.

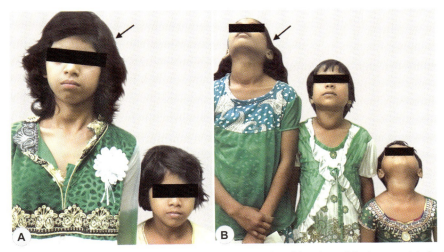

Figs. 3A and B: Two different families with RTH. The index case was the elder sister (black arrows) in both these families.

TABLE 2: Differential diagnoses and patterns of TFT in patients with elevated TH (T4 and/or T3) with normal/high TSH.							
	TT4	FT4 (ED)	TT3	rT3	T3:rT3	TSH	SHBG
RTH-β	High	High	High/Normal	High	Normal	Normal/High	Normal
RTH-α	Normal/Low	Normal/Low	Normal/High	Normal/Low	High	Normal/High	Normal/High
TSPA	High	High	High	High	Normal	High/normal	High
MCT8 mutation	Normal/Low	Low	High	Low	High	Normal/High	High
SBP2 mutation	High	High	Low	High	Low	Normal/high	High
TBG excess	High	Normal	High	High	Normal	Normal	Normal/High
FDH	High	Normal/High	Normal/High	High	Low	Normal	Normal

(FDH: familial dysalbuminemic hyperthyroxinemia; MCT8: monocarboxylate transporters 8; RTH-α: resistance to thyroid hormone-α; TBG: thyroxine-binding globulin; TSPA: thyroid-stimulating hormone-secreting pituitary adenoma; SBP2: selenocysteine insertion sequence binding protein 2).

Diagnosis

The diagnosis of RTH is suspected on the basis of typical TFT. The closest differential diagnosis of RTH is TSPA. Possible differential diagnoses and the pattern of TFT have been summarized in **Table 2**. The diagnosis is confirmed by mutational analysis of the *TRHB* gene. In 14% of families, RTH-β occurs in the absence of identified mutations in the *THRB* genes (non-TRβ–RTH). If genetic study of the *TRHB* gene is not possible, a standardized diagnostic protocol, using short-term administration of incremental doses of LT3 has been suggested to diagnose TRH-β. Adult patients are given LT3 50 µg/day for 3 days, followed by 100 µg/day for 3 days and 200 µg/day for another 3 days in two divided doses, administered 12 hours apart; and increment in serum TSH is measured after intravenous administration of TRH. In addition, changes in serum cholesterol, creatine kinase, SHBG, and ferritin in response to incremental dose of LT3 from baseline are also evaluated.

In contrast to RTH-β, high degree of clinical suspicion is required to diagnose RTH-α, as TSH in RTH-α is normal (usually within the upper half of the reference range). There is a trend for serum T4 and rT3 to be low and T3 to be high; however, in most of these patients TH concentrations are within reference range. T3/rT3 ratio is consistently high and is a good laboratory biomarker for underlying RTH-α, particularly in children with clinical features suggestive of congenital hypothyroidism and normal TSH. The diagnosis of RTH-α is made through mutational analysis of *TRHA* gene.

Treatment

Treatment of RTH is challenging and no specific treatment, which fully and specifically corrects the underlying defect, is available. In most cases of RTH-β, PRTH in particular, the RTH is more severe in the pituitary than in the peripheral tissues, and the partial tissue resistance to TH is adequately compensated for by an increase in TH secretion from the hyperactive thyroid gland. Thus, many such patients do not require therapy except for symptomatic treatment with a β-blocker to ameliorate tachycardia. In GRTH variety of RTH-β, peripheral tissues are relatively more resistant than the pituitary and the compensation of the defect by endogenous TH is incomplete. In such patients, judicious administration of supraphysiologic doses of LT4 is indicated.

Infants and children with failure to thrive, large goiter, retarded bone age, and TSH level above the upper limit of the reference range should be treated with exogenous TH. Since the dose varies greatly among cases, it should be individualized by assessing tissue responses. LT4 should be given in incremental doses and basal metabolic rate (BMR), nitrogen balance, serum SHBG, and osteocalcin be monitored at each dose; development of a catabolic state is an indication of overtreatment. Children should also be monitored with bone age and growth velocity. Suraphysiologic doses of LT3, given as a single dose every other day, is successful in reducing goiter size without causing side effects. The dose is increased until TSH and thyroglobulin (Tg) are suppressed and reduction in goiter size is observed. LT3 has also been used with some success in the treatment of refractory ADHD. Treatment with ATD or thyroid gland ablation should be avoided. Pregnant women with RTH-β carrying a normal fetus should have FT4, which is not >50% the upper limit of normal in order to prevent low birth weight in the newborn.

Among the different TH analogs used to alleviate symptoms of apparent TH excess in RTH, TRIAC (3,5,3'-triiodothyroacetic acid) has been used most widely. It exhibits 2- to 3-fold higher selectivity for TRβ than TRα in vitro. It has greater affinity, potency, and activity for TRβ than T3 and it exerts predominantly pituitary and hepatic thyromimetic effects, target tissues that are relatively refractory to TH in RTH-β. A daily dose of 1.4–2.8 mg is generally used. In view of the spontaneous variation in thyrotoxic symptoms in RTH, periodic cessation of therapy, and reevaluation of the clinical status of the patient is advisable. Other TH analogs with greater selectivity for TRβ compared to TRα are GC-24 (40-fold), Eprotirome (22-fold), MB07344 (15-fold), Sobetirome (10-fold), KB141 (8-fold) among others. TRβ selective Thyromimetics (GC1, MG-3196) have been developed and may have utility in treating some abnormalities (dyslipidemia) in RTH. HY1, an analog of GC1, has also been found to be effective in RTH-β. The majority of children with RTH-α are treated with LT4.

CELL MEMBRANE THYROID HORMONE TRANSPORTER DEFECT

A number of transport proteins belonging to different families of solute carriers transport TH across cell membrane. The list includes monocarboxylate transporters (MCT) of which MCT8 and MCT10 are specific TH transporters; members of the organic anion–transporting polypeptide (OATP) family of which OATP1B1 and OATP1B3 are exclusively expressed in liver and efficiently transport the sulfated iodothyronines (T4S, T3S, and rT3S) and OATP1C1, which is localized preferentially in brain capillaries and shows a high specificity and affinity for T4; L-amino acid transporters (LAT), among which LAT1 and LAT2 transport TH; multidrug resistance-associated proteins; Na$^+$/taurocholate co-transporting polypeptide (NTCP) and fatty acid translocase. Of all these transport proteins, MCT8 mutation is relatively common. The disease is inherited as X-linked recessive trait and known as Allan–Herndon–Dudley syndrome.

MCT8 demonstrates tissue-specific differences in substrate (T4 or T3) specificity. MCT8 knock out mice demonstrate moderate elevation in thyroid gland activity as evidenced by about 1.5-fold rise in intrathyroidal TT4 and TT3 concentrations together with an increase in follicle diameter. Measurement of TH in circulation in these mice (elevated T3 and low T4) suggests a pivotal role of MCT8 in mediating thyroidal T4 efflux. In contrast MCT8 mediates T3 transport across the blood-CSF barrier and entry of T3 inside the neurons from the astrocytes and tanycytes.

Clinical Features

Truncal hypotonia and feeding problems are the most common early signs, appearing within the first 6 months of life. Flaccidity typically then progresses to limb rigidity leading to spastic quadriplegia and majority of the patients are unable to walk, stand, or sit independently. There is gross impairment of psychomotor development including speech. Dystonia and purposeless movements are common and characteristic. Facial dysmorphism includes decrease in facial creases, ptosis, thickening of the nose and ears, long and cup-shaped ears with upturned earlobes, open mouth, and tented upper lip. Poor weight gain and muscle wasting are common and result from dysphagia and increased metabolism due to the thyrotoxic state of peripheral tissues. CNS myelination is delayed in the first 2 years of life, which normalizes in the subsequent years. Combination of clinical features and myelination defect has been referred to as Pelizaeus–Merzbacher–like disease (PMLD).

Diagnosis

The ratio of T3 to rT3 is characteristically high with normal TSH mimicking RTH-α. The tissue markers are altered suggesting high serum T3 levels on peripheral tissues (low cholesterol, high SHBG). Administration of incremental doses of LT3, using the protocol devised for the study of patients with RTH-β, showed reduced pituitary sensitivity to the hormone.

Treatment

Treatment is largely supportive. Supraphysiological dose of LT4 combined with propylthiouracil (PTU), a specific inhibitor of type 1 deiodinase (D1) to prevent T3 production and thereby prevent hypermetabolic state, has been tried to increase the availability of TH to the brain. Thyromimetic drugs like 3,5,3'-triiodothyroacetic acid (TRIAC), its precursor tetraiodothyroacetic acid (TETRAC), and 3,5-diiodothyropropionic acid (DITPA) that binds with equal affinity to TRα and TRβ, but with almost 100-fold lower affinity compared to T3 and seems to be effectively transported into brain in absence of MCT8, have also been tested.

THYROID HORMONE METABOLISM DEFECT

Mutations in the *SBP2 (SECISBP2)* gene encoding selenocysteine insertion sequence-binding protein 2, *TRU-TCA1-1* gene encoding the selenocysteine transfer RNA (tRNASec), having a role in selenoprotein synthesis and mutation in the selenocysteine synthase *(SEPSECS)* genes lead to inherited defect in TH metabolism.

Clinical Features

Delayed motor milestones, short stature, and delayed bone age are the major manifestations.

Diagnosis

The characteristic thyroid test abnormalities in subjects with *SBP2* gene mutations are high total and free T4, low T3, high rT3, and a normal or slightly elevated serum TSH. Serum concentrations of selenium, selenoprotein P, and other selenoproteins are reduced.

Treatment

Three treatment options are available namely selenium, TH, and vitamin E.

UNUSUAL ETIOLOGIES OF EXOGENOUS THYROID HORMONE EXCESS

Rare etiologies of exogenous TH excess include surreptitious ingestion of LT4 as Munchausen syndrome, intake of over-the-counter medicines or herbal preparations for weight loss, occupational exposure to cosmetic creams containing iodine and to THs or veterinary LT4 preparations, and consumption of inappropriate amount of beef as hamburger or sausage contaminated with bovine thyroid. Occupational exposure to TH excess usually involves a group of individuals working together and sharing the same workspace. Ingestion of contaminated beef may present as community outbreak of thyrotoxicosis, the so called "hamburger thyrotoxicosis" as encountered in Midwest United States in mid-1980s and in Nebraska in 1984 or recurrent/persistent thyrotoxicosis in an individual with/without affecting the family members.

Clinical Features

Patients demonstrate variable degree of thyrotoxicosis without goiter and exophthalmos.

Diagnosis

Diagnosis of exogenous TH ingestion requires a very high index of clinical suspicion. Serum TSH is invariably suppressed with varying elevation of serum T3 and T4, depending on the ingested preparation. Technetium or radioactive iodine uptake is low or undetectable mimicking thyroiditis. Low or undetectable Tg, in absence of detectable anti-Tg antibody, is helpful to differentiate exogenous TH ingestion from thyroiditis; Tg is elevated in the latter. In presence of detectable anti-Tg antibody, serum Tg is unreliable and fecal T4 levels may be utilized to confirm exogenous TH source. Fecal T4 level is approximately 1 nmol/g in normal healthy subjects, is mildly increased in GD or thyroiditis (about 2 nmol/g), and is markedly elevated following exogenous TH intake (over 12 nmol/g).

Treatment

Exogenous TH is discontinued, and symptomatic thyrotoxicosis should be treated with β-blockers. Massive overdose of TH is managed with gastric lavage and induced emesis. Activated charcoal (prevents absorption of TH) and cholestyramine (binds TH, decreases enterohepatic circulation and increases fecal excretion) may also be tried. Iodinated radiocontrast agents, iopanoic acid, and ipodate sodium are also helpful as they decrease conversion of T4 to T3. Plasmapheresis and exchange transfusion may be used as last resort if all the above measures fail to control thyrotoxicosis. Antithyroid agents have no role in the management of exogenous TH-induced thyrotoxicosis.

THYROTOXICOSIS DUE TO FUNCTIONAL METASTATIC THYROID CARCINOMA

Thyrotoxicosis due to metastatic DTC or metastatic anaplastic thyroid carcinoma is extremely rare. Most of the thyroid carcinomas, if not all, are associated with normal/elevated TSH due to inefficient TH production within the relatively dedifferentiated thyroid follicular cells. However, thyrotoxicosis may be encountered in presence of an extremely large tumor burden and widespread metastasis in patients with follicular thyroid carcinoma or rarely in papillary thyroid carcinoma. A significantly large volume of thyroid tissue within the metastatic foci may secrete enough TH to cause thyrotoxicosis. Rarely, such metastatic foci are truly hyperfunctional and cause TH excess in absence of large tumor burden. Though thyrotoxicosis and thyroid carcinoma are often detected simultaneously in such cases, cancer diagnosis may precede the development of thyrotoxicosis by many years. Many such patients have concomitant GD and thyrotoxicosis is attributed to circulatory TSH receptor autoantibody (TRAb) acting upon TSH receptors over the tumoral cells. In addition, activating mutations of the TSH receptor gene, that activates the cAMP and/or the IP3 pathways have also been reported.

Diagnosis

Such patients often have preferential elevation of T3 compared to T4 due to increased expression of D1 and D2 deiodinases by the tumor, with suppressed TSH and high Tg. Differentiating thyrotoxicosis due to LT4 overdose from functional metastases in a postoperative patient with DTC is challenging. In an athyreotic patient, undetectable Tg (in absence of undetectable anti-Tg antibody) points toward LT4 overdose. Withdrawal of LT4 for several weeks followed by TSH measurement and whole-body iodine scan should be advised if Tg is elevated or anti-Tg antibody is detected. Suppressed TSH, absent uptake in the thyroid bed, but iodine uptake by the functional metastatic tissues confirm functioning metastatic tumor.

Hyperfunctioning thyroid gland must be ruled out in patients having intact thyroid gland or residual thyroid tissue postsurgery before establishing a definitive diagnosis of hyperfunctioning metastatic thyroid carcinoma. The expression of sodium-iodide symporter (NIS) in primary thyroid tumor and metastatic foci may or may not be different; hence iodine uptake pattern on whole body scan is often variable in presence of residual thyroid tissue.

Treatment

Other than using antithyroid agents to achieve euthyroidism, management of patients with thyrotoxicosis resulting from metastatic thyroid cancer is similar to that for patients with non-functional thyroid carcinoma. From limited data, survival rates are similar to those for patients with metastatic follicular thyroid cancer who do not have thyrotoxicosis.

RARE FORMS OF DESTRUCTIVE THYROIDITIS

Anaplastic thyroid carcinoma (ATC) has the worst prognosis and the highest mortality among all thyroid cancers. On rare occasions, rapidly growing aggressive ATC destroys thyroid follicular cells, releases preformed THs and mimics painful SAT. The thyroid gland is enlarged, tender and patients often have compressive symptoms and cervical lymphadenopathy.

In recent years immune checkpoint inhibitors have been used widely in different cancers. The key agents are antibodies against programmed cell death receptor 1 (PD-1) (pembrolizumab, nivolumab), programmed death receptor ligand (PD-L1) (atezolizumab, avelumab, durvalumab, cemiplimab), and antibodies against cytotoxic T-lymphocyte–associated antigen 4 (CTLA-4) (ipilimumab, tremelimumab). Use of these agents has resulted in painless thyroiditis. About 16–36% of patients, treated with immune checkpoint inhibitors demonstrate antithyroid peroxidase antibody positivity. Monoclonal antibody against CD52, alemtuzumab, and interferon alpha has also been reported to cause painless destructive thyroiditis.

STRUMA OVARII

These are ovarian tumors, usually cystic monodermal teratomas, with thyroid tissue occupying at least 50% of the tumor volume. These rare tumors, comprising 1% of all ovarian tumors and 1–4% of ovarian teratomas, are usually encountered in areas with iodine deficiency with peak incidence at around 50 years of age. Less than 10% of such tumors are bilateral and <5% are malignant, of which 5–25% metastasize. Benign tumors are histologically indistinguishable from normal thyroid tissue. Features of classic papillary thyroid carcinoma, follicular thyroid carcinoma, and follicular variant of papillary thyroid carcinomas are encountered in 44%, 30%, and 26% of malignant SO, respectively. Molecular alterations, including RAS and PAX8-PPARγ mutations, have also been described in malignant SO. Some of these tumors co-secrete other hormones (somatostatin, chromogranin, serotonin, glucagon, insulin, gastrin, or calcitonin) and associated with carcinoid syndrome. Functioning, apparently normal intracardiac thyroid tissue has also been reported and termed struma cordis.

Clinical Features

Women, with SO, usually present to gynecologists with pelvic pain, abdominal mass, or vaginal bleeding with/without ascites. Thyrotoxicosis, either overt or subclinical, is unusual (due to poor synthesis or iodination of Tg) with 5–15% of cases present with typical signs and symptoms of thyrotoxicosis without goiter.

Diagnosis

The usual pattern of TFT in SO is elevated TH (T3>T4), suppressed TSH, and non-suppressed Tg. Whole body iodine scan reveals minimal or absent thyroidal uptake with uptake in the pelvis. Structural imaging with computed tomography (CT) or MRI demonstrates multilocular cystic ovarian mass(es) with variable signal intensity. CA-125 is elevated both in benign and malignant lesions.

Treatment

Surgical resection (salpingo-oophorectomy) is the treatment of choice once euthyroidism is restored with ATD, and extent of surgical resection depends on local invasion and fertility issues. Malignant SO should be offered radioactive iodine ablation postsurgery. Such patients need to undergo total thyroidectomy before iodine ablation. Thyroidectomy also helps to rule out primary thyroid carcinoma with ovarian metastasis. Women with malignant SO should be followed up long-term with interval serum Tg and whole-body iodine scan.

THYROTOXICOSIS DUE TO TROPHOBLASTIC TUMORS

Gestational thyrotoxicosis, mediated by human chorionic gonadotropin (hCG), is encountered in 2–3% of pregnant women during 9–12 weeks of gestation, coinciding with the period of pregnancy with highest concentration of hCG. In addition, 7–57% of patients with trophoblastic tumors, either hydatidiform moles or choriocarcinomas, have thyrotoxicosis. Other rare etiologies of hCG-mediated thyrotoxicosis are hyperplacentosis, a nonneoplastic condition with enlarged placenta and very high serum hCG concentration and recurrent gestational thyrotoxicosis due to TSH-receptor activating mutation, a condition associated with hyperemesis gravidarum in every pregnancy with possible autosomal dominant inheritance. Both these conditions remit promptly after delivery of the placenta.

Human chorionic gonadotropin molecule in women with normal pregnancy and women with hyperemesis gravidarum complicated with gestational thyrotoxicosis have high sialic acid content, while hCG in hydatidiform moles contains less sialic acid, making it a more potent thyroid stimulator, albeit with shorter circulatory half-life. Serum hCG concentration correlates with serum T3, T4, and FT4 concentrations. Thyrotoxic patients with trophoblastic tumors have a lower serum T3:T4 ratio than do patients with thyrotoxicosis caused by GD.

Clinical Features

Nausea, vomiting, and toxemia of pregnancy occur commonly in molar pregnancy and may obscure the symptoms and signs of thyrotoxicosis. Abnormal vaginal bleeding is common. Thyroid gland is normal in size or mildly enlarged, and there is no orbitopathy. Signs and symptoms of metastatic choriocarcinoma depend on the sites and extent of metastasis.

Diagnosis

Such patients have high free and total THs with suppressed TSH. Trophoblastic tumors secrete comparatively less estrogen than normal placental tissue, hence degree of rise in serum TBG concentrations is less in women with a molar pregnancy than in normal pregnant women. Thyroid radioiodine uptake, if performed, is increased.

CONSTITUTIVE ACTIVATION OF TSH RECEPTOR

McCune–Albright syndrome, caused by somatic activating mutations of the *GNAS1* gene encoding the α-subunit of the trimeric GTP-binding protein ($G_s\alpha$) that stimulates adenyl cyclase, is characterized by a triad of café au lait macules **(Figs. 4A and B)**, polyostotic fibrous dysplasia, and peripheral sexual precocity. At least two of these three features must be present to establish the diagnosis. About 19% patients of MAS develop hyperthyroidism. Thyroid may be diffusely enlarged or show nodularity.

Rarely activating mutation of the TSH receptor gives rise to familial thyrotoxicosis, a condition known as hereditary toxic thyroid hyperplasia (HTTH), sometimes called Leclère's disease. The disease is characterized by autosomal dominant inheritance, variable age of onset (from infancy to adulthood, even within a given family), hyperplastic goiter of variable size, and absence of autoimmunity.

ELEVATED TH FOLLOWING MEDICATION USE

An excess of iodine through dietary intake (kelp, sushi, seaweeds), drugs (topical iodine preparations, potassium iodide, expectorants, amiodarone), or other iodine-containing compounds (radiographic contrast agents) can lead to thyrotoxicosis through increased TH synthesis, particularly in presence of underlying thyroid autonomy, a condition known as Jod–Basedow phenomenon.

Several drugs interfere with binding of THs to the serum transport proteins or serum concentrations of the transport proteins. Alterations in circulatory levels of transport proteins do not usually affect actual free hormone concentrations; total T4 and T3 concentrations are mostly altered. Inhibition of protein binding results in reductions in serum total T4 and T3 concentrations, but free TH concentrations are elevated. However, inhibition of TH-binding to the transport proteins requires very high drug concentrations, hence often not encountered in clinical practice.

Salicylates and other nonsteroidal anti-inflammatory drugs displace T4 and T3 from their binding sites in TBG and transthyretin (TTR). Furosemide, when used orally at a dose of at least 100 mg or given intravenously in very large doses, inhibits protein binding of T4 and elevates circulatory FT4 concentration. A transient increase in free T4 has also been observed with heparin and enoxaparin use. Heparin activates lipoprotein lipase and thereby releases nonesterified fatty acids (NEFA) from triglycerides. NEFA subsequently displaces thyroid hormone from the binding proteins resulting in an increased measured level of free hormone. Serum FFA levels of at least 2.5–3 mEq/L is necessary to effectively displace thyroid hormone from the binding proteins; hence such situations are more often encountered in patients receiving intravenous lipid infusions or undergoing hemodialysis. In vitro activation of lipoprotein lipase is possible with even low doses of heparin but can be minimized by rapid and careful handling of blood samples and by avoiding repeated freezing and thawing. It has been recommended to delay free T4 measurements for 10 hours after a dose of enoxaparin to avoid erroneous interpretation of TFT.

CONCLUSION

Clinicians should be familiar with relatively uncommon causes of TH excess. These rare entities represent diagnostic and therapeutic challenges to the treating physician. Laboratory artifacts and medication use (NSAIDS, heparin, high dose frusemide, and biotin) often give rise to falsely

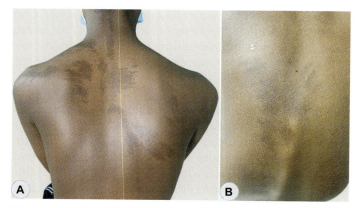

Figs. 4A and B: Café au lait spots with irregular margins (coast of Maine appearance) in two boys with McCune–Albright syndrome.

elevated THs and such interference needs to be ruled out in any asymptomatic patients. True in vivo TH excess leads to signs and/or symptoms of thyrotoxicosis; however, some of the rare etiologies of TH excess is associated with combined signs/symptoms of both hyperthyroidism and hypothyroidism (TRH-β) or only hypothyroidism (RTH-α and TH transport and metabolism defects). A detailed family history, thorough clinical examination, and careful interpretation of the abnormal TFT often help to suspect a particular diagnosis. Failure to identify a particular disease may result in therapeutic misadventure, such as inappropriate thyroidectomy or radioiodine treatment in patients with TSPA or unnecessary pituitary surgery in patients with RTH.

SUGGESTED READINGS

1. Refetoff S, Weiss RE, Usala SJ. The syndromes of resistance to thyroid hormone. Endocr Rev. 1993;14(3):348-99.
2. Refetoff S, Bassett JH, Beck-Peccoz P, Bernal J, Brent G, Chatterjee K, et al. Classification and proposed nomenclature for inherited defects of thyroid hormone action, cell transport, and metabolism. Thyroid. 2014;24(3):407-9.
3. Beck-Peccoz P, Lania A, Persani L. Thyrotropin-induced Thyrotoxicosis. In: Braverman LE, Cooper DS (Eds). The Thyroid a Fundamental and Clinical Text. 11th edition. Philadelphia: Wolters Kluwer; 2021.
4. Hershman JM. Trophoblastic Tumors. In: Braverman LE, Cooper DS (Eds). The Thyroid a Fundamental and Clinical Text. 11th edition. Philadelphia: Wolters Kluwer; 2021.
5. Chakraborty PP, Goswami S, Bhattacharjee R, Chowdhury S. BMJ Case Rep. 2019;12(4):e226087.

15 CHAPTER

Thyroid-associated Orbitopathy

Jubbin Jagan Jacob

INTRODUCTION

About 50% of patients with Graves' disease (GD) develop clinical symptoms involving the eyes called thyroid-associated orbitopathy/ophthalmopathy (TAO) or Graves'-associated ophthalmopathy (GAO) or thyroid eye disease (TED) or just Graves' ophthalmopathy (GO). TAO is the most common extrathyroidal manifestation of GD. To date there are no effective strategies to reliably prevent the development of TAO. Recent improvements in the understanding of the molecular mechanisms involved in the development of TAO have expanded the possibility of more targeted therapy. This chapter summarizes the current understanding of pathophysiology of TAO and the currently available evidence-based treatment options.

EPIDEMIOLOGY

Half the patients with GD develop clinical symptoms of TAO. These symptoms include increased tearing, photophobia, dry and gritty sensation in the eye, retro-orbital pressure sensation, and double vision. Among them, 3–5% of patients develop severe forms of TAO with intense pain and inflammation of the eye, sight-threatening corneal ulceration, and compressive optic neuropathy. Subclinical TAO is diagnosed by magnetic resonance imaging (MRI) of the orbits and can demonstrate extraocular muscle (EOM) thickening in over 70% of patients with GD. There is some suggestion that Asians (7.7%) have a much lower prevalence of TAO with GD compared to Caucasians (42%). A paper from Lucknow looking at prevalence of TAO among North Indian patients with GD (n = 235) revealed that 28% of patients with GD had clinical evidence of eye disease. A majority (83%) was mild in severity with moderate-to-severe TAO reported in 15% of patients and sight-threatening TAO only seen in 2% of patients.

True incidence studies of TAO are difficult to come by. Currently, there are three studies that have estimated the population-based incidence of TAO. The oldest study from Minnesota, United States estimated the incidence of TAO to be 16 per 100,000 population/year in women and 2.9 per 100,000 population/year in men over a period of 15 years. A more recent study from Sweden covering a population of 3.5 million suggested an overall incidence of TAO of 4.2 cases/100,000 population/year with incidence of moderate-to-severe TAO of 0.05 cases per 100,000/year. Lastly, a registry-based study from Denmark suggested incidence rates of 1.61/100,000 population/year in women and 0.54 cases/100,000 population/year in men. These significant differences between the population-based Minnesota study and the registry-based Denmark study might reflect the difficulties in identification of patients with milder TAO in registry studies and also a temporal decrease in the smoking rates in western population over the last three decades. As with GD, women constitute majority of the patients with TAO. However, men are more likely to suffer from severe eye disease. The female-to-male ratio is reported to be 9.3:1, 3.2:1, and 1.4:1 in mild, moderate and severe TAO, respectively.

RISK FACTORS

Factors that increase the risk and severity of TAO include the gender and age of the patient, any form of tobacco use, type of treatment prescribed for hyperthyroidism including the rapidity with which euthyroidism is achieved, genetic background of the patient, ongoing oxidative stress, and titers of serum thyroid-stimulating hormone receptor antibodies (TR-Ab). Among Indian patients smoking increased the risk of development of TAO by 3.9-fold. The evidence for the various risk factors and possible strategies to minimize harm is summarized in **Table 1**.

PATHOGENESIS

There is close relationship between the onset of Graves' related hyperthyroidism and TAO. Regardless of which is clinically manifest first the other manifests itself within 18 months in almost four out of five patients. In view of this close temporal relationship, it was postulated very early that

TABLE 1: Risk factors associated with TAO and ways to minimize risk.		
Risk factor	**Evidence**	**Minimizing risk**
Smoking	• Smokers have increased risk of TAO than nonsmokers • Dose-dependent risk of smoking on development of TAO • Poor response to treatment for TAO among smokers • Cessation of smoking improves symptoms and outcomes in TAO	Encourage all patients with GD with or without TAO to stop smoking
Thyroid functional status	• Hyperthyroidism associated with worse TAO • Untreated hypothyroidism also associated with worse TAO • Euthyroidism associated with better outcomes in TAO	Appropriate treatment of patients with TAO to achieve and maintain euthyroidism
Radioactive iodine (RAI) treatment	Treatment of RAI can result in progression of TAO especially in smokers	• Encourage cessation of smoking among patients planned for RAI treatment • Pretreat selected patients with steroids prior to RAI treatment
Oxidative stress	Increase in oxidative stress associated with an increase in TAO	• Antioxidant therapies • Selenium supplementation in mild TAO
Thyroid stimulating hormone-receptor antibody (TR-Ab)	• Patients with TAO have higher TR-Ab titers than those without TAO • TAO severity correlates with the titers of TR-Ab	Antithyroid drugs have potential to decrease TR-Ab titers because of their immunomodulating properties
Dyslipidemia	• Serum total cholesterol and LDL cholesterol levels correlated with presence and severity of TAO • Use of statins associated with decreased risk of development of TAO	Correct any hypercholesterolemia in patients with GD preferably with a statin

(GD: Graves' disease; LDL: low-density lipoprotein; TAO: thyroid-associated orbitopathy)

the TR-Ab which is responsible for stimulation of follicular cells to produce excess thyroid hormones is also responsible for the orbital disease. Most signs and symptoms of TAO arise from soft tissue enlargement within the retro-orbital bony space leading to an increase in retro-orbital pressure within the bony cavity. The soft tissue expansion behind the orbit is related to an expansion of the extra-orbital muscles, inflammatory cells, and adipose tissue. Younger patients tend to have more adipocyte expansion and older patients have more EOM enlargement. Sight is threatened when there is protrusion of the globe anteriorly because of the increased retro-orbital pressures leading to the inability of the eyelids to cover the cornea or when enlarged muscles at the apex of the orbital cavity compress the optic nerve. Muscle edema and enlargement is also responsible for restrictive diplopia.

Electron microscopy of the expanded muscle fibers reveals that this is primarily caused by the accumulation of a granular material within the muscle tissue consisting mainly of collagen fibrils and glycosaminoglycans (GAGs) predominantly hyaluronan. These proteins are extremely hydrophilic and accumulate many times their weight in water and further contribute to the muscle enlargement and edema. Despite the accumulation of hyaluronan and the separation of fibers, individual muscle fibers within the muscles are generally intact. Additionally, there is focal and diffuse infiltration of the ocular muscles and the orbital adipose tissue with mononuclear cells consisting mainly of CD4+ T-cells with smaller numbers of B-cells, plasma cells, and macrophages.

The molecular mechanism underlying this orbital soft tissue expansion has only recently become clearer. For reasons which are still unclear there is a failure of T-cell tolerance to the thyroid-stimulating hormone (TSH) receptor on the thyroid follicular cells. The internalized receptor peptide within the antigen presenting cell is presented along with major histocompatibility complex II (MHC-II) antigen to helper T-cells. These T-cells then become activated and interact with B-cells via the CD154-CD40 bridge leading to differentiation of the B-cells to plasma cells which in turn lead to the secretion of TR-Ab.

Within the orbit, the orbital fibroblasts appear to be the primary target in TAO. Elevated expression of TSH receptors is seen in the orbital fibroblasts of patients with GD. Circulating TR-Ab interact with the TSH receptors on the orbital fibroblasts (**Fig. 1**) once they gain access to the orbit. A subgroup of fibroblasts then starts differentiation into. Another subgroup of fibroblasts produces hyaluronan which is deposited within the EOMs. Additionally, stimulation of the insulin-like growth factor-1 receptor (IGF-1R) also expressed on the orbital fibroblasts results in the secretion of interleukin-16 (IL-16) and regulated upon activation normal T-cell expressed and secreted (RANTES) both of which enhance recruitment of CD4+ T-cells within the orbit.

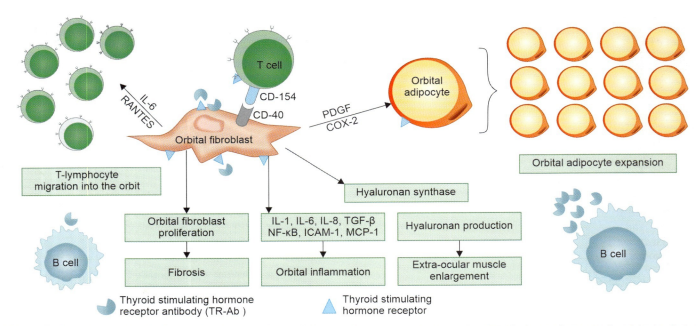

Fig. 1: TAO is triggered by binding and activation of orbital fibroblasts by autoantibodies called TR-Ab directed against thyroid-stimulating hormone receptor (TSHR), which is highly expressed on the fibroblasts, adipocyte, and muscle cells in the orbit. TR-Ab and insulin-like growth factor-1 (IGF-1) increase secretion of regulated upon activation normal T-cell expressed and secreted (RANTES) and interleukin 16 (IL-16), which elevates further T-cell migration into the orbit. This process also induces fibroblast activation, proliferation, and secretion of chemokines, inflammatory cytokines, as well as increased hyaluronic acid production and adipogenesis. Adipogenesis is induced by interleukin-1β (IL-1β) through an increase of cyclooxygenase-2 (COX-2). Platelet-derived growth factor (PDGF) increases the TSHR expression on orbital fibroblasts and plays also an adipogenic role.

(ICAM-1: intercellular adhesion molecule-1; IL-1: interleukin-1; MCP-1: monocyte chemoattractant protein-1; NF-κB: nuclear factor kappa B; TAO: thyroid-associated orbitopathy; TGF-β: transforming growth factor-beta)

CLINICAL PRESENTATION

Most patients with TAO have thyroid dysfunction in the form of hyperthyroidism. Hyperthyroidism usually presents simultaneously with TAO but on occasion TAO may precede or antecede hyperthyroidism by over 18 months. About 5% of patients may present with TAO and continue to be euthyroid even after 18 months. In 10% of patients, TAO is associated with autoimmune hypothyroidism.

Lid retraction is the most common clinical sign associated with TAO **(Fig. 2)**. This is due to a combination of sympathetic stimulation of Müllers' muscles, contraction of the levator muscles and scarring of the fascia around the lacrimal gland. Clinically, mild lid retraction may be demonstrated by lid lag when the upper eye lid lags behind eyeball movements on downward pursuit. Lagophthalmos (incomplete eyelid closure) is common and associated with exposure symptoms of foreign body sensation and photophobia. Corneal exposure symptoms of grittiness, tearing, and pain interfere with daily activities and impair quality of life (QoL) in patients with TAO. Extraorbital muscle involvement may produce bothersome diplopia either episodically, on lateral gaze or constantly. Even with mild disease the lid retraction and exophthalmos produce cosmetic problems and hamper social relationships.

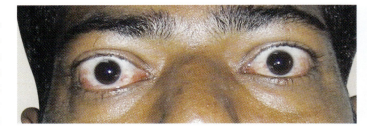

Fig. 2: Clinical picture showing upper as well as lower eyelid retraction (the most common clinical finding) in a patient with thyroid-associated orbitopathy (TAO).

Unilateral involvement is not unusual **(Fig. 3)** and presents with no issues with diagnosis when associated with hyperthyroidism. Rarely, when it is associated with euthyroidism determination of TR-Ab titers may help in the diagnosis. Other conditions which cause unilateral and bilateral exophthalmos include Cushing's syndrome, idiopathic myositis, orbital pseudotumor, primary or metastatic orbital tumors, and cavernous sinus fistulas. When in doubt orbital imaging helps in narrowing down the differential diagnosis.

Sight is threatened when muscle swelling at the orbital apex causes pressure on the optic nerve leading to dysthyroid optic neuropathy (DON) or there is breakdown of the cornea

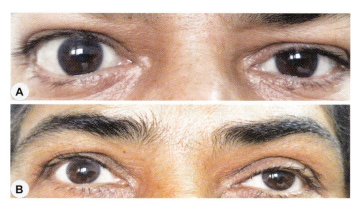

Figs. 3A and B: Mild thyroid eye disease with unilateral eyelid retraction and no clinical activity. Patient A had no evidence of thyroid dysfunction and was diagnosed based on elevated thyroid-stimulating hormone receptor antibody (TR-Ab) levels.

secondary to incomplete eyelid closure. Assessment of vision includes checking visual acuity, color vision assessments, and visual field assessments. Careful visual assessments help in picking up early signs of sight-threatening DON.

EVALUATION AND CLASSIFICATION

Treatment decisions in TAO depend on the inflammatory activity (clinical activity), duration of eye disease, and severity of eye disease. Anti-inflammatory and immunosuppressive therapy is less effective once the disease has been present for >18 months. A complete evaluation would need both assessment of clinical activity and severity of eye disease.

Activity

Activity is best assessed by the clinical activity score (CAS). Details of the traditional seven item CAS are given in **Box 1**. A score of ≥3/7 is considered to be consistent with active TAO. Additionally, three more items included in the box are useful to assess progression over a period of 1–3 months.

Severity

Severity of the TAO is best assessed by an ophthalmologist and requires measurement of the degree of exophthalmos and lid width. Additionally soft tissue assessments, vision assessments, corneal integrity assessments, and assessment of EOM functions are mandatory. The EUGOGO (European Group on Graves' Orbitopathy) classification of severity as mild, moderate-to-severe, and sight-threatening TAO is well validated in clinical and research studies. Any evidence of either DON (decrease in visual acuity, changes in color vision, papilledema on fundoscopy or apical crowding on imaging) or corneal breakdown (globe subluxation, corneal opacity, or lagophthalmos) or both indicates *sight threatening or very severe TAO* and needs to be managed as an emergency. Clinical differentiation between mild and moderate-to-severe TAO is given in detail in **Table 2**.

BOX 1: Components of the clinical activity scoring (CAS).
- Spontaneous retrobulbar pain
- Pain on attempted upward or downward gaze
- Redness of eyelids
- Redness of the conjunctiva
- Swelling (edema) of the eyelids
- Swelling (edema) of the caruncle or plica
- Conjunctival edema (chemosis)

Additional items on follow up over 1–3 months add up to a modified 10 item score
- Increase in exophthalmos by ≥2 mm
- Decrease in eye movements in any direction of gaze by ≥8°
- Decrease in visual acuity ≥1 line on the Snellen chart

Note: The clinical activity score is calculated by adding up 1 point for the presence of any of the above characteristics. Scores can range from 0 to 7. A score of 0–2 indicates inactive thyroid-associated orbitopathy (TAO) and a score of 3–7 indicates active TAO.

TABLE 2: Assessing severity of TAO.

Characteristic	Mild	Moderate to severe
Eyelid retraction (mm)	<2	≥2
Exophthalmos (mm)	<3	≥3
Soft tissue involvement	Mild	Moderate to severe
Diplopia*	None or intermittent	Inconstant or constant
Corneal involvement	None or mild	Moderate

*Intermittent diplopia occurs when patient is fatigued or on waking up in the morning. Inconstant diplopia occurs at extremes of gaze while constant diplopia occurs on looking straight ahead or down.

Note: Sight-threatening (very severe) thyroid-associated orbitopathy (TAO): Patients with dysthyroid optic neuropathy and/or corneal breakdown.

TABLE 3: Assessing severity of thyroid-associated orbitopathy (TAO) using NOSPECS scoring system.

Scores	NOSPECS classification	Features
0	N	No symptoms or signs
1	O	Signs but no symptoms
2	S	Soft tissue involvement
3	P	Proptosis (exophthalmos)
4	E	Extraocular muscle involvement
5	C	Corneal involvement
6	S	Sight loss or visual impairment

Other scoring systems including the popular NOSPECS system **(Table 3)**, VISA (vision, inflammation, strabismus, and appearance), total eye score allow better quantification but have of late been superseded by the EUGOGO classification.

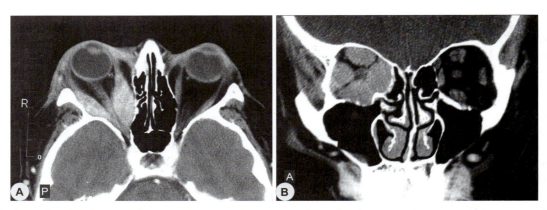

Figs. 4A and B: (A) Axial and (B) Coronal. Computed tomographic images of the orbit showing enlargement of the extraocular muscles with sparing of tendons in the right orbit.
Courtesy: Dr Milind Naik MD, Ophthalmic Plastic Surgery Service, LV Prasad Eye Institute, Hyderabad.

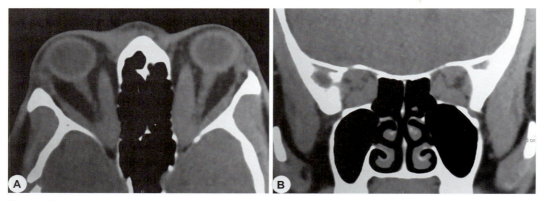

Figs. 5A and B: (A) Axial and (B) Coronal. CT scan of the orbit showing crowding and enlargement of the extraocular muscles around the optic nerve at the apex of the both orbits in a patient with dysthyroid optic neuropathy.
Courtesy: Dr Milind Naik MD, Ophthalmic Plastic Surgery Service, LV Prasad Eye Institute, Hyderabad.

Imaging: The imaging modality of choice to assess TAO is computed tomography (CT) of the orbit. CT is better in identifying EOM enlargement compared to MRI. CT findings include evidence of muscle belly enlargement **(Fig. 4)** with characteristic sparing of the tendons in older patients and evidence of adipose tissue expansion with proptosis seen more in younger patients **(Fig. 5)**. Crowding around the optic nerve at the apex of the orbit by enlarged muscle is seen in sight-threatening DON **(Fig. 5)**.

MEDICAL MANAGEMENT

Surveys from Europe have demonstrated a decrease in the incidence of TAO as well as an improvement in severity over the last three decades. These improvements have come with reduction in smoking habits, early control of thyroid dysfunction in patients with GD, better interaction between the physician, and the ophthalmologist leading to early treatment for TAO. Specialized multidisciplinary thyroid eye clinics are best suited to handle moderate-to-severe TAO, patients with unstable hyperthyroidism and TAO, current smokers with TAO, and those with high TR-Ab levels. Most patients with mild TAO can be managed in primary care.

General Measures to Reduce Risk

- All patients with GD should be urged to quit smoking. Smoking increases risk of development of TAO and also increases the severity of the disease. Current smokers have poor response to immunosuppressive treatments. Cessation of smoking leads to better outcomes in TAO.
- Early and adequate control of thyroid dysfunction is important as both untreated hyperthyroidism and hypothyroidism is associated with negative impact on TAO. Difficult to control hyperthyroidism or brittle hyperthyroidism is best treated by an endocrinologist than in primary care.

- Radioactive iodine (RAI) has been shown to cause progression in 15% of patients with TAO or de novo occurrence of TAO in patients with no preexisting eye disease. Current smoking compounds these risks further. For prevention of RAI-associated occurrence or progression of TAO three short-term steroid regimens is proposed. These include:
    o Original oral regimen using oral prednisolone at a dose of 0.3–0.5 mg/kg/day gradually tapered and withdrawn over 3 months. This should be the regimen used in patients with high risk of progression including current smokers.
    o Low-dose oral prednisolone regimen of 0.1–0.2 mg/kg/day given and tapered over 6 weeks can be used in milder cases.
    o Low-dose intravenous (IV) methylprednisolone once a week over 4 weeks requires day care admission weekly for 4 weeks.
- High cholesterol levels have emerged as a new risk factor for TAO in the last decade. A large retrospective cohort suggested that the use of statins was associated with decreased occurrence of TAO. Though controlled clinical trials are lacking statin therapy should be considered in patients with TAO and hypercholesterolemia.

Local Measures

Dry eye is frequent in patients with TAO because of decreased palpebral width, lagophthalmos, decreased blink rates, exophthalmos, lid lag, and altered osmolality of the tear film. This can be treated with artificial tears during daytime and use of ophthalmic gels and ointments during sleep. Other night time measures could include taping of the eyelids and use of swimming goggles. Botulinum toxin injected into the levator muscle can help reduce the palpebral width.

Treatment of Mild TAO

Majority of patients with TAO have a mild form of the disease. Most patients have spontaneous improvement in symptoms and few go on to progress to moderate and severe TAO. However, even patients with mild eye disease may suffer significant reductions in QoL when assessed with TAO-specific QoL questionnaires. Corneal exposure symptoms can be minimized by the use of sunglasses (for photophobia) when outdoors and use of lubricants and ointments for grittiness and dryness of the eye. Head elevation at night during sleep can reduce periorbital edema in patients with mild active disease.

Selenium supplementation was shown to improve QoL, decrease soft tissue signs, and slow progression of mild TAO compared to pentoxifylline in a randomized controlled trial (RCT) from Europe. Selenium appears to be a safe drug for use in mild TAO with no major side effects though further trials are required to firmly establish its efficacy especially in areas where there is no preexisting selenium deficiency.

The dosing of selenium supplementation includes:
- Sodium selenite 200 µg once daily for 6 months
- Selenomethionine 100 µg once daily for 6 months

The benefits were seen to persist for 6 months after cessation of supplementation. There is no role for selenium supplementation in moderate-to-severe TAO.

Diplopia with mild active TAO can be managed expectantly with patching or with the use of Fresnel prisms. Once disease activity has ceased remnant diplopia can be managed with ground in prisms and/or rehabilitative strabismus surgery.

Most patients with mild TAO do not require any therapy. A small minority of patients may experience profound impact on QoL even with mild disease. These patients may benefit from low-dose immunosuppressive therapy for active disease and rehabilitative surgery for inactive disease after appropriate counseling.

Moderate-to-severe TAO

The natural history of untreated moderate-to-severe TAO includes an active inflammatory phase which can last 18–24 months followed by a plateau and slow remission leading to signs and symptoms consisting of residual disease after 24–36 months since onset. In patients with moderate-to-severe eye disease, the goal of therapy is to intervene early to shorten the duration and severity of the active phase of the eye disease (**Fig. 6**). Additional goals include improving subjective and objective eye manifestations and limit residual disease. Therapy is most effective if treated within the first year of development of disease.

Efficacy of immunosuppressive therapy is between 50 and 80% and rarely leads to a complete remission. Residual disease requires rehabilitative surgery. *Glucocorticoids (GCs)* are the most commonly used first-line medications for TAO. Two RCTs have shown superiority of IV GCs when directly compared with high-dose oral GCs. Intravenous GC was also associated with lower side effects and better tolerability. There are four reported cases of acute hepatic failure in clinical trials with the use of IV GCs and hence liver functions should be monitored when IV GCs are administered. Primary efficacy of the GCs is in reducing the activity score in TAO and they have minimal effects on proptosis, lid aperture, or diplopia. A common dosage strategy is using 500 mg of IV methylprednisolone weekly for 6 weeks and 250 mg of methylprednisolone for another 6 weeks leading to a total cumulative dose of 4.5 g. Dose higher than this is associated with hepatotoxicity. Direct orbital administration of GCs may reduce side effects but studies have been disappointing in terms of efficacy. Details of first-line therapy are summarized in **Flowchart 1**.

Failure to respond to first-line therapy entails choosing one of six possible second-line therapies including higher dose IV GCs, oral prednisolone with cyclosporine or azathioprine, orbital radiotherapy, rituximab, tocilizumab, and teprotumumab.

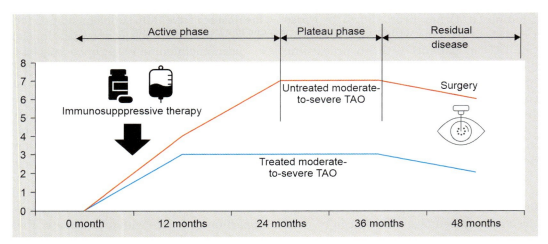

Fig. 6: The natural history of untreated TAO (in red) including active phase, plateau phase, and residual disease. Natural history of a patient with thyroid-associated orbitopathy (TAO) treated early and appropriately with immunosuppressive agents shown in blue with reduced duration and severity of active phase and less residual disease.

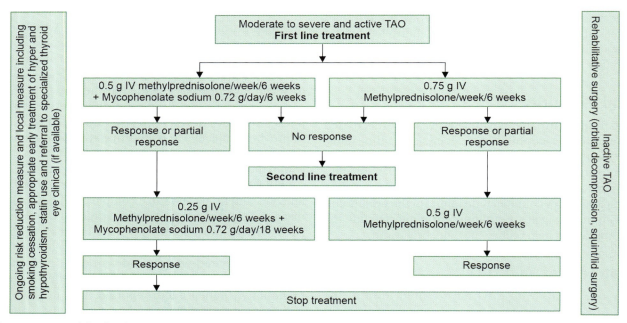

Flowchart 1: Protocol for first-line management of patients with moderate-to-severe active thyroid-associated orbitopathy (TAO) based on the 2021 consensus statement of the European Group on Graves' Orbitopathy (EUGOGO) widely accepted on both sides of the Atlantic.

Rituximab was the first biological agent to be used in the second-line treatment of moderate-to-severe TAO. It was found to be slightly more effective than IV GCs in a head-to-head randomized control trial. The doses used in this trial was (IV methylprednisolone 7.5 g and two different dosing schedules of rituximab, one 1,000 mg into two doses 2 weeks apart and a second dosing schedule of one single dose of 500 mg. Even those on the lower dose did better than IV GCs.

Teprotumumab was recently approved in the United States as a new targeted biological agent for TAO. Teprotumumab is an IGF-1R antagonist and is considered a key receptor in the pathogenesis of TAO. Though the drug is currently not available in India the dosing has been summarized in **Flowchart 2**.

Orbital radiotherapy though popular in the last decade has been shown to have only modest improvements in EOM mobility. Case series suggest a 60% response rate but patients with exophthalmos and lid retraction have poor responses. The standard dose of radiotherapy is the use of 20 Gy/eye divided into 10 doses of 2 Gy each over a period of 2 weeks. Half of this dose is found to be equally effective. Orbital radiation is relatively contraindicated in younger patients (age <35 years) because of the risk of secondary

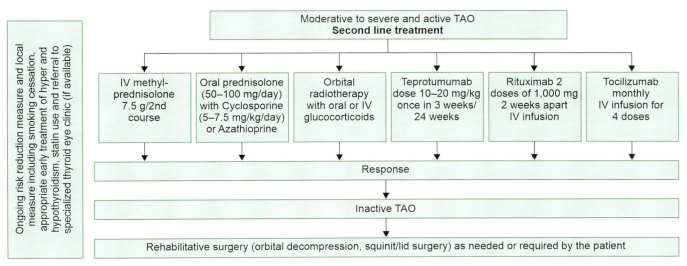

Flowchart 2: Protocol for second-line management of patients with moderate-to-severe active thyroid-associated orbitopathy (TAO) who do not respond to first-line management based on the 2021 consensus statement of the European Group on Graves' Orbitopathy (EUGOGO).

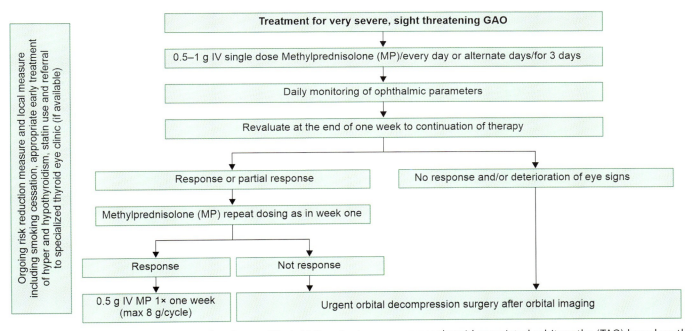

Flowchart 3: Protocol for management of patients with sight threatening, very severe thyroid-associated orbitopathy (TAO) based on the 2021 consensus statement of the European Group on Graves' Orbitopathy (EUGOGO).

malignancy and in patients with significant retinal disease due to diabetes mellitus or hypertension.

Sight Threatening TAO

Sight can be threatened in 5% of patients with TAO. Intravenous GCs are more effective than emergency orbital decompressive therapy but is associated with higher side effects. There is no established treatment regimen for GCs in sight-threatening TAO but a common initial regimen is using pulses of 1 g of IV methylprednisolone on three consecutive days. If there is no change in clinical condition in 1–2 weeks after IV GC then emergency decompressive surgery is the next therapy of choice **(Flowchart 3)**.

Surgical therapy: Patients with moderate-to-severe TAO but inactive disease requires rehabilitative eye surgery (for example, orbital decompression, lid procedures, strabismus surgery, and cosmetic procedures), the details of which are beyond the scope of this chapter.

CONCLUSION

Eye disease accompanying GD appears to be less common among Indians. Majority of patients with TAO have self-limited mild disease which requires no intervention. Selenium supplementation may improve QoL in patients with mild disease in addition to local measures. Intravenous

GC in doses of 4.5 g/12 weeks is the treatment of choice for active disease which is moderate to severe. Sight-threatening TAO is treated with IV pulse therapy of methylprednisolone and/or emergency decompressive surgery. Orbital surgery for rehabilitation remains the therapy of choice for inactive disease.

SUGGESTED READINGS

1. Bartalena L, Tanda ML. Clinical practice. Graves' ophthalmopathy. N Engl J Med. 2009;360:994-1001.
2. Bahn RS. Graves' Ophthalmopathy. N Engl J Med. 2010;362: 726-38.
3. Bartalena L, Piantanida E, Gallo D, Lai A, Tanda ML. Epidemiology, Natural History, Risk Factors, and Prevention of Graves' Orbitopathy. Front Endocrinol (Lausanne). 2020;11:615993.
4. Khong JJ, McNab AA, Ebeling PR, Craig JE, Selva D. Pathogenesis of thyroid eye disease: review and update on molecular mechanisms. Br J Ophthalmol. 2016;100(1):142-50.
5. Bartalena L, Kahaly GJ, Baldeschi L, Dayan CM, Eckstein A, Marcocci C, et al. The 2021 European Group on Graves' orbitopathy (EUGOGO) clinical practice guidelines for the medical management of Graves' orbitopathy. Eur J Endocrinol. 2021;185(4):G43-G67.

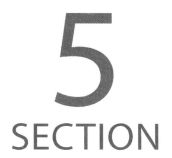

SECTION 5

Goiter, Thyroid Nodules and Thyroid Cancer

CHAPTER 16

Simple or Nontoxic Goiter

Sushil Kumar Gupta, Sabaretnam Mayilvaganan

INTRODUCTION

Nontoxic goiter is one of the most common thyroid disorders encountered in clinical practice. It is also referred as simple goiter. It is defined as an enlargement of thyroid gland which is not the result of an inflammatory or neoplastic process and biochemically euthyroid.

What size of gland constitutes enlargement is matter of debate. Normal size of thyroid gland depends on multiple factors, most importantly iodine intake, thiocyanates exposure, selenium intake, etc. Generally, a thyroid gland should be no larger than 12–18 mL in adult women, and 19–25 mL in adult men, depending on the reference population investigated and as assessed by ultrasonography. Thyroid lobe dimensions in healthy subjects change from birth into adulthood: the length (L) is 1.8–2.0 cm in newborns and 4.0–6.0 cm in adults, while the anteroposterior (AP) dimension measures 0.8–0.9 cm in newborns and 1.3–1.8 cm in adults.

Goiter is categorized into diffuse enlargement or nodular, solitary nodular, or multinodular thyroid. It needs to be emphasized that size of nodular thyroid can be within the normal range of size of thyroid.

ETIOLOGY

It is well accepted fact that it is a complex disease, with clinical phenotype representing the net effect of many contributing genetic and environmental factors. The thyroid gland can enlarge due to a variety of physiological or pathological stimuli. Goiter during adolescence and pregnancy are two causes of a physiological goiter. The most common cause of simple goiter is iodine deficiency. Globally, iodine deficiency affects an estimated 2.2 billion people. The prevalence and incidence of goiter are based on the degree of iodine deficiency. With mild iodine deficiency, the incidence of goiter is 5–20%. With a moderate deficiency, the prevalence increases to 20–30%, and with severe iodine deficiency, the incidence increases to >30%. Regional variation in the iodine status imparts considerable differences in the prevalence of goiter among populations, with a clear inverse correlation with the dietary iodine intake. Long-standing iodine deficiency leads to prolonged elevation of serum thyrotropin [thyroid-stimulating hormone (TSH)] levels, inducing hyperplasia and hypertrophy of thyrotrophs, increasing iodine uptake, trapping and compensatory increase and normalization of circulatory thyroid hormones. With duration, iodine deficiency induces high oxidative stress load within the thyrocyte, leading to an increase in spontaneous mutation rate, and eventually formation of thyroid nodules. Development of nodules may lead to autonomy and finally overproduction of thyroid hormones.

Primary factors involved in development of nodular disease are: (a) heterogeneity of function and growth among polyclonal normal follicular cells probably due to genetic and acquisition of new heritable qualities by replicating epithelial cells and (b) functional and structural abnormalities in hyperplastic goiter. Secondary factors are: (a) elevated TSH due to iodine deficiency, natural goitrogens, inherited dyshormonogenesis, (b) smoking, (c) certain drugs, (d) other thyroid-stimulating factors, and (e) endogenous factors (gender).

Naturally, occurring goitrogens in diet are a significant aggravating factor in presence of mild to severe iodine deficiency. Various naturally occurring goitrogens are flavonoids (millet, soybeans), cyanogenic glucosides (cassava, sweet potato, sorghum), and glucosinolates (cruciferous vegetables, e.g., cabbage, cauliflower, broccoli, turnips), iodine excess (seaweed, kelp), deficiency of vitamin A, iron, and selenium play a significant role in select situations.

Rarely, inherited defects in thyroid hormone synthesis and resistance to thyroid hormone action can result in simple or nodular goiter. Other thyroid-stimulating factors, e.g., epidermal growth factor, insulin-like growth factor, fibroblast growth factor, cytokines, acetylcholine, prostaglandins, vasoactive intestinal peptide, etc. have been shown to play a role in pathogenesis.

Family and twin studies, and linkage studies in past few years have shown significant role of genetic factors in pathogenesis of nodular goiter. Familial goiter has an autosomal dominant inheritance. Children of parents with goiter have a significant risk of developing goiter compared to nongoitrous parents. Gene-gene interaction and various polymorphism of various genes can have synergistic effect on development of goiter. Twin studies demonstrate more concordance rate in monozygotic times than in dizygotic times. Mutations and polymorphisms in genes for thyroid peroxidase (*TPO* gene), thyroglobulin (*TG*), sodium iodide symporter gene (*SCL5A5*), Pendred syndrome gene (*SCL26A4*), iodotyrosine deiodinase (*DEHAL 1*), thyroid oxidase 2 gene 3 (*DUOX2*), and thyrotrophic receptor (*TSHR* gene), can all have a role. Genome-wide linkage studies have shown a candidate locus, MNG1 on chromosome 14q31 in a Canadian and German family with euthyroid goiter, linkage to a second locus MNG2 (Xp22) in an Italian family, and loci on chromosome 18, 2q, 3p, 7q, 8p, etc. Simple goiter is polygenic, with no single gene being either necessary or sufficient for disease development. The pronounced sex difference in prevalence of thyroid disease often 5–10 times more common in females is puzzling. Theoretically, a skewed X-chromosome inactivation (XCI) pattern which is probably genetically determined and the resultant tissue chimerism could offer a new approach to female preponderance of thyroid disorders. A small increase in iodine intake is supposedly reducing the incidence of simple goiter.

Summarily, there are several etiologic factors in simple and nodular goiter, and some of them act synergistically. The end result is diffuse enlargement and later heterogeneously functioning thyroid follicles. The function may turn autonomous and results in hyperthyroidism.

PATHOLOGY

In early phase, there is a hyperplasia with considerable variation in follicle size. Later, gland contains nodules of various size with normal homogenous parenchymal structure in intervening areas. Frequently, nodules undergo degeneration and a cyst is found. There can be evidence of recent or old hemorrhage, calcification, fibrosis, and lymphocytic infiltration. Sometimes, 4–17% of these nodules have microscopic foci of papillary carcinoma.

NATURAL HISTORY

Simple goiter is physiological during puberty and pregnancy, especially in area of iodine deficiency. It usually regresses but may persist if iodine deficiency continues. If nodular goiter develops, it persists for prolonged period and probably for whole life. It can increase progressively in size and can cause compressive symptoms in neck and upper mediastinum. The goiter remains euthyroid but it can be autonomously functioning resulting in thyrotoxicosis, usually in later years of life **(Fig. 1)**.

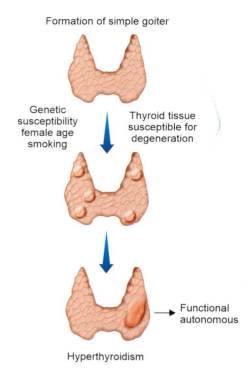

Fig. 1: Pathogenesis of simple goiter.

SYMPTOMS

Goiter can be asymptomatic and come to notice incidentally by the patient or any family member. Sometime the size of the goiter is almost 2–3 times of normal size by the time it comes to attention. It can be diffuse enlargement or a prominent single nodule or a predominant nodule in a multinodular goiter.

Patient may present with compressive features, e.g., globus sensation, dysphagia, irritant cough, change in voice, chocking sensation, respiratory distress, etc. Even large goiter may have no compressive symptoms while small goiter can have pressure symptoms. With increasing use of ultrasound in clinical practice, goiter is discovered while undergoing ultrasound for some other indication. The spontaneous growth is difficult to predict, can be up to 20% yearly. The risk of malignancy is around 2–5% depending on patient and nodule characteristics. The spontaneous development of hypothyroidism is rarely seen.

Pain is a rare complaint and it occurs because of spontaneous hemorrhage into a nodule. Some nodules being located in the lower part of the neck may compress trachea, esophagus, nerves, and blood vessels. It may cause upper airway obstruction by displacing or narrowing the trachea but respiratory symptoms can be few. Very rarely patient can have stridor. To an extent the severity of tracheal compression correlates with goiter volume. Compression of esophagus can result in swallowing difficulties sometimes dysmotility of hyoid bone, tilting of epiglottis, or bolus retention in pharynx can cause swallowing difficulty. Many patients may present with voice fatigue and voice straining **(Figs. 2 to 4)**.

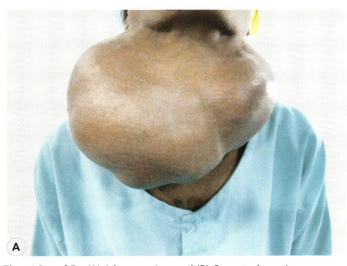
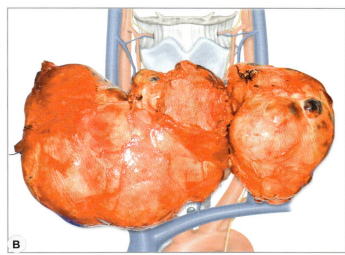

Figs. 2A and B: (A) A large goiter and (B) Operated specimen.

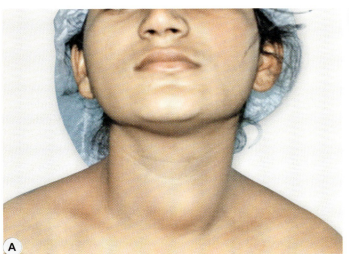
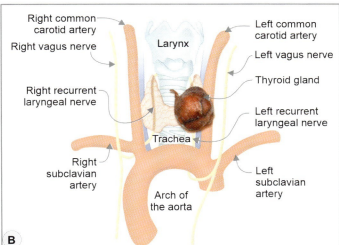
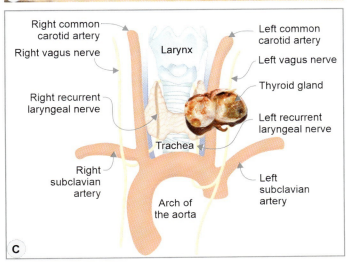

Figs. 3A to C: (A) A small solitary thyroid nodule (STN) and (B and C) Specimen and cut surface.

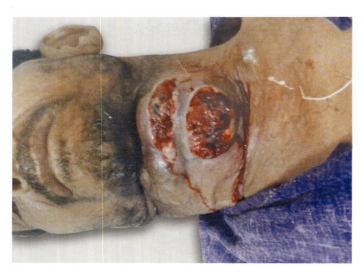

Fig. 4: Bleeding and ulcerated malignant goiter.

CLINICAL EXAMINATION

The clinical examination is primarily focused on assessment of compressive features of goiter, possibility of malignancy, functionality (thyrotoxicosis), and in last cosmetic.

The thyroid gland becomes visible and palpable when it doubles in size. Thyroid is inspected from front while palpated by many methods. Various methods for palpations are: (a) from behind—both thumbs on occiput, palpate with four fingers; (b) Pizzillo method: patient's hands behind occiput, extend neck backward and should be used in obese subjects with short neck; (c) Lahey's method: thyroid is pushed to opposite side from front to palpate each lobe; (d) Crile's method: to feel the thyroid with thumb while patient swallows.

A note of its size and extent, consistency, nodularity, mobility, tenderness, and local temperature is made. It is important to focus on a large nodule or rapidly enlarging nodule. Kocher's test for stridor in a goiter is elicited for features of tracheal compression ("scabbard" trachea) and possibility of tracheomalacia. Cervical and pretracheal lymph nodes should be examined for enlargement. Tracheal deviation and carotid pulsation must be noted. Sometimes goiter grows and descends in upper mediastinum. It can be detected by observing dull percussion note on the manubrium sterni. A large retrosternal goiter with compression of superior vena cava may results in facial congestion, cyanosis, and respiratory distress. Pemberton maneuver is to demonstrate the presence of latent pressure in the thoracic inlet. The patient is asked to elevate both arms (usually 180° anterior flexion at the shoulder) until the forearms touch the sides of the face for 1 minute. A positive Pemberton's sign is marked by the presence of facial congestion and cyanosis, as well as respiratory distress after approximately 1 minute.

It is important to explore the features suggestive of malignancy. The high-risk factors of malignancy are extremes of age (<20 or >70 years), male gender, size >4 cm, recent rapid growth (may suggest anaplastic carcinoma or lymphoma), family history of thyroid malignancy, or genetic disorders such as syndrome of MEN type 2, familial polyposis coli and Cowden syndrome, history of exposure to radiation to head and neck region (e.g., previous treatment of Hodgkin's disease affecting neck), palpable cervical or pretracheal lymphadenopathy, change in voice, or appearance of dysphagia. Most important clinical features in patients with thyroid nodules warranting urgent referral are a nodule that is very firm or hard, nodule fixed to adjacent structures, or presence of cervical lymphadenopathy. Compressive symptoms (dysphagia, dyspnea), foreign body sensation in the throat, hoarseness or voice change, and stridor are soft signs of malignancy.

Features suggestive of thyrotoxicosis should be explored in every case of goiter. Thyrotoxicosis can be asymptomatic or can present with varied catabolic features in absence of adrenergic symptoms. The predominant catabolic features, e.g., weight loss, loss of appetite, marked muscle weakness, tachycardia without tremors, apathy, depression, etc. can be suggestive of malignancy but can be due to thyrotoxicosis as confirmed by thyroid function tests.

Cosmetic assessment is a personal statement by the patient but it needs consideration while planning treatment.

INVESTIGATIONS

Investigation for simple or nontoxic goiter are directed for evaluation of the functional status of gland, morphological evaluation for defining the characteristics for malignancy or compressive features, and at-times functional imaging in select situations.

Various surveys of endocrinologists and thyroidologists in American, European, and Latin American Associations reveal the preference for estimations of various components of thyroid functions. Serum TSH and FT4 are preferred by all but European surveys show adding total T3 as wall in view of coexisting mild iodine deficiency. Antithyroid peroxidase and thyroglobulin antibodies are measured routinely as autoimmunity may coexist with goiter. Further, positive antibodies may represent chronic autoimmune thyroiditis.

Some of groups in India measure urinary iodine excretion for identifying iodine deficiency as the cause; it is useful if it is a diffuse goiter with negative thyroid autoantibody profile. Rarely serum calcitonin is done in routine work up of a simple goiter if there is no wheezing, flushing, and diarrhea.

Diagnostic morphological imaging includes, stepwise, high-resolution ultrasonography (HR-USG) and occasionally elastography, computerized tomography (CT), and magnetic resonance imaging (MRI). HR-USG is the initial step for defining the size, volume, and echotexture of thyroid gland, defining characteristic of nodule as per TIRAD (Thyroid Imaging Reporting And Data system criteria) and characteristic of cervical lymphadenopathy.

USG thyroid has made a paradigm shift in the evaluation of thyroid disorders because of its wide availability, low cost, easy applicability in office practice, and vast experience in defining TIRAD classification for low and high risk of malignancy in the thyroid nodule. Hypoechogenicity, microcalcification, indistinct borders and increased nodular flow (on Doppler studies) in thyroid nodule, and presence of lymphadenopathy are sonographic marker of malignancy and the nodule should be subjected to fine-needle aspiration biopsy and cytology (FNAB/FNAC). Ultrasound elastography can provide information regarding malignant risk in nodule, however, with moderate sensitivity (75%) and specificity (73%).

Computed tomography and MRI provide high resolution of goiter and are specifically useful in defining substernal goiter, their extent and presence of compressive features on neighboring structures, e.g., trachea and upper airway, esophagus, and large vessels.

Isotope imaging by scintigraphy has a limited role in the evaluation; however, it is vital in evaluation of possible dyshormonogenetic goiter. Positron emission tomography has limited role in evaluation except in select situation of medullary thyroid carcinoma.

Fine-needle Aspiration Biopsy and Cytology

Fine-needle aspiration biopsy and cytology should be considered in all patients of nodule goiter with ultrasound assessment of the high risk of malignancy. All nodules with TIRAD classification of three and above should undergo FNAB and the cytology should be performed with BATHESDA criteria.

Liquid biopsy of thyroid nodule: Recent publications have highlighted the role of liquid biopsy of thyroid nodule for diagnosis of thyroid malignancy.

TREATMENT

The treatment of simple goiter is primarily the following:
- Iodine supplementation
- Levothyroxine (L-T4) suppressive therapy
- Radioiodine treatment (alone or preceded by recombinant thyrotropin)
- Surgery

Iodine Supplementation

Iodine supplementation is useful only in the situation of iodine deficiency and in the early stage of goiter. It has limited value in late stages when transition to nodular stage has arrived. A major issue with iodine supplementation is precipitation of thyrotoxicosis (Jod–Basedow phenomenon). Summarily, iodine supplementation is required for correction of iodine deficiency at the level of the community rather than the individual.

L-T4 Suppressive Therapy

Levothyroxine suppressive therapy is used extensively in diffuse goiter both in Europe, USA, and Latin America but has a limited role in nodular goiter. L-T4 suppressive therapy in diffuse goiter results in reduction of goiter by 20–40% after 3–6 months of therapy; however, the beneficial effect is reversible after stopping of treatment. The efficacy of treatment depends on the degree of TSH suppression. Long-term L-T4 suppressive therapy in nodular goiter results in volume reduction is a subgroup of nodules but effectively prevented the appearance of new nodules. A meta-analysis of six prospective controlled studies concluded four of six studies favor treatment with L-T4.

Radioiodine Ablation of Goiter

Radioiodine administration leads to reduction of size of thyroid gland and substernal extension of thyroid with the risk of long-term primary hypothyroidism. Radioiodine ablation of small sized simple non-nodular goiter is generally recommended due to long-term risk of primary hypothyroidism. Radioiodine therapy in multinodular goiter leads to reduction of thyroid volume by 30–40% with long-term risk of primary hypothyroidism ranging from 10 to 60%.

In recent years, pretreatment with recombinant TSH (0.01/0.03 mg 24 hours before 131-I administration) results in increased uptake of 131-I in the goiter and allows with lower dose of 131-I to induce volume reduction. There is marked improvement in airway obstruction in subjects with substernal goiter. There is risk of transient hyperthyroidism and potential risk of transient increase in size by 15–25% in first week after treatment. There is no long-term added risk of thyroid malignancy.

Surgery

The goal of thyroid surgery in simple goiter is to alleviate the pressure symptoms, and prevent recurrence. Hemithyroidectomy and near total/total thyroidectomy are widely used operative procedures. Now instead of open thyroidectomy endoscopic and robotic thyroidectomy are in vogue especially for cosmetic indications. Surgical indications for simple goiter are: cancer suspicion, large goiter, substernal goiter, compressive symptoms, no or low I-131 uptake, and sometimes cosmetic and patient preference.

CONCLUSION

Simple goiter is usually related to iodine deficiency. However, other causes need to be ruled out by systematic evaluation. Any nodule in thyroid should be evaluated to rule out malignancy. Prevention of iodine deficiency by community intervention can reduce the incidence of simple goiter remarkably.

SUGGESTED READINGS

1. Hegedüs L, Brix TH, Paschke R. Etiology of simple goiter. Thyroid. 2009;19(3):209-11.
2. Brix TH, Hegedüs L. Genetic and environmental factors in the aetiology of simple goiter. Ann Med. 2000;32(3):153-6.
3. Studer H, Ramelli F. Simple goiter and its variants: euthyroid and hyperthyroid multinodular goiters. Endocr Rev. 1982 Winter;3(1):40-61.
4. Brix TH, Kyvik KO, Hegedüs L. Major role of genes in the etiology of simple goiter in females: a population-based twin study. J Clin Endocrinol Metab. 1999;84(9):3071-5.
5. Böttcher Y, Eszlinger M, Tönjes A, Paschke R. The genetics of euthyroid familial goiter. Trends Endocrinol Metab. 2005;16(7):314-9.
6. Knudsen N, Laurberg P, Perrild H, Bülow I, Ovesen L, Jørgensen T. Risk factors for goiter and thyroid nodules. Thyroid. 2002;12(10):879-88.
7. Schlumberger MJ, Filetti S, Hay ID. Nontoxic goiter and thyroid neoplasia. Larsen PR, Kronenberg HM, Melmed D, Polonsky KS (Eds). Williams Textbook of Endocrinology. Philadelphia: WB Saunders; 2003. p. 13.
8. Bahn RS, Castro MR. Approach to the patient with nontoxic multinodular goiter. J Clin Endocrinol Metab. 2011;96(5):1202-12.
9. Freitas JE. Therapeutic options in the management of toxic and nontoxic nodular goiter. Semin Nucl Med. 2000;30(2):88-97.
10. Bonnema SJ, Bennedbæk FN, Ladenson PW, Hegedüs L. Management of the nontoxic multinodular goiter: a North American survey. J Clin Endocrinol Metab. 2002;87(1):112-7.
11. Hegedüs L, Bonnema SJ, Bennedbaek FN. Management of simple nodular goiter: current status and future perspectives. Endocr Rev. 2003;24(1):102-32.
12. Agarwal A, Agarwal S, Tewari P, Gupta S, Chand G, Mishra A, et al. Clinicopathological profile, airway management, and outcome in huge multinodular goiters: an institutional experience from an endemic goiter region. World J Surg. 2012;36(4):755-60.
13. Gaitan E, Nelson NC, Poole GV. Endemic goiter and endemic thyroid disorders. World J Surg. 1991;15(2):205-15.
14. Biban BG, Lichiardopol C. Iodine Deficiency, Still a Global Problem? Curr Health Sci J. 2017;43(2):103-11.
15. Talukder MI, Naher N, Karim SM, Hasan KM, Khan SI, Rahman AK. Clinico Pathological Analysis of Nodular Goiter: A Retrospective Study. J Surg Res. 2022;5:80-91.
16. Pelizzo MR, Toniato A, Piotto A, Pagetta C, Ide EC, Boschin IM. The surgical treatment of the nodular goiter. Ann Ital Chir. 2008;79(1):13-6.
17. Al-Saig TH, Al-Omary MS, Zuhair M. Non toxic goiter: Cytology, Histological Analysis: a study in Mosul. Iraqi J Comm Med. 2011;24(4):325-0.
18. Abdella MR, Al-Ahmer MM, Khidr HM. Recurrent nodular goiter: predictors of recurrence and outcome after reoperation. AAMJ. 2014;12(1).
19. La Gamma A, Letoquart JP, Kunin N, Chaperon J, Mambrini A. Nodular goiter. Retrospective analysis of 608 cases. J Chir (Paris). 1993;130(10):391-6.
20. Gutiérrez MT, Gómez J, Taibo MA, Barrios B, Escobar A, Iturburu I. Development and outcomes of the surgical management of multinodular goiter. Cir Esp. 2006;80(2):83-9.
21. Bukhari U, Sadiq S. Histopathological audit of goiter: A study of 998 thyroid lesions. Pak J Med Sci. 2008;24(3):442.
22. Jiang Y, Gao B, Zhao J, Zhang S, Guo L, Tian W, et al. Diagnosis and surgical treatment of giant goiter. Int J ClinExp Med. 2017;10(1):548-5.

CHAPTER 17

Nodular Thyroid Disease

Krishna G Seshadri

INTRODUCTION

An abnormal growth of the thyroid gland is called *goiter*. A thyroid nodule may be defined as a discrete lesion within the thyroid gland that is radiologically distinct from the surrounding gland. Goiters can be diffuse or nodular. Nodules can be solitary or multiple.

Palpable thyroid nodules are reported in approximately 5% of women and 1% of men in iodine sufficient areas (ISA). Up to 50% of patients with a palpable single nodule will demonstrate additional nodules on ultrasonography. If a high resolution ultrasound (USG) were used up to 68% of randomly selected individuals may have nodules—more in women and increasing with age in both sexes. There is a linear increase in prevalence from almost none at age 15–50% by age 65. New nodules appear with an incidence of 1 per 10,000 per year with an estimated lifetime risk of development of a nodule of up to 10%. Up to 60% of thyroid glands will have nodules at autopsy.

PATHOPHYSIOLOGY

The principal causes of thyroid nodules are summarized in **Table 1**. Thyroid nodules are the clinical manifestation of a myriad of pathologic processes. Non-neoplastic nodules are the result of glandular hyperplasia arising spontaneously or following partial thyroidectomy. Hashimoto's thyroiditis may present with a nodular feel, but does not represent an example of true nodule formation.

TABLE 1: Classification of thyroid nodules.

Adenomas	Malignant tumors	Others
• Follicular 　○ Colloid variant 　○ Embryonal 　○ Fetal 　○ Hürthle cell variant • Teratoma	• Differentiated adenocarcinoma 　○ Papillary 　○ Follicular • Medullary carcinoma • Undifferentiated	• Lymphoma • Squamous cell epidermoid carcinoma • Fibrosarcoma • Mucoepithelial carcinoma • Metastatic tumor

Risk Factors

Worldwide, iodine deficiency (ID) is the most common cause of nodular thyroid disease (NTD). The prevalence of NTD correlates inversely with population iodine intake. In iodine deficient areas (IDA) up to 40% of women and up to 30% of men have nodules. The prevalence increases with age—peaking at age forty in IDA. In addition, nodules appear to be more frequent in enlarged glands. In IDA thyroid autonomy correlates with increased prevalence of nodules. Thyroid autonomy is rare in iodine sufficient areas. Correction of iodine insufficiency leads to reduction in thyroid autonomy.

Smoking increases thiocyanate levels which compete with iodine for uptake and organification. Particularly in IDA smoking is associated with an increase in NTD. Radiation exposure is associated with increase in both benign and malignant thyroid nodules. NTD is up to 15-fold more frequent in women.

Goitrogens which can be naturally occurring substances or drugs can cause enlargement of the gland by blocking or impeding a specific step in thyroid hormone synthesis. These include flavonoids (millets, soy beans, and *Babassu coconut*), cyanogenic glucosides that can be metabolized to thiocyanates (cassava, sweet potato, and *Sorghum*) and glucosinolates (cruciferous vegetables—cabbage cauliflower, broccoli, and turnips). Seaweed can induce goiter through iodine excess. Iron and selenium deficiency when associated with low nutritional iodine can impair thyroid hormone synthesis and cause thyroid enlargement.

A strong genetic disposition for goiters and NTD is evident. In the presence of a condition such as iodine deficiency, defects in genes involved in thyroid hormone synthesis could predispose to the development of goiter and subsequent nodular transformation. The genes that encode the proteins involved in thyroid hormone synthesis such as the thyroglobulin-gene (*TG*-gene), the thyroid peroxidase-gene (*TPO*-gene), the sodium-iodide-symporter-gene (*SLC5A5*), the *Pendred syndrome*-gene (SLC26A4), the *thyroid stimulating hormone-receptor*-gene

(*TSH-R-gene*), the iodotyrosine deiodinase (DEHAL 1) and the thyroid oxidase 2 gene3 (DUOX2) are convincing candidate genes in familial euthyroid goiter. Genome wide linkage analysis has identified a candidate locus multinodular goiter (MNG1) on chromosome 14q31 involving a dominant pattern of inheritance with high penetrance in two families. A second locus Xp22 (MNG2) with an X-linked autosomal dominant pattern has also been associated with euthyroid goiters. Other candidate loci include 2p, 3p (dominant), 7q, and 8p.

Molecular Genetics

Thyroid neoplasms are clonal cell populations. Thyroid tumors result from changes in gene expression patterns that are important for cellular regulatory processes such as growth, differentiation, deoxyribonucleic acid (DNA) duplication, mismatch repair, and apoptosis. Tumor development begins with a somatic mutation that confers a growth advantage. Gain of function of genes involved in the growth stimulation and loss of function mutations of genes involved in growth inhibition, cell cycle checkpoints or cell survival are the principal genetic changes that are observed. Specific etiologic factors are involved and cause point mutations and chromosomal rearrangements. Other changes include alteration in gene expression patterns, dysregulation of miRNAs and aberrant gene methylation. In thyroid cancer this includes the activation of the MAPK and PI3K signaling pathways which appear to be crucial for tumor initiation and progression.

Gene expression profiles of benign functioning and nonfunctioning thyroid nodules in the same gland are similar—the modulated genes belonging to the same biological pathways. A greater number of genes are expressed in functioning nodules. Upregulation of cyclin D1 and cyclin dependent kinase inhibitor1 is seen in both functioning and nonfunctioning nodules suggesting feedback control of proliferation. Complement components are down regulated suggesting silencing of the innate immune response. It appears the increased proliferation rate, is similar for both functioning and nonfunctioning nodules.

Thyroid stimulating hormone is an important facilitator of tumor growth and mitosis. There appears to be an association with higher levels of TSH and the risk of thyroid cancer in thyroid nodules. *BRAF* (see below) requires TSH simulation to transform thyroid cells and initiate tumor development. Gain of function somatic mutations of the TSH receptors (TSHR) are observed in up to 82% of autonomously functioning thyroid nodules (AFTN) but are generally not associated with malignant transformation. Interestingly, constitutive activation of the TSHR is seen in 60% of functioning nodules in multinodular goiters. Downstream to the TSHR, mutations in the components of the cyclic adenosine 3′,5′-monophosphate (cAMP) signal cascade can function as oncogenes. Activating point mutations of Gsα are associated with autonomously functioning thyroid nodule (AFTN).

While defective iodide transport and organification are implicated in nonfunctioning nodules the molecular event accounting for the proliferative advantage in these nodules is poorly understood. No specific gene mutation has been described yet in nonfunctioning nodules. A minority of these nodules however harbor gene mutations that are seen in malignant follicular neoplasms (N-RAS, H-RAS, K-RAS mutations, or RET rearrangements).

Peroxisome proliferator-activating receptors (PPARs) are nuclear receptors that bind to DNA as heterodimers with retinoid X receptors. Mutations of PPAR-γ are seen in approximately 35% of patients with follicular cancer, a small proportion of follicular variants of papillary thyroid carcinoma (PTC) and follicular adenomas. These mutations result in the fusion of the DNA-binding domain of the thyroid transcription factor PAX8 to domains A to F of PPAR-γ. PAX8/PPAR-γ positive tumors are present in younger patients and appear to be smaller and show solid growth pattern and greater vascular invasion. Mutations in RAS are found in thyroid follicular cell-derived tumors including follicular carcinomas, follicular adenomas, and follicular variants of PTC. RAS mutations are associated with tumor dedifferentiation and less favorable prognosis, metastasis (particularly bone) on the one hand and encapsulated follicular variant of PTC (an indolent tumor) on the other hand. RAS mutations and PAX8/PPAR-γ are never found together indicating two distinct pathways of tumorigenesis.

A detailed discussion on the molecular pathogenesis of thyroid carcinoma is seen in Chapter 18.

Pathogenesis

Multinodular goiter (MNG) could conceivably result from a defect in any step of thyroid hormone synthesis and resistance to thyroid hormone action (inherited or otherwise). In both the serums, TSH would be elevated and goiter would result from prolonged stimulation.

Cells that form a follicle possess widely differing qualities with regard to thyroid hormone synthesis. Thus, there is heterogeneity of growth and function even within a follicle. New cells may acquire qualities hitherto not present due to somatic mutations that can alter growth and function but not necessarily lead to malignant transformation. For example, constitutive activation somatic mutations are seen in both toxic adenomas and toxic MNGs.

Nodular thyroid disease (NTD) may be considered as the response of the thyroid gland to chronic low-grade intermittent stimulus. Goiter formation may be viewed as a process of global activation of epithelial cell proliferation in the thyroid where accepted risk factors such iodine deficiency smoking female sex, etc., interact with and or trigger the genetic susceptibility, iodine deficiency, autoimmunity or nutritional goitrogens. TSH stimulation as a consequence of iodine deficiency for instance causes growth (hyperplasia) of the gland; at some point, the requirement for thyroid hormone reduces, resulting in a quiescent phase. It is postulated that a repetition of the growth and resting phases results in the formation of a multinodular goiter. The initial lesion appears to be hyperplasia with discrete nodules appearing over time. By the time the goiter is well-developed TSH production rates are normal or even suppressed.

Subsequent nodule formation is a result of focal increase in thyroid epithelial cell proliferation—the most common stimulus being somatic cell mutations. In animal models of hyperplasia an increase in functional activity, an increase in thyroid cell number occurs. This likely increases the number of mutation events. In addition there is increased H_2O_2 production and free radical formation which damage genomic DNA and cause mutations. A high mutation rate and high replication rate prevents mutation repair; it also affects genes that are essential for thyroid physiology. Growth factor expression [insulin-like growth factor-1 (IGF1), transforming growth factor β1 (TGF-β1), or epidermal growth factor] is increased in the proliferating thyroid facilitating cell division, clone formation and proliferation. Synergistic interactions with TSH facilitate growth. Small clones with activating mutations can further proliferate if they achieve self-stimulation. They could form small foci which further develop into nodules. This mechanism is also able to explain nodule formation in TSH secreting pituitary adenomas, nodular Grave's disease, and acromegaly.

Most nodules are functionally inactive, leading to the classic "cold" appearance on functional imaging. This may be due to a specific defect in iodide transport. The sodium iodine syntroper (NIS) appears to be under-expressed in both benign and malignant cold nodules. Some nodules appear to have intact iodide transport but lack peroxidase. These nodules appear hot on technetium ($^{99}TcO_4$) but cold on iodine. Thyroid autonomy (TA) as measured by impaired TRH response to TSH is a consequence of gradual increase in the number of cells with relatively autonomous hormone synthesis. This appears to develop in a proportion of patients with NTD but not in diffuse goiters. The degree of TA appears to be proportional to the size of the gland and is likely to be an increase in the number of cells having TA. Such autonomy appears over time and could possibly be prevented by TSH suppression.

In summary, functional iodine deficiency or other risk factors increase TSH leading to diffuse goiter formation. Nodule formation is a consequence mostly of acquisition of somatic mutations which achieve the ability to self-stimulate forming foci that lead to nodules. Some nodules develop autonomy over time leading to the development of toxic multinodular goiter (TMNG).

CLASSIFICATION

Benign nodules have been histologically distinguished by the presence of a capsule—(i) with a capsule—true adenomas or (ii) without—adenomatous. The World Health Organization (WHO) has defined morphological criteria. Malignant nodules can be papillary, follicular, medullary, and anaplastic; these are discussed at length in chapter.

Adenomas are characterized by orderly architecture and few mitosis with no lymphatic or vascular invasion. Necrosis is common in nodules resulting in cyst formation. Most nodules grow slowly reflecting the long time taken by thyroid cells to divide. They may increase in pregnancy; new nodules may also develop in pregnancy.

Functionally, nodules are classified based on uptake on scintiscan as—(i) cold (ii) hot or, (iii) normal. Depending on iodine sufficiency in the area up to 85% of nodules may be cold, 10% normal, and up to 5% may be hot. Often nodules with more than one function are present in the same gland and their collective function determines if the gland is euthyroid or toxic multinodular. A gland which is euthyroid with respect to function is simply called Multinodular goiter (MNG), the gland which is thyrotoxic with respect to function is called TMNG. In a particular gland this nomenclature is not static. Over time MNG can evolve into TMNG through progressive acquisition of independence from TSH leading to thyroid autonomy.

About 10% of follicular adenomas are "hot" and produce sufficient thyroxine to cause subclinical or overt thyrotoxicosis. Autonomously functioning nodules are more common in areas with a high prevalence of endemic goiters. Activating TSH receptor mutations appear to be common in AFTN; some patients have mutations in the stimulatory GTP binding protein subunit. AFTN is discussed in greater detail in Chapter 8.

PROGRESSION

Growth of nodules is variable. In iodine sufficient areas (ISA), growth, in up to a third of benign nodules has been reported with the majority remaining unchanged or even reducing in size. Greater increase in size has been reported in IDA. In a 15-year follow-up of solitary thyroid nodules (STN) from Japan, 13% of nodules demonstrated increase in size; 34% were unchanged, in 23% there was reduction in size; in 30% the nodule was no longer palpable. Nodules that increased over time were predominantly solid while those that disappeared were predominantly cystic. The pace of growth is heterogenous. It is unclear if nodule growth alone is associated with increased risk of malignancy while traditionally it has been an important clinical indicator.

Progression to hyperthyroidism in MNG can occur and correlates with the nodule size and volume. In contrast to Graves' disease (GD) thyrotoxicosis develops insidiously often preceded by a prolonged period of subclinical thyrotoxicosis characterized by low to suppressed TSH and normal free T3 (FT3) and free T4 (FT4) concentrations. Over 12.2 years of follow up, up to 10% of patients with MNG developed thyrotoxicosis in an iodine sufficient area. Nodule size >3 cm predicted a 20% risk of progression over 6 years. Other factors influence this progression such as genetic predisposition, somatic mutations, and iodine intake. In AFTN progression to toxicity occurred at a rate of up to 4.1% per year.

THYROID CANCER

Thyroid cancers are uncommon and account for <0.5% of cancer deaths. However, the incidence of thyroid cancer is increasing rapidly and currently appears to be the most rapidly increasing malignancy among men and women in the general population. This appears to be a worldwide phenomenon. The mortality rates appear to be unchanged largely reflecting the fact that the increase is primarily in early stage papillary carcinoma. In part this increase may be attributed to greater use of imaging since the early 1990s. Thyroid carcinoma (TC) is more common in women than men, the ratio highest after puberty declining thereafter. The median age of occurrence is 49 years. There are significant ethnic variations. The most common histologic type is PTC. There is a case to be made for low risk for carcinoma in MNG. For a more detailed discussion see Chapter 18 on thyroid cancer.

■ The Clinical Approach to Nodular Thyroid Disease

The clinician's approach to NTD to be—(i) primarily to distinguish the small number of nodules that harbor a malignancy from the majority that do not, (ii) to determine thyroid function and ensure appropriate management of resultant thyrotoxicosis, and (iii) to determine if there is compression of locoregional structures that require intervention.

Most thyroid nodules are benign. Significant bias confounds malignancy estimates in most series. A prevalence of up to 6% of all nodules may be a realistic estimate. At autopsy up to 36% of thyroid glands will harbor malignant nodules which are under 1 cm (microcarcinomas); many but not all of them will have an indolent course.

Most nodules are detected incidentally. Symptoms of growth and invasion such as dysphagia dystonia and stridor are rare in solitary nodules. Bleeding into the nodule occurs rarely and presents with increase in size pain and tenderness or uncommonly as transient thyrotoxicosis.

A detailed history and physical examination is invaluable in the clinical approach and is focused upon stratifying the risk for malignancies. Nodules in the young (<20 years), the elderly (>65 years) or in men have an increased likelihood of malignancy **(Table 2)**. Between 4 and 8% of patients with

TABLE 2: Clinical risk stratification of thyroid nodules.

Risk for cancer	Clinical features
Low	No suspicious symptoms or signs
Moderate	• Age <20 or >60 years • History of head or neck irradiation in childhood • Family history of thyroid cancer or familial syndromes with thyroid cancer • Exposure to nuclear fall out • Male sex • Nodule detected on 18F fluorodeoxyglucose positron emission tomography (18F-FDG PET) or sestamibi
High	• Rapid tumor growth • Very firm nodule • Fixation to adjacent structures • Vocal cord paralysis • Nontender lateral lymphadenopathy

PTC will have a family history of the same tumor. Papillary thyroid carcinoma is also increased in patients with familial tumor syndromes. Medullary cancer of the thyroid (MTC) can be familial, especially as part of the multiple endocrine neoplasia 2 (MEN2) syndrome. Exposure to head and neck radiation or total body irradiation for bone marrow transplant (especially in childhood), or nuclear fallout are other risk factors.

Heavy smoking (>20 PPD) appears to confer risk for goiter and nodule formation in areas of iodine deficiency. Obesity, alcohol consumption (especially in women) appears to increase the risk of nodule formation. An association with uterine fibroids is noted. Oral contraceptive and statin use appear to confer some protection.

It is unclear if the size of the nodule confers an increased risk of malignancy. The risk of malignancy also appears to be independent of the number of nodules. Rapid growth of the nodule and signs of fixity to the surrounding structures are suggestive of higher risk. Change in voice due to compression or infiltration of the recurrent laryngeal nerve and presence of nontender cervical lymphadenopathy confer a higher risk. Nodules that are incidentally discovered on 18F fluorodeoxyglucose positron emission tomography (18FDG-PET) have up to a 30% risk of malignancy; some studies suggest a higher risk of malignancy in nodules identified on technetium 99m (Tc99m) sestamibi scans used in cardiac and parathyroid imaging. These are summarized in **Table 2**.

Symptoms related to thyroid gland and nodule growth are caused by compression in the neck and upper thoracic cavity including the trachea and esophagus. They are usually insidious and become pronounced when there is an intrathoracic extension. Dyspnea, stridor, and cough are symptoms of tracheal compression. This is exacerbated by assumption of a recumbent position. Substantial growth into the anterior mediastinum can cause obstruction of the thoracic inlet resulting in a condition known as "the thyroid cork phenomenon." The Pemberton's maneuver in which raising the arms above the head results in dyspnea, stridor, distension of neck veins, or facial plethora, is suggestive of thoracic inlet obstruction by a MNG. Respiratory distress may be present in up to 85% of patients referred for surgery for a substernal goiter. Flow volume loops are consistent with upper airway obstruction in up to a third of patients. Stridor may develop initially on exertion but later at rest. Acute exacerbations of symptoms may occur with respiratory infection or hemorrhage into a nodule or cyst. Esophageal compression is seen with large intrathoracic goiters. Vocal cord paralysis and Horner's syndrome when present should alert the possibility of malignancy.

A detailed discussion on thyrotoxicosis can be found in Chapter 12.

Thyroid-stimulating Hormone

Measurement of serum TSH is essential in all patients with NTD. A suppressed TSH (with elevated FT4 and FT3) is indicative of thyrotoxicosis. A radionuclide scan is recommended in this instance and will help determine if the nodule is—(i) autonomously functioning with suppression of the surrounding gland (hot), (ii) a nonfunctioning area in a gland with Grave's disease (cold), or (iii) having the same function of the surrounding gland (warm). When available a radioiodine scan is preferred. While both Tc99m and I131 or I123 are taken up by the thyroid, only radioiodine is organified and stored in the thyroid follicles. While most benign and almost all malignancies appear "cold" on radioisotope scans, up to 5% of thyroid cancers are discordant viz., they take up pertechnetate but not radioiodine. Patients with nodules that are functioning on Tc99m should undergo radioiodine imaging to confirm if they are concordant.

Higher TSH values appear to confer a greater risk of malignancy. When the TSH is >5.5 mU/L for instance the prevalence of malignancy was 29.7% versus a prevalence of 2.8% with TSH concentration of <0.4 mU/L. A higher TSH was also associated with a more advanced stage of cancer when diagnosed.

Serum thyroglobulin can be elevated in many thyroid diseases including benign MNG; it does not help differentiate benign from malignant disease. Its use is not recommended.

Calcitonin

Some studies have suggested the routine use of calcitonin in patients with nodules as a screen for medullary thyroid cancer. Calcitonin is superior to FNAC in detecting MTC. Calcitonin levels above 60 are typically indicative of MTC; levels between 10 and 60 are inconclusive. Basal calcitonin is plagued by confounders including drug interference (chronic proton pump inhibitor, β-blocker, and glucocorticoid use) and other conditions including hypergastrinemia, neuroendocrine tumors, renal insufficiency, DTC, thyromegaly, and autoimmune thyroiditis. Pentagastrin stimulation, when available, appears to improve the reliability of calcitonin measurements. There are no high level evidence or consensus that recommends the routine use of calcitonin at this time.

IMAGING

Ultrasound

Thyroid ultrasonography (USG) is the tool that guides diagnosis, risk stratification, further workup, and follow up of patients with NTD. An ultrasound should be performed in all patients with a suspected thyroid nodule. In up to 23% of patients USG detect an additional nodule; ironically in up to 16% of patients no nodule may be detected. This includes patients who have a nodule detected by another imaging procedure [computed tomography (CT), magnetic resonance imaging (MRI), or 18FDG-PET scan].

Both lobes of the thyroid and isthmus should be examined in transverse and sagittal views. The USG should evaluate the homogeneity of the thyroid parenchyma, gland size, location of the nodule(s), size (in three dimensions—width, depth, and height) composition (solid, cystic, or mixed), echogenicity, margins presence and size of calcifications, shape (if taller is >wider) and vascularity. The USG should also evaluate the central (level VI) and lateral compartments for the presence of lymph nodes (level II to IV).

Several USG features have been identified in multivariate analysis as associated with malignancy, specifically papillary cancer of the thyroid (PTC) **(Table 3) (Figs. 1A to D)**. These include the presence of microcalcifications, nodule hypoechogenicity when compared with strap muscles, irregular margins (infiltrative microlobulated and spiculated), shape taller than white on transverse view, central vascularity and twinkling on B flows imaging. While hypoechogenicity is associated with increased risk of malignancy—it is not specific; more than half of hypoechoic nodules are benign. Nodules that are markedly hypoechoic are associated with increased risk of malignancy. Taller than wider shape in transverse or longitudinal imaging is seen in up to 12% of nodules and is associated with increased risk of malignancy. This finding has a specificity of up to 94%; its utility is more in nodules <1 cm. Irregular margins are a marker of malignancy but are not sensitive since 33–93% of malignancy have a smooth or regular border. Extension of the nodule through the capsule into the adjacent tissue is a feature of malignancy. Small <1 mm punctate echogenic foci (especially that lack the comet tail artifact) represent microcalcifications and are suggestive of PTC. Lymph node examination is valuable when present. A hilum may be nonvisualized in both benign and malignant processes; the presence of hilum excludes malignancy.

Follicular thyroid cancer (FTC) has somewhat different features. They are more often iso or hyperechoic, noncalcified, round with greater anteroposterior (AP) dimensions and regular smooth margins. Follicular variant of papillary thyroid carcinoma (FVPTC) has similar dimensions. These nodules must be aspirated and monitored. Lesions <2 cm have low metastatic rates. Medullary cancer of the thyroid (MTC) has some features of PTC on USG but also is known to vary presenting with relatively large nodules, aspect ratio of less than one and mixed echogenicity and increased intranodular blood flow.

Similarly, there are features on USG that are associated with a low risk of DTC. A spongiform appearance defined as the aggregation of multiple microcystic components in >50% of the nodule is strongly suggestive of a benign nodule. Other USG features include hyperechogenicity, large coarse calcifications, peripheral calcifications, puff pastry appearance, and comet tail shadowing.

Several risk stratification systems (RSS) have been developed by many professional organizations. Their purpose is twofold—(i) homogenize the result of USG reports by using a quantitative cancer risk estimation approach—this allows better communication of results between clinicians and with patients and (ii) provide guidance on fine needle aspiration (FNA). Each scoring system has its own lexicon (most of them are similar). It is important to note that the RSS were derived predominantly from a population with papillary thyroid cancer (PTC) thus introducing a selection bias. Each of the RSS has an estimated risk of malignancy that has been validated prospectively in different cohorts.

Risk stratification systems can be broadly classified into pattern based and point based scoring systems. In the ATA guidelines European EU TIRADS and the Korean K TIRADS the clinician assigns a nodule to one of several predetermined patterns or determines how many suspicious features are present. No numerical value is assigned to them. The ACR TI-RADS first introduced in 2017 places nodules in one of five increasing risk levels by assigning specific point values to ultrasound features. At each level ACR TIRADS provides precise cut-offs that determine management recommendations. This approach ensures that no nodule is unclassified; the ATA system for instance would leave as much as 17.9% of nodules as unclassified. ACR TIRADS FNAC cut-off are higher than the other scores **(Tables 4 and 5)**.

In addition to echogenic patterns each RSS uses its own size cut offs to determine if FNAC is required. Most of the systems agree on >10 mm as the FNA threshold off for highly suspicious nodules. The threshold for the intermediate risk nodules vary 10 mm in the ATA and K TIRADS and 15 mm in the ACR and EU TIRADS. For low suspicion nodules the threshold varies from 15 mm for the ATA and K TIRADS, 20 mm for the EU TIRADS and 25 mm for the ACR TIRADS. Most RSS do not recommend FNAC for very low suspicion nodules.

The overall diagnostic performance of RSS (ATA, EUTIRADS, K-TIRADS and ACR TIRADS) appears to be comparable (predominantly cytology based studies). Interobserver variation appears to be similar for these systems. It is higher for high and intermediate suspicion nodules than for lower mildly suspicious ones **(Table 6)**.

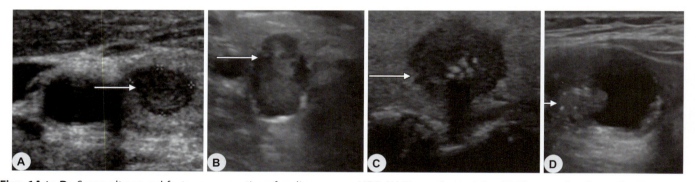

Figs. 1A to D: Some ultrasound features suggestive of malignancy on USG. (A) Hypoechogenicity; (B) Shape wider than taller than wider; (C) Irregular margins; and (D) Punctate echogenic foci.

TABLE 3: Characteristic features of malignancy in thyroid nodules.

Sonographic characteristics	Sensitivity (%)	Specificity (%)	Positive predictive value (%)	Negative predictive value (%)	Accuracy (%)
Microcalcification	59.2	85.8	70.7	79.8	77.4
Irregular or microlobulated margin	55.1	83	60	80	74.2
Marked hypoechogenicity	26.5	94.3	68.4	73.5	72.9
More tall than wide	32.7	92.5	66.7	74.8	73.5

TABLE 4: Comparison of features of malignancy used in commonly used risk scoring systems.

Characteristics of malignancy	ACR TIRADS	ATA	EuTIRADS	K TIRADS
Hypoechoic	Y	Y	Y	Y
Markedly hypoechoic	Y	N	Y	Y
Taller than wider	Y	Y	Y	Y
Irregular shape	Y	Y	Y	Y
Punctate echogenic foci	Y	Y	Y	Y
Macrocalcifications	Y	N		Y
Peripheral calcifications	Y			
Rim calcifications with extrusion		Y		
Irregular margins	Y	Y	Y	Y
Invasion of parenchyma	Y			Y
Intranodular vascularization		Y		Y

The diagnostic odds ratio for the ACR TIRADS system is higher than for other systems. Using a RSS reduces the rate of unnecessary FNACs by up to 53.4%. The percentage of benign nodules that would have received a recommendation for FNAC was lowest for ACR TIRADS followed by ATA and K TIRADS. The ACR TIRADS system identified >50% of biopsies as unnecessary and with a lower false negative rate. This is in part due to the differences in size threshold for FNAC between the various RSS. The percentage of missed carcinomas is low (ACR TIRADS 2.25 ATA 4.1%). The obverse of this is that the diagnosis of a small portion of carcinomas will be postponed and they will be picked when they eventually grow and reach the threshold for FNAC. This strategy does not increase morbidity for most of the patients since the majority would be papillary carcinomas that are of low or intermediate risk. One third of all MTC have USG features considered low suspicion in many of the RSS.

Caution: The clinical background and experience should be used along with guidelines in the clinical setting to avoid missing more aggressive and non-PTC malignancies.

TABLE 5: Comparison of fine needle aspiration threshold among commonly used risk scoring system.

ACR TIRADS		ATA		EuTIRADS		K TIRADS	
Category	Threshold for FNAC (mm)	Category	Threshold for FNAC (mm)	Category	Threshold for FNAC (mm)	Category	Threshold for FNAC (mm)
One benign	No FNAC	Benign	No FNAC	One no nodule	No FNAC	1	No FNAC
Two not suspicious	No FNAC	Very low suspicion	>20	Two benign	No FNAC	2	>20
Three mildly suspicious	>25	Low suspicion	>15	Three low risk	>20	3	>15
Four moderately suspicious	>15	Intermediate suspicion	>10	Four intermediate risk	>15	4	>10
Five suspicious	>10	High suspicion	>10	Five high risk	>10	5	>10

TABLE 6: Comparison of projected risk of malignancy and validation in commonly used risk scoring systems.

ACR TIRADS			ATA			EuTIRADS			K TIRADS		
Category	Risk of malignancy (%)	Validation	Category	Risk of malignancy (%)	Validation	Category	Risk of malignancy (%)	Validation	Category	Risk of malignancy (%)	Validation
One benign	0	0.3	Benign	<1		One no nodule	0	0	1	0	0
Two not suspicious	0	1.5	Very low suspicion	<3	2	Two benign	0	0.5	2	0	0
Three mildly suspicious	<5	4.8	Low suspicion	5–10	8	Three low risk	2–4	5.9	3	7.8	3.5
Four moderately suspicious	5–80	9.1	Intermediate suspicion	10–20	11	Four intermediate risk	6–17	21.4	4	25.4	19
Five suspicious	>80	35	High suspicion	70–90	100	Five high risk	26–87	76.1	5	79.3	73.4

In India, a law that has been enacted to discourage sex determination in the fetus restricts the office use of USG by endocrinologists. Therefore, an RSS that has widespread acceptance by radiologists would be practical to use. The author uses the ACR TIRADS for this among other reasons.

The use of artificial intelligence and machine learning in classifying nodules either independently or as an add on the existing RSS is an interesting development. Feature based machine learning (ML) as well as deep learning algorithms have been used. Using a genetic algorithm and training an AI TIRADS has been developed that has the same form as the original ACR TIRADS but different point values for some features. AI TIRADS higher specificity than ACR TIRADS. Overall deep learning algorithms appear to have accuracy and specificity that approaches that of experienced radiologists. Radiomics is a promising method that seeks to extend AI application beyond differentiation between benign and malignant. Radiomics models can predict the aggressiveness of thyroid carcinoma and have the potential to determine tumor phenotypes and presence of gene mutations.

Ultrasound elastography (USE) has been suggested as a useful adjunct to Ultrasound. Elastography provides a reproducible assessment of tissue stiffness which is increased in malignant nodules. There are two main elastography techniques—(1) strain elastography (SE)—which evaluates the degree of tissue deformation induced by manual compression or acoustic forces, and in which tissue deformation is parallel to the direction of the force and (2) shear wave elastography (SWE), in which a push beam is created and tissue displacement is perpendicular to the direction of the force. Despite initial promise, its performance appears to be variable and is affected by multiple factors. When available a high risk USE adds a cautionary note for increased malignancy in otherwise benign appearing nodules. Contrast enhanced ultrasound evaluates tumor microvascularization and thus identifies malignant neoplasms. Both USE and CEU have not found widespread acceptance.

Imaging for Retrosternal Extension and Tracheal Compression

Neither CT nor MRI has the advantages over ultrasound when it comes to visualization of thyroidal architecture. However, their strength is in their ability to diagnose and assess the extent of substernal goiter and compression of the trachea and esophagus better than other modalities. Both modalities provide planimetric volume estimations. The utility of CT is limited by exposure to ionizing radiation. Both modalities provide no information of functionality and are poor predictors of malignancy.

RADIONUCLIDE IMAGING

Radionuclide imaging is seldom used today in the evaluation of thyroid nodules. Its continued use is predominantly in autonomously functioning thyroid nodules which must be suspected the TSH is suppressed (see above). Some authorities recommend ^{123}I scintigraphy in a subset of nodules with follicular neoplasm cytology if the TSH is in the low normal range. Some AFTN especially those with diameter <2.5 cm may have this cytology but do not produce sufficient thyroxine to suppress TSH. These appear "hot" in scintigraphy. The risk of carcinoma is low in this subset of patients.

FINE NEEDLE ASPIRATION

Fine needle aspiration of the thyroid is the confirmatory procedure of choice in thyroid nodules. FNA reduces the number of unnecessary surgeries and at this time is most accurate among tests or combinations of tests to determine if a nodule requires surgery or not. Ultrasound guided FNA with real time visualization of needle placement decreases false negative rates. A 23–27 gauge needle is used with or without local anesthesia. In experience hands adequacy of sample is seen in up to 97% of aspirates (see below). The capillary action technique in which no suction is applied appears to have lower nondiagnostic rates. Complications are rare. The occasional patient may have mild pain radiating to the jaw or ear for a day or two. Infection is uncommon. Seeding of carcinoma cells in the needle track has been reported in two patients who have had large needle biopsies and one who had a fine needle biopsy. Tg levels may be elevated for a few days after FNAC. In experienced hands false negatives are low with an estimated frequency of up to 3.7%.

Both clinical and sonographic features are used to determine if FNAC is required. Fine needle aspiration is recommended predominantly based on the thresholds recommended based on the RSS used by the clinician. Sonographic features suggestive of malignancy must be the determining factor for which nodule requires FNAC since the malignancy may not be in the dominant nodule in over a third of patients. In the presence of suspicious lymph nodes nodules of any size must be aspirated. The lymph node itself may be aspirated first and the nodule subsequently. Patients with multiple nodules should be evaluated in the same fashion as those with solitary nodules. If the TSH is low in a patient with MNG then an radionuclide scan (iodine is preferred) may be obtained and compared with the USG.

■ Cytology

The diagnostic groups reported under the six-tiered 2017 version of Bethesda system for reporting thyroid cytopathology have gained widespread acceptance **(Table 7)**. An adequate specimen is defined as composed of at least six groups of cells each having 10–15 cells. When this is not present the FNAC is deemed inadequate or nondiagnostic. Approximately 5% of all aspirations in

TABLE 7: The Bethesda scoring system.		
Bethesda class	Diagnostic category	Cancer risk (%)
I	Nondiagnostic	5–10
II	Benign	0–3
III	Atypia of undetermined ACUS or follicular lesion of undetermined significance (FLUS)	10–30
IV	Follicular neoplasm or suspicious for follicular lesion	25–40
V	Suspicious for malignancy	50–75
VI	Malignant	97–99

Source: Ali SZ, Cibas ES. The Bethesda System for Reporting Thyroid Cytopathology: Definitions, Criteria, and Explanatory Notes. Berlin: Springer; 2017.

experienced hands will fall into this category. Several factors contribute to nondiagnostic specimens including nodule components and FNAC technique.

Adequate specimens are categorized as benign, malignant, or indeterminate with the latter being divided into three specific categories each correlating with a different malignancy risk.

Category II benign (BII) is the most commonly assigned category (60–70% of all aspirates) and has a malignancy rate of <3%. This category also includes aspirates that include lymphocytic and subacute thyroiditis.

The indeterminate categories include atypia of undetermined significance (BIII), follicular or Hürthle cell neoplasms (BIV), and suspicious for malignancy (BV) **(Table 6)** BIII has a range of malignancy 5 and 48%. Aspirates are typically sparsely cellular samples arranged in microfollicles with mild nuclear changes or an abundance of Hürthle cells. Noninvasive follicular thyroid neoplasm with papillary-like nuclear features (NIFTP) tumors were initially categorized in BIII. Aspirates categorized as BIV are hypercellular and arranged in a microfollicular or trabecular pattern amidst scant colloid. Malignancy rates are 10–40% and often follicular carcinoma or follicular variant of PTC. Molecular testing is often required in BIII and BIV lesions to guide further decision making (see below). BV has a malignancy rate of 60–75%. Bethesda category VI (BVI)—malignant has malignancy rate of 97–99%. Cytologic findings include large cells, prominent nucleoli, nuclear grooves and inclusions, psammoma bodies, and cells arranged in papillae.

2–3% of benign nodules as determined by FNAC will subsequently prove to be malignant. Conversely the same amount of malignant nodules on FNAC will prove to be benign. Large studies show a high degree of concordance between the system and pathology especially in the definitively benign and the definitively malignant categories with variability in the intermediate categories. Despite limitations the adaptation of the system allows clinicians to explain malignancy risk better to patients.

Molecular Testing

Molecular testing for known RNA and DNA mutations appear to improve the diagnostic accuracy of FNA when added to cytologic evaluation. Approximately 70% of carcinomas will harbor one or some of the following mutation—the Harvey rat sarcoma viral oncogene homolog (H-Ras), neuroblastoma rat sarcoma viral oncogene homolog (N-Ras), Kirsten rat sarcoma viral oncogene homolog (K-Ras), rearranged during transfection/PTC1 (RET/PTC1), Ret/PTC2, Ret/PTC3, v-Raf murine sarcoma viral oncogene homolog B1 (*BRAF*), and paired box gene 8-peroxisome proliferator-activator receptor c (Pax8-PPARc). These mutations when identified enhance the specificity of FNAC but are not sensitive as a detection tool.

In clinical practice the need for a molecular testing is required in nodules where a definite diagnosis of benign or malignant cannot be clearly achieved by clinical exam USG and cytology. In practice these are nodules that have received Bethesda classification of either III, IV, or V (BIII, BIV, and BV). This indeterminate category falls into a malignancy risk between 5 and 75% and represents up to 40% of all FNACs. At the lower end of the spectrum which is atypia undetermined significance (AUS) follicular lesion of undetermined significance (FLUS), a test is required with characteristics to rule out disease, i.e., has high negative predictive value (NPV). An ideal rule out test will have the NPV of Bethesda II (BII) cytology (96.3%). At the higher end of the spectrum, a test is required with characteristics to rule in disease, i.e., high positive predictive value. An ideal "rule in" will have the positive predictive value of Bethesda VI (BVI) cytology (98.6%) **(Fig. 2)**.

According to the predominant ability to exclude or confirm a malignancy, the molecular panels are classified as "rule-in" or "rule-out" tests. Considering a cancer prevalence range of 20–40%, a robust "rule-out" test would require a negative predictive value of at least 94% and a minimum sensitivity of 90%, while for a desirable test to predict or "rule-in" malignancy, an optimal standard should have a positive predictive value of at least 60% and an specificity above 80%. A "rule out" test will perform better in a low risk USG category of TIRADS 3 or cytologic category Bethesda III or IV. Sonographically high-risk such as TIRADS 4 and higher or cytologic category such as Bethesda V would benefit more from a "rule-in" test, in which case a positive test result would decrease the risk of completion surgery.

Molecular testing utilizes alterations in thyroid cancer—these include—(i) recurrent somatic mutations (single nucleotide variants, insertions, and deletions) and (ii) gene fusions in hotspots within oncogenes, tumor suppressor genes as well as large scale chromosomal copy number alterations. It offers a gradient of cancer risk estimates based on the type of genetic alteration detected. The detection of driver alterations such as the *BRAF* V600E mutation and chromosomal rearrangements involving *RET*

ALK or *NTRK* genes are diagnostic of cancer. Detection of mutations in the RAS gene family (*HRAS*, *KRAS*, and *NRAS*), *BRAF* K601E mutation, *PAX8-PPARG* gene fusion, and gene fusions involving thyroid adenoma associated (*THADA*) gene are specific for neoplasia. In addition to these gene and microRNA (miRNA) expression profiles can be obtained—these can be considered as readouts of the cumulative and complex genetic epigenetic and possible environmental influence on cells.

This strategy allows the test results to be stratified into (i) high probability of malignancy in which therapeutic thyroidectomy as the next step is indicated (ii) intermediate probability where diagnostic lobectomy as the next step to further classify the nodule is indicated, and (iii) low probability where the cancer risk is similar to benign aspirates and therefore clinical follow-up is sufficient. Three platforms commercially available in the US use a combination of genotyping and mRNA or miRNA expression profiling. These are briefly discussed. At the time of writing these are not available in India **(Table 8)**.

■ The Afirma Gene Expression/Sequencing Classifier

The Afirma Gene Expression was developed based on an analysis of the whole genome to identify and isolate candidate genes. It evaluates the expression profile of a large panel of genes and uses machine learning algorithms to classify aspirates as having a benign or suspicious gene expression profile. The initial version introduced in 2012 as the Afirma Gene Expression Classifier (GEC) used microarrays to determine the expression of 166 genes. Based on 24% prevalence of malignancy in Bethesda III and IV lesions an NPV of 95% was obtained.

Currently the platform uses high-throughput RNA sequencing that determines the expression profile of 10,196 genes. Machine learning algorithms are used to classify the genes and the platform is now called the Afirma Gene Sequencing Classifier (GSC). It analyzes expression patterns of 1,115 core genes with the 9,000 genes providing stability to the classifier model. It has seven additional

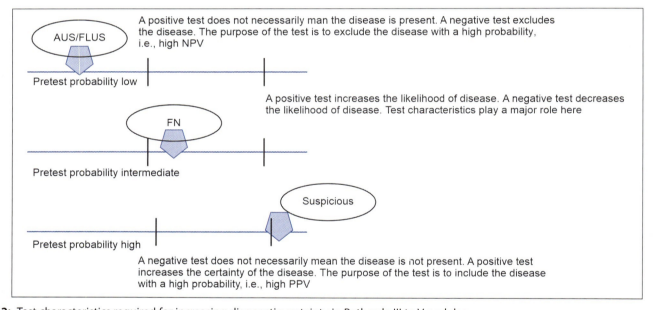

Fig. 2: Test characteristics required for increasing diagnostic certainty in Bethesda III to V nodules.
(AUS/FLUS: atypia (or follicular lesion) of undetermined significance; FN: follicular neoplasm; NPV: negative predictive value; PPV: positive predictive value)

TABLE 8: Performance characteristics of generations of molecular testing in nodular thyroid disease.						
Test	Bethesda category	Sensitivity (%)	Specificity (%)	Cancer (%)	NPV (%)	PPV (%)
Afirma GEC	III–V	92	52	32	93	47
Thyroseq v2	III	91	92	23	89	90
ThygenX/ThyraMIR	III–IV	89	85	32	94	74
Afirma GSC	III–IV	91	68	24	96	47
Thyroseq v3	III–IV	94	82	28	97	66

components to identify parathyroid lesions, MTC, BRAF V600E mutations, RET/PTC1 or RET/PTC3 fusion, and Hürthle cell lesions. When validated with the original set of samples used with GEC, the GSC demonstrated better specificity and positive predictive value with similar sensitivity and NPV of the GEC. Specifically for BIII— sensitivity 92.9%, specificity 70.9%, NPV 96.8 PPV 51; for BIV sensitivity 88.2%, specificity 58.8%, NPV 95.1%, and PPV of 41.7%. Hürthle cell performance was better than the previous GEC.

The GSC has also added mitochondrial transcripts and loss of heterozygosity analysis in order to improve risk stratification in Hürthle cell lesions. The GSC also demonstrated improved performance in Hürthle cell lesions when compared with GEC. The GSC also exports sequence variants that are known to be associated with thyroid cancer in a complementary test called the *Afirma Xpression Atlas*. It currently reports 235 fusions and 905 sequence variants from only the transcribed portions of 593 genes.

Thyroseq v3

Originally a small panel of involving driver mutations and fusion genes involving seven genes (*BRAF, HRAS, KRAS, NRAS, RET-PTC1, RET-PTC3,* and *PAX8-PPARG*), the Thyroseq has evolved into a panel that examines with the help of next generation DNA and RNA sequencing platforms as well as data from several large genomic characterization of thyroid cancers, 12,135 mutations insertions and deletions in 112 genes and over 120 types of gene fusions. Gene expression alterations and chromosomal copy-number alterations (characteristic of Hürthle cell neoplasms) are also examined using RNA and DNA sequencing, respectively. Each genetic alteration is assigned a score between 0 and 2 and the total score is calculated for the sample. A score between 0 and 1 is negative and a score of 2 or more is positive. In a population of Bethesda III and IV nodules with cancer prevalence of 28% Thyroseq v3 had a sensitivity of 94% and a negative predictive value of 97%; it had a 82% specificity of 82% and 66% positive predictive value. A prospective validation of 286 indeterminate samples (BIII and BIV) from ten centers revealed—for BIII sensitivity 91.4%, specificity 84.9%, NPV 97.1%, PPV 64 cancer NIFTP prevalence 23%; for BIV sensitivity 97.1 specificity 75%, NPV 98%, PPV 68% cancer, NIFTP prevalence 35%. Notably all 10 Hürthle cell carcinomas were classified correctly. A recent meta-analysis seems to suggest that Thyroseq v3 has the best overall ability to "rule out malignancy."

ThyGeNEXT/ThyraMIR

This is a two-step classifier. Aspirates with BIII and BIV undergo ThyGeNEXT a targeted DNA and RNA NGS panel that includes hotspot mutations in 10 genes and 38 gene fusions. Adequacy of samples is first determined by a limited gene expression panel that includes NKX2.1 and PAX8. Samples positive for strong driver mutations, e.g., *BRAF* V600E mutation, *BRAF* fusions, RET fusions, TERT promoter mutations, ALK mutations, and fusions have high probability of malignancy and require no further testing. Samples with weak driver mutations—alterations in RAS family genes are considered intermediate probability. These and the samples that are negative for driver mutations are further risk stratified using ThyraMIR. ThyraMIR measures relative expression levels of 10 miRNAs. The results are stratified in three tiers using the combined panels—negative moderate and positive for malignancy. Medullary carcinoma is recognized by upregulation of specific miRNAs (e.g., miR-375) in the ThyraMIR panel.

Plasma Cell Free DNA

In a pilot study, plasma cell free DNA of 67.9 ng/mL was able to discriminate benign from malignant thyroid nodules with a sensitivity of 100% and specificity of 92.3%. This novel approach appears promising and requires validation with prospective multicenter studies.

MANAGEMENT

Author's current approach to NTD is summarized in **Flowchart 1**.

Nondiagnostic Cytology

Nondiagnostic FNAC (Bethesda I) warrants repetition especially with US guidance and if available on site cytology. In patients with repeated nondiagnostic results surgery may be offered if the USG is suspicious or if growth (>20% in two dimensions) is demonstrated on follow-up. A mostly cystic sonographically reassuring nodule can be monitored.

Benign Cytology

When a combination of USG and FNAC are used to guide the diagnosis—a low suspicion on USG and benign cytology (Bethesda II) warrants a strategy of clinical observation. This may be true even of lesions >4 cm where low risk USG and benign cytology appear to confer negligible mortality despite a risk of false negatives (~1.1%). In cytologically benign nodules with high suspicion USG pattern a repeat FNAC within 12 months is warranted. In nodules with low or intermediate suspicion pattern repeat USG is warranted at 12–24 months. The American Thyroid Association advises that nodules with a very low suspicion pattern on USG and benign cytology may not require any subsequent imaging. A nodule that has two benign biopsy results has a likelihood of malignancy that is close to zero and no longer requires USG surveillance. While this is useful for solitary nodules, continued surveillance is required in MNG. Long-term

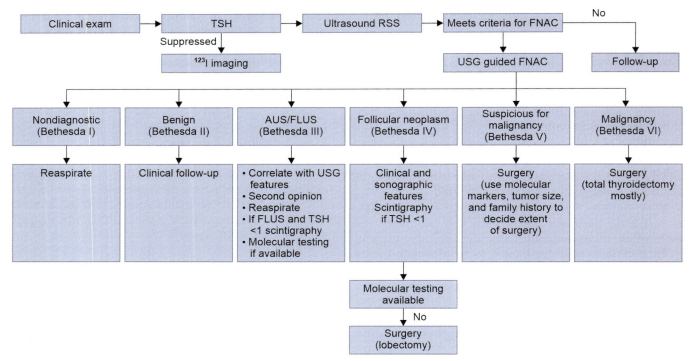

Flowchart 1: Author's current approach to nodular thyroid disease.
(AUS: atypia of undetermined significance; FNAC: fine-needle aspiration cytology; FLUS: follicular lesion of undetermined significance; RSS: risk stratification systems; TSH: thyroid stimulating hormone)

surveillance for nodules that are stable in USG can be lengthened. The ideal monitoring frequency and need for evaluation beyond 5 years is unknown.

A 20% increase in nodule size in at least two dimensions >2 mm in more than two dimensions or a >50% change in volume (measured by the formula 0.52 times the three nodule dimensions) or the development of new suspicious sonographic features warrants repeat aspiration. Based on this criterion only 4–10% of nodules will increase in size over a 18 month period. Suspicious sonographic features rather than size per se appear to predict a malignant cytology in a subsequent aspiration. Malignant nodules demonstrate faster growth rates than benign nodules; faster growth is also associated with more aggressive cancer subtypes. Nodule growth does not necessarily indicate malignancy. In nodules that appear benign on USG, subsequent growth does not appear to influence the low risk of malignancy. Some authorities advocate a selective sampling approach in this setting.

Thyroid suppression is not warranted in benign nodules. Modest reduction in size with TSH suppression has been documented in areas with borderline iodine deficiency but the trade-off has been an increased risk of cardiac arrhythmias and osteoporosis. Surgery may be considered in benign nodules if they are large or cause compression. Laser thermal ablation (LTA) has been applied to being nodules. The procedure is cumbersome but offers a nonsurgical option in some patients who require or desire reduction in nodule size (see below).

Cystic nodules that are cytologically benign can also be monitored. Fluid reaccumulation after aspiration occurs in 60–90% of these patients. If symptomatic these patients may be offered hemithyroidectomy or percutaneous ethanol instillation. This may be an option in predominantly cystic nodules that are benign on cytology (see below).

Nodules that do not meet criteria for aspiration which are classified as low or intermediate risk for malignancy may be followed by USG at 12 months. Longer times may be warranted for spongiform or pure cystic nodules.

Indeterminate Cytology

Atypia of Undetermined Significance/Follicular Lesion of Undetermined Significance

Nodules that are reported as Bethesda III—atypia or follicular lesion of unknown significance (AUS/FLUS) constitute up to 27% of all reported FNACs and have a mean malignancy risk of 16%. The BIII describes a group of FNAC specimens that contain cells with architectural or nuclear atypia that would not qualify it for BII but does not contain enough suspicious features that would warrant a higher class assignment. BIII includes specimens that cannot be classified as benign or as follicular neoplasm because of increased cellularity, atypia, or fixation artifacts. This category was intended for limited use and expected to have a frequency of about 7%. Usage of this category by cytologists has been variable with studies reporting usage up to 27%. When patients in this category underwent surgery, malignancy was seen up to 14.5%.

Reviewing the USG appears to be helpful. The reported cancer risk in BIII lesions and high suspicion sonographic features was between 90 and 100%. The prevalence of at least one suspicious feature on USG in BIII lesions ranged from 18 to 50% and increased the risk of malignancy to 60–90%. It must be noted that the overall malignancy rate in these studies was 40–45%.

Fludeoxyglucose-positron emission tomography (FDG-PET) has been reported to have a high NPV when applied to the diagnosis of cytologically indeterminate thyroid nodules. In a systematic review and meta-analysis of six studies, FDG-PET had a low PPV (39%) and a high NPV (96%) when performed in thyroid nodules with BIII or BIV cytology. This approach is however, not recommended.

Since there is significant interobserver variability in this category one recommended approach is to obtain a second opinion from a high volume cytopathologist. Central cytopathologists from institutions with high volume make fewer indeterminate diagnosis (55% vs. 42%) than community-based cytopathologists In one study, a second opinion for a nodule originally read as indeterminate and subsequently reclassified as benign had an NPV 95%. The second opinion improves diagnostic accuracy from 60 to 74% and avoids diagnostic surgery in 25% of patients.

A repeat FNA may reclassify the lesion into a more definitive diagnosis. A repeat diagnosis recategorizes an AUS lesion into a benign category the majority of the time with an indeterminate diagnosis persisting only a third of the time. Malignancy rates are similar with single BIII and two successive BIII diagnoses. This approach has been recently questioned.

When available the GSC or Thyroseq v3 (see above) are appropriate for use in BIII lesions. They have a high NPV making them high rule out tests. With recent improvements in these platforms their PPV is approaching "rule in status."

As observed above, there is very limited experience for this modality in India. A composite of clinical ultrasound and cytology and patient preference may be used to decide if surgery is required when molecular testing is not available. A pragmatic approach to the diagnosis of AUS/FLUS (BIII) lesions is summarized in **Flowchart 1**.

Follicular Neoplasm

Nodules that are Bethesda IV (follicular neoplasm, suspicious for follicular neoplasm or Hürthle cell neoplasm) describes a cellular aspirate characterized by (i) follicular cells arranged in an altered architectural pattern with cell crowding and/or micro follicle formation and lacking clear features of PTC or (ii) composed exclusively of Hürthle (oncocytic) cells. The majority of tumors are benign follicular adenomas driven by the oncogenic RAS mutation with uncertain malignant potential. The risk for malignancy is intermediate (15–30%). The application of this category has provided a mean prevalence of 10% (1–25%) and mean cancer risk of 26% (14–33%).

Traditionally, diagnostic lobectomy has been used in this category. Molecular markers have added considerably to the diagnostic assessment in this category.

The Thyroseq V3/Affirma GSC and ThyGeNEXT Thyramir have appropriate rule out and improving rule in capability to suggest surveillance or follow up in this diagnostic category. Traditional exceptions to this include populations with unusual prevalence of malignancy or high pretest probability of disease including family history, high-risk sonographic features or prior irradiation. In the presence of these features, the pretest probability will often exceed 50% reducing the NPV to <90%; this would be considered too low to avoid diagnostic thyroidectomy.

The clinical approach to the patient with the BIV lesion is summarized in **Flowchart 1**.

Suspicious For Malignancy

Nodules that are Bethesda V [suspicious for papillary carcinoma (SUSP)] demonstrate cytologic features that are suspicious for malignancy but not conclusive for malignancy. Upto 6% of nodules are in this category with a mean risk of malignancy of 75%. Ultrasound assessment of the neck to discover metastatic nodes and confirmation of malignancy upon aspiration reduces uncertainty in this setting. Molecular testing is able to suggest the extent of surgery. Total thyroidectomy is recommended in the following situations (a) Bethesda V, (b) positive molecular testing, (c) suspicious ultrasound findings, (d) tumor >4 cm, (e) family history of thyroid cancer, and may be considered in the presence of contralateral nodules and coexistent thyrotoxicosis. Lobectomy or hemithyroidectomy may be considered in other indeterminate nodule with intraoperative frozen section and or cytologic assessment identifies between 50 and 80% of thyroid cancers and leads to definitive surgery.

Malignant Cytology

Surgery is recommended in patients with a diagnosis of malignancy in cytology (Bethesda VI) and is discussed in detail in the chapter on management of DTC. Surveillance as opposed to surgery may be an option in patients with papillary microcarcinomas (tumors <1 cm) with no evidence of local regional or distant metastasis since there appears to be a low rate of clinical progression. However, this option is seldom offered to patients outside of Japan.

MANAGEMENT OF MULTINODULAR GOITER

Once malignancy and abnormal thyroid function have been excluded there is seldom an indication to treat NTD unless they cause compression or cosmetic symptoms. Growth prevention interventions other than iodine supplementation in IDA are usually not required. Rapid nodule growth, change in voice are indicators of malignancy and warrant intervention irrespective of cytology. Clinical and USG based follow-up with a periodicity of between 12 and 18 months appears sufficient. FNAC is repeated if there is an increase of >20% in any of the nodule dimensions or an increase of >50% in volume. FNA is also warranted if there is an increase in the risk score of the nodule or if there are new nodules or lymph nodes.

If nodule size is stable, lower frequency of follow up is reasonable. An asymptomatic nontoxic MNG can be clinically followed with no intervention required in the majority of patients. Treatment is reserved for patients with symptoms of compression or if cosmetic disfigurement is a concern.

Thyroid Hormone Suppression

Thyroid hormone suppression has been used widely by clinicians to shrink nodules and reduce nodule growth. Volume reduction is achieved in a third of the patients treated. In four RCTs with durations of follow up from 9 to 24 months and doses ranging from 2.0 to 2.7 μg/kg—up to 30% reduction in volume were seen. The definition of effective reduction in volume size was variable in these studies. In another study of 83 nodules from Italy follow up was extended up to 5 years—volume reduction was 47.6%. Ultrasound detected new nodules in only 7.5% of the treated group (28.5% in the control group). Similar reductions in size over time are reported in trials with single colloid nodules with response seen in a subset of patients. Overall the benefits of modest reduction in nodule size in a small subset of patients must be balanced with adverse effects of TSH suppression. The author does not offer TSH suppression as a choice routinely in single or multiple nodules.

Surgery

Surgery provides relief from compressive symptoms and improves cosmesis. Subtotal thyroidectomy has a recurrence rate of up to 40%. Since reoperation carries with it a 3- to 10-fold increase in recurrent laryngeal damage and hypoparathyroidism, subtotal thyroidectomy is best avoided. Total thyroidectomy achieves a negligible recurrence rate; in experienced hands the risk of permanent recurrent laryngeal nerve injury or hypoparathyroidism is low. Since up to 10% of MNG harbors malignancy, total thyroidectomy obviates the need for completion thyroidectomy.

Radioiodine

Iodine-131 is effective in reducing the volume of euthyroid MNG. It is useful in relieving compression symptoms in the elderly, those who are high risk for surgery or in those who refuse surgery. The response rate is up to 80% with a volume reduction of 40–60% in 1–3 years. Notably there is an improvement in the upper airway obstruction as measured by flow loop volumes. Higher doses may be required with radioiodine uptake is <20%. Pretreatment with low dose (0.3 mg) of recombinant human thyroid-stimulating hormone (rhTSH) can increase the iodine uptake of the gland by up to 74% and facilitates ablation. rTSH may thus reduce the dose of radioiodine required. Various doses of rTSH have been used—the optimal dose is unclear.

I-131 can cause radiation thyroiditis in up to 3% of patients. Transient thyrotoxicosis can be seen in up to 5% of patients. This is greater for patients with rTSH pretreatment. Autoimmune hyperthyroidism is seen to develop in up to 5% of patients. Hypothyroidism occurs in up to 58% of patients 5–8 years after therapy; more in patients with rTSH pretreatment. I-131 may not be suitable in very large MNG. Caution is required in patients with airway compromise because it can cause a transient post treatment increase in volume.

Non/Minimally Invasive Approaches

New technologies are available to safely ablate thyroid nodules without removal of the gland itself. These processes include thermal or chemical ablation of the gland. Chemical ablation using percutaneous ethanol injection (PEI) is effective for cystic nodules. Options for solid nodules include—(i) laser ablation (LTA), (ii) radiofrequency ablation (RFA), (iii) high frequency focused ultrasound (HIFU), and (iv) percutaneous microwave ablation (PMWA).

Percutaneous ethanol injection is effective in pure cysts or predominantly cystic nodules. High purity ethanol is injected which causes coagulative necrosis in cystic nodules and ischemic necrosis in solid nodules. A volume reduction of up to 98.5% has been reported in cystic nodules and up to 73.2% in predominantly cystic nodules. About 5–25% of nodules are refractory. In nodules with >20% sold component PEI is less effective. While PEI has been used for solid nodules it is less effective in this setting; thermal ablation is a better option.

Radiofrequency ablation and LTA both result in significant and stable reduction of nodule volume. RFA uses heat from an energy source and causes coagulation necrosis of the nodule. Volume reduction occurs in the weeks and months following the procedure due to replacement of the nodule by fibrous-scar tissue. The procedure can be repeated if required. The complication rate is 3.5%. Difficulty in future surgery may be an issue. RFA can be used for compressive and aesthetically disfiguring or nodules which are not amenable to surgery or I-131 therapy or based on patient preference. It can be used for autonomously functioning nodules. It has been suggested for use in papillary thyroid microcarcinoma and in loco regional recurrences when surgery or iodine ablation is not feasible or refused by patients. Questions remain about this approach; predominantly an uncertainty about whether cancer cells are completely eliminated. LTA uses similar principles to reduce thyroid nodules. RFA appears to have superior efficacy in nodule shrinkage. Transient thyrotoxicosis has been reported after LTA. Neither voice change nor hypothyroidism have been reported with either modality.

High frequency focused ultrasound has the advantage of not requiring needle puncture. It causes focused thermal coagulation. It is less operator-dependent. However, it has less efficacy for large nodules. Side-effects such as pain, skin redness, subcutaneous swelling, and vocal cord paralysis have been reported and usually transient.

Percutaneous microwave ablation (PMWA) increases the temperature of nodule rapidly through rotation of molecules produced from microwave energy. Significant volume reductions of up to 90% at 1 year have been reported.

Few head-to-head comparisons of these modalities. A small study which compared 3-month outcomes showed a slightly better volume reduction with RFA (50%) than with PMWA (44%) and HIFU (48%).

CONCLUSION

Nodular thyroid disease is common. Most nodules in thyroid glands are benign. The clinicians approach to NTD is to exclude malignancy and manage compressive symptoms. Thyroid USG has emerged as the pivotal test that allows risk stratification and further work-up. Molecular testing has emerged as a useful adjunct to USG and FNA allowing less number of unnecessary surgeries. Nonsurgical alternatives to the management of symptoms have emerged that require further evaluation and integration into clinical care in the appropriate patient.

SUGGESTED READINGS

1. Haugen BR, Alexander EK, Bible KC, Doherty GM, Mandel SJ, Nikiforov YE, et al. 2015 American Thyroid Association Management Guidelines for Adult Patients with Thyroid Nodules and Differentiated Thyroid Cancer: The American Thyroid Association Guidelines Task Force on Thyroid Nodules and Differentiated Thyroid Cancer. Thyroid. 2016;26(1):1-133.
2. Guth S, Theune U, Aberle J, Galach A, Bamberger CM. Very high prevalence of thyroid nodules detected by high frequency (13 MHz) ultrasound examination. Eur J Clin Invest. 2009;39(8): 699-706.
3. Mazzaferri EL. Management of a solitary thyroid nodule. N Engl J Med. 1993;328(8):553-9.
4. Vander JB, Gaston EA, Dawber TR. The significance of nontoxic thyroid nodules. Final report of a 15-year study of the incidence of thyroid malignancy. Ann Intern Med. 1968;69(3):537-40.
5. Delange F, de Benoist B, Pretell E, Dunn JT. Iodine deficiency in the world: where do we stand at the turn of the century? Thyroid. 2001;11(5):437-47.
6. Krohn K, Führer D, Bayer Y, Eszlinger M, Brauer V, Neumann S, et al. Molecular pathogenesis of euthyroid and toxic multinodular goiter. Endocr Rev. 2005;26(4):504-24.
7. Galanti MR, Granath F, Cnattingius S, Ekbom-Schnell A, Ekbom A. Cigarette smoking and the risk of goitre and thyroid nodules amongst parous women. J Intern Med. 2005;258(3):257-64.
8. Medeiros-Neto G, Feingold KR, Anawalt B, Boyce A, Chrousos G, de Herder WW. Multinodular Goiter. In: Endotext [Internet]. South Dartmouth (MA): MDText.com, Inc.; 2000.
9. Knobel M, Medeiros-Neto G. An outline of inherited disorders of the thyroid hormone generating system. Thyroid. 2003;13(8): 771-801.
10. Bignell GR. Familial nontoxic multinodular thyroid goiter locus Maps to Chromosome 14q but does not account for familial nonmedullary thyroid cancer. Am J Hum Genet. 1997;61(5): 1123-30.
11. Agretti P, De Marco G, Ferrarini E, Di Cosmo C, Montanelli L, Bagattini B, et al. Gene expression profile in functioning and non-functioning nodules of autonomous multinodular goiter from an area of iodine deficiency: unexpected common characteristics between the two entities. J Endocrinol Invest. 2022;45(2):399-411.
12. Mayson SE, Haugen BR. Molecular diagnostic evaluation of thyroid nodules. Endocrinol. Metab Clin North Am. 2019;48(1):85-97.
13. Siegel RL, Miller KD, Jemal A. Cancer statistics. CA Cancer J Clin. 2015;65(1):5-29.
14. Farid NR. Molecular basis of thyroid cancer. Berlin: Springer Science & Business Media; 2006.
15. Battista S, Martelli ML, Fedele M, Chiappetta G, Trapasso F, De Vita G, et al. A mutated p53 gene alters thyroid cell differentiation. Oncogene. 1995;11:2029-37.
16. Beckers C, Cornette C. TSH production rate in nontoxic goiter. J Clin Endocrinol Metab. 1971;32:852-4.
17. Arturi F, Russo D, Schlumberger M, du Villard JA, Caillou B, Vigneri P, et al. Iodide symporter gene expression in human thyroid tumors. J Clin Endocrinol Metab. 1983;83(7):2493-6.
18. Demeester-Mirkine N, Van Sande J, Corvilain J, Dumont JE. Benign thyroid nodule with normal iodide trap and defective organification. J Clin Endocrinol Metab. 1975;41(06):1169-71.
19. Hedinger C, Williams ED, Sobin LH. The WHO histological classification of thyroid tumors: a commentary on the second edition. Cancer. 1989;63(5):908-11.
20. Knudsen N, Perrild H, Christiansen E, Rasmussen S, Dige-Petersen H, Jørgensen T. Thyroid structure and size and two-year follow-up of solitary cold thyroid nodules in an unselected population with borderline iodine deficiency. Eur J Endocrinol. 2000;142(3):224-30.
21. Kuma K, Matsuzuka F, Yokozawa T, Miyauchi A, Sugawara M. Fate of untreated benign thyroid nodules: results of long-term follow-up. World J Surg. 1994;18(4):495-8;discussion 499.
22. Kuma K, Matsuzuka F, Kobayashi A, Hirai K, Morita S, Miyauchi A, et al. Outcome of long standing solitary thyroid nodules. World J Surg. 1992;16(4):583-7;discussion 587-8.
23. Gemsenjäger E, Staub JJ, Girard J, Heitz P. Preclinical hyperthyroidism in multinodular goiter. J Clin Endocrinol Metab. 1976;43(4):810-6.
24. Sandrock D, Olbricht T, Emrich D, Benker G, Reinwein D. Long-term follow-up in patients with autonomous thyroid adenoma. Acta Endocrinol (Copenh). 1993;128:51-5.
25. Werk EE, Jr Vernon BM, Gonzalez JJ, Ungaro PC, McCoy RC. Cancer in thyroid nodules. A community hospital survey. Arch Intern Med. 1984;144(3):474-6.
26. Harach HR, Franssila KO, Wasenius VM. Occult papillary carcinoma of the thyroid. A "normal" finding in Finland. A systematic autopsy study. Cancer. 1985;56(3):531-8.

27. Cohen A, Rovelli A, Merlo DF, van Lint MT, Lanino E, Bresters D, et al. Risk for secondary thyroid carcinoma after hematopoietic stem-cell transplantation: an EBMT Late Effects Working Party Study. J Clin Oncol. 2007;25(17):2449-54.
28. Aydin LY, Aydin Y, Besir FH, Demirin H, Yildirim H, Önder E, et al. Effect of smoking intensity on thyroid volume, thyroid nodularity and thyroid function: the Melen study. Minerva Endocrinol. 2011;36(4):273-80.
29. Choi JY, Lee KS, Kim HJ, Shim YM, Kwon OJ, Park K, et al. Focal thyroid lesions incidentally identified by integrated 18F-FDG PET/CT: clinical significance and improved characterization. J Nucl Med. 2006;47(4):609-15.
30. Blum M, Biller BJ, Bergman DA. The thyroid cork. Obstruction of the thoracic inlet due to retroclavicular goiter. JAMA. 1974;227(2):189-91.
31. Boelaert K, Horacek J, Holder RL, Watkinson JC, Sheppard MC, Franklyn JA. Serum thyrotropin concentration as a novel predictor of malignancy in thyroid nodules investigated by fine-needle aspiration. J Clin Endocrinol Metab. 2006;91(11):4295-301.
32. Elisei R, Bottici V, Luchetti F, Di Coscio G, Romei C, Grasso L, et al. Impact of routine measurement of serum calcitonin on the diagnosis and outcome of medullary thyroid cancer: experience in 10,864 patients with nodular thyroid disorders. J Clin Endocrinol Metab. 2004;89(1):163-8.
33. Marqusee E, Benson CB, Frates MC, Doubilet PM, Larsen PR, Cibas ES, et al. Usefulness of ultrasonography in the management of nodular thyroid disease. Ann Intern Med. 2000;133(9):696-700.
34. Kwak JY, Han KH, Yoon JH, Moon HJ, Son EJ, Park SH, et al. Thyroid imaging reporting and data system for US features of nodules: a step in establishing better stratification of cancer risk. Radiology. 2011;260(3):892-9.
35. Maxwell C, Sipos JA. Clinical Diagnostic Evaluation of Thyroid Nodules. Endocrinol Metab Clin North Am. 2019;48(1):61-84.
36. Hoang JK, Middleton WD, Tessler FN. Update on ACR TI-RADS: Successes, Challenges, and Future Directions, From the AJR Special Series on Radiology Reporting and Data Systems. AJR Am J Roentgenol. 2021;216(3):570-8.
37. Moon WJ, Jung SL, Lee JH, Na DG, Baek JH, Lee YH, et al. Benign and malignant thyroid nodules: US differentiation--multicenter retrospective study. Radiology. 2008;247(3):762-70.
38. Moon HJ, Kwak JY, Kim E, Kim MJ. A taller-than-wide shape in thyroid nodules in transverse and longitudinal ultrasonographic planes and the prediction of malignancy. Thyroid. 2011;21(11):1249-53.
39. Tessler FN, Middleton WD, Grant EG, Hoang JK, Berland LL, Teefey SA, et al. ACR Thyroid Imaging, Reporting and Data System (TI-RADS): White Paper of the ACR TI-RADS Committee. J Am Coll Radiol. 2017;14(5):587-95.
40. Leenhardt L, Erdogan MF, Hegedus L. 2013 European thyroid association guidelines for cervical ultrasound scan and ultrasound-guided techniques in the postoperative management of patients with thyroid cancer. Eur Thyroid J. 2013;2(3):147-59.
41. Jeh SK, Jung SL, Kim BS, Lee YS. Evaluating the degree of conformity of papillary carcinoma and follicular carcinoma to the reported ultrasonographic findings of malignant thyroid tumor. Korean J Radiol. 2007;8(3):192-7.
42. Liu MJ, Liu ZF, Hou YY, Men YM, Zhang YX, Gao LY, et al. Ultrasonographic characteristics of medullary thyroid carcinoma: a comparison with papillary thyroid carcinoma. Oncotarget. 2017;8:27520-8.
43. Kwak JY, Koo H, Youk JH, Kim MJ, Moon HJ, Son EJ, et al. Value of US correlation of a thyroid nodule with initially benign cytologic results. Radiology. 2010;254(1):292-300.
44. Russ G, Trimboli P, Buffet C. The New Era of TIRADSs to Stratify the Risk of Malignancy of Thyroid Nodules: Strengths, Weaknesses and Pitfalls. Cancers. 2021;13(17):4316.
45. Grani G, Lamartina L, Ascoli V, Bosco D, Biffoni M, Giacomelli L, et al. Reducing the Number of Unnecessary Thyroid Biopsies While Improving Diagnostic Accuracy: Toward the "Right" TIRADS. J Clin Endocrinol Metab. 2019;104(1):95-102.
46. Wildman-Tobriner B, Buda M, Hoan JK, Middleton WD, Thayer D, Short RG, et al. Using Artificial Intelligence to Revise ACR TI-RADS Risk Stratification of Thyroid Nodules: Diagnostic Accuracy and Utility. Radiology. 2019;292:112-9.
47. Bini F, Pica A, Azzimonti L, Giusti A, Ruinelli L, Marinozzi F, et al. Artificial Intelligence in Thyroid Field—A Comprehensive Review. Cancers. 2021;13(19):4740.
48. Danese D, Sciacchitano S, Farsetti A, Andreoli M, Pontecorvi A. Diagnostic accuracy of conventional versus sonography-guided fine-needle aspiration biopsy of thyroid nodules. Thyroid. 1998;8(1):15-21.
49. Kim MJ, Kim EK, Park SI, Kim BM, Kwak JY, Kim SJ, et al. US-guided fine-needle aspiration of thyroid nodules: indications, techniques, results. Radiographics. 2008;28(7):1869-86;discussion 1887.
50. Lever EG, Refetoff S, Scherberg NH, Carr K. The influence of percutaneous fine needle aspiration on serum thyroglobulin. J Clin Endocrinol Metab. 1983;56(1):26-9.
51. Frates MC, Benson CB, Doubilet PM, Kunreuther E, Contreras M, Cibas ES, et al. Prevalence and distribution of carcinoma in patients with solitary and multiple thyroid nodules on sonography. J Clin Endocrinol Metab. 2006;91(9):3411-7.
52. Ali SZ, Cibas ES. The bethesda system for reporting thyroid cytopathology: definitions, criteria, and explanatory notes. Berlin: Springer; 2017.
53. Olson MT, Clark DP, Erozan YS, Ali SZ. Spectrum of risk of malignancy in subcategories of 'atypia of undetermined significance'. Acta Cytol. 2011;55(6):518-25.
54. Nayar R, Ivanovic M. The indeterminate thyroid fine-needle aspiration: experience from an academic center using terminology similar to that proposed in the 2007 National Cancer Institute Thyroid Fine Needle Aspiration State of the Science Conference. Cancer. 2009;117(3):195-202.
55. Roth MY, Witt RL, Steward DL. Molecular testing for thyroid nodules: Review and current state. Cancer. 2018;124(5):888-98.
56. Seshadri KG. A Pragmatic Approach to the Indeterminate Thyroid Nodule. Indian J Endocrinol Metab. 2017;21:751-7.
57. Nishino M, Bellevicine C, Baloch Z. Molecular tests for risk-stratifying cytologically indeterminate thyroid nodules: an overview of commercially available testing platforms in the united states. Diagn Mol Pathol. 2021;2(2):135-46.
58. Alexander EK, Kennedy GC, Baloch ZW, Cibas ES, Chudova D, Diggans J, et al. Preoperative diagnosis of benign thyroid nodules with indeterminate cytology. N Engl J Med. 2012;367(8):705-15.
59. Patel KN, Angell TE, Babiarz J, Barth NM, Blevins T, Duh QY, et al. Performance of a genomic sequencing classifier for the preoperative diagnosis of cytologically indeterminate thyroid nodules. JAMA Surg. 2018;153(9):817-24.
60. Krane JF, Cibas ES, Endo M, Marqusee E, Hu MI, Nasr CE, et al. The Afirma Xpression Atlas for thyroid nodules and thyroid cancer metastases: Insights to inform clinical decision-making from a fine-needle aspiration sample. Cancer Cytopathol. 2020;128(7):452-9.
61. Nikiforova MN, Lepe M, Tolino LA, Miller ME, Ohori NP, Wald AI, et al. Thyroid cytology smear slides: An untapped resource for ThyroSeq testing. Cancer Cytopathol. 2021;129(1):33-42.
62. Ablordeppey KK, Timmaraju VA, Song-Yang JW, Yaqoob S, Narick C, Mireskandari A, et al. Development and analytical validation of an expanded mutation detection panel for next-generation sequencing of thyroid nodule aspirates. J Mol Diagn. 2020;22(3):355-67.
63. Ciarletto AM, Narick C, Malchoff CD, Massoll NA, Labourier E, Haugh K, et al. Analytical and clinical validation of pairwise microRNA

expression analysis to identify medullary thyroid cancer in thyroid fine-needle aspiration samples. Cancer Cytopathol. 2021;129: 239-49.
64. Dutta S, Tarafdar S, Mukhopadhyay P, Bhattacharyya NP, Ghosh S. Plasma cell-free dna to differentiate malignant from benign thyroid nodules. J Clin Endocrinol Metab. 2021;106(5):e2262-70.
65. Alexander EK. From the Tip to the iceberg below-evolving our molecular understanding of thyroid nodules. J Clin Endocrinol Metab. 2021;106(5):e2357-8.
66. Brauer VF, Eder P, Miehle K, Wiesner TD, Hasenclever H, Paschke R. Interobserver variation for ultrasound determination of thyroid nodule volumes. Thyroid. 2005;15(10):1169-75.
67. Angell TE, Vyas CM, Medici M, Wang Z, Barletta JA, Benson CB, et al. Differential growth rates of benign vs. malignant thyroid nodules. J Clin Endocrinol Metab. 2017;102(12):4642-7.
68. Vriens D, de Wilt JWH, van der Wilt GJ, Netea-Maier RT, Oyen WJG, de Geus-Oei LF. The role of [F-18]-2-fluoro-2-deoxy-d-glucose-positron emission tomography in thyroid nodules with indeterminate fine-needle aspiration biopsy systematic review and meta-analysis of the literature. Cancer. 2011;117(20): 4582-94.
69. Cibas ES, Baloch ZW, Fellegara G, LiVolsi VA, Raab SS, Rosai J, et al. A prospective assessment defining the limitations of thyroid nodule pathologic evaluation. Ann Intern Med. 2013;159(5):325-32.
70. VanderLaan PA, Marqusee E, Krane JF. Clinical outcome for atypia of undetermined significance in thyroid fine-needle aspirations: should repeated fna be the preferred initial approach? Am J Clin Pathol. 2011;135(5):770-5.
71. Haymart MR, Greenblatt DY, Elson DF, Chen H. The role of intraoperative frozen section if suspicious for papillary thyroid cancer. Thyroid. 2008;18(4):419-23.
72. Papini E, Petrucci L, Guglielmi R, Panunzi C, Rinaldi R, Bacci V, et al. Long-term changes in nodular goiter: a 5-year prospective randomized trial of levothyroxine suppressive therapy for benign cold thyroid nodules. J Clin Endocrinol Metab. 1998;83(3):780-3.
73. Snook KL, Stalberg PL, Sidhu SB, Sywak MS, Edhouse P, Delbridge L. Recurrence after total thyroidectomy for benign multinodular goiter. World J Surg. 2007;31(3):593-8;discussion 599-600.
74. Gandolfi PP, Frisina A, Raffa M, Renda F, Rocchetti O, Ruggeri C, et al. The incidence of thyroid carcinoma in multinodular goiter: retrospective analysis. Acta Biomed. 2004;75(2):114-7.
75. Fast S, Nielsen VE, Bonnema SJ, Hegedüs L. Time to reconsider nonsurgical therapy of benign non-toxic multinodular goitre: focus on recombinant human TSH augmented radioiodine therapy. Eur J Endocrinol. 2009;160(4):517-28.
76. Baek JH, Ha EJ, Choi YJ, Sung JY, Kim JK, Shong YK. Radiofrequency versus Ethanol Ablation for Treating Predominantly Cystic Thyroid Nodules: A Randomized Clinical Trial. Korean J Radiol. 2015;16(6):1332-40.
77. Tufano RP, Pace-Asciak P, Russell JO, Suárez C, Randolph GW, López F, et al. Update of Radiofrequency Ablation for Treating Benign and Malignant Thyroid Nodules. The Future Is Now. Front Endocrinol. 2021;12:698689.
78. Hahn SY, Shin JH, Na DG, Ha EJ, Ahn HS, Lim HK, et al. Ethanol Ablation of the Thyroid Nodules: 2018 Consensus Statement by the Korean Society of Thyroid Radiology. Korean J Radiol. 2019;20(4):609-20.
79. Papini E, Gugliemi R, Pacella CM. Laser, radiofrequency, and ethanol ablation for the management of thyroid nodules. Curr Opin Endocrinol Diabetes Obes. 2016;23(5):400-6.
80. Liu YJ, Qian LX, Liu D, Zhao JF. Ultrasound-guided microwave ablation in the treatment of benign thyroid nodules in 435 patients. Exp Biol Med. 2017;242(15):1515-23.

CHAPTER 18

Thyroid Carcinoma

Gazal Bakshi, Sunil Kumar Mishra

INTRODUCTION

Thyroid cancer is the most prevalent endocrine malignancy, accounting for 3–4% of all cancers, with an incidence rate ranking ninth among all cancers in 2020. The incidence of thyroid cancer is on an increasing trend due to increased use of diagnostic imaging and surveillance. Although India currently ranks among the countries with the low thyroid carcinoma incidence average, it is affected by a huge regional variation, with a tenfold difference between lowest and highest incidence areas covered by cancer registries. In view of better access to healthcare between 2006–2008 and 2012–2014, the age-standardized incidence rates for thyroid carcinoma in India increased from 2.5 to 3.5/100,000 women (+37%) and from 1.0 to 1.3/100,000 men (+27%). These results may serve as an alarm for other transitioning countries to prevent over diagnosis. Although incidence is changing but mortality from thyroid cancer has not been affected much over the past five decades. Thyroid cancers exhibit a broad range of clinical behavior—from indolent tumors in most cases, to very aggressive malignancies. Therefore, a proper diagnostic workup is required before treatment is planned.

CLASSIFICATION OF THYROID NEOPLASMS (WHO 2017)

Primary Epithelial Tumors

- Tumors of follicular cells
  - *Benign*: Follicular adenoma
  - Borderline follicular tumors
    - Follicular tumor of uncertain malignant potential
    - Well-differentiated tumor of uncertain malignant potential
    - Noninvasive follicular neoplasm with papillary-like nuclear features (NIFTP)
  - *Malignant*: Carcinoma
    - *Differentiated*: Papillary, follicular, Hürthle cell, and poorly differentiated
    - Undifferentiated (anaplastic)
- Tumors of C cells
  - Medullary carcinoma
- Tumors of follicular and C Cells
  - Mixed medullary-follicular carcinomas

Primary Nonepithelial Tumors

- Malignant lymphomas
- Sarcomas
- Others

Secondary Tumors

Risk Factors

- Idiopathic
- Personal or family history of thyroid cancer
- History of syndromes such as Carney's complex, Cowden disease, and Peutz–Jeghers with a genetic predilection toward the development of thyroid cancer
- Previous radiation exposure (9% of all cases of thyroid cancer and risk increasing linearly at a dose of 20 Gy)

Genetics

Mitogen-activated protein kinase cellular signaling pathway regulates cellular proliferation, differentiation and apoptosis. Most thyroid cancers are found to have mutation in this pathway.

Differentiated thyroid cancer (DTC) and anaplastic thyroid cancer:
- *BRAFT1799A mutation*: The most frequent mutation in thyroid cancer other than medullary cancer. It results in *BRAF* V600E mutant kinase, which is exclusive to papillary thyroid cancer (PTC) and PTC-derived anaplastic thyroid cancer.
- *RAS mutations*: Most frequently in follicular thyroid carcinoma (FTC) and follicular variant PTC.
- *PAX8-PPARγ translocation*: 30% of FTC
- *RET translocations*: 7% of PTC
- *Other translocation genes*: *BRAF*, the *NTRK* gene family, *ALK*, and *THADA*.

- *Phosphatidylinositol-3-kinase or p53 tumor suppressor pathway*: It is most commonly present in association with poorly DTC and anaplastic thyroid cancer.

Medullary Thyroid Cancer
- *RET* proto-oncogene mutations are the most common cause of medullary thyroid cancer (MTC). It can occur sporadically as somatic events or as inherited germline events that exhibit autosomal dominant inheritance as a component of the multiple endocrine neoplasia, type 2A (MEN 2A) and type 2B (2B) syndromes.
- Assessment for a heritable *RET* germline mutation is recommended in all patients with MTC.
- Sporadic Rat sarcoma virus (*RAS)* mutations.

Clinical Presentation
Thyroid Nodules
Thyroid nodules are routinely encountered by clinicians and are rarely malignant. Around 90% are benign and not detected on palpation.

Differentiated Thyroid Cancer
About 95% of thyroid cancers are DTC out of which PTC is the most common. While papillary cancers have the best overall prognosis; follicular thyroid cancer, Hürthle cell thyroid cancer, and poorly-DTCs are high risk cancers. These metastasize to distant sites mostly lungs and bones via the bloodstream whereas PTC metastasizes to cervical lymph nodes and rarely lungs.

Hürthle Cell Neoplasm
Hürthle cell is a mitochondria-rich cell with a distinctive histomorphology that arises in a variety of benign and neoplastic conditions of the thyroid gland. However, unlike FTC, Hürthle cell neoplasm (HCN) exhibits regional spread to cervical nodes and soft tissues in the neck.

Anaplastic Thyroid Cancer
It is a rare form of thyroid cancer (<1%) that usually presents as a rapidly growing large, firm palpable mass in the thyroid with or without cervical adenopathy. Patients develop compressive features and metastasize to the lungs, followed by bones and the brain. It can occur in de novo but usually arises from or coexist with DTC. If a patient with a history of long-standing DTC presents with the aforementioned symptoms anaplastic transformation is to be suspected.

Neuroendocrine C-cell Derived Thyroid Cancer
Medullary thyroid cancer: They arise from parafollicular neuroendocrine cells and are only 1–2 % of all thyroid cancers. They usually present as a thyroid nodule from fourth to sixth decade of life as a solitary nodule. They frequently metastasize via lymphatics. Flushing and diarrhea are suggestive of widespread metastatic disease.

Assessment and Treatment of Thyroid Nodules
Sonographic Features
The 2015 American Thyroid Association guidelines defined risk categories for thyroid nodules based on ultrasonography. Based on these categories they also provide specific recommendations for fine needle aspiration cytology (FNAC) **(Table 1)**.

These include:
- Composition
- Echogenicity
- Shape
- Margin
- Echogenic foci

Fine needle aspiration cytology can be considered based on clinical suspicion and in patients with high risk factors. ATA 2015 guidelines also advised biopsy only for nodules >1 cm.

Fine Needle Aspiration Cytology
There are six diagnostic categories for reporting thyroid cytopathology in Bethesda system. Ultrasonography guided procedure is done and each nodule is categorized as per the cytopathology into the Bethesda System for reporting thyroid cytopathology categories (TBSRTC) **(Table 2)**.

Molecular Diagnostics
In diagnostic categories 3 and 4, the diagnosis of thyroid cancer and its exclusion is not clear. So, molecular diagnostics can be considered in these categories. These include:
- Gene mutation profiling panels
- 167 genes expression classifier

Gene mutation profiling panels have high PPV while 167 genes expression classifier has high negative predictive value (NPV). Therefore, mutation testing is a good rule-in test; by contrast, the gene expression classifier is a good rule-out test. However, more recent molecular diagnostics for thyroid nodules are forthcoming, and molecular approaches will improve the diagnostics of thyroid nodules further. In our country availability and cost limits its use.

Approach and Treatment
After a detailed pretreatment assessment of size, location, number of tumors, lymph nodes, and invasion of surrounding tissues, further treatment and surgical management is planned. Tumor, node, metastasis (TNM) classification and American Joint Committee on Cancer (AJCC) staging are done and further management is planned.

GOITER, THYROID NODULES AND THYROID CANCER

TABLE 1: Thyroid imaging reporting and data system.

TIRADS	Results	Ultrasonographic findings	Risk of malignancy	FNA size cut off (largest dimension)
1	Normal	Normal	–	
2	Benign	• Simple cyst • Spongiform nodule • White knight aspect • Isolated microcalcification	<1	No biopsy
3	Probably benign	• None of high suspicious findings • Isoechogenic • Hyperechogenic	<3	Consider at ≥2 cm
4A	Low suspicious	• None of high suspicious findings • Moderately hypoechogenic	5–10	≥1.5 cm
4B	High suspicious with two or <2 signs	• Taller than wide • Irregular or microlobulated margins • Microcalcification • Marked hypoechogenecity	10–20	≥1 cm
5	High suspicious with ≥3 signs	• Taller than wide • Irregular or microlobulated margins • Microcalcification • Marked hypoechogenecity	>70–90	≥1 cm

(FNA: fine needle aspiration; TIRAD: thyroid imaging reporting and data system)

TABLE 2: Cytology diagnostic categories of the Bethesda system.

Diagnostic category	Cytopathology	Risk of malignancy	Management
1	Nondiagnostic	1–4%	Repeat fine needle aspiration cytology (FNAC)
2	Benign	<3%	Surveillance
3	Atypia of undetermined significance Or Follicular lesion of undetermined significance	1–4%	Surveillance or surgery
4	Follicular neoplasm Or Suspicious for follicular neoplasm	15–30%	Surveillance or surgery
5	Suspicious	60–75%	Surgery
6	Malignant	97–99%	Surgery

TNM (American Joint Committee on Cancer, AJCC/TNM 8th edition)

Primary tumor for papillary, follicular, poorly differentiated, Hürthle cell, and anaplastic thyroid carcinomas:
- *TX*: Primary tumor cannot be assessed
- *T0*: No evidence of primary tumor
- *T1*: Tumor ≤2 cm in greatest dimension limited to the thyroid
  - *T1a*: Tumor ≤1 cm
  - *T1b*: Tumor >1 cm but ≤2 cm
- *T2*: Tumor >2 cm but ≤4 cm in greatest dimension limited to the thyroid
- *T3**: Tumor >4 cm limited to the thyroid or gross extrathyroidal extension (ETE) invading only strap muscles
  - *T3a**: Tumor >4 cm limited to the thyroid
  - *T3b**: Gross extrathyroidal extension (ETE) invading only strap muscles (sternohyoid, sternothyroid, thyrohyoid, or omohyoid muscles) from a tumor of any size
- *T4*: Includes gross ETE into major neck structures
  - *T4a*: Invading subcutaneous soft tissues, larynx, trachea, esophagus, or recurrent laryngeal nerve from a tumor of any size.
  - *T4b*: Invading prevertebral fascia or encasing carotid artery or mediastinal vessels from a tumor of any size.

*All categories may be subdivided—(s) solitary tumor and (m) multifocal tumor (the largest tumor determines the classification).

Medullary thyroid carcinoma
- **TX to T3**: Definitions are similar to the above
- **T4**: Advanced disease
  - *T4a*: Moderately advanced; tumor of any size with gross extrathyroidal extension into the nearby tissues of the neck, including subcutaneous soft tissue, larynx, trachea, esophagus, or recurrent laryngeal nerve.
  - *T4b*: Very advanced; tumor of any size with extension toward the spine or into nearby large blood vessels, invading the prevertebral fascia or encasing the carotid artery or mediastinal vessels.

Regional lymph node
- **NX**: Regional lymph nodes cannot be assessed
- **N0**: No evidence of regional lymph node metastasis
  - *N0a**: One or more cytologic or histologically confirmed benign lymph nodes
  - *N0b**: No radiologic or clinical evidence of locoregional lymph node metastasis
- **N1***: Metastasis to regional nodes
  - *N1a**: Metastasis to level VI or VII (pretracheal, paratracheal, prelaryngeal/Delphian, or upper mediastinal) lymph nodes; this can be unilateral or bilateral disease
  - *N1b**: Metastasis to unilateral, bilateral or contralateral lateral neck lymph nodes (levels I, II, III, IV, or V) or retropharyngeal lymph nodes

Distant metastasis (M)
- **M0**: No distant metastasis
- **M1**: Distant metastasis

AJCC prognostic stage grouping (Tables 3 to 5)
Age is considered as an important factor for differentiated thyroid cancer in prognostic staging. T, N, and M categories as described above not only guide for treatment approach but also predict survival.

TABLE 3: Differentiated thyroid cancer.

	Age at diagnosis <55 years		
Stage I	any T	any N	M0
Stage II	any T	any N	M1
	Age at diagnosis ≥55 years		
Stage I	T1	N0/NX	M0
	T2	N0/NX	M0
Stage II	T1	N1	M0
	T2	N1	M0
	T3a/T3b	any N	M0
Stage III	T4a	any N	M0
Stage IVA	T4b	any N	M0
Stage IVB	any T	any N	M1

TABLE 4: Medullary thyroid cancer.

Stage I	T1	N0	M0
Stage II	T2	N0	M0
	T3	N0	M0
Stage III	T1–T3	N1a	M0
Stage IVA	T4a	any N	M0
	T1–T3	N1b	M0
Stage IVB	T4b	any N	M0
Stage IVC	any T	any N	M1

TABLE 5: Anaplastic thyroid cancer.

Stage IVA	T1–T3a	N0/NX	M0
Stage IVB	T1–T3a	N1	M0
	T3b	any N	M0
	T4	any N	M0
Stage IVC	any T	any N	M1

Major Changes in the AJCC/TNM 8th Edition
Differentiated thyroid cancer
- Age cutoff used for staging was increased from 45 to 55 years at diagnosis.
- Minimal ETE detected was removed from the definition of T3 disease.
- N1 disease no longer upstages a patient to stage III.
- T3a is a new category for tumors >4 cm confined to the thyroid gland.
- T3b is a new category for tumors of any size demonstrating gross ETE into strap muscles.
- Level VII lymph nodes were reclassified as central neck lymph nodes (N1a).
- In DTC, the presence of distant metastases in older patients is classified as stage IVB disease rather than stage IVC disease; distant metastasis in anaplastic thyroid cancer continues to be classified as stage IVC disease.

Anaplastic thyroid cancer
- Unlike previous editions where all anaplastic thyroid cancers were classified as T4 disease, anaplastic cancers will now use the same T definitions as DTC.
- Intrathyroidal disease is stage IVA, gross ETE or cervical lymph node metastases are stage IVB and distant metastases are stage IVC.

TREATMENT
Surgical Approaches
Treatment is decided on the basis of preoperative risk assessment by clinical, imaging, and cytological data.

---
*All categories may be subdivided—(s) solitary tumor and (m) multifocal tumor (the largest tumor determines the classification)

The treatment approaches recommended by the 2015 ATA are more conservative than in the past.

Tumors smaller than 4 cm with no evidence of extrathyroidal extension or lymph node metastasis they can undergo lobectomy. The rate of complications associated with lobectomy is half as compared to total thyroidectomy.

Preoperative findings of lymph node metastases (clinical N1; therapeutic lymph node dissection) or PTC with evidence of gross extrathyroid extension (clinical T4) and distant metastases (clinical M1) should undergo exploration and removal of central and lateral neck lymph nodes.

The common complications of thyroidectomy include hypoparathyroidism, recurrent laryngeal nerve injury, hematoma, and wound infection.

■ Risk Assessment/Active Surveillance

Based on surgical and pathological findings after surgery, the need for radioiodine ablation or thyroid-stimulating hormone (TSH) suppression is considered. TNM staging predicts mortality but does not estimate postoperative persistence or recurrence probability of disease. The revised risk of recurrence proposed in the ATA's 2015 guidelines includes clinical and pathological features **(Table 6)**.

■ Postoperative Monitoring

Postoperative disease status is to be considered in deciding whether additional treatment (e.g., RAI, surgery, or other treatment) may be needed or not. Postoperative serum thyroglobulin (Tg) (on thyroid hormone withdrawal or after TSH stimulation) can help in assessing the persistence of disease or thyroid remnant and predicting potential future disease recurrence. The Tg should reach its nadir by 3–4 weeks postoperatively in most patients. The Optimal Cutoff value for postoperative serum Tg to guide decision-making regarding radioactive iodine (RAI) administration is not known.

■ Radioactive Iodine Ablation and Preparation

After total thyroidectomy, in patients with a high risk of recurrence adjuvant radioactive iodine (I131; usual dose 100–150 mCi) is recommended. In intermediate risk of recurrence, RAI can be considered as per postoperative thyroglobulin levels and iodine scan. In patients with persistent or recurrent RAI-avid disease, 150 mCi or higher dose is required. The side effects of RAI include transient neck pain and swelling, dry mouth and eyes, and secondary malignancy.

For the preparation of RAI there are two suggested approaches.
1. Thyroid hormone withdrawal for 3–4 weeks. Liothyronine may be substituted in the initial weeks if LT4 is withdrawn for 4 or more weeks, and in these circumstances, Liothyronine should be withdrawn for at least 2 weeks. Serum TSH should be measured prior to radioisotope administration to evaluate the degree of TSH elevation and a goal of TSH of >30 IU/mL is generally adopted.
2. Recombinant human thyrotropin is an acceptable alternative to hormone withdrawal for achieving remnant ablation in ATA low risk patients and may be considered in ATA intermediate risk.

A post-therapy whole body scintigraphy (WBS) [with or without single-photon emission computerized tomography

TABLE 6: ATA 2009 risk stratification system with proposed modifications (2015).

ATA low risk	• Papillary thyroid cancer (with all of the following): ○ No local or distant metastases ○ All macroscopic tumor has been resected ○ No tumor invasion of locoregional tissues or structures ○ The tumor does not have aggressive histology ○ No RAI-avid metastatic foci outside the thyroid bed on the first post treatment whole-body RAI scan if performed ○ No vascular invasion ○ Clinical N0 or ≤5 pathologic N1 micrometastases (<0.2 cm in largest dimension) • Intrathyroidal, encapsulated follicular variant of papillary thyroid cancer • Intrathyroidal, well-differentiated follicular thyroid cancer with capsular invasion and no or minimal (<4 foci) vascular invasion • Intrathyroidal, papillary microcarcinoma, unifocal or multifocal, including *BRAF* V600E mutated (if known)
ATA intermediate risk	• Microscopic invasion of tumor into the perithyroidal soft tissues • RAI-avid metastatic foci in the neck on the first post-treatment whole-body RAI scan • Aggressive histology (e.g., tall cell, hobnail variant, and columnar cell carcinoma) • Papillary thyroid cancer with vascular invasion • Clinical N1 or >5 pathologic N1 with all involved lymph nodes <3 cm in largest dimension • Multifocal papillary microcarcinoma with ETE and *BRAF* V600E mutated (if known)
ATA high risk	• Macroscopic invasion of tumor into the perithyroidal soft tissues • Incomplete tumor resection • Distant metastases • Postoperative serum thyroglobulin suggestive of distant metastases • Pathologic N1 with any metastatic lymph node ≥3 cm in largest dimension • Follicular thyroid cancer with extensive vascular invasion (>4 foci of vascular invasion)

(ATA: American Thyroid Association; ETE: extrathyroidal extension; RAI: radioactive iodine)

(SPECT)/computed tomography (CT)] is recommended after RAI remnant ablation or treatment, to inform disease staging and document the RAI avidity of any structural disease.[12]

Thyroid Hormone Suppression Therapy

It is done to suppress TSH and potentially minimize its stimulation of thyroid cancer growth and is recommended in most patients after surgery as per the risk assessment **(Table 7)**.

TABLE 7: TSH goals as per ATA risk stratification.	
Risk stratification	**TSH goal**
ATA high-risk	No >0.1m IU/L
• ATA intermediate-risk category • ATA low risk with detectable Tg levels	Between 0.1 and 0.5 mIU/L
ATA low-risk category with undetectable Tg levels	Between 0.5 and 2.0 mIU/L

(ATA: American Thyroid Association; TSH: thyroid-stimulating hormone; Tg: thyroglobulin)

Response to Therapy

Persistent disease can be detected appropriately by serum thyroglobulin levels and ultrasonography neck rather than diagnostic whole-body ^{131}I scintigraphy.

Guidelines now recommend the selective use of radioactive iodine, based on individual risk, with the lowest activity needed to ensure successful treatment. Response assessment is to be done at each visit and patients are classified accordingly under ATA risks to further plan the treatment **(Table 8)**.

Follow-up

After definitive treatment and risk and response assessment patients require to have a close follow-up. Individualized regular biochemical and imaging modalities are used for monitoring **(Table 9)**.

Treatment of Anaplastic Thyroid Cancer

It is a diagnostic and therapeutic challenge because of the rarity of the disease and cells lose expression of thyroid and epithelial cell markers. An experienced head-and-neck

TABLE 8: Response assessment as per ATA 2015 guidelines.		
Category	**Definitions**	**Clinical outcomes**
Excellent response	Negative imaging And either Suppressed Tg <0.2 ng/mL Or TSH-stimulated Tg <1 ng/mL	• 1–4% recurrence • <1% disease specific death
Biochemical incomplete response	Negative imaging And Suppressed Tg ≥1 ng/mL Or Stimulated Tg ≥10 ng/mL Or Rising anti-Tg antibody levels	• At least 30% spontaneously evolve to NED • 20% achieve NED after additional therapy • 20% develop structural disease • <1% disease specific death
Structural incomplete response	Structural or functional evidence of disease • With any Tg level • With or without anti-Tg antibodies	50–85% continue to have persistent disease despite additional therapy *Disease specific death rates:* • As high as 11% with locoregional metastases • 50% with structural distant metastases
Indeterminate response	• Nonspecific findings on imaging studies • Faint uptake in thyroid bed on RAI scanning • Nonstimulated Tg detectable, but <1 ng/mL • Stimulated Tg detectable, but <10 ng/mL Or • Anti-Tg antibodies stable or declining in the absence of structural or functional disease	50–85% continue to have persistent disease despite additional therapy *Disease specific death rates:* • As high as 11% with locoregional metastases and • 50% with structural distant metastases

(NED: no evidence of disease; RAI: radioactive iodine; TSH: thyroid-stimulating hormone; Tg: thyroglobulin)

TABLE 9: Initial plan based on ATA risk for the first year of follow-up.

Investigation	Low risk	Intermediate risk	High risk
Biochemical Tg, TgAb, and TFT	3–6 months	3–6 months	3–6 months
Imaging: • USG • CECT chest • Imaging of brain, abdomen, and pelvis • FDG PET		• 3–6 months • Consider	• 3–6 months • 6–12 months • Consider • Consider
Diagnostic RAI scan			Consider

(CECT: contrast-enhanced computed tomography; FDG PET: fluorodeoxyglucose positron emission tomography; RAI: radioactive iodine; Tg: thyroglobulin; TgAb: thyroglobulin antibodies; TFT: thyroid function test; USG: ultrasonography)

surgeon should establish whether the tumor is resectable or not. After resection, external beam radiation with combinations of taxanes, with or without platinums, or anthracyclines is recommended. Targeted treatment with BRAF inhibitors, dabrafenib, and mitogen-activated protein kinase kinase (MEK) inhibitor trametinib is under trial. Other drugs being studied are lenvatinib, mechanistic target of rapamycin (mTOR) inhibitors, microtubule inhibitors, and peroxisome proliferator-activated receptor-γ (PPARγ) agonists are also tried.

Treatment of Medullary Thyroid Cancer

All patients suspected of MTC should undergo a detailed ultrasonography and tumor markers measurement such as calcitonin and carcinoembryonic antigen (CEA). The goal of management is complete possible surgical resection. Biochemical testing for pheochromocytoma and hyperparathyroidism for germline *RET* mutation are to be done and adrenalectomy is to be prioritized before thyroidectomy.

THYROID CARCINOMA IN CHILDREN

Thyroid cancer accounts for over 6% of all pediatric cancers and thus is a leading cause of pediatric endocrine cancer. Pediatric thyroid cancer has different clinical presentation, pathophysiology and long-term outcomes but recommendations have been derived from adult guidelines only. They usually present in second decade with female preponderance (6:1) as a thyroid nodule. The most common are PTC (80–90%) followed by FTC (~10%), MTC (3–5%), and rarely ATC and PDTC.

Nodules are usually alarming in pediatric population as more than a quarter thyroid nodules (22–26%) are malignant. Various studies has accounted for up to 40% of pediatric FNACs as Bethesda III and IV.

In children, PTC usually has lymph node metastasis higher risk of recurrence than adults. 15–37% of pediatric PTCs are high risk histologic subtypes. Unlike PTC, follicular carcinoma which is usually minimally invasive and less aggressive in pediatric population when compared to adults.

Treatment

Papillary thyroid cancer and FTC has increased incidence of bilateral (30%) and multifocal (65%) disease therefore, total thyroidectomy is preferred choice.

In children post-thyroidectomy, TSH-stimulated thyroglobulin levels and iodine imaging are recommended for planning adjuvant RAI. Dose adjustment for I^{131} can be done by body weight and body surface area methods but no recommendations have been made.

For MTC use and efficacy of tyrosine kinase inhibitors are extrapolated from the adult population only.

CONCLUSION

In conclusion, thyroid cancers have varied presentation in terms of clinical, biochemical, and histopathological behavior. They range from indolent tumors in most cases with good prognosis, to very aggressive malignancies. Therefore, undertaking a proper diagnostic workup and tailored treatment is of prime importance.

SUGGESTED READINGS

1. Sung H, Ferlay J, Siegel RL, Laversanne M, Soerjomataram I, Jemal A, et al. Global cancer statistics 2020: GLOBOCAN estimates of incidence and mortality worldwide for 36 cancers in 185 countries. CA Cancer J Clin. 2021;71(3):209-49.
2. Mathew IE, Mathew A. Rising thyroid cancer incidence in Southern India: an epidemic of overdiagnosis? J Endocr Soc. 2017;1(5):480-7.
3. Panato C, Vaccarella S, Dal Maso L, Basu P, Franceschi S, Serraino D, et al. Thyroid cancer incidence in India between 2006 and 2014 and impact of overdiagnosis. J Clin Endocrinol Metab. 2020;105(8):2507-14.
4. Nagataki S, Nyström E. Epidemiology and primary prevention of thyroid cancer. Thyroid. 2002;12(10):889-96.
5. Cardis E, Howe G, Ron E, Bebeshko V, Bogdanova T, Bouville A, et al. Cancer consequences of the Chernobyl accident: 20 years on. J Radiol Prot. 2006;26(2):127-40.
6. Cancer Genome Atlas Research Network. Integrated genomic characterization of papillary thyroid carcinoma. Cell. 2014;159: 676-90.
7. Raman P, Koenig RJ. Pax-8-PPAR-γ fusion protein in thyroid carcinoma. Nat Rev Endocrinol. 2014;10:616-23.
8. Santarpia L, El-Naggar AK, Cote GJ, Myers JN, Sherman SI. Phosphatidylinositol 3-kinase/akt and ras/raf-mitogen-activated protein kinase pathway mutations in anaplastic thyroid cancer. J Clin Endocrinol Metab. 2008;93:278-84.

9. Wells SA Jr, Asa SL, Dralle H, Elisei R, Evans DB, Gagel RF, et al. Revised American Thyroid Association guidelines for the management of medullary thyroid carcinoma. Thyroid. 2015;25(6):567-610.
10. Durante C, Costante G, Lucisano G, Bruno R, Meringolo D, Paciaroni A, et al. The natural history of benign thyroid nodules. Jama. 2015;313(9):926-35.
11. Howlader N, Noone AM, Krapcho M, Miller D, Bishop K, Altekruse SF, et al. SEER Cancer Statistics Review, 1975–2013. [Online] Available from http://seer.cancer.gov/csr/1975_2013 [Last accessed December, 2022].
12. Haugen BR, Alexander EK, Bible KC, Doherty GM, Mandel SJ, Nikiforov YE, et al. 2015 American Thyroid Association management guidelines for adult patients with thyroid nodules and differentiated thyroid cancer: the American Thyroid Association guidelines task force on thyroid nodules and differentiated thyroid cancer. Thyroid. 2016;26(1):1-33.
13. Nikiforov YE, Ohori NP, Hodak SP, Carty SE, LeBeau SO, Ferris RL, et al. Impact of mutational testing on the diagnosis and management of patients with cytologically indeterminate thyroid nodules: a prospective analysis of 1056 FNA samples. J Clin Endocrinol Metab. 2011;96(11):3390-7.
14. Hauch A, Al-Qurayshi Z, Randolph G, Kandil E. Total thyroidectomy is associated with increased risk of complications for low- and high-volume surgeons. Ann Surg Oncol. 2014;21(12):3844-52.
15. Brierley JD, Panzarella T, Tsang RW, Gospodarowicz MK, O'Sullivan B. A comparison of different staging systems predictability of patient outcome. Thyroid carcinoma as an example. Cancer. 1997;79(12):2414-23.
16. Hyman DM, Puzanov I, Subbiah V, Faris JE, Chau I, Blay JY, et al. Vemurafenib in multiple nonmelanoma cancers with BRAF V600 mutations. N Engl J Med. 2015;373(8):726-36.
17. Howlader N, Noone AM, Krapcho M, Miller D, Brest A, Yu M, et al. SEER cancer statistics review, 1975-2016. Bethesda, MD: National Cancer Institute; 2019.
18. Francis GL, Waguespack SG, Bauer AJ, Angelos P, Benvenga S, Cerutti JM, et al. Management guidelines for children with thyroid nodules and differentiated thyroid cancer. Thyroid. 2015;25(7):716-59.
19. Karapanou O, Tzanela M, Vlassopoulou B, Kanaka-Gantenbein C. Differentiated thyroid cancer in childhood: a literature update. Hormones. 2017;16(4):381-7.
20. Collini P, Mattavelli F, Pellegrinelli A, Barisella M, Ferrari A, Massimino M. Papillary carcinoma of the thyroid gland of childhood and adolescence: morphologic subtypes, biologic behavior and prognosis: a clinicopathologic study of 42 sporadic cases treated at a single institution during a 30-year period. Am J Surg Pathol. 2006;30(11):1420-6.

CHAPTER 19: Surgery in Differentiated Thyroid Cancers

Abhishek Krishna, Roma Pradhan, Amit Agarwal

INTRODUCTION

A thyroid nodule is defined as a discrete lesion in the thyroid gland which is radiologically distinct from the surrounding parenchyma. Although its incidence increases with age, the increase in its incidence over the last few decades is attributed to widespread use of ultrasound (US) imaging of the neck and increased awareness among the patients as well as healthcare providers. Not all thyroid nodules are cancerous and the incidence of malignancy ranges from 10 to 15%. Thyroid neoplasms are classified as depicted in **Flowchart 1**. A total of 90% are differentiated thyroid cancer (DTC's), ~5% are medullary thyroid cancers (MTC), poorly differentiated thyroid carcinoma (PDTC), and anaplastic thyroid cancer (ATC) are <2%, 1-3% lymphomas and <1% other rare tumors like sarcoma. Thyroid cancer is the most common endocrine malignancy (2.1% of all cancer diagnosis worldwide).

DIFFERENTIATED THYROID CANCER

Differentiated thyroid cancer consists of tumors which arise from the thyroid epithelial follicular cells. They comprise of >90% of total thyroid malignancies. The most common thyroid cancer is papillary thyroid cancer (PTC) 80-85%, followed by follicular thyroid cancer (FTC) 10-15%, Hürthle cell cancer 3-4% and MTC 2%. **Table 1** elucidates the comparative features of the three types of DTC.

- *Etiology and risk factors*: Exact etiology of thyroid cancer (TC) is not known but certain risk factors and somatic and germline mutations have been linked to thyroid cancer. Two environmental factors associated with development of TC are radiation exposure, especially during childhood and iodine deficiency.
- *Radiation*: Exposure to radiation, especially in childhood increases the risk of PTC. The relative risk is cumulative and starts form as low as 0.1 Gy. The latency period after

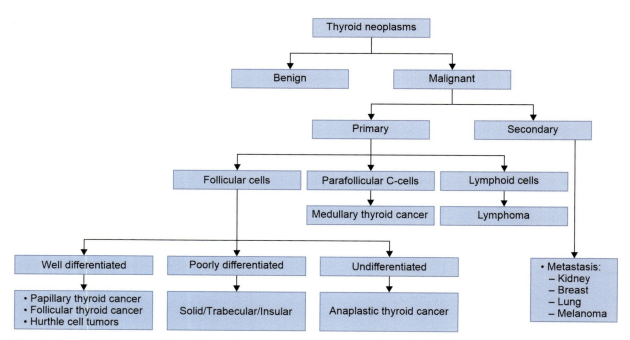

Flowchart 1: Classification of thyroid neoplasm.

Surgery in Differentiated Thyroid Cancers

TABLE 1: Comparative features of three types of differentiated thyroid cancer.

Features	PTC	FTC	MTC
Incidence	85–90%	10–15%	1–2%
Age	Third to fourth decade	Fifth to sixth decade	• *Sporadic*: 40–60 years • *Hereditary*: As early as first year of life
M:F	3:1	3:1	1:1
Clinical presentation	STN/STN with lymph node metastasis	STN/MNG with or without skull metastases	• STN (most common) • MNG with/without lymph node metastasis • Family of MTC
Route of spread	Lymphatic	Hematogenous	Both lymphatic and hematogenous
FNAC	• Diagnostic in >95% • *Well-formed papillae with typical nuclear features*: Grooves/indentations/pseudoinclusions/orphan-Annie nuclei	• Cannot be differentiated between follicular neoplasm and follicular carcinoma • Microfollicular/solid/trabecular pattern with capsular/vascular invasion	• Diagnostic in 75% • Spindle shaped/plasmacytoid cells with salt and pepper appearance of chromatin. Positive staining for calcitonin/chromogranin
Preoperative biochemical marker	None	None	Calcitonin (diagnostic sensitivity >95%) and CEA
Preoperative imaging	• USG neck: Microcalcification and cystic lymph node • CECT neck and thorax (RSE/mets)	• USG neck: No diagnostic feature • CECT neck and thorax (RSE/mets)	• USG neck: No diagnostic feature • CECT neck, and thorax +/− abdomen • Functional imaging (Ga-68 PET CT -mets)

Continued

Continued

Features	PTC	FTC	MTC
Surgical management	• Total thyroidectomy +/− CCLND +/− SLND • *Specimen showing characteristic black LN of PTC*: Both in central and lateral compartments	Total thyroidectomy	• Total thyroidectomy + CCLND +/− SLND • Hereditary MTC show bilateral lesions
Histopathology	Papillary architecture is diagnostic	Capsular and vascular invasion are diagnostic	Intense red staining of amyloid with Congo stain
Postoperative management	RAI according to ATA risk group	RAI according to ATA risk group	Does not concentrate RAI
Prognosis	*Excellent*: 10 years survival >90%	10 years survival rate >85%	10 years survival rate >80%
Postoperative marker	Thyroglobulin	Thyroglobulin	Calcitonin
Follow-up	Clinical examination, Tg/ATG, and USG neck	Clinical examination, Tg/ATG, and USG neck/WBRAI/PET scan	Clinical examination, serum calcitonin and CEA, and CECT/DOTANOC PET scan
Distant metastasis	Lungs and bones (10%)	Bone > lungs (15%)	Lungs, liver, and bone (20%)

(CCLND: central compartment lymph node dissection; CEA: carcinoembryonic antigen; CECT: contrast enhanced computed tomography; mets: metastasis; MNG: multinodular goiter; MTC: medullary thyroid cancer; PET: positron emission tomography; PTC: papillary thyroid carcinoma; RAI: radioactive iodine; SLND: selective lymph node dissection; STN: solitary thyroid nodule; Tg/ATG: thyroglobulin/antithyroglobulin antibody; USG: ultrasonography)

childhood radiation exposure varies between 5 and 10 years and remains high even 40 years after radiation exposure. Also, atomic bomb survivors and persons associated with nuclear accidents are at increased risk of thyroid cancer.
- *Iodine deficiency*: Iodine deficiency is associated with the development of FTC. On the other hand PTC is more common in iodine sufficient areas.
- *Age*: It occurs in two peaks—(1) first/second decade and (2) the second peak after fourth decade.
- *Gender*: 3–4 times more common in females. It is believed that estrogen acts as a stimulus for genomic instability.
- *Family history*: ~5% of nonmedullary thyroid cancers are hereditary. They are associated with familial adenomatous polyposis, Cowden disease, Gardner syndrome, and Carney complex type 1.
- *Genetics*: PTC has been associated with alterations in Mitogen activated protein kinase pathway (MAPK) while in case of FTC; PI3K-AKT pathway is more commonly altered. *BRAF* V600E is the most common mutation in sporadic PTC (36–69%) while RAS mutation is most common in FTC (50%). RET-PTC mutations are associated with PTC especially radiation induced PTC. PAX8/PPARγ mutation is associated with 30–40% of FTC. Hürthle cell carcinoma is associated with mitochondrial DNA mutations and widespread chromosomal losses.

Clinical Features

A thorough clinical history should be taken as most of the patients with TC give a history of asymptomatic long-standing nodule in the thyroid. A history of sudden, rapid growth, features of compression such as dyspnea, orthopnea, dysphagia, hoarseness of voice should create a strong suspicion of malignancy. Family history should also be taken with a pedigree tree of at least two generations. On examination, the nodule size, consistency, surface, and borders should be assessed along with palpation of trachea and carotid. A typical thyroid swelling will move up with deglutition. The lateral neck should be palpated on both sides to look for any evidence of lymphadenopathy. **Table 2** mentions the findings on history and examination which may point toward malignancy.

Diagnostic Work-up

The initial evaluation of a thyroid nodule consists of—serum thyroid-stimulating hormone (TSH), US neck and fine needle aspiration cytology (FNAC).

- *Imaging*: Ultrasound is the imaging of choice for thyroid gland. Before proceeding for cytology the nodule should undergo high resolution ultrasound (USG) with Doppler study to characterize it. Ultrasound is usually performed with 5–12 MHz linear array transducer. Ultrasonographic features of each thyroid nodule are recorded in following categories:
  - *Composition*: Solid, predominantly solid, predominantly cystic
  - *Echogenecity*: Hyper-, iso- or hypoechoic
  - *Margin*: Circumscribed or microlobulated/irregular
  - *Calcification*: Microcalcification, macrocalcification, or mixed calcification
  - *Shape*: Parallel or nonparallel (i.e., taller than wide)

Features suggestive of malignancy include: marked hypoechogenicity, noncircumscribed margin, micro or mixed calcification, and taller than wide. It should be kept in mind that a single USG feature has poor sensitivity for predicting malignancy which is better predicted by a combination of USG features. This is the basis of development of Thyroid Imaging Reporting and Data System (TIRADS) system. The TIRADS categories used are mentioned in **Table 3**.

There are at least five systems of TIRADS. Amongst them The American College of Radiology (ACR)-TIRADS had highest interobserver agreement, a trend to have highest sensitivity and negative predictive value for diagnosis of malignant thyroid nodules.

Other techniques such as contrast-enhanced computed tomography (CECT) neck, magnetic resonance imaging (MRI), and positron emission tomography-computed tomography (PET-CT) may also be used depending upon indications. Contrast-enhanced computed tomography neck and thorax is done in cases of retrosternal extension, locally advanced thyroid cancer and bulky neck nodes.

- *Fine needle aspiration cytology (FNAC)*: FNAC can be blind or US guided. Thyroid FNAC is further classified according to Bethesda classification **(Table 4)**.
- *Indirect/direct laryngoscopy*: To assess the status of vocal cords before surgery.
- *X-ray neck*: X-ray of the neck anteroposterior (AP) and lateral views are taken to assess for tracheal shift, narrowing, calcifications, and retrotracheal extension.

TABLE 2: Findings suspicious of malignancy.

History	• Male gender • Long standing neck swelling • Rapid progression • History of radiation exposure • Family history of thyroid cancer
Clinical examination	• Hard or very firm nodule • Irregular surface/borders • Compressive symptoms (mentioned in text) • Cervical lymphadenopathy • Nodule >4 cm

TABLE 3: TIRADS categories.

TIRADS category	Scoring	Classification	Risk of malignancy	Recommendations
TR1	0 points	Benign	0.3%	No FNA required
TR2	2 points	Not suspicious	1.5%	No FNA required
TR3	3 points	Mildly suspicious	4.8%	• ≥1.5 cm follow-up, ≥2.5 cm FNA • Follow-up: 1, 3, and 5 years
TR4	4–6 points	Moderately suspicious	9.1%	• ≥1.0 cm follow-up, ≥1.5 cm FNA • Follow-up: 1, 2, 3, and 5 years
TR5	≥7 points	Highly suspicious	35%	• ≥0.5 cm follow-up, ≥1.0 cm FNA • Annual follow-up for up to 5 years

(FNA: fine needle aspiration; TIRADS: Thyroid Imaging Reporting and Data System)

TABLE 4: Bethesda system for reporting of thyroid cytopathology and risk of malignancy in each category with management.

Diagnostic category	Bethesda 2007	Bethesda 2017 (when NIFTP was taken as malignancy)	Bethesda 2017 (when NIFTP was not taken as malignancy)	Management
I: Nondiagnostic	1–4%	5–10%	5–10%	Repeat FNAC
II: Benign	0–3%	0–3%	0–3%	Follow-up
III: Atypia of undetermined significance (AUS)/follicular lesion of undetermined significance (FLUS)	5–15%	10–30%	6–18%	• Repeat FNAC • Molecular testing • Lobectomy
IV: Follicular neoplasm	15–30%	25–40%	10–40%	• Molecular testing • Lobectomy
V: Suspicious of malignancy	60–75%	50–75%	45–60%	Lobectomy/total thyroidectomy
VI: Malignant	97–99%	97–99%	94–96%	Total thyroidectomy

(FNAC: fine needle aspiration cytology; NIFTP: noninvasive follicular thyroid neoplasm with papillary like nuclear features)

- *Staging*: American Joint Committee on Cancer (AJCC)/tumor, node, and metastasis (TNM) staging and American Thyroid Association (ATA) are used. The AJCC/TNM staging system predicts survival while the ATA risk stratification system is used to predict recurrence.

Papillary Thyroid Carcinoma

Classical PTC tends to have an indolent clinical course and occurs in iodine sufficient areas. M:F ratio is 3:1 with the mean age of presentation being 34–40 years. Although children and adolescents are more likely to have an advanced disease at the time of diagnosis (80% have nodal metastasis and 15–20% have pulmonary metastasis), they generally have excellent outcomes. Papillary thyroid carcinoma can be multifocal and spread via lymphatic route and clinically palpable neck nodes are present in approximately one-third of patients at presentation. Distant metastasis generally involves lung and bone and it is present in approximately 5% of patients at the time of initial diagnosis.

Histologically, PTC is characterized by well-formed papillae with fibrovascular core and distinct nuclear features such as nuclear grooving, pseudo inclusions, indentations. The chromatin is eccentrically placed which gives the central portion of the nucleus relatively pale and empty look (Orphan Annie eye nuclei). Psammoma bodies (laminated calcific spherules) are present in nearly one third to half cases of PTC. There are numerous histologic variants of PTC of which classic and follicular variants have a good prognosis while tall cell, hobnail, solid, and diffuse sclerosing have a relatively poor prognosis.

Total thyroidectomy with removal of the involved lymph nodal compartment (selective lymph node dissection) is considered as treatment of choice for PTC as they are generally bilateral (30–85%) and multifocal (>30%) and also so that thyroglobulin (Tg) could be monitored for recurrence during follow-up. Adjuvant radioactive iodine (RAI) is indicated in ATA high risk and can be considered in ATA intermediate risk tumors. After surgery patient has to be kept on lifelong thyroxine suppression according to the risk of recurrence. Complications such as recurrent laryngeal nerve paralysis and permanent hypoparathyroidism are extremely rare (<1% and <2–3% respectively) in the hands of an experience endocrine surgeon. However, temporary nerve paresis and transient hypocalcemia do occur and are managed conservatively.

Recently, targeted therapy in the form of tyrosine kinase inhibitors (sorafenib, lenvatinib, and sunitinib) have been used in adjuvant setting in case of a metastatic disease which could not be resected and in neo adjuvant setting in an attempt to make an inoperable tumor operable.

- *Initial follow-up from postoperative surveillance to 2 years*:
  This includes:
  - Initial risk stratification
  - Voice assessment within 2 weeks postoperative to 4 weeks
  - High resolution USG neck
  - Serum thyroglobulin (Tg) with thyroglobulin antibodies (Tg Ab)
  - Whole-body scan (WBS) as and when indicated
- *Subsequent follow-up (FUP)*: As patient progresses through the first 2 years of postoperative period restratification is done based on response to initial therapy.
  - Concept of dynamic FUP: Michael Tuttle from MSKCC conceptualized the system of dynamic risk stratification whereby it is recommended that the initial risk-stratification should not be considered to be rigid or absolute and they should be continuously modified during the follow-up. This concept takes into account the biology of the disease (i.e., response to initial therapy, development of recurrence, etc.)

and thus the intensity of FUP can be individualized in terms of labeling the patient as cured or prescribing particular biochemical or imaging tests and their timing.

Papillary Thyroid Microcarcinoma

Papillary thyroid microcarcinoma are <10 mm or less in maximal diameter. They are generally incidentally discovered lesions due to the advancement in US (high resolution USG) hence an increase in its incidence recently. It has an excellent long-term prognosis. Surgical options include lobectomy/total thyroidectomy. Prophylactic lymph node dissection is not indicated. Active surveillance can also be adopted for incidentally detected PMC.

Follicular Thyroid Cancer

It is the second most common histologic subtype of DTC representing 10–15% of all thyroid cancers. It is seen in iodine deficient regions and M:F ratio is 3:1. It is generally unifocal and unicentric with hematogenous route of spread. However, distant metastasis may be present at initial diagnosis in 15–27% of the patients, the most common sites being bone and lungs. It is difficult to differentiate between the follicular adenoma and carcinoma on cytopathology and complete histopathological examination of the specimen is required which shows capsular and vascular invasion in case of FTC. Histologically, FTC is generally encapsulated with diffuse microfollicular pattern. Based on foci of vascular invasion, it can be classified as minimally invasive (<4 foci of invasion) or widely invasive (>4 foci). Surgical management and follow-up of FTC is largely similar to PTC.

Hürthle Cell Carcinoma

Hürthle cell carcinoma is an uncommon tumor of the thyroid gland. The age of presentation is between 50 and 60 years and M:F ratio is 3:1. It spreads by both lymphatic and hematogenous route and is associated with increased mortality and poorer prognosis. Histologically, it comprises of oncocytic cells (also known as oxyphil/Hürthle cells) which are large polygonal cells characterized by abundant eosinophilic, granular cytoplasm due to accumulation of mitochondria. Surgical management and follow-up is similar to PTC.

Medullary Thyroid Carcinoma

Medullary thyroid carcinoma accounts for about 2–5% of all thyroid malignancies. The distinctive feature of MTC as compared to other thyroid malignancies is its strong genetic predilection with 25% occurring as hereditary MTC with germline mutation in RET proto-oncogene while 75% occurs in sporadic form. 25% of the hereditary MTC's are associated with syndromes multiple endocrine neoplasia type 2 (MEN2) **(Table 5)** while the remaining 75% are known are familial MTC (FMTC). These tumors arise from neuroendocrine parafollicular C-cells which are mainly concentrated at the junction of upper one-third and lower two-thirds of the thyroid lobes.

TABLE 5: MEN2A and MEN2B syndromes.

MEN2A	MEN2B

ATA considers four variants of MEN2A:
• *Classical MEN2A*: MTC (70–95%)
   ○ Pheochromocytoma (50%)
   ○ Primary hyperparathyroidism (13–30%)
• MEN2A and cutaneous lichen amyloidosis
• MEN2A and Hirschsprung's disease
• FMTC
	• MTC (100%)
	• Pheochromocytoma (50%)
	• *Nonendocrine*:
	   ○ Mucosal ganglioneuromas
	   ○ Intestinal ganglioneuromas
	   ○ Thickened corneal nerves
	   ○ Decreased lacrimation
	   ○ Marfanoid habitus

Genetics of MTC

Rearranged during transfection (RET) proto-oncogene is a receptor tyrosine kinase which transducer growth and differentiation signals. It has 21 exons which encodes for a transmembrane receptor tyrosine kinase. It has an extracellular domain, a transmembrane domain and an intracellular tyrosine kinase domain. RET protein activation normally requires binding of a ligand to its extracellular domain which leads to dimerization of RET protein and leads to signal transduction. In the presence of RET mutation there is ligand independent dimerization of RET which leads to its constitutive activation and relay of growth and proliferation signals in the tissues.

The germline mutation has a strong genotype-phenotype correlation. Mutations in the exons 10 and 11 (codons 609, 611, 618, 620, 634) of the extracellular domain of RET leads to MEN2A syndrome. The most common mutation in MEN2A is exon 11 (c634). Mutations in the exons 16 and 15 (codons M918T and A883F respectively) of the intracellular tyrosine kinase domain of RET leads to MEN2B syndrome. 95% of the mutations occur in exon 16 (M918T) while 5% in exon 15 (A883F). The timing of surgery in hereditary MTC patients varies according to the risk categories given by ATA **(Table 6)**. MEN2B is more lethal than MEN2B and >90% of MEN2B patients have a de novo germline mutation.

Clinical Presentation

The commonest presentation of MTC is a solitary thyroid nodule with or with cervical lymphadenopathy. Hereditary MTC presents at a much younger age as compared to sporadic MTC which generally presents between fourth and sixth decade. 70% of the patients with MTC who have a palpable neck swelling on presentation also have cervical metastasis while 10% have distant metastasis. Elevation of serum calcitonin levels is the most characteristic feature of MTC and can be used as a diagnostic as well as prognostic

TABLE 6: ATA risk stratification of MTC and timing of prophylactic surgery.

ATA risk level	Codon mutations	Timing of prophylactic surgery
Highest (HST)	M918T	<1 year of age
High (H)	C634 and A883F	<5 years of age
Moderate (MOD)	609, 611, 618, 620, 768, 790, 791, 804, and 891	When serum calcitonin gets elevated/parents preference

marker. Few patients may also present with paraneoplastic syndrome with symptoms such as diarrhea and flushing (due to elevated calcitonin levels), Cushing's syndrome [ectopic adrenocorticotropic hormone (ACTH) secretion], cholestasis and hypercoagulability. The most common sites of metastasis are liver, lung and bone, so patients with metastatic MTC may present with clinical features related to involvement of these organs. Hereditary MTC patients may present with features of MEN2A/2B syndrome as described in **Table 5**.

Evaluation and Diagnosis

Apart from the routine evaluation of a thyroid nodule as described under DTC, the following tests need to be performed in case of a confirmed diagnosis of MTC:
- *Genetic testing*: All patients diagnosed as MTC on FNAC should undergo RET mutation testing even if it is apparently sporadic.
- *Serum calcitonin and CEA*: It is used as a diagnostic as well as prognostic marker. Calcitonin >500 pg/mL warrants metastatic evaluation.
- *PET scan*: PET scans are less sensitive in detecting MTC metastasis and should not be used during initial work up.
- *Screening for pheochromocytoma and hyperparathyroidism*: It should be done in all patients with MTC with 24 hours urinary metanephrines and normetanephrines and serum calcium, phosphate, and intact parathyroid hormone (PTH) assay.

Surgical Management

Surgical management is the most effective therapy for MTC and the first surgery is the most crucial one. So, patients should be referred to specialized endocrine surgeon for management. The minimum surgery recommended is total thyroidectomy with central compartment lymph node dissection. Lateral lymph node dissection is controversial, however if a suspicious node is found during surgery it should be sent for frozen section histology and if positive, formal lateral compartment lymph node dissection should be done. Few groups have also suggested compartmental lymph node dissection based on the preoperative calcitonin levels.

In case of hereditary MTC, if the patient is found to have a pheochromocytoma then it should be operated first, while for hyperparathyroidism, selective parathyroidectomy could be done at the time of surgery for MTC.

Follow-up

Postoperatively patients have to be started on thyroxine replacement and serum calcium levels have to be monitored. Radioactive iodine (RAI) could not be used in MTC as these tumors are of neuroendocrine origin and do not concentrate RAI. Clinical examination and estimation of serum calcitonin and carcinoembryonic antigen (CEA) have to be done at 3 months and if normal, every 6–12 months thereafter. MTC is considered to be an indolent disease and the reported 10 year survival rate ranges from 69 to 89%.

Management of Metastatic Medullary Thyroid Carcinoma

Based on the calcitonin levels and the symptoms, patients with persistent/recurrent lymph nodal disease should be managed by compartment based neck dissections. If the calcitonin doubling time is >2 years, the patient is said to have a stable disease and in such cases redo surgery should be entertained only if required. External beam radiotherapy (EBRT) has been employed for residual and nodal disease but it does not increase overall survival outcomes.

There has been no effective systemic chemotherapy regimen for MTC. Patients with isolated liver or lung metastasis may be considered for metastatectomy. EBRT is given for bone metastasis. Peptide receptor radionucleotide therapy (PRRT) with Lu-177 or I-131 MIBG therapy have been shown to have partial response and may be tried to limit disease progression. Vandetanib and cabozantinib have been approved by US FDA for treatment of advanced MTC and are considered as first line tyrosine kinase inhibitors (TKI) for metastatic MTC. Recently, RET-specific tyrosine kinase inhibitor (TKI) selpercatinib was approved by US FDA for RET mutation positive MTC. Currently, a phase 3 trial (LIBRETTO-531) is going on to compare selpercatinib with vandetanib and cabozantinib.

CONCLUSION

Papillary thyroid cancers have an excellent prognosis and >95% 10 year survival rate when treated early and adequately with a combination of surgery and RAI. Follicular thyroid carcinomas have a relatively worse prognosis, most commonly metastasize to bones and bone metastasis may be the presenting complaint in few patients. Sporadic MTC's have a relatively worse prognosis than hereditary ones. All patients diagnosed as MTC should undergo RET mutation testing to rule out hereditary syndromes.

SUGGESTED READINGS

1. Haugen BR, Alexander EK, Bible KC, Doherty GM, Mandel SJ, Nikiforov YE, et al. 2015 American Thyroid Association management guidelines for adult patients with thyroid nodules and differentiated thyroid cancer: the American Thyroid Association Guidelines Task Force on Thyroid Nodules and Differentiated Thyroid Cancer. Thyroid. 2016;26(1):1-133.
2. Yassa L, Cibas ES, Benson CB, Frates MC, Doubilet PM, Gawande AA, et al. Long-term assessment of a multidisciplinary approach to thyroid nodule diagnostic evaluation. Cancer. 2007;111(6):508-16.
3. Cibas ES, Ali SZ. The 2017 Bethesda system for reporting thyroid cytopathology. Thyroid. 2017;27(11):1341-6.
4. Jemal A, Siegel R, Ward E, Hao Y, Xu J, Thun MJ. Cancer statistics, 2009. CA Cancer J Clin. 2009;59(4):225-49.
5. Ferlay J, Soerjomataram I, Dikshit R, Eser S, Mathers C, Rebelo M, et al. Cancer incidence and mortality worldwide: sources, methods and major patterns in GLOBOCAN 2012. Int J Cancer. 2015;136(5):E359-86.
6. Schneider AB, Sarne DH. Long-term risks for thyroid cancer and other neoplasms after exposure to radiation. Nat Clin Pract Endocrinol Metab. 2005;1(2):82-91.
7. Busnardo B, De Vido D. The epidemiology and etiology of differentiated thyroid carcinoma. Biomed Pharmacother. 2000;54(6):322-6.
8. Li JJ, Weroha SJ, Lingle WL, Papa D, Salisbury JL, Li SA. Estrogen mediates Aurora-A overexpression, centrosome amplification, chromosomal instability, and breast cancer in female ACI rats. Proc Natl Acad Sci USA. 2004;101(52):18123-8.
9. Stansifer KJ, Guynan JF, Wachal BM, Smith RB. Modifiable risk factors and thyroid cancer. Otolaryngol Head Neck Surg. 2015;152(3):432-7.
10. Liu Z, Hou P, Ji M, Guan H, Studeman K, Jensen K, et al. Highly prevalent genetic alterations in receptor tyrosine kinases and phosphatidylinositol 3-kinase/akt and mitogen-activated protein kinase pathways in anaplastic and follicular thyroid cancers. J Clin Endocrinol Metab. 2008;93(8):3106-16.
11. Penna GC, Vaisman F, Vaisman M, Sobrinho-Simoes M, Soares P. Molecular markers involved in tumorigenesis of thyroid carcinoma: focus on aggressive histotypes. Cytogenet Genome Res. 2016;150(3-4):194-207.
12. Dottorini ME, Vignati A, Mazzucchelli L, Lomuscio G, Colombo L. Differentiated thyroid carcinoma in children and adolescents: a 37-year experience in 85 patients. J Nucl Med. 1997;38(5):669-75.
13. Miyauchi A, Ito Y, Oda H. Insights into the Management of Papillary Microcarcinoma of the Thyroid. 2018;28(1):23-31.
14. Grani G, Lamartina L, Durante C, Filetti S, Cooper DS. Follicular thyroid cancer and Hürthle cell carcinoma: challenges in diagnosis, treatment, and clinical management. Lancet Diabetes Endocrinol. 2018;6(6):500-14.
15. Baloch ZW, LiVolsi VA. Our approach to follicular-patterned lesions of the thyroid. J Clin Pathol. 2007;60(3):244-50.
16. Lim H, Devesa SS, Sosa JA, Check D, Kitahara CM. Trends in Thyroid Cancer Incidence and Mortality in the United States, 1974-2013. JAMA. 2017;317(13):1338-48.
17. Wells SA Jr, Asa SL, Dralle H, Elisei R, Evans DB, Gagel RF, et al. Revised American Thyroid Association guidelines for the management of medullary thyroid carcinoma. Thyroid. 2015;25(6):567-610.
18. Traugott AL, Moley JF. The RET Protooncogene. Cancer Treat Res. 2010;153:303-19.
19. Miyauchi A, Matsuzuka F, Hirai K, Yokozawa T, Kobayashi K, Ito Y, et al. Prospective trial of unilateral surgery for nonhereditary medullary thyroid carcinoma in patients without germline RET mutations. World J Surg. 2002;26(8):1023-8.
20. Moley JF. Medullary thyroid carcinoma: management of lymph node metastases. J Natl Compr Canc Netw. 2010;8(5):549-56.
21. Choi HS, Kim MN, Moon CH, Yoon JY, Ku HR, Kang GW, et al. Medullary thyroid carcinoma with ectopic adrenocorticotropic hormone syndrome. Endocrinol Metab (Seoul). 2014;29(1):96-100.
22. Machens A, Dralle H. Biomarker-based risk stratification for previously untreated medullary thyroid cancer. J Clin Endocrinol Metab. 2010;95(6):2655-63.
23. Hundahl SA, Cady B, Cunningham MP, Mazzaferri E, McKee RF, Rosai J, et al. Initial results from a prospective cohort study of 5583 cases of thyroid carcinoma treated in the united states during 1996. US and German Thyroid Cancer Study Group. An American College of Surgeons Commission on Cancer Patient Care Evaluation study. 2000;89(1):202-17.
24. Modigliani E, Cohen R, Campos JM, Conte-Devolx B, Maes B, Boneu A, et al. Prognostic factors for survival and for biochemical cure in medullary thyroid carcinoma: results in 899 patients. The GETC Study Group. Groupe d'étude des tumeurs à calcitonine. Clin Endocrinol. 1998;48(3):265-73.
25. Martinez SR, Beal SH, Chen A, Chen SL, Schneider PD. Adjuvant external beam radiation for medullary thyroid carcinoma. J Surg Oncol. 2010;102(2):175-8.
26. Maghsoomi Z, Emami Z, Malboosbaf R, Malek M, Khamseh ME. Efficacy and safety of peptide receptor radionuclide therapy in advanced radioiodine-refractory differentiated thyroid cancer and metastatic medullary thyroid cancer: a systematic review. BMC cancer. 2021;21(1):1-4.
27. Makis W, McCann K, McEwan AJ. Medullary thyroid carcinoma (MTC) treated with 177Lu-DOTATATE PRRT: a report of two cases. Clin Nucl Med. 2015;40(5):408-12.
28. Koehler VF, Adam P, Frank-Raue K, Raue F, Berg E, Hoster E, et al. Real-world efficacy and safety of cabozantinib and vandetanib in advanced medullary thyroid cancer. Thyroid. 2021;31(3):459-69.
29. Wirth LJ, Sherman E, Robinson B, Solomon B, Kang H, Lorch J, et al. Efficacy of selpercatinib in RET-altered thyroid cancers. New England J Med. 2020;383(9):825-35.
30. Liu Y, Liu X, Chen X, Zhou L, Gao X, Yu H. Follicular thyroid carcinoma presenting with multiple skull metastases on CT and MRI: A case report and literature review. Radiol Case Rep. 2021;16(11):3260-5.
31. Nervo A, Ragni A, Retta F, Gallo M, Piovesan A, Liberini V, et al. Bone metastases from differentiated thyroid carcinoma: current knowledge and open issues. J Endocrinol Invest. 2021;44(3):403-19.

CHAPTER 20

Surgery in Poorly Differentiated and Anaplastic Thyroid Carcinoma

Himagirish K Rao, Chinnu Mariam, Ajay Tom Francis

INTRODUCTION

Poorly differentiated thyroid cancer (PDTC) is a rare, but aggressive form of thyroid cancer and a main cause of death from nonanaplastic follicular cell-derived thyroid cancer. According to the World Health Organization (WHO) classification, PDTC appears as a distinct entity. It has been classified as an intermediate between well-differentiated thyroid cancer (WDTC) and the fully dedifferentiated anaplastic thyroid cancer (ACT) by virtue of its distinct morphological and behavioral characteristics.

The lesions arise from thyrocytes. Although they do not take up stains on immunohistochemistry (IHC), they can produce thyroglobulin. The avidity of these tumors to radioactive iodine (RAI) is ambiguous. On histopathology, these tumors exhibit insulae, nests or trabeculae of tumor cells. The cells have large nuclei with scanty cytoplasm **(Fig. 1)**. There may be occasional pleomorphic cells. Coagulative tumor necrosis is another characteristic of PDTC **(Fig. 2)**. Extrathyroidal involvement and lymphovascular invasion is common **(Fig. 3)**.

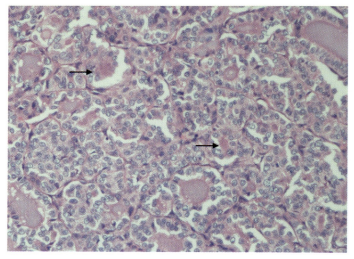

Fig. 2: Foci of coagulative necrosis within the tumor (arrows).

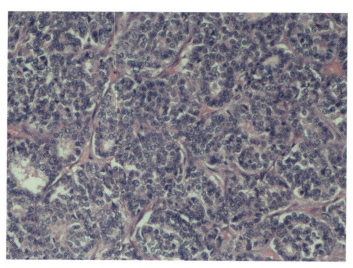

Fig. 1: High power photomicrograph of poorly differentiated thyroid cancer (PDTC) showing tumor cell nests and insulae.

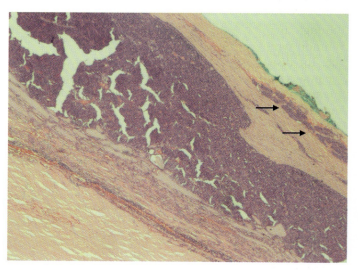

Fig. 3: Capsular invasion of poorly differentiated thyroid cancer (PDTC) focus (arrows).

MANAGEMENT

Although the name suggests guarded prognosis, substantial improvements in outcome can be achieved with appropriate recognition and treatment.

Fine needle aspiration cytology (FNAC) is fairly reliable in the diagnosis of PDTC. In about 75% of the cases, extrathyroidal involvement is seen at diagnosis. Tracheal involvement can be confirmed on laryngoscopy. Preoperative evidence of vocal cord paralysis is a reliable indicator of invasion. Detailed regional and distant radiological work-up is advisable, including neck ultrasound and contrast-enhanced compute tomography (CECT) of the neck and chest. Preoperative knowledge of the extent of disease allows appropriate planning of the extent of surgery, which might involve extensive resections of the trachea and esophagus as well. In case of involvement of the RLN, intraoperative nerve monitoring (IONM) will aid preservation of the nerve on the other side.

With detailed preoperative work-up, the patient as well as the surgeon can be better prepared for any eventuality on the operating table. It aids more complete and safe resection with very little chance of tumor retention. Studies have shown that completeness of tumor resection will improve the outcome substantially.

It is advisable to consider postoperative radioiodine ablation in all patients, since the potential for RAI uptake is high and the treatment is generally safe. In patients with T3M0 disease and T4N1 disease, external beam radiotherapy (XRT) is advisable, especially if the resection has been incomplete with gross retention of tumor. In addition, there is emerging evidence that application of an intense chemotherapy regimen (methotrexate and vinblastin, Adriamycin and bleomycin) in inoperable tumors will render these tumors operable and improve the overall outcome.

ANAPLASTIC THYROID CARCINOMA

Although anaplastic thyroid carcinoma (ATC) is the least common type of thyroid cancer, it is the most aggressive type. The disease-specific mortality approaches 100%, with 1 year survival rate of approximately 20%. Given its poor prognosis, it is vital that we develop strategies to allow early detection or even prevent progression of disease to ATC. Anaplastic thyroid carcinoma appears to be associated with prior or coexisting differentiated thyroid cancer (DTC) (*TP53* and *TERT* promoter mutations), goiter, iodine deficiency, obesity, and type B blood group. A stepwise approach to diagnosis and management is outlined underneath (**Box 1**).

Anaplastic thyroid carcinoma generally presents with a rapidly enlarging neck mass with aero digestive pressure symptoms, Horner syndrome or tendency to aspirate due to vocal cord dysfunction. Extensive local invasion and distant metastases are seen in 15–50% of patients at presentation.

> **BOX 1: Key steps in the management of anaplastic thyroid cancer.**
>
> - Expeditious and accurate establishment of diagnosis
> - Attain multidisciplinary team engagement and coordination (involve surgeons, radiation and medical oncologists, endocrinologists, and palliative care teams to arrive at patient tailored treatment options for best care)
> - *Determine extent of disease*:
>   - Staging, to classify as stage IVA, IVB, IVC (**Annexure A**)
>   - Ascertain extent of local invasion
> - Undertake patient counseling to create individualized patient goals of care
> - *Evaluation of surgical options*: The primary goals in stages IVA and IVB anaplastic thyroid carcinoma (ATC) are complete resection with adjuvant definitive-intention therapy. And in IVC, the limited benefit resulting from surgery must be carefully tempered in consideration of other available palliative approaches, including radiation and systemic therapy
> - *Surgical decision making*:
>   - Asses the feasibility of R0/R1 (**Annexure B**) resection (with intention to cure) or palliative/debulking surgery based on local tumor invasion of the larynx, trachea, esophagus, and status of the major vessels of the neck
>   - Ascertain extent of surgical resection and reconstruction in order to balance surgical morbidity with expected benefits within the context of patient-anticipated prognosis and individualized goals of care
> - *Nonsurgical management decision-making*: (Adjuvant/neoadjuvant chemoradiation, palliative radiotherapy, systemic chemotherapy, targeted therapy including molecular and immunotherapy, etc.)
> - *Keep palliative/end-of-life care discussions in the foreground*: Given the dire prognosis of ATC, especially if stage IVC, realistic presentation of anticipated prognosis is critical in allowing sound patient decisions within their individual goals of care

Cytology and Pathology

It is possible to diagnose ATC in up to 60% of cases when the aspirate is highly cellular. However, core biopsy enables better cellular yield and permits broader spectrum of genomic and molecular testing. Ultrasound (USG) guidance improves diagnostic accuracy, especially in the presence of necrosis or inflammation. Characteristic features include high mitotic count [>1/high-power field (HPF)], atypical mitoses, high Ki-67 index, high degree of proliferation and extensive capsular, extrathyroidal, and vascular invasion. Rarely, heterogeneous elements such as malignant bone and cartilage may be seen. Immunohistochemical confirmation is essential in most cases, unless the diagnosis is absolutely unequivocal. The various markers and consistency of their association in various thyroid malignancies are enlisted below (**Table 1**). The pathological spectrum is highly variable and there are many variants of ATC described, including sarcomatoid or spindle, squamoid, rhabdoid, paucicellular, angiomatoid and lymphoepithelial. Preoperative diagnosis is advisable as far as possible as surgical resection maybe inappropriate in some differentials.

With regards to molecular diagnosis, mutations seen in ATC are nonspecific (*BRAF* V600E and RAS in DTC a precursor for ATC; TP53 and TERT in ATC) and molecular analysis is not very beneficial for the diagnosis, but genetic profiling is recommended nevertheless to facilitate decisions related to the use of targeted therapies.

Initial Evaluation for Staging, Tests, and Procedures

The plan for evaluation and management of ATC is outlined underneath **(Table 2; Figs. 4 and 5)**.

TABLE 1: Panel of routine immunohistochemical markers for the evaluation of suspected anaplastic thyroid cancer and expected results compared with its differentials.

IHC marker	DTC	PTDC	ATC	MTC	SCC	Lymphoma
Pan-cytokeratins	+++	+++	+++	+++	+++	–
Thyroglobulin	+++	+/–	–	–	–	–
Thyroid-transcription factor 1	+++	+/–	–/+	+/–	–	–
BRAF V600E	+/–	–/+	–/+	–	–	–
PAX8	+++	+++	+/–	+/–	–	+/–
Ki-67	<5%	5–30%	>30%	<20%	>30%	Variable
Chromogranin	–			+++		–
Calcitonin	–	–		+++/–		–
CEA	–	–	–	+++	–	–
p53	– (rare+)	+/–	+/–	–	+/–	+/–
CD45, other lymphoid markers	–	–	–	–	–	+++

+ Indicates relative positive staining.
– Indicates negative staining.
+/– Indicates variable positivity.

TABLE 2: Plan for evaluation of anaplastic thyroid carcinoma.

Laboratory tests: CBC with differential	*Inference and reasoning*:
	To look for:
	• Anemia
	• *Leukocytosis*:
	  ○ Due to active infection
	  ○ Due to lymphokine secretion by tumor
	• Adequacy of platelets

• Comprehensive chemistry panel (electrolytes, calcium, blood urea nitrogen, creatinine, glucose, and liver tests) • Coagulation panel	• To ascertain functional status and operative fitness • ATC can be associated with humoral hypercalcemia of malignancy and hypoparathyroidism due to invasion
Thyroid function tests (TSH and free thyroxine), TG/TG antibody	Large tumors have compromised thyroid function and rarely ATC presents with thyrotoxicosis

Imaging:
• High resolution USG of neck
• 18F-FDG PET/CT (preferred whole body)
• CT of neck, chest, abdomen, and pelvis with contrast
  Or
  MRI (acceptable if PET unavailable—and as needed for surgical decision-making)
	• Imaging should not delay therapeutic intervention
	• To evaluate central and lateral lymph node basins
	• To ascertain stage of ATC to decide on operative or nonoperative management
	• To assess resectability, extent and type of surgery based on tumor extent and invasion

Continued

Continued

Recommended and if clinically indicated tests: • MRI of brain with and without contrast • Bone scan (if PET CT not available)	If clinical symptoms suggestive of metastasis is present (e.g., for brain—neurological deficit, headache, etc.)
Procedures: • Laryngoscopy, also esophagoscopy and bronchoscopy as indicated • BRAF assessment by IHC	• *Airway assessment*: Endoscopy of larynx, subglottic up to trachea—if stridor/dyspnea/hoarseness of voice/CV paralysis symptoms are present • *Esophagoscopy*: If dysphagia is present to rule out mass effect and intraluminal extension • *Bronchoscopy*: If imaging shows extension beyond trachea

(ATC: anaplastic thyroid cancer; CBC: complete blood count; CV: cerebrovascular; CT: computed tomography; FDG PET: fluorodeoxyglucose-positron emission tomography; IHC: immunohistochemistry; MRI: magnetic resonance imaging; TG: thyroglobulin; TSH: thyroid-stimulating hormone; USG: ultrasonography)

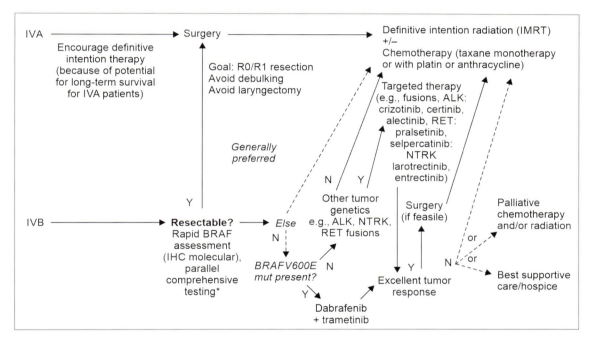

*Bridge chemotherapy.

Fig. 4: Management algorithm for stage IVA and IVB.
Dashed arrows depict circumstances where competing therapeutic options may be of consideration.
(ALK: anaplastic lymphoma kinase; IMRT: intensity modulated radiation therapy; NTRK: neurotrophic tyrosine receptor kinase gene fusion; RET: rearranged during transfection)

Surgical Management

Surgical decision-making is primarily based on differentiating between confined disease and metastatic disease, defining the extent of local invasion and characterization of the structures involved. If the imaging suggests intrathyroid disease and possibility of R0/R1 resection, surgical resection is strongly recommended as it is independently associated with better overall survival. In systemic disease, palliative resection of the primary tumor can be considered to avoid progressive aerodigestive compromise.

Total or near-total thyroidectomy with therapeutic central and lateral neck node dissection is considered optimal. There is no role for prophylactic neck dissection in ATC. Radical resection (including laryngectomy, tracheal resections, esophageal resections, and/or major vascular or mediastinal resections) is generally not recommended, given the poor prognosis. The impact of postoperative wound healing on the time frame for initiation of adjuvant chemoradiation should be considered prior to radical resections. Due to the aggressive nature of ATC, the risk of early recurrence and/or metastasis and/or mortality is significant if systemic therapy is unduly delayed. It is preferable to initiate adjuvant therapy within 2–3 weeks of surgery.

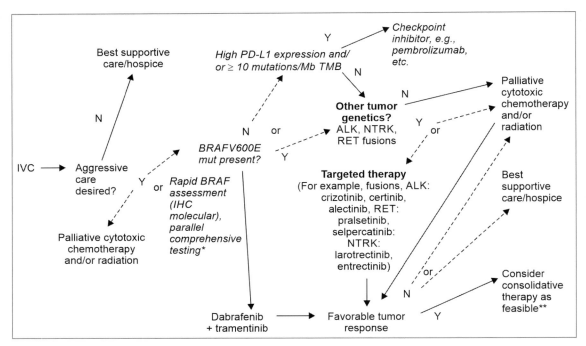

*Bridge chemotherapy.
**Consolidate.

Fig. 5: Management algorithm for stage IVC.
(ALK: anaplastic lymphoma kinase; IMRT: intensity modulated radiation therapy; NTRK: neurotrophic tyrosine receptor kinase gene fusion; RET: rearranged during transfection; Rx refers to focal therapy for residual macrometastatic disease; TMB: tumor mutational burden)

Nonsurgical Management

Modalities of nonsurgical management include radiotherapy with/without concurrent chemotherapy, systemic chemotherapy, and targeted therapies.

Radiation

External beam radiotherapy (EBRT) or intensity-modulated radiation therapy (IMRT) can increase short-term survival, improve local control and can also be used for palliation. Standard fractionation IMRT is to be considered if R0 or R1 resection is successful and even in patients with unresectable but nonmetastatic disease with good performance status.

Chemotherapy

Therapy with taxanes (paclitaxel or docetaxel) with/without anthracyclines (doxorubicin) or platinum (cisplatin or carboplatin) is recommended in patients treated with radiation for locoregionally confined ATC (stages IVA or IVB). In unresectable or advanced disease, early initiation of cytotoxic chemotherapy can be used as a potentially bridging approach until targeted therapies might be available.

Targeted Therapy

In patients with *BRAF* V600E-mutated stage IVC and in unresectable stage IVB disease, initiation of *BRAF/MEK* inhibitors (dabrafenib with trametinib) is recommended. Also, checkpoint (PD-L1 and PD1) inhibitors can be considered first-line therapy in the absence of other targetable alterations in the context of a clinical trial.

Metastatic Disease

Systemic therapy as described above is the first line of treatment, but if a particular metastasis is symptomatic or has progressed despite systemic therapy, treatment may be individualized to metastatic locations. For example, in patients with symptomatic thoracic metastases are quite common (pleura/chest wall, mediastinal nodes, and endobronchial lesions) palliative radiotherapy is advised. In patients with brain metastases with clinical features of neurologic involvement or compression, dexamethasone (4–16 mg/day) and chemoradiotherapy is recommended. For symptomatic or threatening bone metastases—but without structural compromise or threatened spinal cord compression in need of surgical remediation, palliative radiotherapy is to be initiated along with periodic intravenous bisphosphonate infusions or subcutaneous RANK ligand inhibitor.

Prognosis

Ascertaining prognostic factors can help risk-stratify patients to guide treatment. According to studies some good prognostic factors observed were younger age (<65 years), lesser comorbidities, absent nodal disease, absence of metastasis, primary tumor confined to the thyroid, smaller tumor size (<6 cm), and genetic mutations with available targeted therapy, e.g., *BRAF* V600E mutation.

Annexure A
TNM Staging
All ATCs are stage IV (AJCC 8th edition):
- Stage IVA lesions (T1-T3a, N0, and M0) are still localized within the thyroid gland and have not definitely spread to lymph nodes (N0) or to distant sites (M0).
- In stage IVB ATC, the primary tumor has grown outside/through the thyroid capsule (T3b and T4) and/or is involving locoregional lymph nodes (∓N1), but it has not spread to distant sites (M0).
- In stage IVC (any T, any N, and M1), the tumor has spread to distant site(s).

Annexure B
Extent of resection:
- *R0*: Complete resection with negative microscopic margins
- *R1*: Complete resection of all grossly visible tumors but with involved surgical resection margins (microscopically involved resection margins)
- *R2*: Resection in which gross cancer was left in place (macroscopically involved resection margins)

CONCLUSION

Although poorly differentiated thyroid carcinoma suggests a disease with guarded prognosis, the outcome can be promising if diagnosed early enough and treated appropriately. A high index of suspicion, especially when patients present with rapidly progressive symptoms and features of extrathyroid spread, will help early diagnosis. Even so, in most cases, the disease is advanced at diagnosis, necessitating radical and extensive surgery which may include resection of adjacent organs. Adjunctive treatment with radioactive iodine ablation holds promise.

Anaplastic thyroid carcinoma represents the extreme end of the disease spectrum with reported disease-specific mortality of 100% and 1 year mortality of 20%. Extrathyroid involvement at diagnosis is universal. Although extensive surgery is not preferred due to the bleak prognosis, thyroidectomy with central node dissection may help debulk the disease and mitigate aerodigestive tract morbidity in selected patients. Treatment is largely palliative. Since it invariably succeeds pre-esixting DTC, diagnosis of DTC is vital in improving outcomes.

SUGGESTED READINGS

1. Walczyk A, Kopczyński J, Gąsior-Perczak D, Pałyga I, Kowalik A, Chrapek M, et al. Poorly differentiated thyroid cancer in the context of the revised 2015 American Thyroid Association Guidelines and the Updated American Joint Committee on Cancer/Tumor-Node-Metastasis Staging System (8th edition). Clin Endocrinol (Oxf). 2019;91(2):331-9.
2. Sanders EM Jr, LiVolsi VA, Brierley J, Shin J, Randolph GW. An evidence-based review of poorly differentiated thyroid cancer. World J Surg. 2007;31:934-45.
3. Sobrinho-Simões M, Carcangiu ML, Albores-Saavedra J, Tallini G, Santoro M, Volante M, et al. Poorly differentiated carcinoma: an incubating entity. In: DeLellis RA, Lloyd RV, Heitz PU (Eds). Tumours of Endocrine Organs, Pathology & Genetics, World Health Organization Classification of Tumours. Lyon: IARC Press; 2004. pp. 73-6.
4. Volante M, Collini P, Nikiforov YE, Sakamoto A, Kakudo K, Katoh R, et al. Poorly differentiated thyroid carcinoma: The Turin proposal for the use of uniform diagnostic criteria and an algorithmic diagnostic approach. Am J Surg Pathol. 2007;31(8):1256-4.
5. Hiltzik D, Carlson DL, Tuttle RM, Chuai S, Ishill N, Shaha A, et al. Poorly differentiated thyroid carcinomas defined on the basis of mitosis and necrosis: a clinicopathologic study of 58 patients. Cancer. 2006;106(6):1286-95.
6. Randolph GW, Kamani D. The importance of preoperative laryngoscopy in patients undergoing thyroidectomy: voice, vocal cord function, and the preoperative detection of invasive thyroid malignancy. Surgery. 2006;139(3):317-62.
7. Are C, Shaha AR. Anaplastic thyroid carcinoma: biology, pathogenesis, prognostic factors, and treatment approaches. Ann Surg Oncol. 2006;13(4):453-64.
8. Neff RL, Farrar WB, Kloos RT, Burman KD. Anaplastic thyroid cancer. Endocrinol Metab Clin North Am. 2008;37(2):525-38,xi.
9. Landa I, Ibrahimpasic T, Boucai L, Sinha R, Knauf JA, Shah RH, et al. Genomic and transcriptomic hallmarks of poorly differentiated and anaplastic thyroid cancers. J Clin Invest. 2016;126(3):1052-66.
10. Kitahara CM, McCullough ML, Franceschi S, Rinaldi S, Wolk A, Neta G, et al. Anthropometric factors and thyroid cancer risk by histological subtype: pooled analysis of 22 prospective studies. Thyroid. 2016;26(2):306-18.
11. Zivaljevic V, Slijepcevic N, Paunovic I, Diklic A, Kalezic N, Marinkovic J, et al. 2014 Risk factors for anaplastic thyroid cancer. Int J Endocrinol. 2014:815070.
12. Bible KC, Kebebew E, Brierley J, Brito JP, Cabanillas ME, Clark TJ Jr, et al. 2021 American Thyroid Association Guidelines for Management of Patients with Anaplastic Thyroid Cancer. Thyroid. 2021;31(3):337-86.
13. Thompson LD, Wieneke JA, Paal E, Frommelt RA, Adair CF, Heffess CS. A clinicopathologic study of minimally invasive follicular carcinoma of the thyroid gland with a review of the English literature. Cancer. 2001;91(3):505-24.
14. Eilers SG, LaPolice P, Mukunyadzi P, Kapur U, Wendel Spiczka A, et al. Thyroid fine-needle aspiration cytology: performance data of neoplastic and malignant cases as identified from 1558 responses in the ASCP Non-GYN Assessment program thyroid fine-needle performance data. Cancer Cytopathol. 2014;122(10):745-50.
15. Iwai H, Ohno Y, Aoki N. Anaplastic thyroid carcinoma with humoral hypercalcemia of malignancy (HHM): an autopsy case report. Endocr J. 2004;51(3):303-10.

16. Ryken TC, McDermott M, Robinson PD, Ammirati M, Andrews DW, Asher AL, et al. The role of steroids in the management of brain metastases: a systematic review and evidence-based clinical practice guideline. J Neurooncol. 2010;96(1):103-14.
17. Heymann RS, Brent GA, Hershman JM. Anaplastic thyroid carcinoma with thyrotoxicosis and hypoparathyroidism. Endocr Pract. 2005;11(4):281-4.
18. Kebebew E, Greenspan FS, Clark OH, Woeber KA, McMillan A. Anaplastic thyroid carcinoma. Treatment outcome and prognostic factors. Cancer. 2005;103(7):1330-5.
19. Glaser SM, Mandish SF, Gill BS, Balasubramani GK, Clump DA, Beriwal S. Anaplastic thyroid cancer: prognostic factors, patterns of care, and overall survival. Head Neck. 2016;38 (Suppl 1):E2083-90.

SECTION 6

Thyroid Disorders in Women

CHAPTER 21

Thyroid and Reproduction

Gagan Priya

INTRODUCTION

Thyroid hormones have a pivotal role in maintaining reproductive health and fertility. Alterations in thyroid function can manifest with reproductive symptoms such as menstrual irregularities, oligoanovulation, hyperandrogenism, polycystic ovaries, and ovarian cysts in women; and decreased libido, erectile dysfunction (ED), and semen abnormalities in men. Thyroid dysfunction and thyroid autoimmunity (TAI) has also been strongly associated with infertility and adverse pregnancy outcomes such as recurrent miscarriage, preterm birth, pregnancy-induced hypertension (PIH), low birth weight (LBW), and postpartum thyroiditis. Treatment of thyroid dysfunction has the potential to improve reproductive outcomes.

THYROID AND REPRODUCTIVE HEALTH IN WOMEN

Triiodothyronine (T3) mediates its effects on the hypothalamic-pituitary-gonadal (HPG) axis in women at multiple levels, as summarized in **Table 1**. Thyroid hormone receptors (TRs) are abundantly expressed in the female reproductive tract including oocytes, granulosa cells, cumulus cells, stromal cells, endometrial cells, and placental trophoblasts where T3 exerts direct effects. Reproductive tissues also express various deiodinases involved in the conversion of thyroxine (T4) to T3 and to inactive metabolites. Additionally, thyroid hormones regulate the secretion and effect of other hormones involved in reproductive function such as gonadotropin-releasing hormone (GnRH), follicle stimulating hormone (FSH), luteinizing hormone (LH), estrogen, prolactin, kisspeptin, and leptin and regulate the hepatic production of sex hormone binding globulin (SHBG).

Thyroid hormones have an important role in the regulation of menstrual cycle by modulating the pulsatile secretion of GnRH, LH, and FSH, as well as, regulating the action of FSH and LH on ovaries. T3, therefore, regulates ovarian follicle development, ovulation and steroid hormone

TABLE 1: Effects of thyroid hormones on the female reproductive tract.

Organ	Effect of thyroid hormones
Hypothalamus and pituitary	• Regulate the pulsatile secretion of GnRH, LH, and FSH • Regulate the secretion of prolactin (effect of TRH) • Modulate the function of leptin and kisspeptin
Ovaries	• Modulate the action of FSH and LH • Regulate follicle development and facilitate ovulation • Increase proliferation of granulosa cells and reduce apoptosis • Stimulate aromatization of steroid hormones and estrogen secretion by granulosa cells • Inhibit excess androgen production by theca cells
Uterus	• Facilitate decidualization of the endometrium in preparation for implantation • TSH increases the expression of LIF is involved in implantation • Modulate the anchoring of the fetal-placental unit
Placenta and embryo	• Promote angiogenesis and placental invasion by increasing the expression of metalloproteinases, fetal fibronectin and integrins • Promote proliferation and differentiation of trophoblastic cells • Promote differentiation of embryonic cells • Regulate endocrine functions of placenta—stimulate secretion of placenta hormones (hPL, hCG, SHBG, progesterone, and estradiol) • Regulate inflammatory and immunological activity • Regulate fetal growth and neurological development
Liver	Regulate the secretion of SHBG affecting the concentration of SHBG-bound steroid hormone levels

(FSH: follicle stimulating hormone; GnRH: gonadotropin releasing hormone; hCG: human chorionic gonadotropin; hPL: human placental lactogen; LH: luteinizing hormone; LIF: leukemia inhibitory factor; SHBG: sex hormone-binding globulin; TRH: thyrotropin releasing hormone; TSH: thyroid stimulating hormone) secretion. T3 also affects uterine function by modulating uterine responsiveness to estrogen.

Further, T3 as well as TSH are important in implantation and decidualization, which is vital for anchoring of the fetal-placental unit. The endometrium expresses both thyroid peroxidase (TPO) and thyroglobulin (Tg), suggesting local production of thyroid hormones at the maternal-fetal interface. TRs are also abundantly expressed in the villous placenta. During early pregnancy, maternal thyroid hormones are involved in proliferation, differentiation and survival of trophoblast cells, and in maintenance of their immune, angiogenic, and endocrine functions. Maternal thyroid hormones cross the placenta and play a pivotal role in regulating fetal growth and neurodevelopment.

To summarize, thyroid hormones are involved in all phases of reproduction including follicle development, ovulation, implantation, decidualization, placental vascularization and function, maintenance of pregnancy and fetal growth and development.

HYPOTHYROIDISM AND REPRODUCTIVE HEALTH IN WOMEN

Hypothyroidism, overt or subclinical, is one of the most common endocrine disorders in women during the reproductive age and may impact reproductive health.

Hormonal Alterations

While gonadotropin levels are normal, the pulsatile secretion of LH and FSH is altered reflected by a blunted LH response to GnRH. Serum SHBG levels are lower, with reduced total estrogen and testosterone and increased free concentrations. The clearance of steroid hormones may also be reduced. Serum prolactin may be significantly elevated in women with overt or subclinical hypothyroidism (SCH) due to stimulation of pituitary lactotrophs by elevated thyrotropin-releasing hormone (TRH) and pituitary vasoactive intestinal peptide (VIP).

Menstrual Disturbances

Hypothyroidism is associated with a reduced number of growing follicles and increased follicular atresia leading to oligoanovulation. Reduced responsiveness of the uterus to estrogen may result in reduced endometrial thickness. The luteal phase is often prolonged due to reduced catabolism of progesterone. Therefore, menstrual irregularities are almost three times more common in women with hypothyroidism than the general population. These include oligomenorrhea (most common), polymenorrhea, metrorrhagia, and menorrhagia. Menorrhagia results from estrogen breakthrough bleeding due to anovulation and decrease in hemostatic factors (factors VII, VIII, IX, and XI). The severity of menstrual disturbance may correlate with the severity of hypothyroidism but a consistent relationship has not been observed as menstrual abnormalities are reported in women with SCH as well.

Sexual maturation may be delayed in girls with hypothyroidism resulting in delayed puberty. However, overt hypothyroidism (OH) has also been linked with precocious puberty. Hyperprolactinemia may result in galactorrhea, hypogonadotropic anovulation, oligomenorrhea, and reduced fertility due to the inhibition of pulsatile secretion of GnRH and LH.

Hypothyroidism may also contribute to hyperandrogenism due to reduced metabolic clearance of androstenedione, increased peripheral aromatization, and reduced SHBG levels resulting in increased free testosterone. Thyroid dysfunction should be excluded in women presenting with features of polycystic ovary syndrome (PCOS). Hypothyroidism is also associated with increased risk of ovarian cysts due to alterations in HPG axis, hyperprolactinemia and the effect of elevated TSH on FSH receptors in the ovaries.

Treatment with levothyroxine (LT4) has been shown to normalize the LH response to GnRH, reduce prolactin levels, improve menstrual disturbances, and increase the chances of spontaneous fertility.

Sexual Dysfunction

Few case-control studies report decreased Female Sexual Function Index (FSFI) scores across all domains in women with OH compared to controls and these improve with LT4 replacement. The effect of SCH is less clear with some studies reporting a decrease in FSFI scores.

HYPOTHYROIDISM AND FERTILITY IN WOMEN

Maternal hypothyroidism has been associated with risk of infertility and adverse pregnancy outcomes and several factors may play a role **(Fig. 1)**. However, there is limited data on the incidence of infertility in women with hypothyroidism. Most published studies provide data on the prevalence of thyroid dysfunction in women attending infertility clinics. In one study, 4% of the women undergoing evaluation for infertility had elevated TSH.

Overt Hypothyroidism

Overt hypothyroidism has been strongly associated with increased risk of infertility, miscarriage, premature delivery, LBW, fetal distress, perinatal death, PIH, placental abruption, and postpartum hemorrhage. Maternal OH may also affect fetal neurocognitive development and is considered a preventable cause of mental retardation in the offspring. Treatment with LT4 has been consistently shown to improve reproductive and pregnancy outcomes in these women.

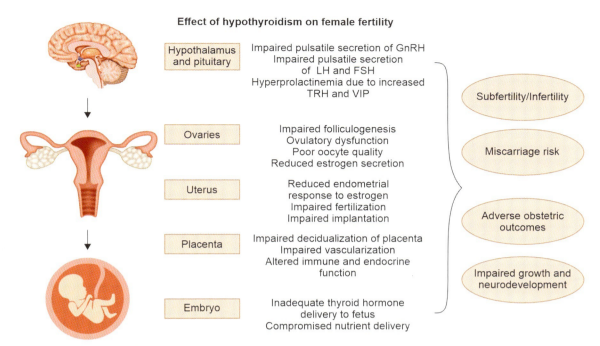

Fig. 1: Effect of hypothyroidism on female fertility.

(FSH: follicle stimulating hormone; GnRH: gonadotropin releasing hormone; LH: luteinizing hormone; TRH: thyrotropin releasing hormone; VIP: vasoactive intestinal peptide)

Note: Hypothyroidism is associated with disturbed GnRH pulsatile secretion, hyperprolactinemia, altered estrogen effect and metabolism, and defects in hemostasis. Anovulation/ovulatory dysfunction is common and oocyte quality may also be affected. Fertilization, implantation of the embryo and decidualization of the placenta may also be compromised resulting in reduced implantation rates and increased risk of embryonic loss. Further, thyroid hormones have a significant role in maintaining the health and function of the fetoplacental unit. Hypothyroidism may result in compromised placental development, reduced proliferation and increased apoptosis of trophoblasts, and endocrine and immunological changes at the maternal-fetal interface. Changes in placental vascularity can lead to miscarriage and compromised transport of nutrients and metabolites to fetus resulting in fetal growth restriction.

Subclinical Hypothyroidism

Subclinical hypothyroidism is present in almost 4–8% women during the reproductive age. An association between SCH and infertility was suggested in several retrospective and uncontrolled studies but this has remained a subject of controversy. Some studies suggest an increased prevalence of SCH in infertile couples and higher TSH levels are reported in women with ovulatory dysfunction undergoing evaluation for infertility. A serum TSH above the upper limit of normal (ULN) or >4 mIU/L is associated with increased risk of infertility, miscarriage, placental abruption, PIH, preeclampsia, preterm birth, premature rupture of membranes and LBW. However, the evidence linking borderline TSH values (2.5–4.0 mIU/L) with adverse outcomes is debatable. Retrospective data indicate that reproductive outcomes are similar in women with TSH <2.5 mIU/L or 2.5–4.0 mIU/L when thyroid autoantibodies are negative.

The effect of LT4 treatment on fertility in women with SCH has been evaluated in a few studies. In a large retrospective cohort, Maraka et al. reported a significant reduction in miscarriage risk with LT4 when baseline TSH was ≥4.1 mIU/L, but no benefit in women with TSH 2.5–4.0 mIU/L. Nazarpour et al. also reported a significant reduction in preterm birth with LT4 in women with TSH ≥4.0 mIU/L, irrespective of antithyroid peroxidase antibody (TPOAb) status. Other studies have reported no difference in neurocognitive outcomes with LT4 in the offspring of mothers with SCH.

Treatment Considerations

It is prudent to detect and treat OH with LT4 in women planning pregnancy, to a preconception TSH target of <2.5 mIU/L. Thyroid-stimulating hormone should also be monitored as soon as pregnancy is confirmed and the dose appropriately increased to maintain trimester-specific TSH targets. Most women with hypothyroidism need an increment of 25–30% in LT4 dose to meet the increased demands of pregnancy.

There is a greater risk of early pregnancy loss in untreated women with SCH and this risk is reduced with LT4 therapy. Moreover, some of these women may progress to OH during pregnancy and LT4 therapy prior to pregnancy may prevent this. Considering that there are minimal risks of low-dose (25–50 μg) LT4 therapy, SCH should be treated with LT4 when the TSH is above the ULN or >4.0 mIU/L, irrespective of TAI in women planning pregnancy. LT4 is not recommended in women planning spontaneous conception when TSH is <4.0 mIU/L if there is no TAI.

TABLE 2: Who should be screened for thyroid dysfunction before or during pregnancy?	
Category	Risk factor
Personal characteristics	• Age >30 years • Body mass index >40 kg/m² • Residing in area of moderate/severe iodine deficiency
Medical history	• Past history of thyroid disease • Presence of goiter • Known thyroid autoimmunity • Symptoms of thyroid dysfunction • Presence of other autoimmune diseases • Previous head/neck irradiation or thyroid surgery • Use of amiodarone, lithium or recent administration of iodinated contrast
Obstetric history	• Infertility • Past history of pregnancy loss or preterm delivery • Recurrent miscarriage • Multiple prior pregnancies (≥2)
Family history	• Family history of thyroid disease • Family history of other autoimmune diseases

Routine screening of women for thyroid dysfunction prior to spontaneous conception or during pregnancy remains a debated area. A case-finding approach based on risk factors **(Table 2)** is recommended by the Endocrine Society and the American Thyroid Association (ATA).

In women who are not on LT4 therapy, it is important to ensure adequate iodine intake. The World Health Organization (WHO) and ATA recommend daily iodine intake of 150 μg for women planning pregnancy and 250 μg for pregnant and lactating women.

Hypothyroidism in Women Undergoing Assisted Reproduction

There is increasing interest in understanding the impact of hypothyroidism in women undergoing in vitro fertilization (IVF). Elevated serum TSH is a significant predictor of fertilization failure with most studies reporting that IVF outcomes were suboptimal when serum TSH was >4 mIU/L. Treatment with LT4 was associated with significant increase in the number of good quality embryos, increase in implantation rates and live birth rate (LBR) as well as a decrease in miscarriage rate. While the evidence supporting LT4 treatment is more robust in women with TSH >4 mIU/L, clinical outcomes did not differ in women with TSH <2.5 mIU/L and those with TSH 2.5–4.0 mIU/L. Therefore, women planning assisted reproduction treatment (ART) should be treated with LT4 if they have OH or SCH (TSH above the ULN or >4.0 mIU/L) to a preconception TSH target of <2.5 mIU/L. Treatment benefits are unclear in women with TSH between 2.5 and 4.0 mIU/L if they do not have TAI.

THYROID AUTOIMMUNITY AND FERTILITY

The relationship between autoimmunity and reproductive dysfunction has been an area of great interest. TAI has a high prevalence in women of reproductive age group, with studies reporting that 5–15% of women may have antithyroid antibodies. The prevalence of TAI, as assessed by positive TPOAb or antithyroglobulin antibodies (TgAb), seems to be particularly high in women attending fertility clinics. Most of these women may not have overt thyroid dysfunction even though some studies report that the median serum TSH was slightly higher compared to controls. The prevalence of TAI is significantly higher in women who are older or have endometriosis, PCOS, ovulatory dysfunction and premature ovarian failure (POF). The mean serum TSH was also higher in women with PCOS with greater prevalence of OH and SCH compared to controls.

Thyroid autoimmunity may affect conception and has been linked to adverse pregnancy outcomes. In an analysis of 31 studies of euthyroid women with recurrent miscarriages or infertility, TAI was associated with a threefold increased risk of miscarriages and twofold increased risk of preterm birth. The risk of spontaneous miscarriage, recurrent miscarriage, placental abruption, preeclampsia, preterm delivery, and fetal loss was higher in TPOAb-positive women in some studies. TAI is also linked to the risk of postpartum thyroiditis and progression to OH.

Mechanisms of Risk

Thyroid autoimmunity affects conception, especially when it is associated with thyroid dysfunction. Several mechanisms have been suggested to explain this association including hypothyroidism, subtle thyroid hormone deficiency, generalized autoimmunity and a direct cytotoxic effect of antithyroid antibodies on the ovaries and developing embryo **(Fig. 2)**. Subfertility could also be due to conditions associated with TAI such as older age, endometriosis, PCOS or POF. Dosiou et al. proposed a two-stage model of the effect of TAI on fertility in women. In early stages, when TPOAb titers are low, the main effect may be via a hostile immune environment in the ovary with TPO as the direct antigen. LT4 therapy is unlikely to have any beneficial effect as the thyroid response to hCG stimulation is adequate. It would be pertinent to explore the role of immunomodulatory therapies at this stage. With the progression of TAI, the thyroid reserve is impaired and may lead to unmasking of subtle thyroid hormone deficiency especially during controlled ovarian hyperstimulation (COH). LT4 is likely to have beneficial effects at this stage.

Treatment Considerations

The obvious question is whether LT4 would improve fertility and pregnancy outcomes in women with TAI. Early evidence emerged from small studies. In a meta-analysis of two studies of euthyroid TPOAb-positive women, LT4 led to significant

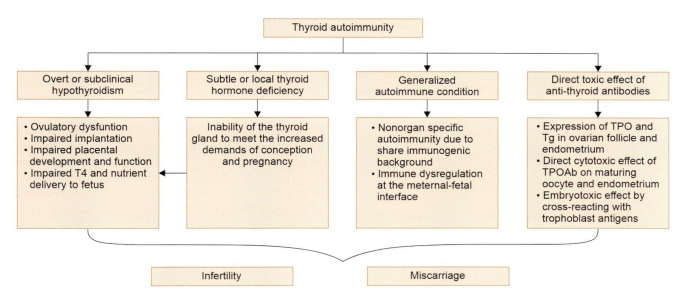

Fig. 2: Thyroid autoimmunity and female reproductive health—mechanisms of increased risk.

Note: Thyroid hormones are essential for the maintenance of reproductive health; thyroid autoimmunity is the most common cause of hypothyroidism (overt or subclinical) and this has been associated with increased risk of infertility, miscarriage, and adverse pregnancy outcomes due to decreased availability of thyroid hormones in reproductive tissues. In women with normal thyroid function tests, it is hypothesized that locally available T3 concentrations in reproductive tissues may be lower. Additionally, these women may have subtle thyroid dysfunction and thyroid gland may be unable to adapt to the increased physiological demands of pregnancy. Thyroid autoimmunity could be a marker of a more generalized autoimmune state with impaired cellular and humoral immune response. Dysregulated activity of the immune system at the maternal-fetal interface is detrimental to the establishment of an appropriate anti-inflammatory environment resulting in risk of early pregnancy loss. A direct effect of anti-thyroid antibodies has also been proposed. TPOAb have been demonstrated in ovarian follicular fluid; antibody-mediated cytotoxicity in the growing follicle may damage the maturing oocyte. The endometrium also expresses thyroid peroxidase and thyroglobulin and a direct effect of TPOAb and TgAb is plausible. Thyroid antibodies may also have embryotoxic effect on trophoblast limiting its invasion and development of fetus. Murine models suggest that thyroid antibodies cross-react with trophoblast antigens and lead to fetal wastage and low fetal and placental weight.

reduction in miscarriage and preterm birth. In a Cochrane review of four studies that evaluated the effect of LT4 in TPOAb-positive women who were euthyroid or had SCH, LT4 led to improvement in LBR in women with SCH, but not in euthyroid women. There was no effect on miscarriage in either group. However, the quality of evidence was graded to be low.

The recent TABLET (Thyroid AntiBodies and LEvo-Thyroxine) trial included 952 TPOAb-positive euthyroid women with history of miscarriage or infertility across several centers in the UK. These women were randomized to 50 µg LT4 versus placebo prior to conception. There was no difference in LBR, preterm birth or neonatal outcomes. The T4LIFE trial also reported no difference in LBR or other outcomes with LT4 versus placebo in euthyroid TPOAb-positive women with history of recurrent miscarriages. Due to the lack of benefit with LT4 seen in more recent studies which strictly included euthyroid TPOAb-positive women (with TSH <2.5 mIU/L), it is likely that the effect of TAI is largely driven by underlying subtle hypothyroidism. This would also explain the benefit seen with LT4 in earlier studies which included women with borderline high TSH values.

In light of the current evidence, it seems reasonable to screen women with history of infertility and miscarriage with both TSH and TPOAb. OH or SCH (TSH >4.0 mIU/L) should be treated with LT4 prior to conception to maintain a TSH <2.5 mIU/L, irrespective of TPOAb status. However, for those women with TSH <4.0 mIU/L, TPOAb can be used to guide treatment; TPOAb-positive women with TSH 2.5–4.0 mIU/L may potentially benefit from LT4 with reduction in miscarriage and preterm birth. However, the benefits of treating euthyroid TPOAb-positive women (with TSH <2.5 mIU/L) have not been established.

Studies evaluating the use of glucocorticoids in women with TAI are small, heterogenous, and have shown conflicting results. Similarly, there is scant evidence to support the use of intravenous immunoglobulins (IVIGs). The effect of selenium supplementation has also been evaluated in the SERENA study; while there was a reduction in TPOAb titers, no benefit was seen on maternal or fetal outcomes. The ATA recommends against the use of these agents.

Thyroid Autoimmunity and Assisted Reproduction

In women undergoing IVF, TAI has been associated with lower fertilization and pregnancy rates and higher miscarriage rates. Antithyroid antibodies are considered to be an independent marker for the failure of ART and associated with lower oocyte fertilization. In addition, COH may itself affect thyroid function as the marked rise in estradiol (E2) levels leads to an increase in thyroxine-binding globulin (TBG), resulting in a need for increased production of thyroid hormones. This may potentially unmask underlying subtle thyroid dysfunction. A significant increase in serum TSH and decrease in FT4 after COH, especially in women with TAI, correlated with the increase in E2 and TBG levels in several studies. The postconception serum TSH was higher after COH compared to spontaneous pregnancy suggesting the need to appropriately up-titrate the dose of LT4.

However, in a meta-analysis of 14 studies evaluating the effect of TAI on IVF and intracytoplasmic sperm injection (ICSI) outcomes in euthyroid women, no difference was seen in number of oocytes retrieved or embryos transferred, clinical pregnancy rate, miscarriage rate or LBR per cycle. Similarly, no difference in LBR or miscarriage rate was seen after intrauterine insemination (IUI) in TPOAb-positive versus negative women.

Recent studies have evaluated the effect of LT4 in women undergoing IVF/ICSI who have TAI with normal thyroid function. The Pregnancy Outcomes Study in Euthyroid Women with Thyroid Autoimmunity after Levothyroxine (POSTAL) randomized 600 Chinese women with TAI undergoing IVF to LT4 or placebo. There was no difference in miscarriage or LBR in women with TSH <2.5 mIU/L or between 2.5 and 4.0 mIU/L. A recent meta-analysis reported a significant decrease in miscarriage rate but not in clinical pregnancy, LBR or preterm birth, compared to placebo or no treatment.

Women undergoing ART should be screened for thyroid dysfunction (TSH) and TAI (TPOAb) prior to IVF. LT4 should be initiated in all women if they have OH or SCH to reduce the risk of miscarriage. TPOAb-positive women should be treated if serum TSH ≥2.5 mIU/L and LT4 may be considered for those with TSH <2.5 mIU/L. In women who are already on LT4 replacement, the dose of LT4 should be titrated to maintain serum TSH <2.5 mIU/L. In case LT4 is not initiated and the woman conceives, TSH should be closely monitored every 4 weeks till midpregnancy in TPOAb-positive women. The ATA recommends that TSH should be monitored before or 7–14 days after COH. If TSH is elevated after COH and women do not achieve pregnancy, TSH should be repeated after 2–4 weeks for further decision. In case of pregnancy, any TSH elevation should be treated as per pregnancy guidelines.

GUIDELINE RECOMMENDATIONS

We summarize the guidelines of the American Society of Reproductive Medicine (ASRM) 2015, ATA 2017 and European Thyroid Association (ETA) 2021 in **Table 3**. **Flowchart 1** depicts an algorithm for the management of thyroid dysfunction and TAI in women planning pregnancy.

THYROTOXICOSIS AND REPRODUCTIVE HEALTH IN WOMEN

Hyperthyroidism affects approximately 1% of women in the reproductive age, with Graves' disease (GD) being the most common cause. The effects of thyrotoxicosis on female reproductive health are less well understood.

Hormonal Alterations

Sex hormone binding globulin levels are increased, resulting in two- to threefold increased estrogen levels compared to euthyroid women. Thyrotoxicosis is also associated with increased synthesis and reduced clearance of androgens (androstenedione and testosterone). The mean serum LH in both follicular and luteal phases is higher and decreases within a few weeks of treatment with antithyroid drugs. No alterations in prolactin levels have been reported.

Menstrual Alterations

Thyrotoxicosis is associated with irregular cycles, increased follicle atresia and ovarian cysts. An increased incidence of oligomenorrhea and amenorrhea was reported as early as 1840 by von Basedow. Hyperthyroidism may also lead to hypomenorrhea, polymenorrhea, and anovulation. Smoking aggravates the development of menstrual disturbances in women with hyperthyroidism. When hyperthyroidism occurs before puberty, it may result in delayed sexual maturation and menstruation.

Sexual Dysfunction

In small studies, women with hyperthyroidism were reported to have significantly worse FSFI scores with improvements seen after 3 months of treatment with antithyroid drugs.

Fertility

Hyperthyroidism has been linked with reduced fertility in some studies with prevalence of infertility varying from 2.1 to 5.8%. In one study, 50% of women with GD had subfertility. However, most women with hyperthyroidism remain ovulatory and the association of thyrotoxicosis with subfertility is not robust. Placental morphogenesis may be affected with increased proliferative activity of trophoblasts and altered oxidative state of the endometrium. Untreated severe hyperthyroidism can lead to early pregnancy loss and adverse maternal-fetal outcomes [PIH, LBW, intrauterine growth restriction, stillbirth, thyroid storm, and congestive heart failure (CHF)] but subclinical hyperthyroidism has not been associated with adverse pregnancy outcomes. It is advisable to achieve a stable euthyroid state prior to conception. There is lack of data about the outcomes of ART in women with hyperthyroidism.

THYROID AND REPRODUCTIVE HEALTH IN MEN

Thyroid hormones exert myriad effects on different testicular components, including Leydig cells, Sertoli cells, and germ cells via both genomic and nongenomic

TABLE 3: Guideline recommendations for the treatment of hypothyroidism and thyroid autoimmunity in women planning pregnancy.

	ASRM 2015 guidelines for women with infertility	ATA 2017 guidelines for diagnosis and management of thyroid disease during pregnancy	ETA 2021 guidelines for women planning ART
Screening before pregnancy	• Recommend TSH testing in all infertile women attempting pregnancy with ART • Measure TPOAb if TSH >2.5 mIU/L	• Does not recommend universal screening of all women planning conception • Screen all women at high risk (Table 2) with TSH • Screen women undergoing IVF with both TSH and TPOAb	• Recommend screening all women with infertility prior to ART with TSH and TPOAb • If TSH >2.5 mIU/L and TPOAb is negative, consider screening for TgAb
Overt hypothyroidism	Treatment with LT4 to maintain a TSH <2.5 mIU/L, irrespective of TAI	Strongly recommend LT4 to maintain TSH <2.5 mIU/L in all women planning pregnancy	Prompt treatment independent of TAI, to maintain TSH <2.5 mIU/L
Subclinical hypothyroidism (TSH > ULN or >4.0 mIU/L)	Treatment with LT4 to maintain TSH <2.5 mIU/L	Recommend LT4 therapy to maintain TSH <2.5 mIU/L prior to pregnancy, especially if undergoing IVF/ICSI	Prompt treatment independent of TAI, to maintain TSH <2.5 mIU/L
Mild TSH elevation (TSH 2.5–4.0 mIU/L)	• Consider TPOAb testing • Consider treatment with LT4 (25–50 µg) especially if TPOAb positive to maintain TSH <2.5 mIU/L or monitor and initiate LT4 if TSH >4.0 mIU/L	Consider LT4 (25–50 µg) if TPOAb positive as there may be potential benefits compared to minimal risk	• Consider treatment with LT4 (25–50 µg) if TAI is present to maintain TSH <2.5 mIU/L on a case-by-case basis • Do not recommend treatment if TAI is absent, but monitor TSH after COH
Euthyroid (TSH <2.5 mIU/L)	Consider TPOAb testing if there are risk factors and treat with low-dose LT4 (25–50 µg) if TPOAb positive	• Does not recommend LT4, if TPOAb negative • No recommendation for TPOAb positive women attempting natural conception • May consider LT4 (25–50 µg) in women with history of pregnancy loss or those undergoing IVF/ICSI if TPOAb positive given its potential benefit compared to minimal risk • If LT4 is not started in TPOAb or TgAb positive women, TSH should be monitored at the confirmation of pregnancy and every 4 weeks till midpregnancy	• Do not recommend treating euthyroid women with or without TAI • Monitor TSH after COH, if TAI is present

(ART: assisted reproductive technology; COH: controlled ovarian hyperstimulation; ICSI: intracytoplasmic sperm injection; IVF: in vitro fertilization; TAI: thyroid autoimmunity; TgAb: anti-thyroglobulin antibodies; TPOAb: thyroid peroxidase antibody; TSH: thyroid stimulating hormone; ULN: upper limit of normal)

mechanisms, as enlisted in **Table 4**. Thyroid hormones also regulate the redox status of testis which is considered vital for spermatozoa health, via effects on enzymes such as glutathione peroxidase, γ-glutamyltransferase, and catalase.

The prevalence of OH/SCH and hyperthyroidism is higher in men attending infertility clinics. Altered thyroid function (hypothyroidism as well as thyrotoxicosis) may affect male reproductive health, spermatogenesis and semen quality **(Table 5)** and these improve with achievement of euthyroid state.

RADIOIODINE THERAPY AND REPRODUCTION

Radioiodine-131 ablation (RAIA) is often used as definitive therapy for hyperthyroidism (GD and toxic nodular goiter) and for remnant thyroid gland ablation in differentiated thyroid cancer. There have been concerns about its potential mutagenic effects on the gonads, especially in children, adolescents and young adults. The dose of RAIA used for hyperthyroidism is typically low (5–15 mCi) and carries

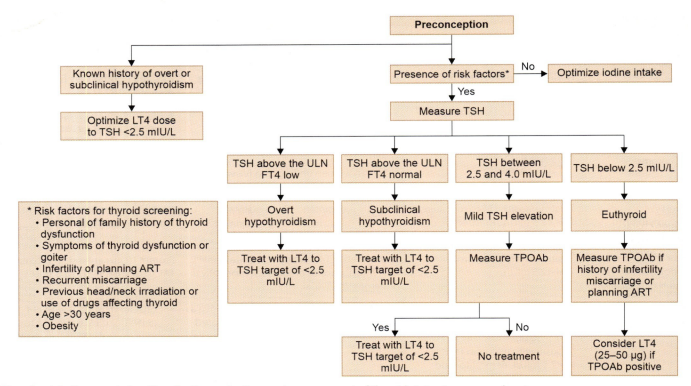

Flowchart 1: Proposed algorithm for the evaluation and management of thyroid status in women planning pregnancy.
(ART: assisted reproductive technology; FT4: free thyroxine; LT4: levothyroxine; TPOAb: thyroid peroxidase antibody; TSH: thyroid-stimulating hormone; ULN: upper limits of normal)

TABLE 4: Effects of thyroid hormones on various cell types within the testis.		
Cell type	**Effect type**	**Effect of thyroid hormones**
Sertoli cells	Genomic	• Reduced proliferation • Increased differentiation • Regulate their number at puberty • Adhesion to gonocytes
Leydig cells	Genomic	• Acute—stimulate LH-mediated steroidogenesis • Chronic—inhibit steroidogenesis
Germ cells	Genomic	Development and differentiation
Sperm cells	Nongenomic	Enhance cyclic AMP synthesis to improve flagellar movements of spermatozoa
(AMP: anti-müllerian hormone; LH: luteinizing hormone)		

little risk. However, much higher doses are used in thyroid cancer (100–150 mCi) and may have deleterious effects on reproductive health due to higher cumulative dose absorbed by the gonads. Further, it may take a few months to achieve a euthyroid state following RAIA.

Several studies have reported no effects of RAIA on reproductive function in men with hyperthyroidism. A transient initial decline in serum testosterone was followed by return to normal. Sperm quality, in fact, was found to be improved within 1 year of therapy. However, with RAIA for thyroid cancer, few reports suggest that there may be transient impairment of testicular function with increase in FSH and fall in inhibin B and sperm count for 1–3 years. No long-term effect on fertility is reported unless the cumulative dose exceeds 400 mCi.

Radioiodine-131 ablation may result in transient amenorrhea in some women but does not seem to affect fertility or pregnancy outcomes or birth rate in population-based studies. Some studies report a transient decrease in anti-müllerian hormone (AMH) with nadir at 3 months and then partial recovery at 1 year.

For individuals who have undergone RAIA, ATA recommends that women should wait for 6 months and men for 120 days and a stable euthyroid state should be attained before conception.

CONCLUSION

Normal thyroid function is important to maintain reproductive health and fertility in both women and men. Both hypothyroidism and hyperthyroidism can manifest with a wide range of reproductive abnormalities, especially in women where reproductive dysfunction may be the presenting feature. Even mild thyroid dysfunction and TAI can contribute to infertility and adverse pregnancy outcomes. For women with history of infertility and recurrent miscarriage or those attempting pregnancy with ART, it is important to evaluate for thyroid dysfunction and TAI and treatment with LT4 should be individualized based on risk factors, TSH value and presence of TAI. Treatment of OH, SCH, and hyperthyroidism is warranted to optimize the reproductive potential of men as well.

TABLE 5: Effects of thyroid dysfunction on male reproductive health.

	Hypothyroidism	Hyperthyroidism
Hormonal changes	• Blunted LH and FSH response to GnRH stimulation • Exaggerated response of testosterone to hCG stimulation • Decreased SHBG • Decreased total testosterone • Decreased free testosterone • Elevated prolactin	• Increased SHBG • Increased total testosterone • Normal free testosterone • Increased total and free estradiol • Exaggerated LH and FSH response to GnRH stimulation • Blunted testosterone response to hCG stimulation
Symptoms	• Decreased libido • Erectile dysfunction • Delayed ejaculation	• Decreased libido • Erectile dysfunction • Premature ejaculation • Gynecomastia
Semen characteristics and sperm quality	*Animal studies*: • Arrest of spermatogenesis resulting in reduced number of live sperms • Reduced progressive sperm motility • Decreased volume of testis and accessory glands • Delayed sperm transit through the epididymis *Human studies*: • Altered semen quality • Teratozoospermia (abnormal sperm morphology) • Reduced sperm motility • Reduced secretion of accessory glands (epididymis and vas deferens) with low ejaculate volume • Reduced concentration of fructose, fucose, and sialic acid in semen	*Rodent studies*: • Delay in spermatogenesis with maturation arrest • Reduced sperm motility • Reduced testis weight *Human studies*: • Reduced semen volume and quality • Asthenozoospermia (reduced sperm motility) in 50% • Oligozoospermia (reduced sperm count) in 40% • Teratozoospermia

(FSH: follicle stimulating hormone; GnRH: gonadotropin releasing hormone; hCG: human chorionic gonadotropin; LH: luteinizing hormone; SHBG: sex hormone binding globulin)

SUGGESTED READINGS

1. Krassas GE, Poppe K, Glinoer D. Thyroid function and human reproductive health. Endocr Rev. 2010;31(5):702-55.
2. Silva JF, Ocarino NM, Serakides R. Thyroid hormones and female reproduction. Biol Reprod. 2018;99(5):907-21.
3. Dosiou C. Thyroid and Fertility: Recent Advances. Thyroid. 2020;30(4):479-86.
4. Unuane D, Velkeniers B. Impact of thyroid disease on fertility and assisted conception. Best Pract Res Clin Endocrinol Metab. 2020;34(4):101378.
5. Maraka S, Ospina NM, O'Keeffe DT, Espinosa De Ycaza AE, Gionfriddo MR, Erwin PJ, et al. Subclinical hypothyroidism in pregnancy: a systematic review and meta-analysis. Thyroid. 2016;26(4):580-90.
6. Nazarpour S, Ramezani Tehrani F, Simbar M, Azizi F. Thyroid dysfunction and pregnancy outcomes. Int J Reprod BioMed. 2015;13(7):387-96.
7. Alexander EK, Pearce EN, Brent GA, Brown RS, Chen H, Dosiou C, et al. 2017 Guidelines of the American Thyroid Association for the Diagnosis and Management of Thyroid Disease During Pregnancy and the Postpartum. Thyroid. 2017;27(3):315-89.
8. Thangaratinam S, Tan A, Knox E, Kilby MD, Franklyn J, Coomarasamy A. Association between thyroid autoantibodies and miscarriage and preterm birth: meta-analysis of evidence. BMJ. 2011;342:d2616.
9. Akhtar MA, Agrawal R, Brown J, Sajjad Y, Craciunas L. Thyroxine replacement for subfertile women with euthyroid autoimmune thyroid disease or subclinical hypothyroidism. Cochrane Database Syst Rev. 2019;6(6):CD011009.
10. Dhillon-Smith RK, Middleton LJ, Sunner KK, Cheed V, Baker K, Farrell-Carver S, et al. Levothyroxine in Women with Thyroid Peroxidase Antibodies before Conception. N Engl J Med. 2019;380(14):1316-25.
11. van Dijk MM, Vissenberg R, Fliers E, van der Post JAM, van der Hoorn MP, de Weerd S, et al. Levothyroxine in euthyroid thyroid peroxidase antibody positive women with recurrent pregnancy loss (T4LIFE trial): a multicentre, randomised, double-blind, placebo-controlled, phase 3 trial. Lancet Diabetes Endocrinol. 2022;10(5):322-29.
12. Venables A, Wong W, Way M, Homer HA. Thyroid autoimmunity and IVF/ICSI outcomes in euthyroid women: a systematic review and meta-analysis. Reprod Biol Endocrinol. 2020;18(1):120.
13. Wang H, Gao H, Chi H, Zeng L, Xiao W, Wang Y, et al. Effect of Levothyroxine on Miscarriage Among Women With Normal Thyroid Function and Thyroid Autoimmunity Undergoing In Vitro Fertilization and Embryo Transfer: A Randomized Clinical Trial. JAMA. 2017;318(22):2190-8.
14. Rao M, Zeng Z, Zhao S, Tang L. Effect of levothyroxine supplementation on pregnancy outcomes in women with subclinical hypothyroidism and thyroid autoimmuneity undergoing in vitro fertilization/intracytoplasmic sperm injection: an updated meta-analysis of randomized controlled trials. Reprod Biol Endocrinol. 2018;16(1):92.
15. Practice Committee of the American Society for Reproductive Medicine. Subclinical hypothyroidism in the infertile female population: a guideline. Fertil Steril. 2015;104(3):545-53.
16. Poppe K, Bisschop P, Fugazzola L, Minziori G, Unuane D, Weghofer A. 2021 European Thyroid Association Guideline on Thyroid Disorders prior to and during Assisted Reproduction. Eur Thyroid J. 2020;9(6):281-95.
17. Jannini EA, Ulisse S, D'Armiento M. Thyroid hormone and male gonadal function. Endocr Rev. 1995;16(4):443-59.
18. La Vignera S, Vita R. Thyroid dysfunction and semen quality. Int J Immunopathol Pharmacol. 2018;32:2058738418775241.

CHAPTER 22

Hypothyroidism and Pregnancy

Rajesh Rajput, Ashish Sehgal, Vasundhara Rajput

INTRODUCTION

Hypothyroidism is not uncommon in women of reproductive age group, particularly during pregnancy and the puerperal period. Many studies that have screened women for thyroid dysfunction during pregnancy have shown prevalence of overt and subclinical hypothyroidism to be 0.3–0.5% and 2–3% of all pregnancies respectively. The causes of hypothyroidism during pregnancy are not different compared to the nonpregnant state. In geographic areas with prevalent iodine deficiency, this deficiency itself is the most common cause of hypothyroidism, while in iodine replete areas, Hashimoto's thyroiditis is more common. Other relatively less common causes include overtreated hyperthyroidism, pituitary and hypothalamic diseases, postradioactive ablation, and post-total thyroidectomy hypothyroidism.

HYPOTHYROIDISM AND PREGNANCY: NORMAL PHYSIOLOGY

Pregnancy represents a stress test for the thyroid gland. This is because of many reversible physiological changes in maternal thyroid axis that characterize normal pregnancy. These include increase in levels of thyroid-binding globulin (TBG) starting from the 7th week of gestation, increased renal iodine clearance because of increased glomerular filtration rate (GFR), the requirement of transplacental transfer of levothyroxine (LT4) and iodine for normal development of fetal brain, particularly in the first trimester, and, placental deiodinase-mediated degradation of maternal thyroid hormones. These changes necessitate synthesis of increased amounts of T3 and T4 hormones from the maternal thyroid gland. Subclinical or overt hypothyroidism results when maternal thyroid is unable to compensate for these increased physiologic demands of the pregnant state.

EFFECT OF HYPOTHYROIDISM ON PREGNANCY OUTCOMES

Untreated overt hypothyroidism is detrimental for both mother and fetus. Maternal complications of untreated hypothyroidism include preeclampsia, placental abruption, postpartum hemorrhage, and miscarriage. Subclinical hypothyroidism, particularly when thyroid peroxidase (TPO) antibodies are positive, has also been linked to adverse pregnancy outcomes—spontaneous abortion and pretermlabor.

FETAL AND NEONATAL CONSEQUENCES OF MATERNAL HYPOTHYROIDISM

Fetal thyroid gland develops by the end of first trimester and starts producing thyroid hormones only by the 16th week of gestation. However, fetal brain and neuropsychological development has an obligatory requirement of thyroid hormones throughout the gestation period. Hence, the early phases of brain development that occur in first and second trimester, including neuronal multiplication, migration, and architectural organization, are completely dependent on transplacental transfer of maternal thyroid hormones. If there is untreated overt hypothyroidism in first trimester, it can lead to serious adverse outcomes ranging from decrease in IQ to irreversible frank mental retardation.

The later phases of brain development that include glial cell multiplication, migration, and myelinization occur during the third trimester of pregnancy, through the first 3 years of life. During this time fetal thyroid gland is functional and hence maternal hypothyroidism during the later part of pregnancy leads to less severe and partially reversible brain damage.

AUTOIMMUNE THYROID DISEASE AND PREGNANCY

Pregnancy is a hyperestrogenemic and hyperprogesteronemic state, with relatively higher serum progesterone levels. Progesterone is known to supress both humoral and cellular immune response. This, along with many other not well known mechanisms results in relative immune tolerance during the gravid state. This reverts back to normal in the postpartum period, hence the increased chances of thyroiditis during this period.

Thyroid autoimmunity during pregnancy, as evidenced by elevated thyroid peroxidase antibody (TPO-Ab) levels, has been documented to be associated with adverse fetal outcomes, even in the presence of biochemical maternal euthyroidism. The reasons for this are not clearly known. It is thought that thyroid autoimmunity probably is part of a more widespread immune imbalance that results in reduced immune tolerance toward the fetus. Other plausible explanations include advanced maternal age as seen in TPO-Ab-positive women and the inability of the ailing thyroid to respond to the increased thyroid hormone demands of pregnancy despite the fact that TPO-Ab titers fall with advancing gestation. Consequent to this, as many as half of antenatal women have subnormal T4 levels during the second and third trimesters, necessitating the need for monitoring thyroid function so that timely LT4 replacement can be initiated. Whether all TPO-Ab-positive women need to be treated is not clear presently, but thyroid-stimulating hormone (TSH) >2.0 mIU/L in the presence of TPO titers >12,500 U/mL before 20 weeks of gestation increases the likelihood of progression to overt hypothyroidism as gestation advances, hence these women should be monitored during pregnancy and the postpartum period. Intriguingly, many studies have shown beneficial effects of LT4 replacement in such women irrespective of baseline thyroid function status.

DIAGNOSIS

Normal upper limit of TSH in pregnancy has been a subject of debate since a long time. Normative TSH reference range during pregnancy varies widely between different geographic locations and populations, likely attributable to differences in the iodine status between populations as well as the TSH assays used in studies. Trimester-specific reference intervals for thyroid function test (TFT) in pregnant women should be established after using rigorous exclusion criteria, i.e., any history of chronic illness, goiter on physical examination, thyroid illness in the past or present, consuming thyroid medications (current and past), family history of thyroid illness, presence of anti-TPO, poor obstetrics history included three or more abortions. Rajput et al. in their cross-sectional study involving 1,430 pregnant women had shown that 2.5th–97.5th percentiles for FT3, FT4, and TSH were 2.53–4.54 pg/mL, 0.88–1.78 ng/mL, and 0.37–3.69 µIU/mL in the first trimester; 2.0–4.73 pg/mL, 0.91–1.78 ng/mL, and 0.54–4.47 µIU/mL in the second trimester; 2.01–4.01 pg/mL, 0.83–1.73 ng/mL, and 0.70–4.64 µIU/mL in the third trimester of pregnancy, respectively. Mean TSH increased and mean FT3 decreased significantly with the progression of gestational period. FT4 decreased from trimester first to third, but the decrease was nonsignificant from second to third trimester. Similar observations were made by Marwaha et al. in their cross-sectional study involving 541 pregnant Indian women. The 5th and 95th percentiles values for FT4 (pmol/L) 12.0–19.45, 9.48–19.58, 11.32–17.7; FT3 (pmol/L) 1.92–5.86, 3.2–5.73, 3.3–5.18; and TSH (mIU/L) 0.6–5.0, 0.44–5.78, 0.74–5.7 in first, second, and third trimester, respectively. It is hence not possible to clearly establish a universal TSH cut off beyond which LT4 replacement should be started. ATA 2017 guidelines recommend that whenever possible, population and trimester-specific TSH reference range should be defined. When that is not possible, TSH reference from similar representative population, and using same assay should be used to guide decision making for starting LT4 replacement. If both above are not available, then upper reference limit of 4 mIU/L may be used.

Ideally free T3 and T4 levels should be ascertained in pregnancy because total T3 and T4 levels are altered in pregnancy owing to the physiological increase in circulation TBG levels due to estrogenic stimulation of the liver. If free thyroid hormone assays are not available, total T3, and T4 assays may be used, but to interpret the results, the upper reference range needs to be increased by 5% per week from the 7th through 16th week, after which the upper reference range needs to be increased by 50% throughout the remaining gestation period. One simple way to do that is to multiply the normal nonpregnant range for total T4 by a factor of 1.5 during the pregnancy. Hypothyroidism is diagnosed in presence of normal or low FT4 or total T4 levels and elevated TSH levels.

TREATMENT

The drug of choice for treatment of hypothyroidism during pregnancy, whether subclinical or overt, is LT4. The dose of this replacement depends on the trimester of pregnancy when hypothyroidism is diagnosed, and also upon the severity of hypothyroidism. For newly diagnosed overt hypothyroidism, LT4 should be started at dosage of 2 µg/kg body weight, which is a slightly higher dose than what is used in nonpregnant women. LT4 has to be taken on empty stomach at least 30 minutes before anything else is consumed. Moreover, any iron/calcium supplementation should not be taken for at least 4 hours after ingesting LT4. If these precautions are not followed, the absorption of LT4 may decrease by as much as 20–30% resulting in poor control of hypothyroidism as well as requirement of an injudicious increase in dosage of LT4. Thyroid function should be rechecked after 4 weeks and dose of LT4 should

TABLE 1: Suggested starting dose of LT4 based on initial TSH level.

Baseline TSH levels	LT4 dosage
TSH <10 mIU/L	Increase LT4 by 50 µg/day
TSH 10–20 mIU/L	Increase LT4 by 75 µg/day
TSH >20 mIU/L	Increase LT4 by 100 µg/day

(LT4: levothyroxine; TSH: thyroid-stimulating hormone)

be adjusted as needed to keep TSH within the population and trimester-specific TSH reference range for the given TSH assay. For previously diagnosed hypothyroid women becoming pregnant, the need for LT4 increases by as much as 30–50% during gestation. Hence the dose of LT4 should be increased depending on their baseline thyroid function test **(Table 1)**.

Thyroid function test should be reassessed at least 4 weeks after any LT4 dosage modification. Once thyroid function is in normal range for pregnancy, repeat thyroid function test should be done every 6 weeks. The recommended mean intake of iodine during pregnancy and lactation is approximately 250 µg/day.

AMERICAN THYROID ASSOCIATION 2017 RECOMMENDATIONS

In 2017, American Thyroid Association (ATA) published its recommendations highlighting the role of thyroid function tests, hypothyroidism, thyrotoxicosis, thyroid antibodies, and miscarriage/preterm delivery, thyroid nodules and cancer, postpartum thyroiditis, recommendations on screening for thyroid disease during pregnancy, and areas for future research. The specific recommendations relating to hypothyroidism and pregnancy are summarized in **Box 1**.

WHETHER TO SCREEN ALL PREGNANT WOMEN FOR HYPOTHYROIDISM

There can be two approaches for screening pregnant women for hypothyroidism—universal screening and risk factor-based case finding. Though several studies have documented brain developmental abnormalities ranging from mild decrease in IQ to frank mental retardation in children born to women who had subclinical to overt hypothyroidism during pregnancy, at this time there is no general consensus regarding screening all women for hypothyroidism during pregnancy. ATA 2017 guidelines also mention that currently there is not sufficient evidence to recommend universal screening. These guidelines however highlight 11 risk factors any of which if present necessitate screening the antenatal woman for thyroid dysfunction. If the TSH is initially normal, no further monitoring is typically required. The 11 risk factors include history of hypothyroidism/hyperthyroidism or current features of thyroid dysfunction, known TPO-Ab positivity or presence of a goiter, history of head or neck radiation or prior thyroid surgery, age >30 years, type 1 diabetes mellitus (T1DM) or other autoimmune disorders, history of pregnancy loss, preterm delivery, or infertility, multiple prior pregnancies, family history of autoimmune thyroid disease, morbid obesity [body mass index (BMI) >40 kg/m^2], use of amiodarone or lithium, or recent administration of iodinated radiologic contrast and residing in an area of known moderate to severe iodine insufficiency.

Postpartum Thyroiditis

Postpartum thyroiditis is thyroiditis that occurs in women within first year after the delivery. It occurs in approximately 5–10% of women but the incidence can be greater in certain high-risk women **(Box 2)**.

BOX 1: ATA recommendation for hypothyroidism during pregnancy.

- To treat maternal hypothyroidism, use of triiodothyronine, desiccated thyroid, or other thyroid preparations is strongly recommended against
- Oral levothyroxine is indicated for women with overt hypothyroidism [thyroid-stimulating hormone (TSH) >10], which is associated with greater risks for fetal loss and premature birth
- Women who are already receiving thyroid replacement therapy should increase their dose by 25–30% when they become pregnant
- Women with TSH 2.5–10 mIU/mL during initial screening should be checked for TPO-Ab titers. For those TPO-Ab-positive and TSH 2.5-upperlimit of the reference range (ULRR), treatment with LT4 may be considered, while such women with TSH-ULRR—10 mIU/mL must be treated with LT4
- For TPO-Ab negative women with TSH 2.5-(ULRR), no treatment is recommended, while treatment may be considered for those who are TPO-Ab negative and have TSH-ULRR—10 mIU/L
- Women with subclinical hypothyroidism in pregnancy who are not initially treated should be monitored for progression to overt hypothyroidism. Serum TSH and free thyroxine (FT4) levels should be measured approximately every 4 weeks until 16–20 weeks' gestation and at least once between 26 and 32 weeks' gestation
- Ideally population and trimester specific TSH reference range should be defined. When that is not possible, TSH reference from similar representative population and using same assay should be used to guide decision making for starting LT4 replacement. If both above are not available, then upper reference limit of 4 mIU/L may be used
- Serum levels of FT4 during pregnancy should be measured with online solid-phase extraction-liquid chromatography, or tandem mass spectrometry on serum dialysate or ultrafiltrate
- Treatment is not needed for women with isolated low FT4 levels

(ATA: American Thyroid Association; TPO-Ab: peroxidase antibody)

> **BOX 2: Women at high risk for postpartum thyroiditis.**
>
> - Women with type 1 diabetes mellitus or other autoimmune disorders
> - Women with a strong family history of autoimmune thyroid disease
> - Thyroid peroxidase antibody-positive
> - Prior episode of postpartum thyroiditis
> - Postpartum depression
> - Women with prior miscarriage

Postpartum thyroiditis is the exacerbation of an underlying autoimmune thyroiditis, aggravated by the postdelivery immunological rebound that follows the progesterone-mediated partial immunosuppression of pregnancy. The various presentations of postpartum thyroiditis include transient hyperthyroidism, transient hypothyroidism, or transient hyperthyroidism followed by transient hypothyroidism. The contemporary description of postpartum thyroiditis includes thyrotoxicosis followed by hypothyroidism but not all women go through both phases; approximately one-third manifests both phases, while one-third has only a thyrotoxic or hypothyroid phase.

The thyrotoxic phase occurs 1–4 months postdelivery, lasts for 1–3 months, and is associated with symptoms including anxiety, insomnia, palpitations, fatigue, weight loss, and irritability. Since these symptoms are often attributed to the postpartum state per se, the thyrotoxic phase of postpartum thyroiditis is often missed. It is much more common for women to present in the hypothyroid phase, which typically occurs 4–8 months after delivery and may last up to 9–12 months. Typical symptoms of this phase include fatigue, weight gain, constipation, dry skin, depression, and poor exercise tolerance. In most women, thyroid function returns to normal within 12–18 months of the onset of symptoms.

Treatment depends on the phase of thyroiditis and the degree of symptoms. Women presenting with thyrotoxicosis may be treated with β-blockers to reduce palpitations and other adrenergic symptoms. As the symptoms improve, the medication is tapered off since the thyrotoxic phase is expected to be transient. Among β-blockers propranolol is recommended by Food and Drug Administration (FDA) as safe drug to be used during lactation. Antithyroid medications are not indicated for the thyrotoxic phase since the thyroid gland per se is not overactive. The hypothyroid phase is treated with LT4 replacement. If the hypothyroidism is mild, and the patient has few symptoms, no therapy may be necessary. If thyroid hormone therapy is begun, treatment should be continued for approximately 6–12 months and then tapered to see if thyroid hormone is required permanently, since 80% of patients will regain normal thyroid function and not require chronic therapy. However, approximately 20% of those that go into a hypothyroid phase will remain hypothyroid and will require continuation of LT4 therapy. In women where LT4 is stopped, serum TSH should be monitored annually for early detection of future hypothyroidism.

Controversy surrounds whether or not to screen for postpartum thyroiditis in all women. The American College of Obstetricians and Gynecologists does not recommend thyroid screening postpartum. The ATA states that the decision regarding screening in women of childbearing should be made jointly between each physician and patient and the American Association of Clinical Endocrinologists recommends postpartum screening in pregnant women known to have high titers of TPO-Ab. In view of these controversies, it is recommended to do selective screening based on risk profile of postpartum women and it should include an antithyroid TPO-Ab titer and TSH level. Women who are euthyroid and antithyroid TPO-Ab-negative require no further follow-up. Antithyroid TPO-Ab-positive women should have a serum TSH performed at 6 and 9 months postpartum.

SUGGESTED READINGS

1. Abalovich M, Amino N, Barbour LA, Cobin RH, De Groot LJ, Glinoer D. Management of thyroid dysfunction during pregnancy and postpartum: an Endocrine Society Clinical Practice Guideline. J Clin Endocrinol Metab. 2007;92(8 Suppl):S1-47.
2. Becks GP, Burrow GN. Thyroid disease and pregnancy. Med Clin North Am. 1991;75(1):121-50.
3. LeBeau SO, Mandel SJ. Thyroid disorders during pregnancy. Endocrinol Metab Clin North Am. 2006;35(1):117-36, vii.
4. Poppe K, Velkeniers B, Glinoer D. Thyroid disease and female reproduction. Clin Endocrinol (Oxf). 2007;66(3):309-21.
5. Cooper DS. Clinical practice. Subclinical hypothyroidism. N Engl J Med. 2001;345(4):260-5.
6. Leung AS, Millar LK, Koonings PP, Montoro M, Mestman JH. Perinatal outcome in hypothyroid pregnancies. Obstet Gynecol. 1993;81(3):349-53.
7. Haddow JE, Palomaki GE, Allan WC, Williams JR, Knight GJ, Gagnon J. Maternal thyroid deficiency during pregnancy and subsequent neuropsychological development of the child. N Engl J Med. 1999;341(8):549-55.
8. Geenen V, Perrier de Hauterive S, Puit M, Hazout A, Goffin F, Frankenne F, et al. Autoimmunity and Pregnancy: theory and practice. Acta Clin Belg. 2002;57:317-24.
9. Thangaratinam S, Tan A, Knox E, Kilby MD, Franklyn J, Coomarasamy A. Association between thyroid autoantibodies and miscarriage and preterm birth: meta-analysis of evidence. BMJ. 2011;342:d2616.
10. Glinoer D. Management of hypo- and hyperthyroidism during pregnancy. Growth Horm IGF Res. 2003;13 (Suppl A):S45-54.
11. Negro R, Formoso G, Mangieri T, Pezzarossa A, Dazzi D, Hassan H. Levothyroxine treatment in euthyroid pregnant women with

autoimmune thyroid disease: Effects on obstetrical complications. J Clin Endocrinol Metab. 2006;91:2587-91.
12. Rajput R, Singh B, Goel V, Verma A, Seth S, Nanda S. Trimester specific reference interval for thyroid hormones during pregnancy at a tertiary care hospital in Haryana, India. Indian J Endocrinol Metab. 2016;20(6):810-5.
13. Marwah RK, Chopra S, Gopalakrishnan S, Sharma B, Kanwar RS, Sastry S, et al. Establishment of reference range for thyroid hormones in normal pregnant Indian women. Int J Obstet Gynecol. 2008;115:602-6.
14. Brent GA. Maternal thyroid function: interpretation of thyroid function tests in pregnancy. Clin Obstet Gynecol. 1997;40(1): 3-15.
15. Alexander EK, Marqusee E, Lawrence J, Jarolim P, Fischer GA, Larsen PR. Timing and magnitude of increases in levothyroxine requirements during pregnancy in women with hypothyroidism. N Engl J Med. 2004;351(3):241-9.
16. Toft A. Increased levothyroxine requirements in pregnancy: Why, when, and how much? N Engl J Med. 2004;351:292-4.
17. Bungard TJ, Hurlburt M. Management of hypothyroidism during pregnancy. CMAJ. 2007;176(8):1077-8.
18. Alexander EK, Pearce EN, Brent GA, Brown RS, Chen H, Dosiou C, et al. 2017 Guidelines of the American Thyroid Association for the Diagnosis and Management of Thyroid Disease during Pregnancy and the Postpartum. Thyroid. 2017;27:315-89.
19. Vaidya B, Anthony S, Bilous M, Shields B, Drury J, Hutchison S, et al. Detection of thyroid dysfunction in early pregnancy: Universal screening or targeted high-risk case finding? J Clin Endocrinol Metab. 2007;92:203-7.
20. Muller AF, Drexhage HA, Berghout A. Postpartum thyroiditis and autoimmune thyroiditis in women of childbearing age: recent insights and consequences for antenatal and postnatal care. Endocr Rev. 2001;22(5):605-30.
21. Lucas A, Pizarro E, Granada ML, Salinas I, Roca J, Sanmartí A. Postpartum thyroiditis: long-term follow-up. Thyroid. 2005;15(10):1177-81.
22. Roti E, Emerson CH. Clinical review 29: Postpartum thyroiditis. J Clin Endocrinol Metab. 1992;74(1):3-5.

CHAPTER 23

Thyroid Excess in Pregnancy

Mohd Ashraf Ganie, Sailesh Kumar Bansiwal

INTRODUCTION

Hyperthyroidism in pregnancy is relatively an uncommon condition with prevalence between 0.1 and 5%. This includes both overt [Graves' disease (GD) accounting for 85% of the cases] and subclinical forms (2–5%). Serum thyroid-stimulating hormone (TSH) below 0.1 mIU/L has been shown to be present in 5% of women by the 11th week of pregnancy. Multiple physiological changes that occur in pregnancy are also known to affect functioning of thyroid gland in many ways that also includes a steep increase in human chorionic gonadotrophin (hCG) during first trimester that in turn stimulates TSH receptor owing to its structural homology. Other changes include increase in thyroxine-binding globulin (TBG), urinary iodine excretion, plasma volume, rise in thyroid hormone degradation by placental type 3 deiodinase, and increase in fetal utilization of maternal hormones.

As a general rule, FT4 transiently rises in the first trimester due to the relatively high circulating hCG concentration, while it decreases in the second and third trimester, albeit still within the normal reference range, FT3 changes broadly parallel the FT4. Hyperemesis gravidarum, which may sometimes require hospitalizations due to dehydration and ketosis, may be associated with gestational thyrotoxicosis. Identification of hyperthyroidism in pregnancy is essential as it leads to unfavorable maternal and fetal outcomes, such as pregnancy-induced hypertension (PIH), maternal congestive heart failure, pregnancy loss, prematurity, low birth weight, stillbirth, intrauterine growth restriction, along with neurobehavioral disorders in offspring in later life. Besides maternal hyperthyroidism TSH receptor antibodies (TRAb) may affect fetus and antithyroid drugs may lead to birth defects and maternal liver injury. Up to 5% of neonates of mothers with GD have hyperthyroidism due to the transplacental passage of maternal stimulating TRAbs (despite of mother being euthyroid or has received previous treatment for GD).

CAUSES OF THYROID HORMONE EXCESS DURING PREGNANCY

The two most common causes of hyperthyroidism in pregnant women are GD, due to thyroid stimulation by thyroid receptor antibodies (TRAbs), and gestational transient thyrotoxicosis (GTT). These two forms may have similar presentation, but a careful past history and physical examination with appropriate laboratory test may be needed to differentiate between the two. Other less frequent causes of thyroid excess in pregnancy may include multiple gestation, trophoblastic disease, hyperplacentosis, hyperreactio luteinalis, toxic multinodular goiter, solitary toxic adenoma, de Quervain's, painless and acute thyroiditis, overtreatment with levothyroxine (LT4), factitious intake of thyroid hormone, struma ovarii, and functional thyroid malignancy metastasis.

PHYSIOLOGY OF MATERNAL AND FETAL THYROID IN PREGNANCY

Major changes in thyroid morphology and physiology are seen during pregnancy making the diagnosis of thyroid dysfunction challenging. During pregnancy there is increase in size (between 10 and 40%) and vascularization of thyroid gland, size can further enlarge in areas of iodine deficiency. During early gestation there is stimulation of thyroid gland by hCG, which is produced by syncytiotrophoblast from the beginning of gestation, peaking at around 9–11 weeks. This leads to increase thyroid hormone production and decrease in serum TSH concentration by the end of the first trimester. During first trimester 15% healthy women may have TSH below the lower limit of reference range, while during second and third trimester TSH may be suppressed in 10% and 5% women respectively. Serum levels of hCG decline after first trimester until 20 weeks, following which it remain stable for the remainder of pregnancy.

Rise in serum estrogen from fourth week of gestation, increase levels and sialylation of thyroid-binding globulin which decreases its hepatic clearance and prolong its half-life from 15 minutes to 3 days in comparison with nonpregnant state. TBG after plateauing at midgestation remains same during the rest of gestation and normalize after delivery. This TBG rise leads to increase in total concentration of total thyroxine (T4) and total triiodothyronine (T3) during first trimester which plateaus in second trimester, at a level 30–100% greater than prepregnancy state. Placenta having high expression of type 3 deiodinase leads to enhanced metabolism of T4 and T3 to reverse T3 and 3,3' T2 respectively thereby modulating the amount of thyroid hormone reaching the fetus. This physiological changes are desirable since thyroid hormones play a vital role in the early embryogenesis primarily neurodevelopment, somatic growth, and tissue differentiation. Since fetal thyroid gland becomes functional only after 8–12 weeks of gestation, maternal T4 levels assume significant importance in the earlier weeks of gestation. Consequently iodine status of mother assumes importance for meeting this increased demand during pregnancy for both mother and fetus.

HYPERTHYROIDISM IN PREGNANCY

Physiological Hyperthyroidism

Gestational Transient Thyrotoxicosis

Gestational transient thyrotoxicosis refers to hyperthyroidism occurring in pregnant women that resolves spontaneously by the end of early gestation and has no evidence of thyroid autoimmunity. GTT is attributed to all conditions (twin, multiple pregnancies, hyperplacentosis, and hydatidiform mole) leading to elevations in serum hCG. It may also be due to circulating hCG isoforms with increased thyrotropic activity and/or prolonged half-life. Symptoms of thyrotoxicosis typically occur by 4–9 weeks of gestation and remit by the end of the first or early second trimester of pregnancy (i.e., parallel to changes in hCG levels). Owing to its short and self-limiting course GTT in general does not require any specific treatment and the milder forms may even go unrecognized. Severe forms occurring in 0.3–1% of pregnancies may, however, be associated with persistent vomiting, weight loss (at least 5% loss of prepregnancy weight), dehydration, ketonuria and serum electrolyte, and acid-base abnormalities (hypochloremic alkalosis, hypokalemia, and hyponatremia). Clinical diagnosis is confirmed by laboratory testing showing absence of serum TRAbs, along with undetectable TSH and increased FT4 levels.

Pathological Hyperthyroidism

This usually occurs in patients with Graves' disease, rarely toxic multinodular goiter or toxic adenoma and thus are independent of serum levels. This pathological form has risks for both mother and the fetus in the form of pre-eclampsia, heart failure in mother, preterm delivery, low birth weight, and may also lead to fetal loss.

Graves' Disease and Pregnancy

There are few scenarios in which GD can occur in pregnancy. GD preexisting active disease may be a relapse in previous remission or may occur first time during pregnancy. Pathogenesis of GD being same as in nonpregnant state occurs by overstimulation of thyroid by TRAbs is likely to remit during the second and third trimesters, and often relapse in the postpartum period like other autoimmune diseases. The physiological immunosuppression that occurs during the later half of pregnancy, aimed at preventing the fetus being recognized as foreign tissue, is the basis of this phenomenon. To safeguard pregnancy outcomes the clinician must have a clear knowledge about the clinical presentation (age, duration, and eye symptoms), physical examination (goiter, dermopathy, and orbitopathy), and biochemical testing in order to differentiate GD from other causes of thyrotoxicosis.

DIAGNOSIS

Diagnosis of hyperthyroidism is challenging in pregnancy as pregnancy itself is a hypermetabolic state and the symptoms (palpitations, heat intolerance) may overlap. Therefore, the initial step should focus to take a proper history (present, medical, and family) and if the patient has had symptoms prior to pregnancy and if signs such as diffuse goiter and orbitopathy are present, a diagnosis of GD can be entertained. Laboratory evaluation should follow with FT3, FT4, and TSH. A low TSH together with high thyroid hormones (FT4, FT3) make thyrotoxicosis. A high free T3 may help us distinguish between hyperemesis gravidarum and hyperthyroid patients as the ratio is not reversed in the former and <15% of hyperemetic women have elevations in FT3. Serum TRAb levels have a diagnostic utility as it crosses the placental barrier and may cause fetal hyperthyroidism, levels over 3–5 times are associated with hyperthyroidism in fetus and newborn and point toward GD.

PREGNANCY OUTCOMES

Pathological hyperthyroidism is associated with adverse outcomes for both mother and fetus. Before the advent of antithyroid drugs (ATDs), only 50% of women with hyperthyroidism were able to conceive, and among them those with poorly or uncontrolled disease had increased frequency of spontaneous miscarriage and premature delivery. Uncontrolled thyrotoxicosis and use of ATD during first trimester are known to increase the risk of congenital malformations (harelip, polydactyly, and imperforate anus). Complications as a result of pathological hyperthyroidism include miscarriage 8–21%, preterm delivery 3–88%, preeclampsia 2–11%, heart failure 3–63%, stillbirth 0–50%, small for gestational age, and thyroid storm during parturition.

TREATMENT

Patients with overt hyperthyroidism require restoration of a euthyroid state because of potential adverse maternal and fetal outcomes. While therapeutic options including ATD and or surgery differ from case to case radioiodine is contraindicated in pregnancy and lactation. In cases where GD precedes pregnancy, restoration of euthyroidism remains of utmost importance. Generally, it is done with ATD and those may continue throughout the pregnancy with minimal risk. Patients choosing a definitive therapy like radioiodine should be advised to postpone the pregnancy by at least 6 months for restoring euthyroidism. For a rapid restoration of euthyroid state surgery can be considered prior to conception. In cases where GD is diagnosed during the pregnancy; ATDs are the only therapeutic option. Surgery may be offered during second trimester in exceptional cases. Radioiodine is absolutely contraindicated as it can lead to congenital hypothyroidism and even teratogenesis. If GD is diagnosed after delivery and possibility of thyrotoxicosis is excluded, it is favorable to start ATD. Infants should not be breastfed due to risk of hypothyroidism. Radioiodine is also not favorable due to its delayed effect. Those who have adverse effects due to ATDs, surgery can be offered. Decision to start ATD, depends on severity of clinical and biochemical hyperthyroidism. In mild GD [with FT4 slightly above upper limit of normal (ULN)], wait and watch approach can be used with frequent monitoring. Pregnant women with GD should be kept in subclinical hyperthyroidism with minimum possible ATD dose. This level will ensure fetal euthyroidism, because FT4 in the mother's serum correlates with fetal FT4 levels in cord blood.

Antithyroid drugs are the first choice for treatment of GD during pregnancy. Propylthiouracil (PTU) and methimazole (MMI) are equally effective in the management of hyperthyroidism during pregnancy. PTU by inhibiting type 1 deiodinase inhibits the conversion of T4 to T3, an effect not seen with MMI. But in comparative studies MMI normalizes serum thyroid hormones faster than PTU. As PTU is a bigger molecule, it crosses the breast epithelium and placenta less readily and therefore preferred in first trimester. MMI can also be used if the patient is having adverse effects with PTU. Initial dose needed to normalize FT4 and TSH rarely exceeds 450 mg and 30 mg for PTU and MMI respectively. It usually takes around 7–8 weeks for normalization of maternal FT4 by both PTU/MMI. Prolonged suppression can be seen for TSH even after normalization of FT4. Studies have showed higher risk of congenital anomalies with MMI, however due to risk of acute liver failure with PTU, its use is limited to first trimester. MMI is preferred in second and third trimester as it is less hepatotoxic.

ANTITHYROID DRUGS: EFFECT ON THE FETUS

We know both maternal TRAb activity and ATD dosage can have effects on fetal thyroid status. TRAb may have both stimulating and blocking effect and can lead to fetal hyperthyroidism and hypothyroidism respectively. ATD may lead to hypothyroidism in fetus after crossing the placenta, as evidenced by elevated cord TSH levels in both PTU (23%) and MMI (14%) treated mothers. There is a strong correlation at term between maternal and cord TRAb levels with development of neonatal hyperthyroidism. All women taking ATDs at relatively high doses (PTU ≥450 mg/day and MMI ≥30 mg/day) should undergo a fetal ultrasound at 26–28 weeks in order to rule out a goiter. Goiter can occur in both hyperthyroidism (stimulating TRAbs) and hypothyroidism (ATDs).

OTHER OPTIONS

For adrenergic symptoms β-blockers can be transiently used while awaiting ATD therapy, but they should be used for short period with caution. Iodides should not be used as it is associated with neonatal hypothyroidism and goiter, however, it could be used transiently in preparation for surgery. Surgery is rarely considered during pregnancy, and if considered is usually performed during the second trimester in order to reduce the ATD dosage. ^{131}I is completely contraindicated in pregnancy and lactation. Because of the presence of ATD in breast milk their use in lactating women is limited. Less amount of PTU appears in breast milk because of its tight protein binding with a milk to serum ratio of PTU (0.67) and that of MMI (1.0). Doses of PTU and MMI 300 mg/day and 20 mg/day respectively are relatively safe during lactation. Mother is advised to take the drug after feeding the baby. No ATD-related adverse effects have been seen in breastfed infants.

CONCLUSION

A close maternal and fetal surveillance is required for management of hyperthyroidism during pregnancy. Treatment is generally needed in pathological hyperthyroidism, while a wait and watch approach can be taken for physiological hyperthyroidism (GTT). Care should be taken to keep the mothers thyroid hormone in check with the minimum doses of ATD in order to prevent fetal complications. Preconception counseling should be done in patients with GD, and pregnancy should be postponed until euthyroidism is achieved, ATDs are generally preferred for achieving this but if a definitive treatment is needed radioiodine and surgery can be offered prior to conception.

TRAb levels may persist for several years after resolution of hyperthyroidism treated by radioiodine or surgery, so a TRAb before conception may be needed in such patients. PTU is usually used in the first trimester followed by MMI in the second and third trimester because of the risk of hepatotoxicity with PTU. Low doses of ATD can be used in a lactating women to control GD without causing ill effects in the fetus.

SUGGESTED READINGS

1. Lazarus JH. Thyroid function in pregnancy. Br Med Bull. 2011;97:137-48.
2. Patil-Sisodia K, Mestman JH. Graves hyperthyroidism and pregnancy: a clinical update. Endocr Pract. 2010;16:118-29.
3. Laurberg P, Andersen SL. Endocrinology in pregnancy: pregnancy and the incidence, diagnosing and therapy of Graves' disease. Eur J Endocrinol. 2016;175(5):R219-30.
4. Brent GA. Maternal thyroid function: interpretation of thyroid function tests in pregnancy. Clin Obstet Gynecol. 1997;40:3-15.
5. Hershman JM. The role of human chorionic gonadotropin as a thyroid stimulator in normal pregnancy. J Clin Endocrinol Metab. 2008;93:3305-6.
6. Kimura M, Amino N, Tamaki H, Ito E, Mitsuda N, Miyai K, et al. Gestational thyrotoxicosis and hyperemesis gravidarum: possible role of hCG with higher stimulating activity. Clin Endocrinol (Oxf). 1993;38:345-50.
7. Krassas GE, Poppe K, Glinoer D. Thyroid function and human reproductive health. Endocr Rev. 2010;31:702-55.
8. Andersen SL, Andersen S, Vestergaard P, Olsen J. Maternal thyroid function in early pregnancy and child neurodevelopmental disorders: a danish nationwide case-cohort study. Thyroid. 2018;28:537-46.
9. Mestman JH. Hyperthyroidism in pregnancy. Best Pract Res Clin Endocrinol Metab. 2004;18:267-88.
10. Cooper DS, Laurberg P. Hyperthyroidism in pregnancy. Lancet Diabetes Endocrinol. 2013;1:238-49.
11. Soldin OP. Guidelines of the American Thyroid Association for the diagnosis and management of thyroid disease during pregnancy and postpartum. Clin Chem. 2011;21:1081-125.
12. Hershman JM. Physiological and pathological aspects of the effect of human chorionic gonadotropin on the thyroid. Best Pract Res Clin Endocrinol Metab. 2004;18(2):249-65.
13. Soldin OP, Tractenberg RE, Hollowell JG, Jonklaas J, Janicic N, Soldin SJ. Trimester-specific changes in maternal thyroid hormone, thyrotropin, and thyroglobulin concentrations during gestation: trends and associations across trimesters in iodine sufficiency. Thyroid. 2004;14:1084-90.
14. Kahric-Janicic N, Soldin SJ, Soldin OP, West T, Gu J, Jonklaas J. Tandem mass spectrometry improves the accuracy of free thyroxine measurements during pregnancy. Thyroid. 2007;17:303-11.
15. Glinoer D. The regulation of thyroid function in pregnancy: pathways of endocrine adaptation from physiology to pathology. Endocr Rev. 1997;18:404-33.
16. Skjoldebrand L, Brundin J, Carlstrom A, Pettersson T. Thyroid associated components in serum during normal pregnancy. Acta Endocrinol. 1982;100(4):504-11.
17. Kurtz A, Dwyer K, Ekins R. Serum free thyroxine in pregnancy. Br Med J. 1979;2(6189):550-1.
18. Roti E, Fang SL, Emerson CH, Braverman LE. Placental inner ring iodothyronine deiodination: a mechanism for decreased passage of T4 and T3 from mother to fetus. Trans Assoc Am Physicians. 1981;94:183-9.
19. De Escobar GM, Obregón MJ, Del Rey FE. Iodine deficiency and brain development in the first half of pregnancy. Public Health Nutr. 2007;10(2):1554-70.
20. Goldman AM, Mestman JH. Transient non-autoimmune hyperthyroidism of early pregnancy. J Thyroid Res. 2011;2011:142413.
21. Ekary AE, Jackson IM, Goodwin TM, Pang XP, Hein MD, Hershman JM. Increased in vitro thyrotropic activity of partially isolated human chorionic gonadotropin extracted from hydatidiform moles of patients with hyperthyroidism. J Clin Endocrinol Metab. 1993;76:70-4.
22. Goodwin TM. Hyperemesis gravidarum. Clin Obstet Gynecol. 1998;41:597-605.
23. Niebyl JR. Nausea and vomiting in pregnancy. N Engl J Med. 2010;363:1544-50.
24. Chan GW, Mandel SJ. Therapy insight: Management of Graves' disease during pregnancy. Nat Clin Pract Endocrinol Metab. 2007;3(6):470-8.
25. Goodwin TM, Montoro M, Mestman JH, Pekary AE, Hershman JM. The role of chorionic gonadotropin in transient hyperthyroidism of hyperemesis gravidarum. J Clin Endocrinol Metab. 1992;75(5):1333-7.
26. Lee RH, Spencer CA, Mestman JH, Miller EA, Petrovic I, Braverman LE, et al. Free T4 immunoassays are flawed during pregnancy. Am J Obstet Gynecol. 2009;200(3):260.e1-6.
27. Peleg D, Cada S, Peleg A, Ben-Ami M. The relationship between maternal serum Thyroid-stimulating immunoglobulin and fetal and neonatal thyrotoxicosis. Obstet Gynecol. 2002;99(6):1040-3.
28. Polak M, Le Gac I, Vuillard E, Guibourdenche J, Leger J, Toubert ME, et al. Fetal and neonatal thyroid function in relation to maternal Graves' disease. Best Pract Res Clin Endocrinol Metab. 2004;18(2):289-302.
29. Gardiner-Hill H. Pregnancy complicating simple goitre and Graves' disease. Lancet. 1929;1:120-12.
30. Momotani N, Ito K, Hamada N, Ban Y, Nishikawa Y, Mimura T. Maternal hyperthyroidism and congenital malformation in the offspring. Clin Endocrinol (Oxf). 1984;20(6):695-700.
31. Mestman JH, Manning PR, Hodgman J. Hyperthyroidism and pregnancy. Arch Intern Med. 1974;134(3):434-9.
32. Sugrue D, Drury MI. Hyperthyroidism complicating pregnancy: Results of treatment by antithyroid drugs in 77 pregnancies. Br J Obstet Gynaecol. 1980;87(11):970-5.
33. Millar LK, Wing DA, Leung AS, Koonings PP, Montoro MN, Mestman JH. Low birth weight and preeclampsia in pregnancies complicated by hyperthyroidism. Obstet Gynecol. 1994;84(6):946-9.
34. Davis LE, Lucas MJ, Hankins GD, Roark ML, Cunningham FG. Thyrotoxicosis complicating pregnancy. Am J Obstet Gynecol. 1989;160(1):63-70.
35. Mitsuda N, Tamaki H, Amino N, Hosono T, Miyai K, Tanizawa O. Risk factors for developmental disorders in infants born to women with Graves disease. Obstet Gynecol. 1992;80(3 Pt 1):359-64.
36. Momotani N, Noh J, Oyangi H, Ishikawa N, Ito K. Antithyroid drug therapy for Graves' disease during pregnancy: optimal regimen for fetal thyroid status. N Engl J Med. 1986;315(1):24-8.
37. Santini F, Chiovato L, Ghirri P, Lapi P, Mammoli C, Montanelli L, et al. Serum iodothyronines in the human fetus and the newborn: evidence for an important role of placenta in the fetal thyroid hormone homeostasis. J Clin Endocrinol Metab. 1999;84:493-8.

38. Mandel SJ, Brent GA, Larsen PR. Review of antithyroid drug use during pregnancy and report of a case of aplasia cutis. Thyroid. 1994;4(1):129-33.
39. Wing DA, Millar LK, Koonings PP, Montoro MN, Mestman JH. A comparison of propylthiouracil versus methimazole in the treatment of hyperthyroidism in pregnancy. Am J Obstet Gynecol. 1994;170(1 Pt 1):90-5.
40. Momotani N, Noh JY, Ishikawa N, Ito K. Effects of propylthiouracil and methimazole on fetal thyroid status in mothers with Graves' hyperthyroidism. J Clin Endocrinol Metab. 1997;82(11): 3633-6.
41. Momotani N, Iwama S, Noh J (Eds). Anti-thyroid drug therapy for Graves' disease during pregnancy: Mildest thyrotoxic maternal free thyroxine concentrations to avoid fetal hypothyroidism. Phoenix, AZ: 77th Annual Meeting of the American Thyroid Association; 2006.
42. Kampmann JP, Johansen K, Hansen JM, Helweg J. Propylthiouracil in human milk. Revision of a dogma. Lancet. 1980;1(8171):736-7.
43. Johansen K, Andersen AN, Kampmann JP, Mølholm Hansen JM, Mortensen HB. Excretion of methimazole in human milk. Eur J Clin Pharmacol. 1982;23(4):339-41.
44. Azizi F, Khoshniat M, Bahrainian M, Hedayati M. Thyroid function and intellectual development of infants nursed by mothers taking methimazole. J Clin Endocrinol Metab. 2000;85(9):3233-8.
45. Mandel SJ, Cooper DS. The use of antithyroid drugs in pregnancy and lactation. J Clin Endocrinol Metab. 2001;86(6):2354-9.

SECTION 7

Thyroid Disorders in Children

CHAPTER 24

Congenital Hypothyroidism

Sunetra Mondal, Pradip Mukhopadhyay, Sujoy Ghosh

INTRODUCTION

Congenital hypothyroidism (CH) is the most common endocrine condition and a preventable cause of mental retardation worldwide. Thyroid hormones play an important role in central nervous system (CNS) maturation, neurogenesis, dendritic and axonal growth, and neurotransmitter synthesis in the antenatal and early postnatal periods. Untreated severe CH, thus, leads to neurological and psychodevelopmental defects including intellectual disability, spasticity, and disturbances of gait and coordination. The global prevalence of CH has increased from one in 6,700 before the advent of universal newborn screening to about one in 2,000–3,000 live births worldwide. The prevalence is reported to be higher in certain ethnicities such as the Asian, Native American, and Hispanic populations. As per data from the Indian Council of Medical Research (ICMR) National Task Force Team on New Born Screening at AIIMS, New Delhi (2007–2012), the prevalence in India is one in 1,130 live births. With universal screening, the devastating permanent neuropsychological disabilities due to untreated congenital hypothyroidism are a thing of the past. Unfortunately, the diagnosis is often late in developing countries like India, with average age at presentation being 4.1 years. The average prevalence of congenital central hypothyroidism is 1:16,000.

ETIOLOGY

Congenital hypothyroidism can be transient or permanent. Temporary CH may normalize within the first few months or years of life. Primary CH results from a defect in the embryologic development of the thyroid gland (dysgenesis), accounting for up to 85% of the cases, or an inborn error of thyroid hormone synthesis (dyshormonogenesis), seen in 10–15% of cases. Though rare, secondary, or central hypothyroidism due to deficiency of thyroid stimulating hormone (TSH), in isolation or as a part of multiple pituitary hormone deficiencies, may also manifest as CH. Peripheral hypothyroidism results from defects of thyroid hormone transport, metabolism, or action (**Box 1**).

> **BOX 1: Etiology of congenital hypothyroidism (CH).**
>
> **Primary CH**
> - *Thyroid dysgenesis*: Aplasia, hemiagenesis, hypoplasia, and ectopic gland
> - *Thyroid dyshormonogenesis*: Due to defects in genes encoding sodium-iodide symporter (*NIS* mutation)
>   - Thyroid peroxidase
>   (Hydrogen peroxide generation or maturation defects—*DUOX2, DUOXA2* gene mutations)
>   - Pendrin
>   - Thyroglobulin
>   - Deiodinase (*DEHAL1, SECISBP2* gene mutation)
> - *Resistance to thyroid stimulating hormone (TSH) binding or signaling*:
>   - TSH receptor defect
>   - G protein defect (Pseudohypoparathyroidism type 1a)
>
> **Secondary (central) CH**
> - Isolated TSH deficiency (due to defects in *TSHB, TRHR, IGSF1, TBL1X,* or *IRS4* genes)
> - Congenital hypopituitarism (multiple pituitary hormone deficiency)
>
> **Peripheral CH**
> - Thyroid hormone transport defect (*MCT8* gene mutation)
> - Thyroid hormone resistance (thyroid hormone receptor beta mutation, less commonly alpha mutation)
>
> **Transient CH**
> - Maternal or neonatal excess iodine exposure
> - Maternal or neonatal iodine deficiency
> - Transplacental transfer of maternal antithyroid drugs
> - Transplacental transfer of maternal TSH receptor blocking—antibody heterozygous DUOX2 or DUOXA2 mutations
> - Congenital hepatic hemangiomas
> - Central neonatal hypothyroidism due to maternal hyperthyroidism

PERMANENT CONGENITAL HYPOTHYROIDISM

Thyroid Dysgenesis

It occurs due to defects in any of the developmental steps necessary for transformation of pluripotent stem cells to functional thyrocytes. Thyroid dysgenesis manifests as a spectrum of abnormalities from athyreosis, hypoplasia, and hemiagenesis to ectopic thyroid without normal thyroid function. Thyroid ectopy results due to block in thyroid migration from foramen caecum to its final position. It accounts for two-thirds of cases of thyroid dysgenesis and is more common in females. Though ectopic thyroid can manifest as CH, but some cases can manifest only during childhood or adolescence during periods of increasing demand for thyroid hormones when the ectopic thyroid with maldeveloped lateral lobes fail to proliferate. Thyroid hypoplasia can rarely result from mutations in the TSH receptor gene or mutations in the Gs alpha resulting in resistance to the action of TSH.

Thyroid Dyshormonogenesis

The presence of goiter in a newborn could point toward defects in thyroid hormonogenesis, which may result from defects in a number of different genes controlling important proteins involved in thyroid hormone synthesis. Iodide is taken up into the thyrocyte by the NIS, which is then released into the follicle by the apical membrane protein SLC26A4. Thyroglobulin (TG) is synthesized and released from the thyrocyte into the follicular lumen. Iodide is oxidized and gets bound to tyrosine residues on TG thus forming mono- and diiodotyrosines (MIT and DIT). These are then coupled to form thyroxine (T4), and to a lesser extent triiodothyronine (T3). These reactions of iodination and coupling are catalyzed by thyroid peroxidase (TPO). These actions of TPO are catalyzed by hydrogen peroxide generated by dual oxidase 2 (DUOX2) and dual oxidase maturation factor 2 (DUOXA2). While T4 and T3 are released into blood, the iodide bound to MIT; DIT is recycled by the iodotyrosine dehydrogenase (IYD/DEHAL1). Mutation in any of these genes can result in thyroid dyshormonogenesis. All these defects are inherited in an autosomal recessive fashion, except DUOXA2, which is autosomal dominant. The most common disorders arise due to TPO mutations, while the most severe mutation is due to defects in TG mutations.

Secondary or Central Hypothyroidism

Central congenital hypothyroidism commonly arises as a part of combined pituitary hormone deficiency, occurring due to structural defects of the hypothalamo pituitary region or transcription factors. These can be classified as CPHD without pituitary malformations (mutation in POU1F1, PROP1), CPHD with pituitary malformation (isolated pituitary stalk interruption syndrome) or syndromic CPHD (septo-optic dysplasia, holoprosencephaly, Arnold–Chiari malformations). The latter has associated midline defects, midbrain, or cerebellar defects, optic nerve problems along with manifestations of CPHD. In the past few years, a number of different genes have been identified, the defects in which could result in isolated TSH deficiency. These include TSHB, TRHR, TBL1X, IRS4, and IGSF1.

Peripheral Defects in Thyroid Hormone Metabolism

Mutations in genes encoding monocarboxylate transporter 8 (MCT8) impair the entry of T3 into neurons, and result in an X-linked hypothyroidism associated with mental retardation, also known as Allan–Herndon–Dudley syndrome.

Peripheral resistance to the action of thyroid hormone occurs due to mutations in genes encoding for thyroid hormone receptor beta (TR beta). These are dominantly inherited and affected individuals are only rarely hypothyroid. Due to mild elevation of circulating T3 and T4 are mildly elevated and TSH levels are often nonsuppressed (within normal range), these infants are not detected on neonatal screening tests.

TRANSIENT CONGENITAL HYPOTHYROIDISM

Causes of transient CH include iodine deficiency, transplacental passage of maternal TSH-binding inhibitory antibodies, and maternal exposure to radioiodine, iodine or antithyroid drugs, neonatal iodine exposure, liver hemangiomas (expressing large amounts of type 3 iodothyronine deiodinase leading to consumptive type of hypothyroidism) or mutations in DUOX2 (THOX2) and DUOXA2. Another scenario is a false positive screening test due to premature TSH estimation (on the first day of life) due to physiological TSH surge. Similarly, a transiently low T3 syndrome can be seen in premature and sick neonates due to a syndrome akin to adult nonthyroidal illness. In the study by Nair et al., thyroid hormone supplementation could be discontinued at 3 years in 50% of children diagnosed with CH. In these cases, it is better to institute T4 replacement until it becomes apparent that the dose need not be increased in order to curtail the TSH levels or till the child is 3 years old, when it is safe to stop therapy for 4–6 weeks to assess need for continued replacement.

CLINICAL FEATURES

Symptoms of CH are mostly subtle. Points in history should include period of gestation, maternal hyperthyroidism, maternal intake of antithyroid drugs, maternal iodine deficient diet or inadvertent radioactive iodine treatment during pregnancy. An infant with overt CH may be born post-term, with birth weight greater than the 19th percentile

TABLE 1: Syndromic associations of congenital hypothyroidism (CH).

Extrathyroidal manifestations (syndrome)	Candidate gene
Deafness (Pendred's syndrome)	SLC26A4/PDS TBL1X (central CH)
Cleft palate, "spiky hair" (Bamforth–Lazarus syndrome)	FOXE1 (previously TTF-2)
Kidney agenesis or other genitourinary malformation	PAX8
Choreoathetosis, neonatal respiratory distress due to surfactant deficiency (brain–lung–thyroid syndrome)	NKX2-1 (previously TTF-1)
Cardiac defects	NKX2-5
Short stature, obesity, hypocalcemia	GNAS
Glaucoma, polycystic kidneys, hepatic fibrosis, neonatal diabetes	GLIS3
Septo-optic dysplasia	HESX1, SOX2, SOX3, and OTX2
Macroorchidism, delayed puberty, increased BMI, and fat percentage, acromegaloid facies	IGSF1

and have delayed physiological jaundice, poor feeding, hoarse cry, umbilical hernia, macroglossia, and cold or mottled skin. They can have a wide posterior fontanelle >5 mm in maximum diameter. Goiter can be present in infants with transient hypothyroidism due to maternal Graves' disease or antithyroid drug intake, iodine exposure to mother or infant, severe maternal iodine deficiency or thyroid dyshormonogenesis. Rare clinical manifestations include bradycardia and hypotonia with delayed reflexes.

Congenital Malformations

Distinct clinical phenotypes can provide a clue to the underlying gene mutation as summarized in **Table 1**.

SCREENING

Neonatal screening programs for CH have successfully eliminated the profound deleterious consequences of thyroid hormone deficiency on growth and neurodevelopment outcomes, and are one of the most cost-effective screening programs worldwide. Unfortunately, only 25% of infants worldwide are born in areas with universal screening programs. Ironically, most of the areas without neonatal screening programs also have endemic iodine deficiency. Since primary CH is several folds more common than central CH, the initial priority of neonatal screening for CH focuses on the detection of all forms and severity of primary CH. The first CH screening program in India was undertaken at BJ Wadia Hospital, Mumbai in 1982 using cord blood TSH followed by postnatal DBS T4 in 1984. A number of controversial areas exist till date regarding screening strategies, types of samples, and assay methods for CH screening, which have been summarized in **Table 2**. A screening strategy appropriate for the Indian settings is outlined in **Flowchart 1**. Normative data for Indian preterm infants may be used to interpret data available for premature babies **(Table 3)**. If DBS is used as a screening method, TSH is assayed using immunofluorescence or colorimetric neonatal TSH kit (e.g., Perkin Elmer® or Biorad®) at a centralized laboratory.

DIAGNOSTIC EVALUATION

An approach to establishment of etiologic diagnosis in CH is outlined in **Flowcharts 2A and B**. However, diagnostic studies are not necessary to start treatment though findings do have prognostic and help separate transient from permanent cases facilitate the choice of genetic tests required. Ultrasonography and nuclear scintigraphy have complimentary roles in the diagnostic evaluation of CH. Scanning with 10–20 MBq (0.27–0.54 mCi) of ^{99m}Tc is favored as it can be done in 20 minutes in contrast to scintigraphy with 1–2 MBq (0.027–0.054 mCi) of I^{123} that takes several hours, is more expensive and less widely available. However, I^{123} is mandatory for a perchlorate discharge test. A discharge of > 10% after 2 hours administration indicates an organification defect. Though ultrasonography is highly observer-dependent and sometimes misdiagnose non-thyroidal tissue in thyroid fossa as a hypoplastic thyroid, in resource limited settings, it can be the first line imaging and guides the need for scintigraphy. Color flow Doppler can detect ectopic thyroid tissue in up to 90% of cases. Serum thyroglobulin (TG) levels can reflect the amount of thyroid tissue and with proper assay can be an important tool in the diagnostic algorithm. There is a role for urinary iodine estimation in areas of endemic iodine deficiency. Absence of epiphyses around the knees on X-rays indicates severe prenatal hypothyroidism. The diagnostic algorithms to a case of CH in set-ups with and without scintigraphy facilities are outlined in **Flowcharts 2A and B** respectively.

Role of Genetic Testing

Targeted genetic testing by newer techniques such as comparative genomic hybridization (CGH) array, next-generation sequencing (NGS) of gene panels (targeted NGS), or nontargeted whole exome sequencing (WES) can be performed to arrive at a genetic diagnosis for cases of CH. Genetic testing can give a confirmatory diagnosis for CH. Apart from its role in genetic counseling and research settings, a genetic diagnosis can help identify cases of transient and permanent hypothyroidism very early in life and thus obviates the need for discontinuation and retesting later in life for permanent cases. Also, identification of mutated genes related to particular syndromes can guide the screening for associated extrathyroidal malformations **(Table 1)**. Presence of syndromic features should guide

THYROID DISORDERS IN CHILDREN

TABLE 2: Comparison of different methods and strategies for neonatal screening for congenital hypothyroidism and recommendations by recent guidelines.

Type of sample		Guidelines
Cord blood sample	**Postnatal sample**	
Collected from placental end of cord	Collected after 72 hours (D3–D5), rarely 48 hours after birth	*ISPAE 2018, ESPE-ESE 2021*: Either cord blood or postnatal day, 3–day, 5 samples
Advantages: • No effect of physiologic TSH surge • Painless sampling of large quantity of blood • Allows screening of early discharged cases • Report ready before discharge, parents can be counseled	**Advantages:** • Allows screening of other inborn errors of metabolism such as CAH and disorders dependent on feeding (e.g., galactosemia, PKU) • Less need for training or logistics • Recommended for NBS in special situation (as described in the text)	
Disadvantages: • Metabolic disorders which depend on feeding may not be tested • Round the clock personnel need to be trained, not just morning shift • Result may be affected by perinatal factors such as birth asphyxia	**Disadvantages:** • False positive screen in case of early discharge • Painful • Special assay system required if measured on dried blood filter paper sample by heel prick	

Screening strategy				Guidelines
T4	**TSH**	**Primary T4, backup TSH**	**Simultaneous T4, TSH**	
• Identifies primary and central CH • US, Israel	• Most sensitive for primary CH; • Most commonly used; • Can detect mild/compensated CH; • Most cost-effective • ISPAE	• TSH is measured from the same DBS for those samples with T4 in the lowest percentiles (from 3–20%) for that day —> if TSH > cut-off, neonates are recalled for confirmatory venous samples • Very low false positive and recall rates • Netherlands	Best strategy	*ISPAE 2018*: Primary TSH *ESPE-ESE 2021(18)*: • Primary TSH most sensitive • If resources available, simultaneous TSH + Total/free T4
• Misses mild CH – important in ectopic thyroid • False positive in TBG deficiency, preterm and sick neonates	• Misses central TSH • Delayed TSH rise in some infants, so preterm • False positive if drawn < 48 hours	Costly	Not cost-effective	

Type of assay		Guidelines
Cord blood or postnatal heel prick filter paper DBS	**Cord blood or venous postnatal sample**	*ISPAE 2018*: TSH measured from a DBS should be expressed in whole blood units. Serum units may be derived by multiplying the whole blood units value by 2.2
• Transported to a central NBS laboratory • Filter paper sample requires special equipment and assay kits • Only small amount of serum is available from a filter paper punch	• Sent to a routine laboratory in a plain vacutainer • ELISA or chemiluminescence methods at routine laboratories	

Special subgroups

- *Preterm, LBW, sick infants*: Second specimen at ~ 10–14 days of age
- *Down syndrome*: TSH measurement at the end of neonatal period
- *Twins*: Second screening for same sex affected twins; F/U nonaffected twin for possible delayed TSH rise
- *Clinical suspicion, normal screening, or family history*: Further evaluation, irrespective of screening results

(CAH: congenital adrenal hyperplasia; D3: day 3 after birth; D5: day 5 after birth; DBS: dried blood sample; ELISA: enzyme linked immunosorbent assay; ESE: European Society for Endocrinology; ESPE: European Society for Pediatric Endocrinology; F/U: follow-up; ISPAE: Indian Society for Pediatric and Adolescent Endocrinology; LBW: low birth weight; NBS: newborn screening; PKU: phenylketonuria)

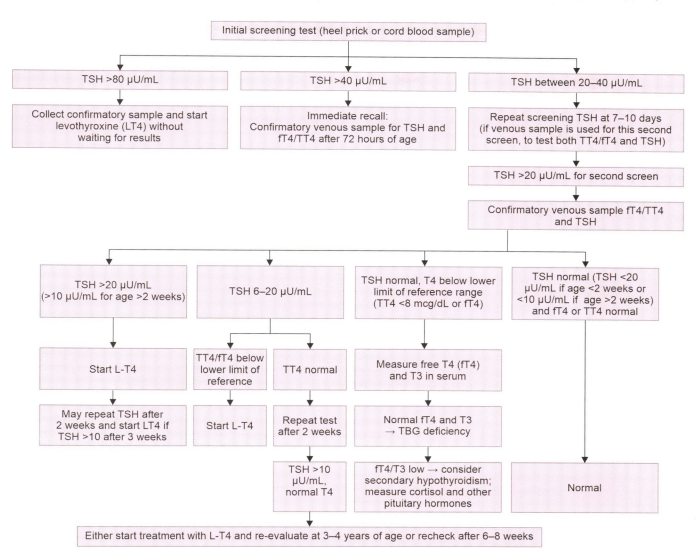

Flowchart 1: Algorithm for confirmatory diagnosis and treatment after screening at birth.
(TSH: thyroid stimulating hormone)
Source: Modified and adapted from ISPAE 2018 and ESE-ESPE 2021 guidelines.

TABLE 3: Normative data for thyroid function parameters for preterm babies at 3–7 days of life and 4 weeks.										
Parameters (n = 102)	Day 3–7 (percentile)					4 weeks after birth (percentile)				
	2.5th	25th	75th	97.5th	Median	Median	2.5th	25th	75th	97.5th
TSH (µIU/mL)	1.69	3.72	8.28	26.45	5.02	2.87	0.07	1.68	4.17	13.97
T3 (ng/dL)	66	128	185	264	152	98	45	77	122	200
T4 (µg/dL)	6.6	10.3	15.0	22.0	12.8	11.2	5.4	9.1	14.7	21.7
Free T4 (ng/dL)	0.76	1.16	1.77	3.10	1.38	1.33	0.81	1.20	1.67	2.39
(TSH: thyroid stimulating hormone)										

testing for responsible genes. In nonsyndromic cases, the choice of panel of genes to be tested would depend on findings on imaging and other biochemical findings **(Flowcharts 2A and B)**. Though most genetic cases are thyroid dyshormonogenesis, certain forms of dysgenesis and central CH too are inherited. Genetic counseling should focus on explaining the inheritance pattern and the risk of recurrence based on the patient's CH subtype, family history, and, if known, the (genetic) etiology.

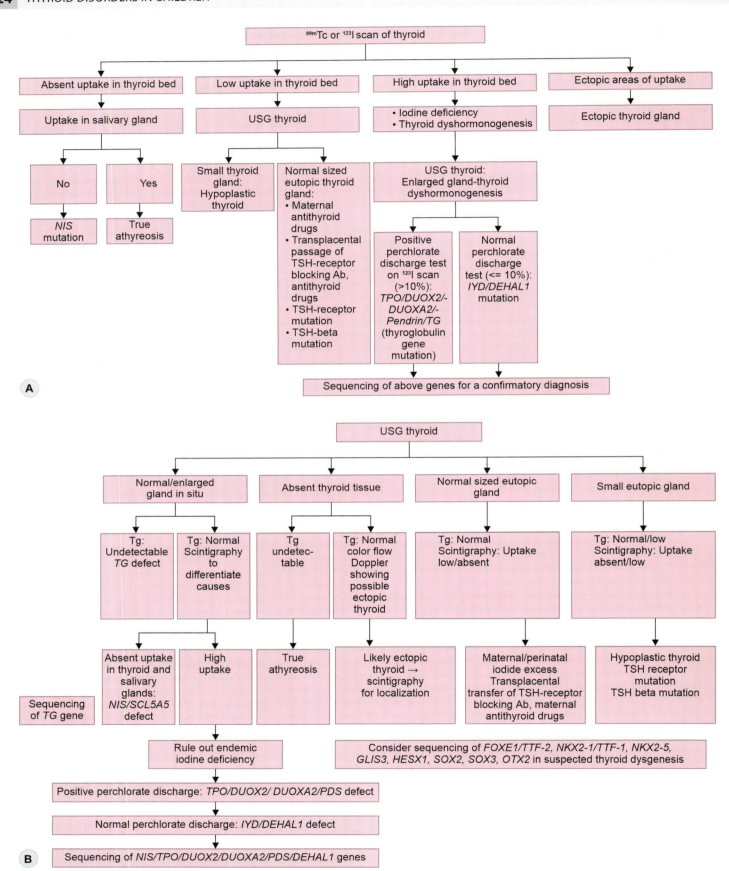

Flowcharts 2A and B: Diagnostic algorithm for congenital hypothyroidism in clinical set-ups where thyroid scintigraphy is available (A) or not available (B).

(^{123}I: iodine-123; ^{99m}Tc: technetium-99m; Tg: thyroglobulin; USG: ultrasonography)

ENDEMIC CRETINISM

Endemic cretinism occurs in regions of severe iodine deficiency and manifests in two major clinical patterns, myxedematous and neurological, or sometimes with combined features of both. Severe maternal iodine deficiency in early gestation results in impaired brain development and permanent neurologic sequelae. Those who subsequently develop goiter can compensate for the T4 deficiency and develop as neurologic cretins with manifestations including mental retardation, deaf mutism, squint, and cerebral diplegia. Those who have thyroid gland atrophies go on to become myxedematous cretin due to severe and persistent hypothyroxinemia with severe growth retardation and myxedematous features. Endemic cretinism is now reduced widely in India due to nationwide iodine-fortification of salt.

TREATMENT AND MONITORING

The goal of therapy is to rapidly restore and maintain clinical and biochemical euthyroidism as soon as possible so that these children develop physically and mentally to the best of their genetic potential. Levothyroxine (L-T4) administered orally is the treatment of choice. A brand rather than a generic formulation is recommended.

L-T4 must be started within the first 2 weeks of life and immediately after confirmatory test results in infants identified in a second screening test. L-T4 is taken in the morning, before feeding, and it should be administered in the same time daily, avoiding nutritional supplements such as soy protein formulas or drugs that interfere with LT4 absorption.

The recommended initial L-T4 dose set forth by most guidelines for CH is 10–15 µg/kg/day. Infants with severe CH, defined by a very low pretreatment fT4 (<5 pmol/L) or total T4 with elevated TSH should receive the highest doses. Those with mild CH (fT4 >10 pmol/L with elevated TSH) should receive lower initial dose (~ 10 µg/kg/day) and those infants with fT4 concentrations within the normal age-specific reference interval should be started on an even lower dose (from 5–10 µg/kg). The dose requirement decreases to 4–5 µg/day by 5 years due to decreased rate of T4 turnover. Monitoring the children clinically and biochemically is important at frequent intervals **(Table 4)**.

RE-EVALUATION OF CONGENITAL HYPOTHYROIDISM

Re-evaluation of the thyroid axis is recommended in cases where no etiological diagnostic assessment was carried out during early infancy. Permanent CH can be assumed if:
- Thyroid gland is absent/ectopic
- Dyshormonogenesis has been demonstrated as the cause (except DUOXA2) or

TABLE 4: Goals and monitoring of treatment of CH.	
Biochemical goals	• Serum fT4 or total T4 levels in the upper range of normal during the first year of life • TSH is to be kept in the age-specific reference range • TSH may remain elevated for prolonged period during infancy due to alteration of feedback system • If TSH > or within age-specific reference and patient is asymptomatic, fT4 > ULN may be acceptable without change in LT4 dose • Reduction in dose only if TSH suppressed or fT4 high with signs of over-treatment (jitteriness/ tachycardia)
Frequency of follow-up	• First follow-up examination 1–2 weeks after the start of L-T4 treatment (1 week for doses > = 50 µg/day) then, • Every 2 weeks until TSH levels are normalized • After normalization of T4/Free T4; every 1–3 months, until age of 12 months • Between 1–3 years; regular evaluations every 3–6 months until growth is completed • More frequent monitoring if questionable compliance or abnormal values are obtained • 4–6 weeks after any change in L-T4 dose or L-T4 formulation
Adverse events	• For children with preexisting cardiac insufficiency, L-T4 should be introduced at 50% of the target dose with slow increment • Growth deceleration could indicate overtreatment —> bone age estimations • Risks of benign intracranial hypertension, attention-deficit-hyperactivity disorder and rarely, craniosynostosis with overdosage —> symptoms to be explained to parents/caregivers
Additional aspects	• Neurocognition including psychomotor, language development, and school progression, behavior, memory, hearing and visuospatial skills to be evaluated • Adequately treated infants have normal growth, puberty, fertility, and bone health • Lifestyle interventions encouraged to maintain optimal weight • If planning pregnancy —> optimization of LT4 treatment; counseling regarding need for higher doses of LT4 during pregnancy, target TSH <2.5 mU/L throughout gestation; lower to preconception dose post-pregnancy • Primary CH due to dyshormonogenesis may develop goiter and nodule, TSH to be targeted in lower part of reference, periodic ultrasound. Suspicious nodules on USG —> evaluation with fine needle aspiration

(CH: congenital hypothyroidism; TSH: thyroid stimulating hormone; ULN: upper limit normal; USG: ultrasonography)

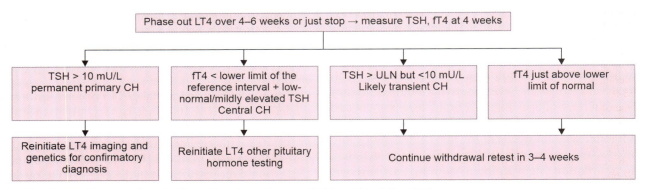

Flowchart 3: Protocol for re-evaluation for permanence of congenital hypothyroidism (CH).
(TSH: thyroid stimulating hormone; ULN: upper limit normal)

- If at any time during the first year of life, TSH rises above 20 mU/L.

Reevaluation is usually done after the age of 3 years, though earlier reevaluation may be indicated in newborns in whom thyroid peroxidase or TSH receptor antibodies are detectable in the blood; and when an eutopic, normally sized gland is found. A protocol to phase off LT4 for reevaluation is outlined in **Flowchart 3**. If a child with eutopic thyroid gland requires an LT4 dose <3 μg/kg/day at the age of 6 months, then reevaluation may be done this early.

ANTENATAL DIAGNOSIS AND TREATMENT

Antenatal diagnosis of CH should be considered if a goiter is discovered on routine fetal ultrasound, if there is a family history of dyshormonogenesis or known defects of genes involved in CH with potential germ line transmission. If fetal thyroid measurement values based on diameter or perimeter are above the 95th percentile, the mother and fetus should be referred to a specialized center for antenatal treatment. Ultrasound at 20–24 weeks of gestation should be used to detect fetal goiter or absence of thyroid tissue. Clinical scenario and ultrasound give the diagnosis in most cases. If unclear, for assessment of thyroid function, cordocentesis, rather than amniocentesis should be done. In cases of large fetal goiter with hydramnios and/or tracheal occlusion, if the mother is hypothyroid, she should be treated, while for the euthyroid mother, fetal treatment by intra-amniotic T4 injections is recommended at a dose of 10 μg/kg estimated fetal weight every 15 days with monitoring of goiter size.

CONCLUSION

Universal screening for CH can help eliminate globally the debilitating consequences of untreated CH. Screening and diagnostic algorithms should be tailored depending on resources. Timely institution of LT4 with appropriate monitoring is indicated in all cases of CH.

SUGGESTED READINGS

1. van Trotsenburg P, Stoupa A, Léger J, Rohrer T, Peters C, Fugazzola L, et al. Congenital hypothyroidism: a 2020–2021 consensus guidelines update–an ENDO-European reference network initiative endorsed by the European Society for pediatric endocrinology and the European Society for endocrinology. Thyroid. 2021;31(3):387-419.
2. Desai MP, Sharma R, Riaz I, Sudhanshu S, Parikh R, Bhatia V. Newborn screening guidelines for congenital hypothyroidism in India: recommendations of the Indian Society for Pediatric and Adolescent Endocrinology (ISPAE)—Part I: screening and confirmation of diagnosis. Indian J Pediatr. 2018;85(6):440-7.
3. Sudhanshu S, Riaz I, Sharma R, Desai MP, Parikh R, Bhatia V. Newborn screening guidelines for congenital hypothyroidism in India: recommendations of the Indian Society for Pediatric and Adolescent Endocrinology (ISPAE)—Part II: Imaging, treatment and follow-up. Indian J Pediatr. 2018;85(6):448-53.
4. Mondal S, Mukhopadhyay P, Ghosh S. Clinical approach to congenital hypothyroidism. Thyroid Res Pract. 2017;14(2):45.
5. LaFranchi SH. Approach to the diagnosis and treatment of neonatal hypothyroidism. J Clin Endocrinol Metab. 2011;96:2959-67.
6. Prabhu S, Mahadevan S, Jagadeesh S, Suresh S. Congenital hypothyroidism: recent Indian data. Indian J Endocrinol Metab. 2015;19(3):436-7.
7. Virmani A, Menon PS, Karmarkar MG, Gopinath PG, Padhy AK. Profile of thyroid disorders in a referral centre in North India. Indian Pediatr. 1989;26:265-9.
8. García M, Fernández A, Moreno JC. Central hypothyroidism in children. Paediatr Thyroidol. 2014;26:79-107.
9. Park SM, Chatterjee VK. Genetics of congenital hypothyroidism. J Med Genet. 2005;42:379-89.
10. Cangul H, Aycan Z, Olivera-Nappa A, Saglam H, Schoenmakers NA, Boelaert K, et al. Thyroid dyshormonogenesis is mainly caused by TPO mutations in consanguineous community. Clin Endocrinol (Oxf). 2013;79:275-81.
11. Kostopoulou E, Miliordos K, Spiliotis B. Genetics of primary congenital hypothyroidism—a review. Hormones. 2021;20(2):225-36.
12. Lauffer P, Zwaveling-Soonawala N, Naafs JC, Boelen A, Van Trotsenburg AP. Diagnosis and management of central congenital hypothyroidism. Front Endocrinol. 2021;12:686317.

13. Stevenson RE, Goodman HO, Schwartz CE, Simensen RJ, McLean WT Jr., Herndon CN. Allan–Herndon syndrome. I. clinical studies. Am J Hum Genet. 1990;47:446-53.
14. Huang SA, Tu HM, Harney JW, Venihaki M, Butte AJ, Kozakewich HP, et al. Severe hypothyroidism caused by type 3 iodothyronine deiodinase in infantile hemangiomas. N Engl J Med. 2000;343:185-9.
15. Delange F, Fisher DA. The thyroid gland. In: Brook CG (Ed). Clinical Pediatric Endocrinology. 3rd edition. London: Blackwell Science; 1995. pp. 397-433.
16. Nair PS, Sobhakumar S, Kailas L. Diagnostic re-evaluation of children with congenital hypothyroidism. Indian Pediatr. 2010;47(9):757-60.
17. Ford G, LaFranchi SH. Screening for congenital hypothyroidism: a worldwide view of strategies. Best Pract Res Clin Endocrinol Metab. 2014;28:175-87.
18. Colaco MP, Desai MP, Ajgaonkar AR, Mahadik CV, Vas FE, Bandivdekar AN, et al. Neonatal screening for hypothyroidism. Indian Pediatr. 1984;21:695-700.
19. Desai MP, Upadhye P, Colaco MP, Mehre M, Naik SP, Vaz FE, et al. Neonatal screening for congenital hypothyroidism using the filter paper thyroxine technique. Indian J Med Res. 1994;100:36-42.
20. S choen EJ, Clapp W, To TT, Fireman BH. The key role of newborn thyroid scintigraphy with isotopic iodide (^{123}I) in defining and managing congenital hypothyroidism. Pediatrics. 2004;114:e683-8.
21. Léger J, Olivieri A, Donaldson M, Torresani T, Krude H, van Vliet G, et al. European Society for Paediatric Endocrinology consensus guidelines on screening, diagnosis, and management of congenital hypothyroidism. Horm Res Paediatr. 2014;81:80-103.
22. Jones JH, Attaie M, Maroo S, Neumann D, Perry R, Donaldson MD. Heterogeneous tissue in the thyroid fossa on ultrasound in infants with proven thyroid ectopia on isotope scan: a diagnostic trap. Pediatr Radiol. 2010;40:725-31.
23. Rastogi MV, LaFranchi SH. Congenital hypothyroidism. Orphanet J Rare Dis. 2010;5:17.
24. Grosse SD, Van Vliet G. Prevention of intellectual disability through screening for congenital hypothyroidism: How much and at what level? Arch Dis Child. 2011;96:374-9.
25. Boyages SC, Halpern JP, Maberly GF, Eastman CJ, Morris J, Collins J, et al. A comparative study of neurological and myxedematous endemic cretinism in western China. J Clin Endocrinol Metab. 1988;67(6):1262-71.
26. Van Vliet G, Diaz Escagedo P. Redefining congenital hypothyroidism? J Clin Endocrinol Metab. 2021;106(3):e1463-5.
27. Matejek N, Tittel SR, Haberland H, Rohrer T, Busemann EM, Jorch N, et al. Predictors of transient congenital primary hypothyroidism: data from the German registry for congenital hypothyroidism (AQUAPE "HypoDok"). European J Pediatr. 2021;180(8):2401-8.
28. Ranzini AC, Ananth CV, Smulian JC, Kung M, Limbachia A, Vintzileos AM. Ultrasonography of the fetal thyroid: nomograms based on biparietal diameter and gestational age. J Ultrasound Med. 2001;20:613-7.
29. Mukherjee D, Mukhopadhyay P, Sen S, Saha B, Ghosh S. Thyroid function in preterm neonates. Unpublished data 2022.

CHAPTER 25

Hypothyroidism in Children

Rashi Agrawal, Nisha Bhavani

INTRODUCTION

Hypothyroidism like in adults is the most common thyroid related illness in children. Hypofunctioning of thyroid gland leading to hypothyroidism is referred to as primary hypothyroidism and any defect in hypothalamic–pituitary–thyroid axis causing decreased production of thyroid hormones is referred to as secondary or central hypothyroidism.

Primary hypothyroidism can be in the form of overt hypothyroidism (OH) or subclinical hypothyroidism (SCH). Among Indian children, the prevalence of SCH and OH has been reported as 6.1% and 0.4% in a study conducted on 39,000 school children by Marwaha et al. Their prevalence of goiter has been reported to be between 16 and 23%.

ETIOLOGY

Autoimmune thyroiditis (AIT): Since iodization of salt became a routine, AIT has become the most common cause of hypothyroidism in children and is also referred to as Hashimoto's thyroiditis or chronic lymphocytic thyroiditis. Like adults AIT is more common in females than in males. In a study conducted among 4,320 school children aged 10–16 years in Delhi by Gopalakrishnan et al., AIT was found in 3.9% girls versus 1.4% boys.

The hallmark of the condition lies in presence of autoantibodies to one or more of thyroid antigens, i.e., antithyroid peroxidase antibody (anti-TPO-Ab) or antithyroglobulin antibody (anti-Tg-Ab). Sensitivity of anti-TPO-Ab in AIT is about 90% and that of anti-Tg is 60–80%. Presence of anti-TPO-Ab is almost a sine qua non in case of AIT. The histopathology is characterized by lymphocytic infiltration, lymphoid germinal centers, and destruction of thyroid follicles. The intrathyroidal lymphocytes are both B and T lymphocytes. B cell activation results in production of anti-TPO-Ab and anti-Tg-Ab which belong to IgG1 and IgG3 subclass and are polyclonal in nature. AIT can present as goitrous and atrophic forms. Goiter formation occurs due to one of the mechanisms mentioned above whereas atrophic thyroiditis is the result of cell-mediated cytotoxicity and apoptosis of follicular cells. Complement-dependent antibody-mediated cytotoxicity may also contribute to thyroid damage. Children with AIT can remain euthyroid for variable periods of time, or develop SCH followed by OH. The rate of development of hypothyroidism from euthyroid state is about 5% per year. Rarely, children can present with transient hyperthyroidism lasting <3 months preceding hypothyroidism known as Hashitoxicosis. This results from release of preformed thyroid hormone during destructive thyroiditis followed by hypothyroidism once stored hormone supply is exhausted.

Syndromes associated with AIT: Children with chromosomal anomalies and other autoimmune diseases such as Down syndrome, Turner syndrome, Klinefelter syndrome, type 1 diabetes mellitus (T1DM), celiac disease, vitiligo, and Addison's disease are more susceptible to AIT and resulting hypothyroidism.

Children with Down syndrome have increased prevalence of both congenital hypothyroidism (CH) and autoimmune hypothyroidism. About 20–30% children with Down syndrome have AIT with concomitant presence of anti-TPO-Ab. These children should be screened at birth and then at 6 months, 12 months, and then annually for AIT and hypothyroidism.

Patients with Turner syndrome who have isochromosome Xq or deletion of Xp are much more susceptible to AIT compared to patients with 45 X chromosomes. Untreated hypothyroidism can contribute to short stature associated with Turner syndrome.

Autoimmunity of thyroid is present in up to 30% children with T1DM and warrants annual screening since these children do not have overt features of hypothyroidism during initial stages of the disease. Hypothyroidism in T1DM can contribute to hypoglycemia.

Autoimmune thyroiditis can also occur as part of syndromes of autoimmunity. While autoimmune polyglandular syndrome (APS) type I is more commonly associated with hypoparathyroidism, adrenal insufficiency, and mucocutaneous candidiasis, about 10% of these patients have hypothyroidism. However, in APS, II, 70% children have chronic AIT which has autoimmune diabetes and adrenal insufficiency as its other major manifestations.

In immunodysregulation polyendocrinopathy enteropathy X-linked (IPEX) syndrome, AIT may present in infancy as part of polyendocrinopathy.

Subacute granulomatous thyroiditis: This condition is a postviral syndrome, also referred to as de Quervain thyroiditis which is characterized by diffuse tender goiter, elevated erythrocyte sedimentation rate, and a transient period of hyperthyroidism followed by hypothyroidism and then recovery. This can be distinguished from suppurative thyroiditis caused by bacterial infections by the absence of fever and leukocytosis. Also suppurative thyroiditis usually does not have a period of hyperthyroidism.

Iodine deficiency or excess: Iodine deficiency remains the most common preventable cause of hypothyroidism and intellectual disability worldwide. Though the prevalence of endemic goiter has reduced drastically after routine fortification of salt and other food products such as dairy by iodine, it still continues to remain as a minor public health concern.

As per the survey conducted by the National Nutrition Monitoring Board (NNMB) in 2000–2001 in rural areas of Kerala, Tamil Nadu, Karnataka, Andhra Pradesh, Maharashtra, Madhya Pradesh, Odisha, and West Bengal, the overall prevalence of total goiter rate (TGR) among 6–12-year-old children was about 4%. The prevalence of goiter was highest in Maharashtra (11.9%) and West Bengal (9%).

Iodine excess on the other hand commonly occurs due to routine use of iodine containing antiseptics in newborn nurseries and intensive care units, and use of iodinated contrast agents for imaging. This can cause transient downregulation of sodium iodide symporter on the luminal aspect of follicular cells leading to transient hypothyroidism known as Wolff–Chaikoff effect. This phase is transient and lasts only until these channels escape the downregulation following which hyperthyroidism ensues, which is known as Jod–Basedow phenomenon.

Post-therapy hypothyroidism: In children with Graves' disease, treated with antithyroid drugs, about half achieve remission by 3 years of therapy and become euthyroid. About 10% of children are rendered hypothyroid with antithyroid drugs alone. Children who require radioiodine therapy or thyroidectomy for control of hyperthyroidism will be rendered hypothyroid permanently requiring lifelong thyroid hormone supplementation.

Infiltrative conditions: Infiltrative disorders which cause deposition of substances or inflammatory cells in the thyroid gland such a cystine crystals in cystinosis, histiocytes in Langerhans cell histiocytosis, iron deposition in hemochromatosis, and thalassemia can give rise to atrophic thyroiditis which is associated with hypothyroidism in children.

Drugs: Several drugs like antithyroid medications, antiepileptics such as phenytoin, phenobarbital, valproate, lithium, immunomodulating agents, and anticancer drugs including interferon α, tyrosine kinase inhibitors (TKIs), immune checkpoint inhibitors (ICIs), and iodine-containing drugs like amiodarone may cause hypothyroidism albeit by different mechanisms.

Late onset congenital hypothyroidism: Some forms of CH owing to thyroid dysgenesis like ectopic thyroid gland and mild forms of dyshormonogenesis can present in childhood as childhood hypothyroidism. Some other forms of CH due to neonatal iodine deficiency or excess and genetic mutations of DUOX2 and DUOXA2 can lead to delayed presentation of CH and is often a transient condition.

Central hypothyroidism: Acquired diseases of the hypothalamic-pituitary axis such as space occupying lesions such as craniopharyngoma and pituitary adenoma, local trauma, hemorrhage, vascular insult, necrosis, central nervous system (CNS) infections, and irradiation to brain can give rise to central hypothyroidism.

Congenital central hypothyroidism can occur as part of a congenital hypopituitarism due to developmental defects of midbrain or optic nerve hypoplasia known as septo-optic dysplasia. Though these defects are congenital, they may become apparent only later in life and hence appear acquired. These defects present as multiple pituitary hormone deficiency. Isolated thyroid-stimulating hormone (TSH) deficiency, on the other hand is caused by mutations in *IGSF1* gene or less commonly in thyroid-stimulating hormone β (TSH-β) subunit or thyrotropin-releasing hormone (TRH) receptor genes.

Certain drugs such as glucocorticoids and dopamine also suppress TSH secretion and hence can give rise to central hypothyroidism like biochemical picture.

Consumption of large quantities of goitrogens belonging to cassava family or green leafy vegetables can produce goiter and hypothyroidism.

Consumptive hypothyroidism: Hypothyroidism can occur in children with large hemangiomas involving the liver due to over expression of deiodinase type 3 enzyme which converts T4 to reverse T3 (rT3) and triiodothyronine (T3) to diiodothyronine (T2). Thus these infants have low T3 and T4 and elevated TSH and progressively increasing requirements of levothyroxine to achieve euthyroid state **(Fig. 1)**.

Thyroid hormone resistance: This is a rare genetic condition characterized by mutation in thyroid hormone receptor β (*THR-β*) gene and thus elevated serum T4 and T3 levels with concomitant normal or high TSH levels. Children with this genetic condition usually present later in life with symptoms of hyper- or hypothyroidism depending on the differential expression of thyroid hormone receptors α and β in different organs. Mutation of thyroid hormone receptor α (THR-α) gene is much less common.

The etiology of hypothyroidism in childhood is listed in **Box 1**.

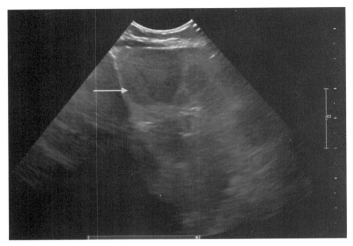

Fig. 1: Presence of liver hemangioma in a 2-month-old baby who presented with abdominal distension and hypothyroidism at 1 month of age.

> **BOX 1: Etiology of childhood hypothyroidism.**
>
> - *Chronic lymphocytic thyroiditis (Hashimoto thyroiditis—goitrous and atrophic)*: Reversible autoimmune hypothyroidism (postpartum, cytokine-induced thyroiditis)
> - *Iodine deficiency or excess*:
>   - Infective: Viral and bacterial infections causing subacute and acute thyroiditis
>   - Infiltrative: Cystinosis, hemochromatosis, thalassemia, and Langerhans cell histiocytosis
> - Post-thyroidectomy
> - *Post-radioablation of thyroid*: External irradiation for head and neck tumors
> - Drug induced (lithium, antithyroid drugs, antiepileptics, iodine-containing drugs, interferon α, aminosalicylic acid, aminoglutethimide, TKI, ICI)
> - *Late onset congenital hypothyroidism*: Goitrogens such as cassava, green leafy vegetables, soybeans, broccoli, cauliflower, cabbage
> - *Central hypothyroidism*: Tumors (meningioma, craniopharyngioma, pituitary adenoma, glioma, metastases)
>   - Trauma, irradiation, and head injury
>   - Vascular insult like stalk interruption, necrosis, and hemorrhage
>   - Infections
>   - Hypothalamic disorders
>   - Drugs: Dopamine, glucocorticoids, LT4 withdrawal
> - *Consumptive hypothyroidism*: Skin or liver hemangiomas overexpressing deiodinase 3
> - Thyroid hormone resistance
>
> (ICI: immune checkpoint inhibitor; TKI: tyrosine kinase inhibitor)

Subclinical Hypothyroidism

Subclinical hypothyroidism defined as TSH above the upper limit of normal with normal T4 and free T4 levels is also called isolated hyperthyrotropinemia. It indicates a compensated mild form of thyroid dysfunction. In children, the problem with TSH levels is that the upper limit varies widely depending on the age of the child and the assays used. So isolated persistent TSH elevation ideally on two separate occasions using different assays many days apart is needed to diagnose SCH in children. SCH can be classified into mild when TSH is between upper limit and 10 mIU/L and severe when its >10 mIU/L. The prevalence of SCH in children varies from 1.7 to 2.9% whereas Indian studies show a prevalence of 6.1–8.4%. Etiology of SCH is similar to that of OH. AIT is the most common cause of SCH in children of which half will progress and rest will either remain static or regress to normal thyroid function. Chances of progression of SCH to OH are more when associated with the genetic syndromes like Downs and Turner, in presence of high titres of anti-TPO-Abs and goiter. The association of SCH with obesity is alluded to subsequent section. Causes of neonatal hyperthyrotropinemia such as DUOX2 and TSHR mutations, pseudohypoparathyroidism, brain-lung-thyroid syndrome, and ectopic thyroid gland can present as SCH in children. Another common cause of SCH in children is the intake of drugs like antiepileptic drugs (AEDs) such as phenytoin, phenobarbital, carbamazepine, and valproic acid which will reverse once AEDs are discontinued. Exposure to radioiodine and external radiotherapy can also cause SCH with a propensity for thyroid cancer in future. Iodine deficiency and iodine excess also are rare causes of SCH in children. Transient increases in TSH can occur due to sleep deprivation, in the periovulatory phase of menstrual cycle and in the recovery phase of sick euthyroid syndrome. False elevations of TSH due to macro-TSH should also be considered in the differential diagnosis of SCH and can be differentiated if TSH measurements are repeated in dilution or after polyethylene glycol (PEG) precipitation.

The major area of uncertainty is to determine whether to treat mild SCH in children. Current data shows that mild SCH does not affect linear growth, bone health, and intellectual outcome although data is controversial regarding neurocognitive functioning in certain domains. However, there is some evidence to show that children with long-standing SCH have an unfavorable cardiometabolic profile such as dyslipidemia, increase in visceral adiposity, and early markers of atherosclerotic cardiovascular disease. But whether treatment with LT4 will reverse this adverse cardiovascular risk is not yet clear.

CLINICAL FEATURES

The clinical presentation depends on the age at onset of hypothyroidism, duration and severity. Children with

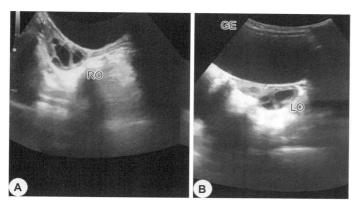

Figs. 2A and B: Van Wyk–Grumbach syndrome: Large multicystic ovaries in a 9-year-old child who presented with premature menarche due to primary hypothyroidism. Height was 3.6 standard deviation score (SDS) and bone age was 6 years.

> **BOX 2: Atypical manifestations of primary hypothyroidism.**
>
> - Kocher–Debre–Semelaigne syndrome
> - Polymyositis like syndrome
> - Slipped capital femoral epiphyses
> - Massive pericardial/pleural effusion
> - Hypothyroid ophthalmopathy
> - Hashimoto's encephalopathy
> - Van Wyk–Grumbach syndrome
> - Pseudotumor cerebri
> - Anemia of chronic disease

untreated hypothyroidism often have faltering of growth with linear growth more affected than weight and hence they appear short and chubby. This should be distinguished from minor TSH elevation that is commonly encountered in children with exogenous obesity where linear growth is unaffected, and TSH elevation is secondary to leptin-mediated stimulation of TRH. While the former needs hormone replacement, TSH tends to normalize in latter by weight loss alone.

The next major effect of hypothyroidism is on puberty. Along with delay in bone maturation, pubertal onset is delayed in children with untreated hypothyroidism. However, some rare cases of isosexual central precocity in both sexes have been reported, also known as Van Wyk–Grumbach syndrome owing to costimulation of follicle-stimulating hormone (FSH) receptors by high TSH levels due to structural homology in both the hormones. It presents as multicystic ovaries in females **(Fig. 2)** and enlargement of testes in males. Thus adequate treatment of hypothyroidism alone will suffice and the need for managing precocity and surgery for the cysts are not needed.

Those girls, who develop hypothyroidism post attainment of menarche can have menstrual irregularities in the form of menorrhagia, polymenorrhea, and rarely oligomenorrhea. If hypothyroidism sets in before 3 years of age which is the phase of brain development, it can have permanent effects on neurodevelopmental outcome. After 3 years, however, this effect is limited though decline in scholastic performance due to lack of concentration and tiredness can be a presenting complaint. Sometimes initiation of treatment of hypothyroidism can worsen the scholastic performance as is seen in children with hyperthyroidism. Symptoms of fatigue, constipation, cold intolerance, decreased appetite, hairfall, and puffiness of face can be encountered quite often in isolation or combination in juvenile hypothyroidism.

There are few atypical manifestations of hypothyroidism, awareness of which can prevent delay in diagnosis and initiation of treatment which are mentioned in **Box 2.**

Physical examination of affected children and adolescents may reveal presence of a goiter which is firm and pebbly in consistency, increased weight for height centiles, coarse facies, bradycardia, cold extremities, and rarely calf muscle hypertrophy known as Kocher–Debre–Semelaigne syndrome. In our experience this muscle hypertrophy can be more generalized and may mimic lipodystrophy syndrome **(Fig. 3)**.

The clinical features of central hypothyroidism are not as pronounced as primary hypothyroidism and may be associated with other features of hypopituitarism such as short stature and delayed puberty. Rare causes of central hypothyroidism like IGSF1 mutation may also be associated with delayed puberty, prolactin deficiency and macro-orchidism.

EVALUATION

Thyroid-stimulating hormone is the most sensitive screening test for hypothyroidism. An elevated TSH should be followed up with free T4 levels if not done simultaneously and a low or normal free T4 level helps in distinguishing SCH from OH. Isolated low T4 levels are suggestive of central hypothyroidism or sick euthyroid syndrome. TSH levels are not helpful in diagnosing central hypothyroidism as it can be low, normal, or mildly elevated with low levels of free thyroid hormones. Thyroid antibodies (anti-TPO, anti-Tg) should be ordered in all cases of acquired primary hypothyroidism owing to >90% positivity rates. Coexistence of TSH receptor antibodies can lead to Hashitoxicosis like picture with varying periods of hyperthyroidism followed by hypothyroidism.

Thyroid imaging in the form of ultrasound is not routinely indicated unless there are palpable nodules which need evaluation. Thyroid scintigraphy is reserved for cases with negative thyroid antibodies and absent eutopic thyroid gland to rule out ectopic thyroid. A radiograph of left hand with wrist for bone age assessment may have to be ordered in children presenting with growth retardation. When central hypothyroidism is suspected, other pituitary axes need to be assessed simultaneously. Since chromosomal anomalies are associated with increased frequency of

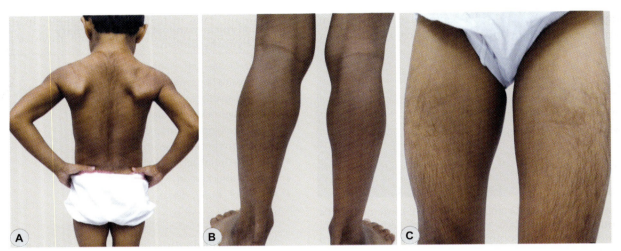

Figs. 3A to C: Presence of muscle hypertrophy in a 9-year-old child.
Courtesy: Dr Ankush Desai, Goa Medical College, Bambolim, Goa, India.

thyroid dysfunction and autoimmunity, it is worthwhile to regularly check thyroid function in children with Down syndrome, Turner syndrome, Noonan syndrome, and Klinefelter syndrome. Obese children needs evaluation for metabolic syndrome as dyslipidemia is commonly associated with hypothyroidism.

TREATMENT

Treatment with oral tablet formulation of levothyroxine remains the gold standard in confirmed cases of hypothyroidism. The age-specific dose of initiation has been mentioned in **Table 1**. Though age and body weight appropriate full dose should be initiated routinely, long-standing and severe cases of hypothyroidism may require lower starting doses than expected doses to the tune of 50%, especially in the peripubertal age to prevent rapid normalization of TSH which can cause accelerated bone maturation along with shorter adult height. Use of gonadotropin agonists in such cases to prevent fusion of epiphyses has been discussed but remains questionable. The dose should be individually titrated to keep TSH in the normal range and FT4 or T4 in the upper half of the reference range. Once daily administration at a fixed time with adequate gap from food (1 hour) and medicines (4 hours) ensures optimal outcomes.

MONITORING AND PROGNOSIS

Thyroid-stimulating hormone levels should not be repeated earlier than 4 weeks after initiation of hormone replacement owing to longer time taken to reach equilibrium. Once biochemical euthyroid state is achieved, thyroid function tests can be repeated 3-6 monthly. Peripubertal adolescents and periconceptional adolescents need to be educated regarding the increased requirement of thyroid hormone replacement during these periods and need

TABLE 1: Age-based dosage of LT4.

Age	LT4 dose (µg/kg)
0–3 months	10–15
3–6 months	8–10
6–12 months	6–8
1–3 years	4–6
3–10 years	3–4
10–15 years	2–4
>15 years	2–3
Adult	1.6

for close monitoring during pregnancy. However, the adolescent females can be reassured that the possibility of congenital defects while the mother is adequately treated is the same as euthyroid mother and the risk of transplacental transfer of maternal antibodies is significantly low. Along with biochemical monitoring, growth monitoring remains central to management of hypothyroidism with regular plotting of growth trajectory at each outpatient visit. If the hypothyroidism is long-standing prior to treatment, the chances of achieving normal adult height are guarded.

Children with SCH may progress to OH over the years and treatment of SCH may be considered if TSH is persistently >10 µIU/mL after elimination of confounding factors such as obesity, use of anticonvulsants, recent recovery from an illness, or chronic exposure to iodine-containing preparations. In cases of TSH between 6 and 10 µIU/mL, treatment may be decided on a case to case basis depending on the clinical picture. Relative indications to treat SCH in children are presence of antithyroid antibodies, goiter with or without nodules and symptomatic patients.

It should be remembered that while most cases of autoimmune hypothyroidism are permanent, up to 15% can have fluctuating levels of thyroid hormones including normalization of thyroid function. Thus in mild cases, a trial off therapy for 4 weeks can be tried after every few years of treatment excluding the critical physiological periods such as puberty or near conception.

CONCLUSION

Hypothyroidism is the most common pediatric endocrinopathy which needs a systematic approach for diagnosis and management. Due to lack of heterogeneity in treatment options, treatment remains fairly simple provided a methodical approach is followed. The need for patient education and sensitization can never be undermined and remains at the core of attaining favorable outcomes with simple cost-effective measures, thus helping a major subset of the community in achieving optimal goals in terms of final adult height, intelligence, and metabolic parameters.

SUGGESTED READINGS

1. Braverman L. Werner and Ingbar's the Thyroid, 11th edition. Philadelphia: Wolters Kluwer Health; 2020. pp. 2118-48.
2. Sperling M, Majzoub J, Menon R, Stratakis C. Sperling pediatric endocrinology, 5th edition. Philadelphia: Elsevier; 2021. pp. 202-19.
3. De Groot L, Jameson L. Endocrinology: Adult and Pediatric, 7th edition. Philadelphia: Elsevier Saunders; 2016.
4. Lifshitz F. Pediatric endocrinology, 5th edition. New York: Informa Healthcare; 2007. pp. 391-414
5. Marwaha RK, Tandon N, Garg MK, Desai A, Kanwar R, Sastry A, et al. Thyroid status two decades after salt iodization: country-wide data in school children from India. Clin Endocrinol (Oxf). 2012;76(6): 905-10.
6. Marwaha RK, Tandon N, Garg MK, Kanwar R, Sastry A, Narang A, et al. Dyslipidemia in subclinical hypothyroidism in an Indian population. Clin Biochem. 2011;44(14-15):1214-7.
7. Salerno M, Improda N, Capalbo D. Management of endocrine disease subclinical hypothyroidism in children. Eur J Endocrinol. 2020;183(2):R13-R28.
8. Pandav CS, Yadav K, Srivastava R, Pandav R, Karmarkar MG. Iodine deficiency disorders (IDD) control in India. Indian J Med Res. 2013;138(3):418-33.
9. Rallison ML, Keating FR, Tyler FH. Occurrence and natural history of chronic lymphocytic thyroiditis in childhood. J Pediatr. 1975;86(5):675-82

CHAPTER 26

Hyperthyroidism in Children, Adolescents, and Neonates

Leena Priyambada

INTRODUCTION

Hyperthyroidism is frequently missed or misdiagnosed in children. A high degree of suspicion and vigilance is important on the part of the primary care physician as the initial features of hyperthyroidism are nonspecific and can be easily missed or misdiagnosed, even for a few months to years. This manual provides important specifics of hyperthyroidism in neonates, children and adolescents.

Hyperthyroidism refers to increased levels of thyroid hormones in the body whereas thyrotoxicosis refers to the clinical features of hypermetabolism caused due to thyroid hormone excess.

EPIDEMIOLOGY

The incidence of hyperthyroidism rises sharply during puberty. There is a strong female predominance (5:1) in adolescence which is not seen in younger children. The true prevalence of childhood hyperthyroidism in children in India is not known.

CAUSES

Hyperthyroidism may be the result of increased thyroid hormone production or release from the thyroid gland. The various causes of hyperthyroidism in children are grouped into three categories and listed in **Table 1**.
- Thyroidal factors (primary hyperthyroidism)
- Central causes (central hyperthyroidism)
- External causes (exogenous hyperthyroidism)

In children, Graves' disease (GD) is the most common cause of hyperthyroidism.

CLINICAL FEATURES

Initial features of hyperthyroidism are nonspecific, progress gradually, and may be attributed to behavioral, gastrointestinal, respiratory, or cardiac disease. The diagnosis may be missed even for a few years. Prompt diagnosis and treatment has a beneficial effect on consequences and duration of disease. The details of the clinical features are described in **Box 1**.

First objective signs may include constant tachycardia, goiter, hyperdefecation/diarrhea, or increased appetite with or without weight loss.

TABLE 1: Causes of hyperthyroidism in children.

Central	Thyroid causes	External
Increased TSH: • TSH producing pituitary adenoma • Pituitary resistance to thyroid hormones	*Increased synthesis of thyroid hormones:* • Graves' disease • Toxic multinodular goiter • Toxic (autonomous) nodule (rare) *Increased release of preformed thyroid hormones:* • Autoimmune thyroiditis (hashitoxicosis, subacute, destructive) • Subacute granulomatous thyroiditis *Genetic:* • Activating *TSHR* gene mutations • Activating somatic GNAS, e.g., McCune–Albright syndrome	*Drug induced:* • Acute ingestion of thyroxine • Iodine-induced hyperthyroidism (e.g., iodine containing contrast agents, amiodarone)

(TSH: thyroid-stimulating hormone; TSHR: TSH receptor)

INVESTIGATIONS AND DIAGNOSIS

Young people with hyperthyroidism may present with varying degrees of thyrotoxicosis.
- *Thyroid function test (TFT):*
    - Thyroid-stimulating hormone (TSH) is suppressed
    - T4/free T4 are raised in overt hyperthyroidism and high normal in subclinical hyperthyroidism

Hyperthyroidism in Children, Adolescents, and Neonates

BOX 1: Clinical features of hyperthyroidism in children.

Nonspecific/Behavioral:
- Fatigability, emotionality, poor concentration, inattention, nervousness, anxiety, mood swings, mania, and worsening handwriting
- Decreasing school performance

Cardiovascular: Increased heart rate, palpitations, and wide pulse pressure

Hypermetabolic state:
- Increased appetite with weight loss and hyperdefecation
- Increased sweating and heat intolerance

Goiter: This may be present in more than half of the children with Graves' disease (GD)
- Variable size, symmetrical, smooth, firm, and homogenous
- Thrill or bruit may be present due to hypervascularity
- Compressive symptoms such as dysphagia and dyspnea (large goiter)
- Large single nodule is suggestive of toxic adenoma and multiple nodules are in toxic multinodular goiter. Hashitoxicosis may be associated with a firm goiter

Eye disease: Eye features are not common in children, and if present suggest GD etiology
- Irritation, foreign body sensation, and pain in the eyes
- Diplopia due to extraocular muscle dysfunction
- Stare, lid retraction, and lid lag are characteristic and may lead to corneal ulceration
- Inflammatory features such as proptosis and periorbital edema are uncommon

Neurologic:
- Tremors are demonstrated in outstretched hands or tongue fasciculations
- Hyperdefecation
- Hyperactive deep tendon reflexes
- Severe headache should raise suspicion for benign intracranial hypertension
- Rarely, moyamoya disease may cause focal neurologic deficits in GD

Skin, nails, and hair:
- Skin is warm (hyperthermia)
- Loosening of nails from nail bed (Plummer's sign), softening of nails, and hair loss
- Vitiligo and alopecia areata. Pretibial myxedema is uncommon in children

Musculoskeletal:
- Decreased bone mineral density and increased fracture risk
- Proximal muscle weakness may be seen

Growth and puberty:
- Mildly accelerated growth and bone maturation
- Oligomenorrhea, secondary amenorrhea, and anovulatory cycles may be seen

- T3 elevations more than T4 may be seen in autonomously functioning nodule, toxic multinodular goiter, or sometimes in the early stages of GD. Elevated free T3 is a more sensitive marker than free T4.

  Elevation of T4 and/or T3 along with suppressed TSH is the key to diagnosis. Uncommonly only T3 may be initially raised (without significantly increased T4) which suppresses TSH.

  Low TSH may also be seen in nonthyroidal illness (sick euthyroidism), but without any elevation in T4 or T3. As a laboratory artefact, suppressed TSH may be seen in children taking biotin. Normal TFTs essentially exclude hyperthyroidism.

  Once hyperthyroidism is confirmed, etiology must be ascertained.

- *Thyroid antibodies*:
  - Thyrotropin receptor antibody (TRAb) is increased in GD. If negative initially, this should be repeated after a few weeks.
  - Thyroid peroxidase antibodies and thyroglobulin antibodies (TPO-Ab and Tg-Ab) are more elevated in Hashimoto's thyroiditis, though they may also be present in GD.

- *Radionuclide scan*: This is useful to delineate the etiology of hyperthyroidism. The various patterns that can be seen are as follows:
  - GD: Diffuse, homogenous increased uptake
  - Hashitoxicosis and destructive thyroiditis: Poor or absent uptake
  - Toxic multinodular goiter: Spotty uptake
  - Autonomous/toxic nodule: Focal increased uptake along with decreased uptake in the rest of the gland.

    Technitium-99m (^{99m}Tc) is generally used though I-123 scans may be used at some centers.

- *Thyroid ultrasonography* (USG) is not routinely required in hyperthyroidism. USG along with Doppler blood flow assessment may be used instead of ^{99m}Tc scintigraphy to avoid radiation exposure. USG may be helpful if thyroid nodules or associated lymph nodes are found on clinical examination.

MANAGEMENT OF HYPERTHYROIDISM

The management will depend upon the cause and severity of hyperthyroidism. Management options for various scenarios of hyperthyroidism in children are described below in detail.

Graves' Disease

Graves' disease is an autoimmune disorder in which stimulating antibodies to the TSH receptor (TRAb acting like TSH agonist) cause increased production of thyroid hormones as well as growth of the thyroid gland. This results in goiter. GD may also be associated with ophthalmopathy as TSH receptors (TSHRs) are present in the orbit as well.

The course may be long and relapsing requiring prolonged treatment.

Graves' disease has a strong genetic predisposition. There should be a high degree of suspicion in children with certain genetic conditions such as Down syndrome, Turner syndrome and in association with other autoimmune conditions such as type 1 diabetes mellitus, vitiligo, and celiac disease.

Diagnosis of GD is aided by the presence of a soft diffuse, vascular goiter, eye signs if present, elevated TRAb, and characteristics on scintigraphy.

Prompt diagnosis and therapy is important as rendering the child euthyroid, by itself, has a beneficial effect on the thyroid autoimmunity. Hyperthyroidism increases autoimmunity and thus TRAb, which further increases the hyperthyroidism.

Medical Management of Graves' Disease
Antithyroid Drugs (ATDs)
Antithyroid drugs are the first-line treatment for hyperthyroidism in children with GD and should be promptly started.

Thionamides, either carbimazole (CBZ) or its active metabolite, and methimazole (MMI) can be used in children and adolescents with GD. They block thyroid hormone synthesis by preventing tyrosine iodination in the thyroglobulin molecule. CBZ is rapidly converted to MMI in the body and is the commonly used ATD in India.

Propylthiouracil (PTU) is no longer recommended in children because of risk of hepatic failure. This should be used exclusively in exceptional circumstances, only for short periods, with close monitoring for signs of hepatic dysfunction. The indications for PTU arise when CBZ or MMI is not tolerated because of severe side effects or rarely, in severe thyrotoxicosis due to acute thyroxine ingestion.

There are two approaches of administering ATDs: Dose titration approach or block and replace approach.

Dose titration approach: In this method, the dose of ATD is titrated against the TFTs to maintain euthyroid state. This is the preferred approach in most cases.
- A starting dose of CBZ of 0.25–0.5 mg/kg/day (MMI*, 0.15–0.3 mg/kg/day) will usually normalize TFT in 4–6 weeks. The dose is then reduced by 25–50% based on the TFTs. Higher doses of 0.75 mg/kg/day of CBZ (MMI: 0.5 mg/kg/day) may be needed in severe cases. Once daily dosing is effective.
- Once control is achieved, a dose of 2.5–5 mg of CBZ/MMI may be sufficient and should be continued for at least 2–3 years.

Block and replace approach: In this method, a high dose of CBZ (0.5–0.75 mg/kg/day) or MMI (0.3–0.5 mg/kg/day) will prevent thyroid hormone production completely, and then levothyroxine is added. A maximum of 1.3 mg/kg of CBZ or 1 mg/kg of MMI can be used if needed. This can be used in severe disease, if the thyroid hormone levels are very fluctuating or the thyroid hormones do not decrease as expected. This approach is associated with more adverse effects, though theoretically they can provide greater stability in thyroid hormone levels.

Monitoring of antithyroid drug therapy (Box 2):
Clinical: Weight and the metabolic rates improve by 3 months. Severe disease, poor compliance, and lower dose may increase time to remission.

Thyroid functions: Most patients become biochemically euthyroid by 4–6 weeks. TFT is measured every 3–6 weeks for the first 3 months, followed by once in 2–3 months when TFTs become stable. The initial 4–6 months ATD dose titrations are guided by the T4/free T4 and T3/free T3 as TSH may remain suppressed for months. TSH is used to titrate ATD dose subsequently. When thyroid hormones (T4/T3) are normalized, the dose is gradually decreased by 25–50% of daily dose.

Full blood count, and liver functions should be done before starting therapy and in appropriate clinical situations such as jaundice, fever, sore throat, and others.

In case of lack of response to therapy, compliance and use of iodine containing substances should be explored. Compliance should be emphasized at every visit.

Adverse effects of antithyroid drugs: Complete blood count should ensure neutrophils >1,000/mm^3 and liver enzymes not more than three times elevated before starting ATD therapy. Minor side effects occur in 10–20% of children, being more prevalent in younger children. These are usually seen in the first 3 months of starting treatment and generally transient.

BOX 2: Monitoring of antithyroid (ATD) drug therapy.
- *Starting dose of ATD:* CBZ—0.25–0.5 mg/kg/day (MMI—0.15–0.3 mg/kg/day)
- Titrate the dose of ATD up or down 25–50% based on T4 and/or T3 levels in the initial 6 months. Beyond 6 months, titrate ATDs based on T4/T3 as well as TSH
- *Clinical:* Vitals, weight gain, growth rate, and other presenting signs and symptoms
- *Biochemical:* TFTs
  - 3–6 weekly in the initial 3–6 months (assess response in terms of thyroid hormones)
  - 2–3 monthly once stable (TSH is used along with thyroid hormones to assess response)
  - Complete blood count (CBC) and liver function test at initiation and in appropriate clinical scenarios
- If there is nonresponse despite CBZ > 1 mg/kg/day or MMI > 0.6 mg/kg/day; check compliance and use of iodine-containing supplements

(CBZ: carbimazole; MMI: methimazole; TFTs: thyroid function test; TSH: thyroid-stimulating hormone)

---

*MMI of 0.6 mg is approximately equivalent to 1.0 mg CBZ.

- Pruritic rash and urticaria (10% of cases) resolve spontaneously if mild. In severe cases as Steven–Johnson syndrome, ATD should be stopped immediately.
- Cholestatic liver dysfunction may be seen. If transaminases rise more than three times the normal, then ATD should be stopped.
- Neutropenia can occur in untreated hyperthyroidism or develop in response to ATD. Agranulocytosis is rare (0.2%) and may develop within the first month of treatment. Families must be counselled to seek help in suggestive clinical cases like fever or severe sore throat. ATD should be temporarily stopped in such cases, and other treatment options may be needed.

Carbimazole/MMI should not be reinitiated if adverse effects are severe.

How long to continue antithyroid drugs: Relapse rates are higher in children than adults. ATDs are recommended for at least 3 years or 5 years and beyond in candidates who have high chances of relapse **(Box 3)**. If TFTs are euthyroid on low dose of ATD, and TRAb undetectable for several months, a trial-off ATDs may be done. If TRAb levels are elevated, remission is unlikely and ATD should not be stopped.

After stopping ATD, clinical monitored and TFTs should be done every 3–4 months initially, then 6 monthly and then annually. Patients who relapse will usually do so within 1 year of stopping ATD. Severe presentation in younger age children is more likely to relapse. TFTs should be monitored for at least 10 years and whenever symptomatic.

The overall remission for pediatric GD is 20–30% (vs. 40–60% in adults) after 2 years of ATDs. Longer duration of ATDs for 3–6 years may offer better chances of remission. The remission rate increases to 43% with 5–6 years and 75% with 9 years of ATD therapy. Very long-term ATDs (>10 years), if tolerated, with monitoring for side effects have also been used for some children with GD.

When to go for definitive treatment in children with GD: Children who relapse may either opt for definitive treatment or can reinitiate ATDs. Very long-term ATDs (>10 years), if tolerated, with monitoring for side effects have been used in children with GD, safely and effectively. Considering that 100% of children will not go into remission even with prolonged ATDs, the decision when to go for definitive treatment after prolonged ATD is a debatable topic and needs to be individualized based on the risk factors, age of the child, wishes of the family, resources, and expertise available. This should be a shared decision between the family and the care providers.

Other Medications
Beta blockers: Propranolol 1–2 mg/kg/day in three to four divided doses, or atenolol (0.5–1 mg/kg/day) in one to two divided doses is indicated for sympathetic symptoms like tachycardia. This is usually needed for the first few weeks and can be stopped when symptoms normalize. Beta blockers are contraindicated in asthma.

Newer therapeutic options including biologics, small molecules, and peptide immunomodulation for B-cell therapies, TSHR targeted therapies, and TSHR peptide desensitization are investigational and not indicated for pediatric GD.

Definitive Treatment of Graves' Disease
Thyroid ablation by radioactive iodine (RAI) or total thyroidectomy is regarded as definitive treatment for GD. Indications for definitive treatment are:
- Contraindication to medical therapy (Serious side effects with ATDs)
- Relapse despite prolonged ATD
- Poorly controlled hyperthyroidism due to lack of compliance
- Large goiter causing obstruction

Definitive treatment, if successful, is associated with lifelong hypothyroidism and needs thyroxine replacements. However, hypothyroidism is considered preferable to hyperthyroidism due to nature of symptoms and ease of management.

Surgical Management of Graves' Disease
Total thyroidectomy is the definitive treatment in children <5 years. Even for 5–10-year-old children, surgery is preferred over RAI. Other indications for surgery are large compressive and nodular goiters and severe GO. Partial or subtotal thyroidectomy is not preferred as there is a risk of recurrence.

Patients need to be euthyroid before surgery to avoid anesthetic complications and thyroid storm. Oral iodine (5–10 drops Lugol's iodine or 1–4 drops of saturated potassium iodide solution three times daily) for 1–2 weeks before surgery would usually normalize free T3 levels. Beta blockers and steroids may be needed before surgery. ATDs are continued till the day of surgery.

Hypocalcemia and recurrent laryngeal nerve damage (transient or permanent) may occur. Patients should be calcium and vitamin D replete before surgery to lower the risk of hypocalcemia. The risk of complications is lower if the surgery is done by a high-volume thyroid surgeon.

Subsequent lifelong thyroid hormone replacements will be necessary.

BOX 3: Predictive markers of relapse of Graves' disease after stopping antithyroid drug (ATD).

- Younger age
- Large goiter
- Lower body mass index (BMI) at onset
- Increased severity of hyperthyroidism
- Higher thyrotropin receptor antibody (TRAb) at onset and stopping treatment
- Shorter duration of ATDs

Radioactive Iodine Treatment of Graves' Disease

Radioactive iodine is taken up and metabolized by the thyrocytes. Emission of beta-radiation damages these thyrocytes, causing apoptosis and thyroid tissue necrosis. This will result in hypothyroidism.

Radioactive iodine dose should be sufficient to cause complete thyroid ablation so that radiation damaged cells do not survive. Persistence of radiation-damaged cells increases the theoretical risk of relapse and future malignancy. RAI activity should ideally be personalized using an activity of 15 MBq I-131 per gram thyroid tissue (thyroid weight measured using ultrasound) or thyroid dosimetry (highest amount of activity that will be administered to the patient to achieve maximum therapeutic outcome without causing harm) delivering at least 300 Gy for complete functional thyroid ablation.

Radioactive iodine is avoided in children younger than 5 years and performed with caution in children 5–10 years age only when surgery is not an option. It is safe and effective in postpubertal adolescents. Active Graves' ophthalmopathy (GO) is a contraindication for RAI. In cases of inactive GO, steroids may be given concurrently to prevent exacerbation. ATDs should be stopped 3–7 days before the procedure.

Achieving hypothyroidism takes weeks to months and ATDs should be continued for at least 3 months postprocedure. TSH levels may take several months to normalize. Lifelong thyroid replacements will be necessary if thyroid ablation is achieved successfully.

Side effects of RAI are rare. There may be thyroid tenderness for a few weeks post-RAI. Short-term side effects such as vomiting, local inflammation, and myxedema have been rarely reported. Although there is a theoretical neoplasia risk and risk of genetic damage to offsprings, long-term follow-ups have not shown much evidence of second malignancies and fertility issues. Benign thyroid nodules ($n = 6$), multinodular benign goiter ($n = 1$) and papillary thyroid carcinoma ($n = 1$) was reported out of 1,283 children and adolescents with GD from 23 studies undergoing RAI. The safety and efficacy of RAI increased with higher doses.

About three-fourths of RAIs is successful. A minority of children have required repeat RAI to achieve hypothyroidism. Smaller thyroid size is associated with more success.

Apart from the contraindications, the choice between RAI and surgery depends on the expertise available and shared decision-making within the multidisciplinary team and the family.

The various therapy options for persistent hyperthyroidism are summarized in **Table 2**.

Graves' Ophthalmopathy in Children

Apart from thyroid, TSHRs are also expressed in the fibroblasts of the orbit. TRAb and the activated T cells result in retro-ocular fibroblast proliferation, inflammation, and excess hyaluronan production which are hydrophilic. This causes bulging of the eyeball forward which further results in extraocular muscles dysfunction.

Graves' ophthalmopathy is present in one-third to two-thirds of cases of GD in children. Girls are more affected. High TRAb and free T4 levels increase the risk of GO.

Eyelid retraction and proptosis are the common symptoms while soft tissue inflammation is uncommon. In children, the GO course is usually mild and treatment is conservative. Remission of hyperthyroidism results in improvement of GO. Artificial tears may be helpful. Steroids may be required in severe cases. Surgical management like lid lengthening and orbit decompression is rarely needed. Children with GO is associated with a more severe course of

TABLE 2: Therapy options for Graves' disease in children.			
Therapy	**Pros**	**Cons**	**Remarks**
Antithyroid drugs (ATDs): • Carbimazole and methimazole • Propylthiouracil (PTU) not recommended in children	• Effective initial treatment • Drug-free euthyroid period after ATDs possible	• Risk of relapse • Adverse effects • Prolonged treatment • Compliance issues	• First-line therapy • Stabilizing before surgery or RAI • Effective as once daily dose • Slow tapering advised • Monitor complete blood count (CBC) and liver function test (LFT)
Surgery (total or near total thyroidectomy)	• Permanent cure • Immediate results • Nodular or large compressive goiters	• Surgical-anesthetic risk • Hypoparathyroidism, recurrent laryngeal (RL) nerve damage risk • Lifelong thyroxine	• Experienced high-volume thyroid surgeon for best results • Replete calcium/vitamin D before surgery
Radioactive iodine (RAI)	• Permanent cure • Alternative to surgery	• CI: Age < 5 years, active Graves' ophthalmopathy (GO) (relative CI: 5–10 years, inactive GO, large goiter) • Takes weeks for effect • Lifelong thyroxine • Theoretical risk of secondary malignancy	• ATDs needed for months post-RAI • Postpuberty

GD. If definitive treatment for GD is required in the presence of GO, thyroidectomy is preferred over RAI.

Thyroid Storm

An acute severe exacerbation of thyrotoxicosis is called thyroid crisis or storm. Significant stressors such as infections (most common), surgery, and RAI can trigger thyroid storm in untreated or poorly controlled GD. This presents as extreme tachycardia, hyperthermia, heart failure, gastrointestinal/hepatic symptoms, extreme anxiety, and altered mental state. The symptoms may be misdiagnosed as acute encephalopathy in the emergency room. Associated fatality rate is high. Recognizing the symptoms and monitoring these children in high care settings is crucial.

Initial resuscitation, cooling blankets, and antipyretics are indicated. Large dose of ATDs an hour before iodine (potassium iodide solution) to stop the release of preformed thyroid hormones, glucocorticoids to stop the peripheral conversion of T4 to T3, intravenous (IV) propranolol for sympathetic blockade will be needed. PTU at 16–30 mg/kg/day is considered more effective than MMI/CBZ. Treatment for triggers, like antibiotics, should be administered. If clinical symptoms do not improve, plasmapheresis should be tried.

Subclinical or Mild Hyperthyroidism

In this, TSH is suppressed but free T4 and free T3 are in the high-normal reference range. This is usually incidentally diagnosed (e.g., TFTs obtained for other reasons) and children are asymptomatic. They do not need treatment but require follow-up TFT testing, sometimes over several months. TFTs may spontaneously normalize, become hypothyroid or progress to overt hyperthyroidism on follow-up. The etiology should be worked up in the meantime.

Hashitoxicosis

Hashitoxicosis is transient. If there are troublesome sympathetic features due to hyperthyroidism such as tachycardia, palpitations, or anxiety; beta blockers are indicated. Some children with thyroiditis may need low-dose ATDs for a few weeks before they turn euthyroid or hypothyroid.

Children with GD will usually progress and will need long-term antithyroid treatment.

Acute Thyroxine Overdose

This is not uncommon in children. A probable estimation of the ingested dose should be made. Due to long half-life of thyroxine, immediate testing may not be representative and TFT should be done at 3–5 days. The symptoms usually appear in 12 weeks, if at all.

If child is asymptomatic close monitoring and observation would be adequate. Beta blockers may be necessary if mild sympathetic symptoms are present. If severe symptoms are present then PTU, steroids and/or cholestyramine may be required. If there is cardiac or neurological compromise, plasmapheresis, or charcoal hemoperfusion may be warranted.

Toxic Thyroid Nodules

Toxic nodules are uncommon in children and show increased focal uptake with the rest of the thyroid gland poor/no uptake in scintigraphy. Malignancy must be carefully looked for in such cases. Surgical management is preferred.

APPROACH TO HYPERTHYROIDISM IN CHILDREN (FLOWCHART 1)

History

To elicit the clinical features consistent with hyperthyroidism and eliminate differential diagnosis. Personal or family history of autoimmunity is corroborative.

Clinical Features

Pulse rate, pulse pressure, warm extremities, details of goiter, brisk reflexes, eye signs, growth, and puberty should be noted. Features suggestive of syndromes like Down syndrome, Turner syndrome, McCune Albright, 22q11.2 deletion syndrome, etc., in which hyperthyroidism may be more common should be looked for.

Investigation

Thyroid function tests, TRAb, and thyroid scintigraphy clinch the diagnosis.

Flowchart 1 provides an approach to hyperthyroidism in children and **Table 3** summarizes the important features of the various causes of hyperthyroidism in children.

NEONATAL HYPERTHYROIDISM

Neonatal hyperthyroidism (NH) usually occurs in children born to mothers with GD. Mothers who have had prior definitive treatment for GD like RAI or thyroidectomy years ago and are now hypothyroid on treatment can also have babies with NH. Some mothers may have undiagnosed GD. A careful maternal history or previously affected sibling is helpful. Maternal GD causes NH due to transplacental passage of maternal TSHR-stimulating antibodies. The fetal thyroid gland axis becomes responsive to TSH and TRAb at about 20 weeks of gestation when maternal TRAbs should be reassessed.

There may also be neonatal hypothyroidism (primary or central) due to the maternal ATD, impaired regulation of the fetal hypothalamic–pituitary–thyroid axis, or maternal TSHR blocking antibodies.

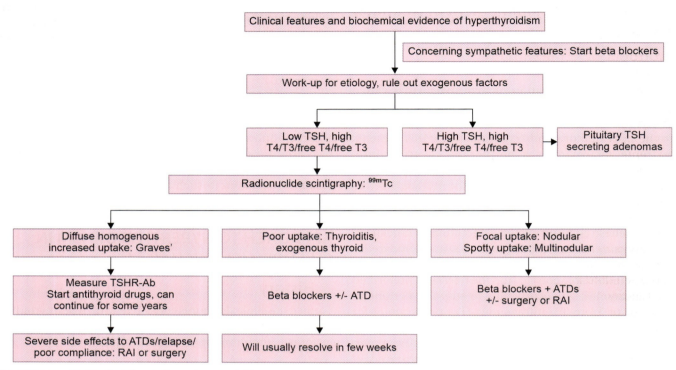

Flowchart 1: Approach to hyperthyroidism in children.
(ATDs: antithyroid drugs; RAI: radioactive iodine; TSH: thyroid-stimulating hormone; TSHR: TSH receptor)

TABLE 3: Summary of hyperthyroid conditions in children.			
Conditions	Tests	Management	Remarks
Graves' disease: Hyperthyroid C/F, long duration of symptoms, goiter with/without eye signs	• TRAb • *Scintigraphy*: Increased homogenous uptake	Start ATD early, continue long, slow taper	• Most common cause of hyperthyroidism in children • Counsel for long-term therapy
Thyroiditis: Hashitoxicosis, destructive—hyperthyroid C/F, firm goiter, no eye signs	• *Scintigraphy*: Poor uptake • *Suggestive*: High TPO/TgAb, absent TRAb	*Observation*: Beta blockers may be needed, rarely ATD	Usually transient, follow-up for hypothyroidism
Toxic thyroid nodule: Nodular goiter, hyperthyroid C/F	*Scintigraphy*: Focal uptake	ATD and early surgery	Careful evaluation for malignancy
Acute thyroxine ingestion: Careful history	TFTs after 3–5 days	• Usually asymptomatic • Close follow-up for 1–2 weeks	• Careful follow-up as delayed rise of TFT and C/F • Prevent future episodes

(ATD: antithyroid drug; C/F: clinical feature; TFTs: thyroid function test; TgAb: thyroglobulin antibody; TPO: thyroid peroxidase; TRAb: thyrotropin receptor antibody)

Other rare causes of NH include topical iodine use, activating mutations of TSHR, somatic activating mutations of GNAS in McCune–Albright syndrome.

Clinical Features of Neonatal Hyperthyroidism

Neonatal hyperthyroidism is present in about 2% of babies born to GD mothers and usually present within the first 2 weeks.

Newborns may be asymptomatic or have unexplained tachycardia, irritability, poor weight gain, goiter, or prominent eyes. There may be prematurity and small for gestational age (SGA). Severe untreated NH may uncommonly cause cardiac failure, liver dysfunction, coagulopathy, craniosynostosis, and neurodevelopmental concerns. Rarely, low platelets, jaundice, and hepatosplenomegaly may mimic congenital infection. NH is usually transient but clinical monitoring is important for the first 2–3 months of life.

Evaluation and Management of Neonatal Hyperthyroidism

Thyrotropin Receptor Antibody

Maternal TRAb levels are recommended at diagnosis of pregnancy and 18–22 weeks in all mothers with present or past history of GD. TRAb levels will be higher after RAI than thyroidectomy. If the TRAb levels are >3.7 times raised than the upper limit or >5 IU/L (also taken as >6 IU/L in some centers), then the risk of NH is high, and the fetus should be closely monitored. Goiter is the earliest and most characteristic sign of fetal hyperthyroidism. Mothers should be on the lowest possible ATDs to maintain free T4 in the high normal pregnancy-specific range.

In the newborn, TRAb should be measured in cord blood at delivery or as soon as possible after delivery. If negative, the risk of neonatal involvement is negligible. TRAb >6.8 IU/L within 0–5 days of life predict neonatal thyroid dysfunction with a sensitivity of 100% and specificity of 94%. TRAb levels if elevated are subsequently assessed along with the TFTs.

Undetectable TRAbs with persistent hyperthyroidism in the neonate is classified as nonautoimmune hyperthyroidism. Rarely neonates may be euthyroid despite high TRAbs and this denotes the presence of both stimulating and blocking antibodies.

Thyroid Function Tests

Cord blood TSH and free T4 reflect fetal thyroid status and do not predict neonatal course. TFTs and TRAbs are repeated on 3, 7–8, and 10–14 days of life. If TRAb are more than four times raised, then TFTs should be repeated every 10–14 days till TRAb disappear. A screening TSH < 0.18 mIU/L on the third postnatal day has been proposed for detecting severe NH with 71% sensitivity, 99% specificity, 81% positive predictive value, and 98% negative predictive value.

Treatment

In symptomatic neonates with suppressed TSH and high free T4, ATD is administered (CBZ 0.4–1.6 mg/kg/day or MMI 0.25–1.0 mg/kg/day) in three divided doses till euthyroidism is achieved. The ATD dose is subsequently titrated to TFTs till TRAb disappears. The ATD requirement is usually transient (approximately for 2–6 weeks). Propranolol (2 mg/kg/day in two or three divided doses) may be required for sympathetic features. Thyroxine may be subsequently required transiently following ATDs in some babies.

In severe cases, Lugol's solution or saturated solution of potassium iodide (SSKI), 1 drop every 8 hours is added to block the release of thyroid hormone. Digoxin is used for cardiac failure with stopping of propranolol. Rarely, prednisone (2 mg/kg/day) is added for immediate inhibition of thyroid hormone secretion. Breastfeeding can be done if PTU or MMI does not exceed 400 mg or 40 mg, respectively.

Isolated TSH suppression or a low normal TSH with high normal free T4 may not need treatment but will warrant follow-up.

Neonatal nonautoimmune hyperthyroidism may need prolonged ATDs. Surgery (total or partial thyroidectomy) may be needed in these cases subsequently.

CONCLUSION

Hyperthyroidism in children can easily be missed and misdiagnosed. High degree of suspicion on the part of the primary care physician is important for diagnosis. GD is the most common cause presenting more during adolescence and in females. Prompt diagnosis and early treatment improves autoimmunity and subsequent course of hyperthyroidism. Long-term ATDs at the lowest dose to maintain euthyroidism offers the best chances of remission. The choice of definitive management between thyroidectomy and RAI should be a shared decision depending on the multidisciplinary expertise available and the family's preference. It is important to educate families regarding the course of illness and improve compliance. Similarly, NH should be looked for in appropriate settings and managed promptly.

SUGGESTED READINGS

1. Mooij CF, Cheetham TD, Verburg FA, Eckstein A, Pearce SH, Léger J, et al. 2022 European Thyroid Association Guideline for the management of pediatric Graves' disease. Eur Thyroid J. 2022;11(1):e210073.
2. Song A, Kim SJ, Kim MS, Kim J, Kim I, Bae GY, et al. Long-term antithyroid drug treatment of Graves' disease in children and adolescents: a 20-year single-center experience. Front Endocrinol (Lausanne). 2021;12:687834.
3. Lutterman SL, Zwaveling-Soonawala N, Verberne HJ, Verburg FA, van Trotsenburg ASP, Mooij CF. The efficacy and short- and long-term side effects of radioactive iodine treatment in pediatric Graves' disease: a systematic review. Eur Thyroid J. 2021;10(5):353-63.
4. Chung SK, Asban A, Hur J, Iyer P, Chen H. Hyperthyroidism symptoms, management, and outcomes in children and adults seeking definitive surgical treatment. Ann Surg. 2021;273(5):e181-2.
5. Yu W, Wu N, Li L, Wang J, OuYang H, Shen H. SIDE effects of PTU and MMI IN the treatment of hyperthyroidism: a systematic review and meta-analysis. Endocr Pract. 2020;26(2):207-17.
6. Vigone MC, Peroni E, Di Frenna M, Mora S, Barera G, Weber G. "Block-and-replace" treatment in Graves' disease: experience in a cohort of pediatric patients. J Endocrinol Invest. 2020;43(5):595-600.
7. Lane LC, Cheetham TD, Perros P, Pearce SHS. New Therapeutic horizons for Graves' hyperthyroidism. Endocr Rev. 2020;41(6):873-84.

8. Kyritsi EM, Kanaka-Gantenbein C. Autoimmune thyroid disease in specific genetic syndromes in childhood and adolescence. Front Endocrinol (Lausanne). 2020;11:543.
9. Zader SJ, Williams E, Buryk MA. Mental health conditions and hyperthyroidism. Pediatrics. 2019;144(5):e20182874.
10. Williams GR, Bassett JHD. Thyroid diseases and bone health. J Endocrinol Invest. 2018;41(1):99-109.
11. Léger J, Oliver I, Rodrigue D, Lambert AS, Coutant R. Graves' disease in children. Ann Endocrinol (Paris). 2018;79(6):647-55.
12. Kourime M, McGowan S, Al Towati M, Ahmed SF, Stewart G, Williamson S, et al. Long-term outcome of thyrotoxicosis in childhood and adolescence in the west of Scotland: the case for long-term antithyroid treatment and the importance of initial counselling. Arch Dis Child. 2018;103(7):637-42.
13. Minamitani K, Sato H, Ohye H, Harada S, Arisaka O. Guidelines for the treatment of childhood-onset Graves' disease in Japan, 2016. Clin Pediatr Endocrinol. 2017;26(2):29-62.
14. Léger J, Carel J-C. MANAGEMENT OF ENDOCRINE DISEASE: arguments for the prolonged use of antithyroid drugs in children with Graves' disease. Eur J Endocrinol. 2017;177(2):R59-R67.
15. Hamed SA, Attiah FA, Abdulhamid SK, Fawzy M. Behavioral assessment of children and adolescents with Graves' disease: a prospective study. PLoS One. 2021;16(4):e0248937.
16. Kaplowitz PB, Jiang J, Vaidyanathan P. Radioactive iodine therapy for pediatric Graves' disease: a single-center experience over a 10-year period. J Pediatr Endocrinol Metab. 2020;33(3):383-9.
17. Namwongprom S, Dejkhamron P, Unachak K. Success rate of radioactive iodine treatment for children and adolescent with hyperthyroidism. J Endocrinol Invest. 2021;44(3):541-5.
18. Pyrżak B, Rumińska M, Witkowska-Sędek E, Kucharska A. Follow-up of thyroid function in children with neonatal hyperthyroidism. Front Endocrinol (Lausanne). 2022;13:877119.
19. Banigé M, Kariyawasam D, Gauthereau V, Luton D, Polak M. Neonatal screening for hyperthyroidism proof of concept. J Clin Endocrinol Metab. 2022;107(4):e1374-81.
20. Benlarbi H, Simon D, Rosenblatt J, Dumaine C, de Roux N, Chevenne D, et al. Prevalence and course of thyroid dysfunction in neonates at high risk of Graves' disease or with non-autoimmune hyperthyroidism. Eur J Endocrinol. 2021;184(3):427-36.
21. van Trotsenburg ASP. Management of neonates born to mothers with thyroid dysfunction, and points for attention during pregnancy. Best Pract Res Clin Endocrinol Metab. 2020;34(4):101437.
22. Samuels SL, Namoc SM, Bauer AJ. Neonatal thyrotoxicosis. Clin Perinatol. 2018;45(1):31-40.

CHAPTER 27

Thyroid Nodules in Children

Shakun Chaudhary, Ashu Rastogi

INTRODUCTION

Nodular thyroid diseases includes solitary thyroid nodule, multinodular goiter, thyroid nodules with preexisting autoimmune thyroid disease (Hashimoto's thyroiditis and Graves' disease), and nonpalpable thyroid nodules. Pediatric thyroid nodules are affected by various hormonal changes during puberty. To maintain the uniformity in definition pediatric age group is taken as <18 years of age. Thyroid malignancy is more common in postadolescent children as compared to younger children. Thyroid malignancy is the eighth most common malignancy in children in this age group and the second most common malignancy in female.

Thyroid nodules are rare in children. However, the risk of malignancy is higher. Children with differentiated thyroid carcinoma (DTC) are more likely to have an extrathyroidal disease, lymph node involvement, and pulmonary metastasis. Furthermore, even with more extensive disease mortality in children is lesser than in adults. Among genetic defects childhood papillary thyroid carcinoma (PTC) is more likely to have gene rearrangements. Due to these differences, separate recommendations are needed in children.

EPIDEMIOLOGY

Prevalence of thyroid nodules is less in children as compared to adults. However, their presence should alarm the physician as when these nodules present, the risk of malignancy in pediatric thyroid nodules is higher when compared to adults (20–22% vs. 5%). The prevalence of pediatric thyroid nodules according to a postmortem series is 1–1.5%. The prevalence is higher in older adolescents and young adults (up to 13%). Previous studies have shown that children <10–15 years of age have a more extensive disease and a higher risk of recurrence. Overall, the prevalence of thyroid nodules is higher in female as compared to male. However, the gender distribution depends upon the age of presentation. In the age group of <15 years female to male ratio is 1.5:1 while it is 3:1 in age group of >15 years. The presence of sex hormones at the onset of puberty has a role to play in this difference in gender distribution.

CAUSATION

Various etiological factors implicated in the development of thyroid nodules in children include radiation exposure, iodine deficiency, preexisting thyroid disease, and genetic syndromes.

Radiation Exposure

External irradiation to the head, neck, and chest is a risk factor for the development of thyroid nodules in children. This association was first noticed by Duffy BJ et al. who found that 36% of children with malignant thyroid nodules had the previous history of radiation exposure. Also, an increased prevalence of thyroid malignancy was found in children who were exposed to the Chernobyl disaster. Among these also younger children had a higher incidence of thyroid malignancy.

Preexisting Thyroid Disease

Both PTC and follicular thyroid carcinoma (FTC) in thyroid nodules have been found to be associated with preexisting thyroid disease. Juvenile autoimmune thyroiditis is associated with more prevalence of thyroid nodules (31.5%). Out of these 9.6% of nodules developed PTC. Hashimoto's thyroiditis is associated with both benign nodules and PTC. Dyshormonogenesis resulting in hypothyroidism is associated with a higher frequency of thyroid nodules and FTC.

Iodine Deficiency

Iodine deficiency areas have a higher prevalence of thyroid nodules as well as FTC.

Genetic Disease

Thyroid nodules are more common in children with a family history of thyroid disorders (41%). Among these familial association is more frequent in children with parafollicular cell malignancy [medullary thyroid carcinoma (MTC)] as compared to follicular cell malignancy (FTC and PTC). Around 20% of the children with MTC have familial cancer-associated RET proto-oncogene mutation. MTC can occur in isolation or as a part of multiple endocrine neoplasia (MEN) syndrome. Besides this familial nonmedullary thyroid cancer occur in Carney's complex, Cowden syndrome, and familial polyposis coli.

WHOM TO SCREEN?

Childhood cancer survivors who have received radiation to head and neck area develop thyroid nodule at an annual rate of 2%. Studies have shown that ultrasonographic (USG) screening of such children can lead to an early detection of thyroid nodules. However, whether this early detection translates into long-term survival benefit is not clear. Hence, present screening recommendation is annual clinical examination of children with high risk for development of thyroid nodules. Ultrasonography should be done only if there are palpable nodules, asymmetric nodules, and/or cervical lymphadenopathy. Also, children with genetic syndromes like familial polyposis coli, non-MTC syndrome, PTEN hamartoma tumor syndrome, etc. have higher prevalence of thyroid nodules. These children should be evaluated at centers of excellence for comprehensive evaluation and genetic counseling.

Children with Hashimoto's thyroiditis have an increased risk of development of thyroid nodules. Any suspicious nodule on clinical examination, thyroid gland asymmetry, or cervical lymphadenopathy should be subjected to USG examination.

CLINICAL EXAMINATION AND INVESTIGATIONS

Thyroid nodules in children can be single or multiple. Multiple thyroid nodules are usually detected on USG. Any child presenting with thyroid nodules should be inquired about time since nodule was first noticed, change in size over time, pain in nodule, family/personal history of thyroid disorder, and compressive symptoms. Clinical examination of thyroid nodule includes assessment of size, site, consistency, borders, tenderness, fixation to overlying skin or underlying structures, and compressive symptoms. Regional lymph node involvement is a feature of both PTC and MTC. Hence, examination of cervical lymph nodes is essential. On palpation, firm to stony hard nodules, fixation to underlying structures, and paralysis of vocal cords are features of malignant thyroid nodule.

EVALUATION

Thyroid Function Test

Thyroid-stimulating hormone (TSH) should be done in all children presenting with thyroid nodule. If TSH is suppressed nuclear scintigraphy should be done, if TSH is not suppressed or nodule is hypofunctioning on nuclear scintigraphy USG followed by fine-needle aspiration biopsy (FNAB) should be performed if needed.

Ultrasonography

All children presenting with thyroid nodule should be subjected to USG to look for characteristics of malignancy in nodule and for assessment of cervical lymphadenopathy. PTC can sometimes present as diffuse thyroid enlargement rather than isolated nodule in children. Hence, children with diffuse thyroid enlargement especially with cervical lymphadenopathy should also be subjected to thyroid USG. In contrary to thyroid nodules in adult, size of thyroid nodule as a criterion for further evaluation is not feasible in children as thyroid volume changes with age and size of thyroid nodule alone does not predict malignancy. Nodules with USG features are likely to be malignant such as:
- Hypoechogenicity
- Microcalcification
- Irregular margins
- Increased vascularity

Moreover, cervical lymphadenopathy should be specifically evaluated in every child with thyroid nodule as it is an important feature of malignancy.

Thyroid Scan

Thyroid scan differentiates between functional and nonfunctional thyroid nodules. Nodules are categorized into hot and cold nodules depending upon iodine trapping function. Cold nodules are considered to carry higher risk of malignancy as compared to hot nodule. The incidence of malignancy in cold nodule ranges from 20 to 60%.

Fine-needle Aspiration Biopsy

Fine-needle aspiration biopsy in children should be performed in a setting with availability of age appropriate anesthesia and pediatric advanced life support monitoring and intervention if needed.

Fine-needle aspiration biopsy is recommended for evaluation of all pediatric nodules with suspicious USG features. All children with hyperfunctioning thyroid nodule are subjected to surgery and hence FNAB is not indicated in hot nodules.

Fine-needle aspiration biopsy complements the diagnosis made by USG and guides regarding need for surgery. Previous studies have shown that fine-needle aspiration cytology (FNAC) decreases the need for surgery by 67 to 43%. FNAB has sensitivity of 60–100% and specificity of 63–100% in adults. Since there are no separate studies for FNAB in children these values hold true for children also. Overall in adults, USG-guided FNAB has been shown to have increased sensitivity and specificity as compared to palpation-guided FNAB. Because of the higher proportion of malignancy in children, potential difficulties in procurement of repeat sample, more proximity with esophagus, trachea, and great vessels in children only USG-guided FNAB is recommended in children. Reporting of cytopathology in pediatric nodules is done according to Bethesda system for reporting thyroid cytopathology as in adults.

Nodules are classified into six categories:
1. Nondiagnostic/Unsatisfactory
2. Benign
3. Atypia of undetermined significance/follicular lesion of undetermined significance
4. Suspicious of follicular neoplasm
5. Suspicious for malignancy
6. Malignant
   Repeated FNAB if needed should be performed after a minimum of 3 months to avoid atypical cellular features arising from reparative process.

Molecular Genetic Studies with Fine-needle Aspiration Biopsy

Role of molecular genetics comes when FNAB is indeterminate. In the setting of indeterminate cytology lobectomy with isthmectomy is performed followed by completion operation if histopathology reveals malignancy. With small neck area in children the risk of complications increases with repeat surgery. This can be reduced if FNAB is complemented with molecular genetic analysis. PTC is associated with BRAF and RET/PTC rearrangement. Around 17% of pediatric nodules are positive for molecular genetics. When molecular genetic analysis is done in children with indeterminate cytology of thyroid nodule presence of BRAF, RAS, RET/PTC, PAX8/PPAR-γ predicted malignancy in all of cases. Therefore, addition of molecular genetic studies to FNAB increases positive predictive value to 100% and sensitivity and specificity to 80% and 100%. However, only presence of genetic mutation has value and negative genetic analysis does not exclude malignancy. Although molecular genetic analysis when complemented with indeterminate FNAB can be very useful; it is not routinely recommended due to lack of sufficient validation.

Calcitonin

Calcitonin is recommended for evaluation of all thyroid nodules in adults. However, reference ranges of calcitonin are not validated in children and prevalence of MTC is also low in children. Hence, routine use of calcitonin for evaluation of thyroid nodules is not recommended.

TREATMENT

Choice of treatment depends upon clinical features, thyroid function test (TFT), USG features, scintigraphy, FNAB, and molecular genetic analysis (if done). Decision regarding treatment should be taken after discussion regarding pros and cons of various treatment options with the parents/guardian of child. Various treatment options according to type of thyroid nodule are as follows:

Nondiagnostic Lesions

In case of nondiagnostic lesions, repeat USG and FNAB is done after 3–6 months. If found to be benign 6–12 monthly USG follow-up is done.

Benign Lesions

Conservative Management

False negative rate for FNAB in studies which included both children and adults is 3–5%. Most of the times it is because of sampling error in large lesions. Benign nodules on FNAB are managed with follow-up USG after 6–12 months. If nodule remains stable on subsequent follow-up with USG every 1–2 years is recommended. If there is significant increase in size of nodule (>50% increase in volume or >20% increase in at least 2 dimensions) or features suspicious of malignancy on subsequent USG repeat FNAB is warranted.

Levothyroxine Suppression Therapy

Formation of nodules in children with radiation exposure has been shown to be reduced by the use of levothyroxine suppression therapy. Also, a few studies have shown reduction in the size of spontaneous nodules after using levothyroxine suppression therapy. However, long-term use of LT4 can be associated with features of hyperthyroidism, bone loss, and increased risk of arrhythmia. Due to safety concerns with long-term use of LT4, routine use of levothyroxine suppression therapy for decreasing size of nodule is not recommended. However, depending upon individual circumstances in children with compressive symptoms and children with radiation exposure levothyroxine suppression therapy can be useful for short term.

Surgery

Surgery is recommended in benign lesions if there is increase in size on subsequent follow-up, development of suspicious USG features, compressive symptoms, cosmetic reasons, and patient/parent choice. Also, surgery is preferable in lesions >4 cm size especially with solid consistency as false negative rate is higher in large lesions. Surgical procedure of choice is lobectomy.

Indeterminate Cytology

Frequency of indeterminate lesion is higher in children as compare to adults (35% vs. 2–25%). Also, risk of malignancy in atypia of undetermined significance/follicular lesion of undetermined significance (AUS/FLUS) (5–15% vs. 28%) and follicular (15–30% vs. 58%) is higher in children as compared to adults. Therefore, definitive surgery (lobectomy with isthmectomy) is recommended in children with indeterminate lesions. Children with nodules with features of malignancy but indeterminate cytology should be subjected to lobectomy. After surgery if histopathological examination shows features of malignancy completion operation (near total or total thyroidectomy) is advocated.

Malignant Lesions

Various treatment options for malignant thyroid nodules are surgery, radioactive iodine ablation (RAIA), and TSH suppressive therapy.

Surgery

All lesions with nodules suspicious of malignancy or malignant on FNAB are subjected to surgery.

- *Papillary thyroid carcinoma*: Surgical approaches for the management of malignant thyroid nodule are near total thyroidectomy and total thyroidectomy. As risk of bilateral and multifocal disease is higher in children total thyroidectomy is the surgical procedure of choice in majority of children. Near total thyroidectomy is indicated only if there is a small unilateral tumor confined to thyroid gland. To define the treatment plan a comprehensive neck USG of whole neck should be done preoperatively. FNAB should be performed in suspicious lateral neck lymph nodes.
    - *Role of central neck dissection and lateral neck dissection*: Disease-free survival (DFS) depends most strongly on presence of metastatic or recurrent locoregional disease. In order to prolong DFS prophylactic central neck dissection (CND) was recommended in children previously at the time of initial surgery. However, it is not clear which subset of patient is likely to have metastatic or recurrent locoregional disease. Although studies have shown higher DFS after prophylactic CND, whether or not this is the effect of postoperative radioactive iodine is not clear. Hence, present recommendation is to perform CND in malignant thyroid nodules with evidence of gross extrathyroidal invasion and/or locoregional metastasis on preoperative staging or intraoperative findings. In patients with no evidence of gross extrathyroidal invasion and/or locoregional metastasis prophylactic CND can be considered depending upon size of tumor (>4 cm), multifocality, and experience of surgeon. For unifocal lesion ipsilateral CND should be performed and decision regarding contralateral CND should be taken intraoperatively. Whenever performed CND should be done by compartment-oriented resection and not by berry picking. Lateral neck dissection should be performed only if there is cytological evidence of lateral neck metastasis.
- *Follicular thyroid carcinoma*: FTC is rare in children. Pediatric FTC is characterized by less advanced disease, less metastasis, and recurrence. For minimally invasive FTC only lobectomy is done. If there are more than three vascular invasions or tumor size is >4 cm total thyroidectomy is done with postsurgery RAIA.
- *Medullary thyroid carcinoma*: MTC is also rare in children. Pediatric thyroid nodule of any size with MTC is managed with total thyroidectomy with bilateral central neck dissection. If there is USG evidence of lateral cervical lymph node involvement FNAB should be done. If malignant lateral neck dissection should be done.

Complications of Surgery

Complications of surgery mainly depend upon surgical expertise. Complications are lesser in the centers performing high-volume surgeries. Risk of complications is higher in children with extrathyroidal extension, lymph node dissection, and repeat surgery. Endocrine complications are more common and include transient or permanent hypoparathyroidism (5–15%). Risk of permanent hypoparathyroidism is <2.5% in high-volume thyroid surgery centers. Risk of hypoparathyroidism and hence need for calcium and calcitriol supplementation can be predicted by postoperative intact parathyroid hormone (iPTH) 10–15 pg/mL and increase in postoperative phosphorus. Risk of hypoparathyroidism is higher in children who undergo total thyroidectomy along with CND. Nonendocrine complications include injury to recurrent laryngeal nerve, spinal accessory nerve, and Horner syndrome. There is no reliable predictor for nonendocrine complications.

Radioactive Iodine Ablation

Previous studies have shown that RAIA along with surgery significantly decreases thyroid bed recurrence as compare to surgery alone. There is a problem in adolescent and young adults with compliance of TSH suppressive therapy. So, previously RAIA was routinely recommended to all children undergoing total thyroidectomy for DTC. Long-term studies after RAIA have shown that routine use of RAIA increases all-cause mortality due to second malignancies in childhood DTC survivors. Present guidelines recommend assessment of patients at 12 weeks. Children are classified into low risk, intermediate risk, and high risk according to extent beyond thyroid gland, nodal involvement, and metastasis. Diagnostic scan along with TSH-stimulated thyroglobulin is done in intermediate- and high-risk category. Radioactive iodine ablation is indicated in case of residual disease, elevated thyroglobulin, unresectable cervical metastasis, and distant metastasis. RAIA is not indicated in low-risk category. Dose of radioactive iodine (RAI) can be empirical or based on body weight. Empirical doses are simple to use. In general, 15-year-old requires five-sixth of adult activity, 10-year-old require one-half of adult activity, and 5-year-old requires one-third of adult activity for similar extent of disease. Dose can also be given according to body weight (1–1.5 mCi/kg).

Adverse Effects of RAIA

Radioactive iodine ablation can have both short-term and long-term effects. Short-term effects include xerostomia, sialadenitis, dental caries, stomatitis, dry eyes, and obstruction of nasolacrimal duct. Sour candy or lemon juice is given after 24 hours along with hydration for 3–5 days to prevent xerostomia. Other effects are risk of gonadal damage (transient in low doses), acute bone marrow suppression, risk of second malignancy, and subsequently all-cause mortality. Risk of second malignancies is higher in younger children.

Thyroid-stimulating Hormone Suppressive Therapy

Thyroid-stimulating hormone suppressive therapy is given to all children undergoing total thyroidectomy. Depending upon risk category target of LT4 suppressed TSH is 0.5–1 mIU/L for low risk, 0.1–0.5 mIU/L for intermediate risk, and <0.1 mIU/L for high-risk category.

AUTONOMOUS THYROID NODULE

Treatment options for autonomous thyroid nodule in adult include surgery, RAIA, and ethanol injection. However, the role of RAIA and ethanol injection is not well defined in children. Also, there are concerns regarding mutagenic effects of iodine on normal thyroid tissue. Moreover, up to one-third of children with autonomous nodules can have incidental DTC. So, all symptomatic autonomous nodules on radioactive scan in children should be subjected to lobectomy. In case of asymptomatic children or subclinical hyperthyroidism wait and watch policy can be exercised but FNAB should be performed if there are suspicious features of malignancy on USG.

CONCLUSION

Majority of pediatric thyroid nodules are benign and can be managed conservatively. Indeterminate nodules in children should be managed with lobectomy followed by completion thyroidectomy if found malignant. Autonomous thyroid nodules in children are managed with lobectomy. Total thyroidectomy remains the mainstay of management of malignant thyroid nodules. There is change in paradigm regarding use of RAIA in recent years. Use of RAIA now depends upon postoperative risk stratification and is recommended in only intermediate-risk and high-risk malignant thyroid nodules.

SUGGESTED READINGS

1. De Luca F, Aversa T, Alessi L, Cama V, Costanzo D, Genovese C, et al. Thyroid nodules in childhood: indications for biopsy and surgery. Ital J Pediatr. 2014;40:48.
2. Gupta A, Ly S, Castroneves LA, Frates MC, Benson CB, Feldman HA, et al. A standardized assessment of thyroid nodules in children confirms higher cancer prevalence than in adults. J Clin Endocrinol Metab. 2013;98:3238-45.
3. Guille JT, Opoku-Boateng A, Thibeault SL, Chen H. Evaluation and management of the pediatric thyroid nodule. Oncologist. 2015;20(1):19-27.
4. Bauer AJ. Thyroid nodules in children and adolescents. Curr Opin Endocrinol Diabetes Obes. 2019;26:266-74.

SECTION 8

Thyroid Disorders in Special Situations

CHAPTER 28

Subclinical Hypothyroidism

Pramila Kalra, Bharathi Kolla

INTRODUCTION

Subclinical hypothyroidism (SCH) is defined as a state of elevated thyroid-stimulating hormone (TSH), triiodothyronine (T3), and thyroxine (T4) concentrations within the population reference range. The incidence of SCH is 3–15%. Decrease in T4 or free thyroxine (FT4) levels lead to stimulation of hypothalamic–pituitary–thyroid axis, resulting in secretion of pituitary thyrotropin.

ETIOLOGY

The etiology of subclinical hypothyroidism is similar to that of overt hypothyroidism and the most common cause of SCH is Hashimoto's thyroiditis. However, a few causes of elevated TSH do not define the concept of SCH. Causes include nonthyroidal illness, assay variability, thyroid hormone resistance, drugs such as metoclopramide, domperidone, and heterophile antibodies or macro-TSH may cause artifactual elevations in serum TSH **(Box 1)**.

Mild elevations in TSH must be persistent for 3–6 months before the diagnosis of SCH is confirmed.

Two to six percent of individuals with SCH progress to hypothyroidism per year. The probable risk factors for progression include—patients with higher TSH elevations, antithyroid peroxidase antibodies (anti-TPO-Abs), female gender, individuals with low-normal FT4 levels, and family history of hypothyroidism.

> **BOX 1: Etiology of subclinical hypothyroidism.**
> - Hashimoto's thyroiditis
> - Iodine deficiency
> - Inadequate levothyroxine replacement for overt hypothyroidism
> - Lithium therapy
> - Postradioactive iodine ablation
> - Few patients with obesity

CLINICAL IMPORTANCE

Thyroid Hormones on Various Organs

The thyroid gland produces iodothyronines, the primary secretory product, an inactive hormone T4. Thyroxine is converted to T3 via type 1 deiodinase in tissues with high blood flow such as the liver and kidneys. Thyroxine is converted to T3 in the brain through type 2 deiodinase by glial cells.

T3 regulates the functioning of various organs at the cellular level.

Heart: Thyroid hormones increase heart rate, cardiac output, and stroke volume through positive inotropic and chronotropic effects. Thyroid hormones increase intracellular calcium within the cardiac myocytes and help increase the force of contraction and speed. As a result, vasculature in the skin, heart, and muscle dilate, decreasing peripheral vascular resistance. In addition, there is an activation of the renin-angiotensin-aldosterone system.

Basal metabolic rate: Thyroid hormones favor the activation of mitochondrial uncoupling proteins, leading to increased heat production and oxygen consumption. There is increased thermogenesis through increased fatty acid uptake and oxidation.

Respiratory: Triiodothyronine stimulates resting respiratory rate and minute ventilation, thereby normalizing arterial oxygen consumption for increased oxidation rates. Triiodothyronine stimulates erythropoietin and hemoglobin production, helping folate, and cobalamin absorption through the gastrointestinal tract.

Growth: Triiodothyronine favors the development of the fetal growth center, linear growth of the bone, endochondral ossification, and maturation of epiphyseal bone. Triiodothyronine also helps in remodeling of adult bone, degradation of fibronectin, and mucopolysaccharides in extracellular connective tissue.

Nervous system: Triiodothyronine stimulates wakefulness and alertness in response to external stimuli. In addition, T3 increases peripheral reflexes, gastrointestinal tone, and motility through stimulation of the peripheral nervous system.

Reproductive system: Thyroid hormone helps stimulate and release growth hormone. It inhibits prolactin release. It favors the regulation of normal reproductive function in both men and women by regulating the ovulatory cycle and spermatogenesis.

For differentiating the mild and severe forms of SCH, TSH of 10 mU/L is considered, with TSH <10 mU/L being mild and TSH >10 mU/L being more severe.

Subclinical Hypothyroidism and Lipids

The thyroid hormone regulates the formation of cholesterol by regulating the activity of the 3-hydroxy-3-methylglutaryl coenzyme an enzyme, and its degradation rate with the help of regulating the expression of the *SREBP2* gene, which is a transcription factor that regulates the activity of low-density lipoprotein (LDL) receptor. The action of thyroid hormone on lipids is through LDL receptors that are expressed at hepatic and peripheral levels. There is increased activity of enzymes like hepatic lipase (HL), lipoprotein lipase (LDL), cholesterol ester transport protein (CTEP), and lecithin–cholesterol acyltransferase (LCAT) which help in the metabolism of lipoproteins and reverse cholesterol transport.

In a cross-sectional epidemiological, nested case-control study, the 5th Tromsø study, which included 5,143 subjects, there was a significant and positive correlation between serum TSH levels and total serum cholesterol and low density lipid-C (LDL-C) levels in both genders. Furthermore, patients with newly diagnosed SCH showed a prominent rise in triglycerides and LDL-C and low HDL cholesterol compared with the control group after adjustment for age and body mass index (BMI). Notably, women with TSH levels higher than 10 mIU/L exhibited a significant increase in LDL.

Another cross-sectional and controlled study that included 49 children with persistent, idiopathic, long-standing (3.2 ± 0.4 years), mild SCH (TSH: 4.5–10 mU/L), waist-to-height-ratio (WHtR) ($p < 0.0001$), atherogenic index ($p = 0.001$), TGs/high-density [triglyceride high-density lipid (HDL)]-cholesterol ratio ($p = 0.01$) and homocysteine levels ($p = 0.002$) were significantly higher and HDL-cholesterol significantly lower ($p = 0.003$) in SCH subjects compared with 49 controls.

Subclinical Hypothyroidism and Hyperthyroidism

In individuals with SCH, there is a significant association with hypertension. A meta-analysis on the association between SCH and systolic blood pressure revealed that SCH was associated with elevated systolic blood pressure, and it was therefore, hypothesized that it might be a potential risk factor for high systolic blood pressure. In addition, hypothyroidism is associated with arterial stiffness and left ventricular diastolic dysfunction. A cross-sectional study assessed the association between thyroid hormone level and cardio-ankle vascular index (CAVI), and left ventricular diastolic function. Eighty-three patients were enrolled with untreated SCH; log N-terminal prohormone of brain natriuretic peptide (NT-proBNP), CAVI, and C-reactive protein (CRP) were found higher in SCH. Thus, high logNT-proBNP may be associated with a raised CAVI in patients with SCH. This state may be a risk factor for cardiovascular (CV) events related to arterial stiffening and left ventricular diastolic dysfunction.

Subclinical Hypothyroidism and Cardiovascular Disease

Thyroid hormones act through various mechanisms in the heart. Thyroid hormones, either elevated or decreased, affect the CV system. Few studies demonstrated that SCH increased CV risk factors, including an altered lipid profile, insulin resistance, oxidative stress, increased vascular stiffness, and endothelial dysfunction.

A meta-analysis which included 35 eligible articles with a total of 555,530 participants showed that SCH was associated with increased cardiovascular death (CVD) and all-cause mortality [relative risk (RR) for CVD = 1.33, confidence interval (CI) 1.14–1.54; RR for all-cause mortality = 1.20 (CI 1.07–1.34)].

A meta-analysis to assess the noninvasive markers of CV risk in SCH with 27 studies, including 1,065 SCH patients and 866 euthyroid subjects, provided evidence of association of SCH with increased arterial stiffness. An increase in epicardial adipose tissue and endothelial dysfunction that is evident by reduced flow-mediated dilatation (FMD) and glyceryl trinitrate (GNT)-induced dilation in SCH patients compared with euthyroid controls was also found.

Young females with SCH had higher QT variability index (QTvi) compared to controls ($p = 0.01$) which may be an indicator of increased CV mortality risk.

Subclinical Hypothyroidism and Brain

Thyroid hormones stimulate the nervous system and increase alertness and wakefulness. Cognitive impairment is associated both with hypothyroidism and hyperthyroidism. Clinical guidelines recommend screening of thyroid functions among patients with cognitive dysfunction. However, there is conflicting data on cognitive impairment in SCH.

Few studies have shown that cognitive impairment is increased fourfold in SCH. Few meta-analyses have demonstrated a relationship between SCH and cognitive impairment only in individuals younger than 75 years of age and with higher TSH concentrations while in older population no correlation with cognition has been shown. These studies are heterogenous as they have used different cut offs for TSH, and many of them have not done very elaborate tests for cognition. Younger patients with SCH have been shown to have delayed visual memory recall and category fluency deficits, which may be suggestive of dysfunction of the prefrontal cortex and temporal lobe in young patients.

In a cross-sectional study, brain volumes were assessed in a population with hyperthyroidism and hypothyroidism with a TSH cut-off of <0.5 and >3.4 mIU/L. It was shown that elevated TSH was associated with decreased total brain volumes, white matter volume, and hippocampal volume, but no association was established with gray matter volume.

Subclinical Hypothyroidism and Psychiatric Illness

The correlation between overt hypothyroidism, mood disorders, and cognitive disorders has been established. In addition, several studies have shown an association between SCH and depression, anxiety, and psychosis.

A cross-sectional study which evaluated the prevalence of depression, and anxiety among patients with SCH, has shown a significant association between SCH and depression and panic attacks.

However, data from National Health and Nutrition Examination Survey (NHANES) have shown no association between SCH and depression in older patients but younger patients did show an association. Therefore, the effect of treatment with levothyroxine (LT4) in this group leading to improvement in depression is controversial.

Hypercoagulation and Insulin Resistance

Subclinical hypothyroidism may cause an elevation of homocysteine, CRP, and increase in arterial stiffness, endothelial dysfunction, and altered coagulation parameters. The other abnormalities reported include the abnormalities in hemostatic parameters, and glucose abnormalities the former being due to the increase in the activity of plasminogen activator inhibitor 1 and factor VII, which suggests that atherosclerosis in SCH may be secondary to hypofibrinolytic and hypercoagulable state.

Subclinical Hypothyroidism and Fertility

Conception and pregnancy require a normal functioning thyroid gland. SCH is seen in 13.9–16% of the population with infertility. Inconclusive data is concluded to suggest that SCH is associated with infertility.

In a large prospective study of >16,000 pregnant women, it was observed that SCH were at higher risk for placental abruption and preterm delivery compared with euthyroid women. The offspring of these women were more likely to have respiratory distress syndrome and be admitted to the neonatal intensive care unit. It has been reported in few studies that compared SCH is associated with miscarriage, preterm delivery, eclampsia, gestational hypertension, intrauterine growth retardation, premature rupture of membranes, and low birth weight. Anti-TPO seems to play a synergistic role with the elevated TSH concentrations in increasing the risk for pregnancy complications.

In a meta-analysis of 18 cohort studies that included 3,995 pregnant women, it was shown that SCH was associated with pregnancy loss and 2.6-fold more likely to suffer a neonatal death compared with euthyroid women, and higher risk of premature rupture of membranes and placental abruption.

Thyroid Hormone and Aging

There is an increase in prevalence of SCH with age ranging from 3 to 16% in individuals above 60 years. Unlike in overt hypothyroidism, SCH is not associated with decline in cognition, or associated with depression, or poor quality of life in elderly. Overall mortality is not increased due to SCH in elderly.

Aging is associated with changes in the pituitary thyroid axis, and there is an increased prevalence of nodular thyroid disease and autoimmune thyroid illness. It was initially hypothesized that aging was associated with a decrease in TSH secretion. However, a survey by NHANES showed that serum TSH was elevated in people without any prior existing thyroid diseases in iodine deficiency. They included 14,376 participants who did not have a history of thyroid disorders and were negative for TPO and thyroglobulin antibodies. It was noted that there was a progressive shift in the TSH curve toward higher TSH values with an increase in age. A longitudinal study included 908 participants, with a mean period of 13 years; the change in TSH was 0.32 mU/L which was significant.

TREATMENT

Why should We Treat Patients with Subclinical Hypothyroidism?

Symptomatic Improvement

Few studies have shown significant improvement in symptoms in euthyroid compared to the subclinical hypothyroid population, especially concerning drier skin, poorer memory, slower thinking, weaker muscles, more significant tiredness, and constipation. In some studies, there has been no improvement in symptoms of the subclinical hypothyroid population treated with LT4, while some have shown significant benefits.

Dosing in SCH varies. Levothyroxine can be started at a dose of 0.5–1 µg/kg/day body weight. Caution should be taken in patients who are elderly and have CV risk factors.

Mood Disturbances/Mental Health

In a few cross-sectional studies, it has been shown that treatment with LT4 has benefited working memory and motor learning. However, there is conflicting data on this, especially in subjects whose TSH is between 3.5 and 10 mU/L. In addition, no studies have shown the benefit of treatment of SCH in a population >65 years, but data in the younger population is controversial.

Goiter and Thyroid Cancer

Subclinical hypothyroidism may be associated with goiter. Increasing TSH levels have shown a positive correlation with the risk of thyroid malignancy. A large study that included 27,914 patients has shown that treatment with LT4 was associated with a lower risk of malignancy. As the frequency of thyroid carcinoma is low and tumors develop slowly, treatment with LT4 to reduce thyroid cancers has not been established yet.

Dyslipidemia

In many studies there was significant positive correlation between SCH and dyslipidemia. In addition, two meta-analyses studies have shown an overall benefit on lipids in SCH treated with LT4.

Data from the Helsinki Heart Study show that in a population with SCH treated with LT4, there was a 7% reduction in LDL-C and 15% reduction in CHD cardiovascular heart disease (CHD).

Cardiovascular System, Heart Failure, and Ischemic Heart Disease

Subclinical hypothyroidism has been associated with increased vascular resistance, arterial stiffness, endothelial dysfunction, atherosclerosis, left ventricular diastolic dysfunction, reduced resting and exertional systolic function, and increased heart failure risk.

Levothyroxine treatment in SCH with patients at increased risk of CHD events has a modest benefit with a good prognosis.

▪ Subclinical Hypothyroidism Treatment in Infertility and Pregnancy

American thyroid association (ATA) suggests a weak recommendation that administration of LT4 may be considered in women who are SCH and planning for conception without any artificial reproductive techniques (ARTs) to prevent the progression to overt hypothyroidism once pregnancy is achieved. The guidelines suggests to consider treatment in all pregnant women with TSH >4 mIU/L or more than population-specific cut offs for TSH (if available) but only in high risk pregnancies or TPO-positive pregnant women between 2.5 and 4 mIU/L.

Evidence from randomized controlled studies shows that LT4 therapy improves pregnancy and miscarriage rates in women with SCH in patients undergoing ARTs. The ATA substantiates treating maternal hypothyroidism to a target TSH level of <2.5 mIU/L. Thyroid test have to be repeated every 4 weeks during the first half of pregnancy followed by once in 6–8 weeks. After delivery, levothyroxine dose has to be reduced to preconception dose, and thyroid tests should repeated at 6 weeks postpartum. For women who initiated LT4 during pregnancy, LT4 could potentially be discontinued, especially when the LT4 dose is <50 µg/day.

Whom should we probably treat?
- Hypothyroid symptoms in younger patients as per indications (<65 years)
- Persistent SCH following hemithyroidectomy
- Patients with diffuse or nodular goiter
- Patients with anti-TPO-Ab positivity
- Women planning for conception or on IVF treatment for pregnancy
- Patients with CV risk factors are at increased risk of CV morbidity
- Younger patients with dyslipidemia without a known cause
- Psychiatric disorders in younger patients
- Patients with cognitive abnormalities with no other attributable cause

Subclinical hypothyroidism is a biochemical diagnosis defined as elevated TSH and normal T4 and T3. Before treating, transient causes of elevated TSH must be ruled out. Confirmation of the diagnosis is required. So TSH, T3, T4, and anti-TPO-Abs must be repeated after 2–3 months before labeling it SCH. Anti-TPO provides additional information regarding the chances of conversion to overt hypothyroidism.

Individuals with anti-TPO-Ab positivity have twofold higher chances of progression to overt hypothyroidism.

European and American Thyroid Association recommend treating SCH if TSH >10 mU/L. European Thyroid Association (ETA) guidelines recommend distinguishing between patients younger and older than 70 years. In individuals >70 years of treatment, recommendations are restricted. Treatment recommendations in individuals with TSH <10 mU/L are based on symptoms suggestive of hypothyroidism, anti-TPO-Ab positivity, age (above or below 70 years), evidence of cardiovascular disease, or associated risk factors. If the symptoms improve after treatment, consider lifelong treatment in individuals with symptoms. If there is no symptomatic improvement, LT4 can be stopped after 3–6 months of treatment. If no treatment is offered, TSH should be monitored every 6–12 months.

The target of the treatment with LT4 is to restore the TSH within the normal range. TSH target should preferably be in the lower half of the reference range in patients younger than 70 years. Treatment targets for individuals aged >70 years are higher. As individuals with SCH have residual thyroid gland functioning, the LT4 dose required to normalize TSH is less than that of overt hypothyroidism.

CONCLUSION

The treatment of SCH is indicated in few scenarios. The improvement in cognition, mood, dyslipidemia, CV morbidity, and cardiac risk factor reduction in younger age group has been seen in few studies with LT4 treatment. The benefit in older age group has not been seen in most of the studies.

SUGGESTED READINGS

1. Vanderpump MP, Tunbridge WM, French JM, Appleton D, Bates D, Clark F, et al. The incidence of thyroid disorders in the community: a twenty-year follow-up of the Whickham Survey. Clin Endocrinol (Oxf). 1995;43(1):55-68.
2. Canaris GJ, Manowitz NR, Mayor G, Ridgway EC. The Colorado thyroid disease prevalence study. Arch Intern Med. 2000;160(4):526-34.
3. Livingston EH. Subclinical Hypothyroidism. JAMA. 2019;322(2):180.
4. Fatourechi V. Subclinical hypothyroidism: an update for primary care physicians. Mayo Clin Proc. 2009;84(1):65-71.
5. Armstrong M, Asuka E, Fingeret A. Physiology, Thyroid Function. In: StatPearls [Internet]. Treasure Island (FL): StatPearls Publishing; 2022.
6. Shahid MA, Ashraf MA, Sharma S. Physiology, Thyroid Hormone. In: StatPearls [Internet]. Treasure Island (FL): StatPearls Publishing; 2022.
7. Abrams JJ, Grundy SM. Cholesterol metabolism in hypothyroidism and hyperthyroidism in man. J Lipid Res. 1981;22(2):323-38.
8. Iqbal A, Jorde R, Figenschau Y. Serum lipid levels in relation to serum thyroid-stimulating hormone and the effect of thyroxine treatment on serum lipid levels in subjects with subclinical hypothyroidism: the Tromsø Study. J Intern Med. 2006;260(1):53-61.
9. Cerbone M, Capalbo D, Wasniewska M, Mattace Raso G, Alfano S, Meli R, et al. Cardiovascular risk factors in children with long-standing untreated idiopathic subclinical hypothyroidism. J Clin Endocrinol Metab. 2014;99(8):2697-703.
10. Cai YF, Shi JP. Meta-analysis on the relationship between subclinical hypothyroidism and the levels of systolic blood pressure. Zhonghua Liu Xing Bing Xue Za Zhi. 2011;32(1):55-9.
11. Masaki M, Komamura K, Goda A, Hirotani S, Otsuka M, Nakabo A, et al. Elevated arterial stiffness and diastolic dysfunction in subclinical hypothyroidism. Circ J. 2014;78(6):1494-500.
12. Moon S, Kim MJ, Yu JM, Yoo HJ, Park YJ. Subclinical Hypothyroidism and the Risk of Cardiovascular Disease and All-Cause Mortality: A Meta-analysis of Prospective Cohort Studies. Thyroid. 2018;28(9):1101-10.
13. Yao K, Zhao T, Zeng L, Yang J, Liu Y, He Q, et al. Non-invasive markers of cardiovascular risk in patients with subclinical hypothyroidism: A systematic review and meta-analysis of 27 case control studies. Sci Rep. 2018;8(1):4579.
14. Kalra P, Yeragani VK, Prasanna Kumar KM. Cardiac autonomic function and vascular profile in subclinical hypothyroidism: Increased beat-to-beat QT variability. Indian J Endocrinol Metab. 2016;20(5):605-11.
15. Pasqualetti G, Pagano G, Rengo G, Ferrara N, Monzani F. Subclinical Hypothyroidism and Cognitive Impairment: Systematic Review and Meta-Analysis. J Clin Endocrinol Metab. 2015;100(11):4240-8.
16. Akintola AA, Jansen SW, van Bodegom D, van der Grond J, Westendorp RG, de Craen AJM, et al. Subclinical hypothyroidism and cognitive function in people over 60 years: a systematic review and meta-analysis. Front Aging Neurosci. 2015;7:150.
17. Kalra P, Kumaraswamy DR, Dharmalingam M, Saini J, Yadav R. Neuropsychological Impairments in Young Patients with Subclinical Hypothyroidism: A Case Control Study. Ann Neurosci. 2020;27(3-4):169-74.
18. Ittermann T, Wittfeld K, Nauck M, Bülow R, Hosten N, Völzke H, et al. High Thyrotropin is Associated with Reduced Hippocampal Volume in a Population-based Study from Germany. Thyroid. 2018;28(11):1434-42.
19. Benseñor IM, Nunes MA, Sander Diniz M de F, Santos IS, Brunoni AR, Lotufo PA. Subclinical thyroid dysfunction and psychiatric disorders: cross-sectional results from the Brazilian Study of Adult Health (ELSA-Brasil). Clin Endocrinol (Oxf). 2016;84(2):250-6.
20. Airaksinen J, Komulainen K, García-Velázquez R, Määttänen I, Gluschkoff K, Savelieva K, et al. Subclinical hypothyroidism and symptoms of depression: Evidence from the National Health and Nutrition Examination Surveys (NHANES). Compr Psychiatry. 2021;109:152253.
21. Duntas LH, Chiovato L. Cardiovascular Risk in Patients with Subclinical Hypothyroidism. Eur Endocrinol. 2014;10(2):157-60.
22. Strickland DM, Whitted WA, Wians FH. Screening infertile women for subclinical hypothyroidism. Am J Obstet Gynecol. 1990;163(1 Pt 1):262-3.
23. Maraka S, Singh Ospina NM, Mastorakos G, O'Keeffe DT. Subclinical Hypothyroidism in Women Planning Conception and during Pregnancy: Who should be Treated and How? J Endocr Soc. 2018;2(6):533-46.
24. Maraka S, Ospina NMS, O'Keeffe DT, Espinosa De Ycaza AE, Gionfriddo MR, Erwin PJ, et al. Subclinical Hypothyroidism in Pregnancy: A Systematic Review and Meta-analysis. Thyroid. 2016;26(4):580-90.
25. Aggarwal N, Razvi S. Thyroid and aging or the aging thyroid? An evidence-based analysis of the literature. J Thyroid Res. 2013;2013:481287.
26. Calsolaro V, Niccolai F, Pasqualetti G, Tognini S, Magno S, Riccioni T, et al. Hypothyroidism in the elderly: who should be treated and how? J Endocr Soc. 2018;3(1):146-58.
27. Bremner AP, Feddema P, Leedman PJ, Brown SJ, Beilby JP, Lim EM, et al. Age-related changes in thyroid function: a longitudinal study of a community-based cohort. J Clin Endocrinol Metab. 2012;97(5):1554-62.
28. Jorde R, Waterloo K, Storhaug H, Nyrnes A, Sundsfjord J, Jenssen TG. Neuropsychological function and symptoms in subjects with subclinical hypothyroidism and the effect of thyroxine treatment. J Clin Endocrinol Metab. 2006;91(1):145-5.
29. Samuels MH, Schuff KG, Carlson NE, Carello P, Janowsky JS. Health status, mood, and cognition in experimentally induced subclinical hypothyroidism. J Clin Endocrinol Metab. 2007;92(7):2545-51.
30. Fiore E, Rago T, Provenzale MA, Scutari M, Ugolini C, Basolo F, et al. L-thyroxine-treated patients with nodular goiter have lower serum TSH and lower frequency of papillary thyroid cancer: results of a cross-sectional study on 27,914 patients. Endocr Relat Cancer. 2010;17(1):231-9.
31. Danese MD, Ladenson PW, Meinert CL, Powe NR. Clinical review 115: effect of thyroxine therapy on serum lipoproteins in patients with mild thyroid failure: a quantitative review of the literature. J Clin Endocrinol Metab. 2000;85(9):2993-3001.

32. Mänttäri M, Huttunen JK, Koskinen P, Manninen V, Tenkanen L, Heinonen OP, et al. Lipoproteins and coronary heart disease in the Helsinki Heart Study. Eur Heart J. 1990;11 Suppl H:26-31.
33. Monzani F, Di Bello V, Caraccio N, Bertini A, Giorgi D, Giusti C, et al. Effect of levothyroxine on cardiac function and structure in subclinical hypothyroidism: a double blind, placebo-controlled study. J Clin Endocrinol Metab. 2001;86(3):1110-5.
34. Alexander EK, Pearce EN, Brent GA, Brown RS, Chen H, Dosiou C, et al. 2017 Guidelines of the American Thyroid Association for the Diagnosis and Management of Thyroid Disease during Pregnancy and the Postpartum. Thyroid. 2017;27(3):315-89.
35. Rao M, Zeng Z, Zhao S, Tang L. Effect of levothyroxine supplementation on pregnancy outcomes in women with subclinical hypothyroidism and thyroid autoimmuneity undergoing in vitro fertilization/intracytoplasmic sperm injection: an updated meta-analysis of randomized controlled trials. Reprod Biol Endocrinol. 2018;16(1):92.
36. Tsakiridis I, Giouleka S, Kourtis A, Mamopoulos A, Athanasiadis A, Dagklis T. Thyroid Disease in Pregnancy: A Descriptive Review of Guidelines. Obstet Gynecol Surv. 2022;77(1):45-62.
37. Garber JR, Cobin RH, Gharib H, Hennessey JV, Klein I, Mechanick JI, et al. Clinical practice guidelines for hypothyroidism in adults: cosponsored by the American Association of Clinical Endocrinologists and the American Thyroid Association. Endocr Pract. 2012;18(6):988-1028.
38. Pearce SH, Brabant G, Duntas LH, Monzani F, Peeters RP, Razvi S, et al. 2013 ETA Guideline: Management of Subclinical Hypothyroidism. Eur Thyroid J. 2013;2(4):215-28.

CHAPTER 29

Thyroid and Obesity: Coexisting Perplexity

Sindhu Sree Rallapalli, Nitin Kapoor

INTRODUCTION

The prevalence of obesity and hypothyroidism, two among the leading noncommunicable endocrine disorders are increasing worldwide. Change in cultural habits, sedentary lifestyles, along with the abundance and ease of high calorie food have rapidly propelled a global pandemic of obesity.

It is one of the key components of metabolic syndrome and enhances the risk for development of type 2 diabetes mellitus (T2DM), dyslipidemia, cardiovascular disease, disability-adjusted life-years (DALYs) and mortality, leading to 4.9% and 7.1% of all global DALYs and deaths in 2015. Similar to obesity, hypothyroidism is also associated with insulin resistance (IR), dyslipidemia, and atherosclerotic diseases across all ages. Hypothyroidism is more prevalent in patients with obesity. Data from India suggests that among individuals with obesity about one-third have overt and subclinical hypothyroidism (SCH) respectively.

Thus, obesity and hypothyroidism are coexisting common illnesses with mutual impact on each other and additive metabolic effects. Hypothyroidism is often implicated in the weight gain due to changes in basal metabolic rate (BMR), total energy expenditure (TEE), and resting energy expenditure (REE), independent of physical activity. And recent studies suggest obesity to as such cause changes in levels of thyroid-stimulating hormone (TSH) and thyroid hormone (TH), rather than simply be the effect of them. Thyroid dysfunction with moderately elevated TSH, elevated T3, and lower T4 is classically described in patients with obesity, more often with metabolically unhealthy obese phenotype. High leptin levels and thyroid autoimmunity might have a role to play.

So the relationship between obesity and hypothyroidism seems bidirectional and understanding this relationship is necessary for clinical application.

EPIDEMIOLOGY

Prevalence of obesity is increasing at an alarming rate. The worldwide prevalence of overweight and obesity has nearly tripled between 1975 and 2016, with 39% of adults aged 18 and above being overweight and 13% obese. The global prevalence of obesity increased from 3.2% in 1975 to 10.8% in 2014 in males and from 6.4 to 14.9% in females. According to National Family Health Survey 5 (2019–2021), prevalence of overweight and obesity in Indian men and women aged 15–49 years was 24% and 23% respectively.

The prevalence of overt and SCH in the general population ranges between 0.1–2% and 4–10%, respectively. Prevalence of hypothyroidism in India is around 11% and South Indians have elevated thyroid peroxidase antibody (TPO-Ab) levels detected in around 9.5% of general population. A population-based Indian study found prevalence of SCH three times more than overt hypothyroidism with female to male ratio of 2:1.

Reports of prevalence of hypothyroidism are variable, in part to variations in iodine intake and thyroid autoimmunity of study population.

Results of a meta-analysis involving 22 studies showed the relative risk of hypothyroidism among individuals with obesity was found to be 1.86 [95% confidence interval (CI) 1.63–2.11, $p < 0.001$] and the relative risk of positive TPO-Ab in individuals with obesity was 1.93 (95% CI 1.31–2.85, $p = 0.001$). Moreover, thyroid dysfunction in women seems 10 times more common than men.

PHYSIOLOGY OF THYROID HORMONES

The weight gain in an individual is the consequence of imbalance between increased energy intake and decreased energy expenditure leading to a positive energy balance.

Thyroid hormones accelerate energy expenditure by upregulating the BMR, thermogenesis and oxygen consumption through direct actions on metabolically active tissues such as the liver, skeletal muscle, heart, and brown adipose tissue (BAT). The catabolic effects of TH on lipid, protein, and glucose metabolism further result in weight loss. The concentrations of thyroxine-binding globulin (TBG), the major transport protein for TH are reduced in obesity which necessitates measurement of free TH,

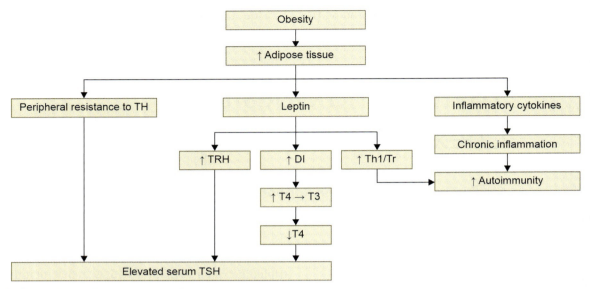

Flowchart 1: Mechanisms of obesity causing hypothyroidism.
(T3: triiodothyronine; T4: thyroxine; TH: thyroid hormone; TRH: thyrotropin-releasing hormone; TSH: thyroid-stimulating hormone)

preferably free T4 (FT4) in evaluating thyroid dysfunction in subjects with obesity.

Multiple mechanisms have described bidirectional relationship between thyroid and obesity. Various theories and mechanisms explain obesity-related elevation of serum TSH as detailed in **Flowchart 1**.

Leptin

Leptin, produced by adipose tissue regulates energy homeostasis by modulating neuroendocrine and behavioral responses to overfeeding, thereby regulating food intake, energy expenditure, and adipose tissue reserves.

A positive correlation between increased serum leptin and TSH levels exists in individuals with obesity, even after adjusting for body mass index (BMI), fat-mass, insulin sensitivity, and other metabolic parameters.

At the central level, leptin promotes expression and synthesis of thyrotropin-releasing hormone (TRH) in the arcuate and paraventricular nuclei of hypothalamus, thereby resulting in raised serum TSH levels.

At the peripheral level, leptin stimulates thyroid deiodinase increasing the conversion of T4 to T3 in peripheral tissues as a compensatory mechanism to increase energy expenditure by increasing free T3 levels. This resultant decreased serum T4 levels leads to compensatory stimulation of the hypothalamus-pituitary-thyroid axis, resetting the central thyrostat at higher level to maintain euthyroid TH range, thereby increasing serum TSH levels.

Leptin may also reduce the expressions of sodium/iodide symporter and thyroglobulin in thyroid cells. On the contrary, with calorie restriction, serum T3 declines significantly as an adaptive response for energy preservation. This adaptive decline in T3 is partly mediated by fall in leptin levels with weight loss and can be reversed with leptin administration.

Some studies showed leptin and TH to share some common downstream action sites leading to additive enhancement of calorigenic metabolism.

Adipocytes also generate a state of peripheral resistance to TH in obesity due to their lower expression of TSH receptors, which can also contribute to an increase in the plasma TSH as a compensatory mechanism.

Autoimmunity

Many studies have shown a positive association between obesity and TPO-Ab. In subjects with obesity, adipokines and inflammatory cytokines like interleukin-1 (IL-1), IL-6, and tumor necrosis factor α released by the adipose tissue induce chronic low-grade immune and inflammatory process. Leptin can further increase the number of T helper-1 (Th1) cells and decrease the function of regulatory T (Tr) cells thereby augmenting autoimmune process. Inflammatory cytokines also inhibit the messenger ribonucleic acid (mRNA) expression of sodium/iodide symporter. Chronic inflammation also modulates the expression and function of deiodinases. As a result, individuals with obesity are more prone to inflammatory and autoimmune processes in the thyroid gland that results in hypothyroidism.

A recent meta-analysis revealed obesity to be associated with a 93% increased risk of developing positive TPO-Ab. TPO-Abs are the hallmarks of Hashimoto thyroiditis which is a common cause of primary hypothyroidism in iodine-sufficient regions. The prevalence of hypothyroidism is higher, by about 20% in individuals with morbid obesity unrelated to BMI or fat mass. On the contrary, raised serum TSH without low TH is seen in most individuals with morbid obesity in the absence of clinical features of hypothyroidism. This phenotype is often not associated with an elevated TPO-Ab. Hence, raised TSH alone (hyperthyrotropinemia, sometimes mislabeled as SCH) is common biochemical entity in patients with morbid obesity and need not be treated always.

Few studies found inconsistent results regarding TSH levels in obesity. These discrepancies may be due to variations in iodine and the smoking status of the study population as smoking is observed to be negatively associated with TSH levels.

Elevated inflammatory markers in obesity also increase the vascular permeability with fluid extravasation in thyroid gland giving rise to a hypoechoic pattern on ultrasonogram without features of thyroid disease or positive TPO-Ab. These alterations in thyroid morphology in patients with morbid obesity are reversible with marked weight loss usually achieved by bariatric surgery.

Both subclinical and overt hypothyroidism can cause weight gain and changes in body composition independent of physical activity. Hypothyroidism-related weight gain is attributed to positive energy balance secondary to decreased BMR, TEE, and REE. There is also expansion of compartments of extracellular water and fat-mass, to a lesser extent of fat-free lean body mass.

One of the hypotheses states that TSH stimulates the release of leptin by adipocytes and leptin stimulates the release of TSH to compensate for the increase in adipocyte mass.

This positive association between hypothyroidism and weight gain is seen across the normal serum ranges of TSH and BMI. Some cross-sectional studies suggest that even a slightly elevated TSH can be considered a risk factor for overweight and obesity.

A study of 2,760 euthyroid young females showed higher prevalence of metabolic syndrome in those with high-normal TSH (2.6–4.5 mIU/L) than those with low-normal TSH (0.3–2.5 mIU/L).

Reversibility

The relationship between hypothyroidism and obesity is thus bidirectional (**Fig. 1**), and to precisely assert the dominant direction is not possible. Several studies suggest obesity to be the primary factor that causes thyroid dysfunction based on the reversion of thyroid dysfunction after weight loss.

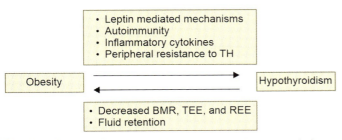

Fig. 1: Bidirectional relationship between obesity and hypothyroidism.
(BMR: basal metabolic rate; REE: resting energy expenditure; TEE: total energy expenditure; TH: thyroid hormone)

Due to the altered thyroid physiology in obesity as described before, a progressive fat accumulation is associated with an increase in TSH, and FT3 irrespective of other metabolic associations. These thyroid alterations revert after weight loss either by bariatric surgery or low calorie diet. Even earlier stages of life-style interventions without much noticeable changes in BMI have shown to reduce TSH, FT3, and TPO-Ab levels, probably secondary to changes in the body composition causing reduction in inflammatory cytokines and their resultant thyroid dysfunction. Patients with SCH have been shown to have normalization of TSH levels with weight loss without further progression to overt hypothyroidism. BMI reductions also reduced thyroid volume, improved thyroid structure, and parenchymal pattern on ultrasonogram.

CLINICAL IMPLICATIONS

The key clinical challenge in clinical practice is to differentiate SCH from elevated TSH secondary to obesity. Furthermore, deranged lipid profile at times may be secondary to either SCH or obesity, thus adding to treatment dilemma. However, it is important not to attribute the entire weight gain in patients with constitutional obesity to elevated TSH. Treatment of overt hypothyroidism itself results in only modest weight loss. Through a study by Valdes et al., normative TSH reference ranges based on BMI have been described and should be used clinically (**Table 1**). The TSH in this study was performed on E170, Roche Diagnostics, Basel, Switzerland.

A study in children with SCH and obesity found that, dietary-behavioral intervention alone contributed to weight loss, irrespective of levothyroxine use. The elevations in TSH and FT3 in obesity are probably compensatory adaptive mechanisms to increase BMR and REE and cause weight loss, analogous to the reduction in TSH and FT3 in anorexia nervosa, to prevent weight loss. These findings suggest that moderately elevated serum TSH is likely a consequence rather than cause of obesity and overweight and thyroxine replacement in expectation of weight loss should be avoided. This complexity of causes and effects make it hard to ascertain effective testing strategies. "Endocrine work-up in obesity" is a new clinical practice guideline released by The European Society of Endocrinology. The guideline recommends that all patients with obesity should be tested for thyroid function which is the only condition for

TABLE 1: TSH cut-offs based on body mass index (BMI).	
BMI (kg/m^2)	Normal TSH range (µIU/mL)
<20	0.6–4.8
20–29.9	0.6–5.5
30–39.9	0.5–5.9
>40	0.7–7.5
(TSH: thyroid-stimulating hormone)	

which it recommends testing without the need for signs and symptoms. Furthermore, untreated hypothyroidism could blight the attempts at losing body weight.

The guideline recommends thyroid screening because of:
- The high prevalence of hypothyroidism in obesity
- Hypothyroidism if left untreated could potentiate weight gain and worsen cardiovascular risk in obesity.
- Assessment is simple, and treatment is inexpensive and safe.
- The testing should initially include TSH, and if TSH is elevated, free T4 and TPO-Abs could be measured if clinically deemed necessary.

Thyroid nodules and cancer: Body mass index is also positively associated with thyroid volume and incidence of thyroid nodules, both benign and malignant. This association is in positive correlation with the degree of IR. Higher visceral fat mass has a stronger association with thyroid cancer since visceral adipose tissue is highly metabolically active and associated with hyperinsulinemia and increased IR. Certain genetic factors also explain this association **(Table 2)**. Five of the obesity-specific genes, *FABP4*, *CFD*, *GHR*, *TNFRSF11B*, and *LTF*, had significantly decreased expression in patients with thyroid cancer. Further research is needed into identification of etiological factors regarding association of obesity with thyroid nodules and cancer.

Fertility outcomes: In women, obesity and autoimmune hypothyroidism both impact female fertility outcomes with/without being associated with polycystic ovarian syndrome. The risk of infertility, miscarriage rates, subfecundity and pregnancy complications are increased in these women. In men, both TH and leptin receptors have been shown on the testes, role of these two hormones in the male reproductive function have been studied. Both these hormones negatively affect spermatogenesis and may cause male infertility. The longer the untreated, persistent hypothyroidism, the greater the damage to the testes.

Selective thyroid receptor β (TRB) agonists: Synthetic TH preparations have been used to facilitate weight loss. Stimulation of BAT in adults, through TH-mediated pathways, has been an attractive pathway for managing obesity. However, TH treatment often results in subclinical hyperthyroidism in most patients without consistent effect on weight loss across the studies, with additive adverse effects on bone and heart. TH acts through two major receptors, (1) thyroid receptor α (TRA) and TRB. Action of TH depends on activated receptor, with TRA-mediating T4 effects on bone, skeletal muscle, heart and brain, and TRB-regulating secretion of TRH/TSH and metabolic effects of T3 in liver, such as lowering of lipids. Adipose tissue expresses both thyroid receptors. Selective TRB agonists are promising drugs for management of dyslipidemia, obesity, and nonalcoholic steatohepatitis (NASH) in euthyroid patients without adverse effects on bones or heart. Further evidence-based human studies are required before attempting their clinical use.

CONCLUSION

- Obesity and hypothyroidism are common public health problems.
- Crosstalk between thyroid and adipose tissue alters the physiological processes involved with obesity and hypothyroidism
- Obesity is positively associated with increased odds of overt hypothyroidism and TPO-Ab positivity even after adjustment for confounding factors.
- A moderately elevated TSH, elevated T3, and a lower T4 is classically described thyroid dysfunction in patients with obesity.
- Isolated, moderately elevated TSH levels in the absence of autoimmunity, or clinical features of hypothyroidism could be regarded as normal in individuals with obesity. BMI-based TSH cut-offs can guide in management.
- Thyroid ultrasonogram, a commonly used diagnostic tool, cannot be reliably used in obese patients for the diagnosis of autoimmune thyroiditis.
- Obesity is associated with increased incidence of thyroid nodules.
- Selective TRB agonists may seem a promising therapy for obesity.

TABLE 2: Genetic syndromes and mutations associated with obesity and thyroid disorders.

Associated with autoimmune thyroid diseases	Associated with central hypothyroidism
• Turner syndrome • Down syndrome • Klinefelter syndrome • DiGeorge syndrome • Williams syndrome • Prader–Willi syndrome • Noonan syndrome • Neurofibromatosis type 1	• Prader–Willi syndrome • *LEPR* mutations • *PCSK1* mutations • *POMC* mutations • *TRHR* mutations • *IGSF1* mutations • ROHHADNET (rapid-onset obesity with hypothalamic dysfunction, hypoventilation, autonomic dysregulation and neural crest tumor) syndrome • Chromosome 6q16 deletions • *SIM1* mutations

SUGGESTED READINGS

1. Aurangabadkar G, Kusuma Boddu S. Hypothyroidism and obesity: Is there a bidirectional link? What is the impact on our clinical practice? Thyroid Res Pract. 2020;17:118-22.
2. Thomas V, Rallapalli S, Kapoor N, Kalra S. Weight gain and Thyroid in women: The coexisting confounder. Recent advances in endocrinology. J Pak Med Assoc. 2022;72(9):1871-3.
3. Sanyal D, Raychaudhuri M. Hypothyroidism and obesity: An intriguing link. Indian J Endocr Metab. 2016;20:554-7.
4. Song RH, Wang B, Yao QM, Li Q, Jia X, Zhang JA. The Impact of Obesity on Thyroid Autoimmunity and Dysfunction: A Systematic Review and Meta-Analysis. Front Immunol. 2019;10:2349.
5. Biondi B. Thyroid and obesity: an intriguing relationship. J Clin Endocrinol Metab. 2010;95(8):3614-7.
6. Al Mohareb O, Al Saqaaby M, Ekhzaimy A, Hamza M, AlMalki MH, Bamehriz F, et al. The Relationship Between Thyroid Function and Body Composition, Leptin, Adiponectin, and Insulin Sensitivity in Morbidly Obese Euthyroid Subjects Compared to Non-obese Subjects. Clin Med Insights Endocrinol Diabetes. 2021;14:1179551420988523.
7. Ylli D, Sidhu S, Parikh T, Burman KD. Endocrine Changes in Obesity. Endotext [Internet]. South Dartmouth (MA): MDText.com, Inc.; 2000.
8. Santini F, Marzullo P, Rotondi M, Ceccarini G, Pagano L, Ippolito S, et al. Mechanisms in endocrinology: the crosstalk between thyroid gland and adipose tissue: signal integration in health and disease. Eur J Endocrinol. 2014;171(4):R137-52.
9. Yan Y, Xu M, Wu M, Wang X, Li F, Zhang J, et al. Obesity is associated with subclinical hypothyroidism in the presence of thyroid autoantibodies: a cross-sectional study. BMC Endocr Disord. 2022;22(1):94.
10. Ríos-Prego M, Anibarro L, Sánchez-Sobrino P. Relationship between thyroid dysfunction and body weight: a not so evident paradigm. Int J Gen Med. 2019;12:299-304.
11. Mahdavi M, Amouzegar A, Mehran L, Madreseh E, Tohidi M, Azizi F. Investigating the prevalence of primary thyroid dysfunction in obese and overweight individuals: Tehran thyroid study. BMC Endocr Disord. 2021;21(1):89.
12. Valdés S, Maldonado-Araque C, Lago-Sampedro A, Lillo-Muñoz JA, Garcia-Fuentes E, Perez-Valero V, et al. Reference values for TSH may be inadequate to define hypothyroidism in persons with morbid obesity: Di@bet.es study. Obesity (Silver Spring). 2017;25(4):788-93.
13. Pasquali R, Casanueva F, Haluzik M, van Hulsteijn L, Ledoux S, Monteiro MP, et al. European Society of Endocrinology Clinical Practice Guideline: Endocrine work-up in obesity. Eur J Endocrinol. 2020;182(1):G1-G32.
14. Chen J, Cao H, Lian M, Fang J. Five genes influenced by obesity may contribute to the development of thyroid cancer through the regulation of insulin levels. PeerJ. 2020;8:e9302.
15. Aiceles V, da Fonte Ramos C. A link between hypothyroidism, obesity and male reproduction. Horm Mol Biol Clin Investig. 2016;25(1):5-13.
16. Baxter JD, Webb P. Thyroid hormone mimetics: potential applications in atherosclerosis, obesity and type 2 diabetes. Nat Rev Drug Discov. 2009;8(4):308-20.
17. Kyritsi EM, Kanaka-Gantenbein C. Autoimmune Thyroid Disease in Specific Genetic Syndromes in Childhood and Adolescence. Front Endocrinol (Lausanne). 2020;11:543.

CHAPTER 30

Nonthyroidal Illness Syndrome

Rakesh K Sahay, Ameya Joshi

INTRODUCTION

Illness or starvation is associated with a series of changes occurring across various body systems. These changes or adaptations depend on duration as well as severity of underlying pathology. Thyroid is also one of the organs affected by these. The thyroid hormone levels undergo a series of changes based on the underlying illness (mainly associated reduction in thyroid hormone levels) and these constitute the spectrum of nonthyroidal illness syndrome (NTIS) or euthyroid sick syndrome. The debate spanning over last few decades still continues whether these changes are a true reduction in thyroid hormones or mere assay artifacts, whether they represent true hypothyroidism and whether this hypothyroidism is an adaptive protective response to illness in order to reduce metabolism to spare calories. Uncertainty also continues about whether this state needs treatment or not, with most advocating against a recommendation which also lacks evidence.

SPECTRUM OF ABNORMALITIES IN NONTHYROIDAL ILLNESS SYNDROME

■ Low T3 States

Isolated low T3 states are probably the earliest adaptation to illness/starvation. It is also associated with increased reverse T3 (rT3). This is the mildest form of NTIS and usually has no clinical features of hypothyroidism.

■ Low T4 (In Addition to Low T3) States

It occurs with further increase in severity of illness (or duration of starvation). This state is usually associated with low or low normal thyroid-stimulating hormone (TSH) and normal/increases rT3 level. This is the most common alteration in thyroid function tests seen in severe forms of illness or prolonged starvation. Rapid development of this is associated with worse prognosis and chances of mortality also worsen with reducing T4 almost reaching 80% with T4 levels below 2 g/dL.

EXPLANATIONS OF NONTHYROIDAL ILLNESS SYNDROME STATE

- Some think that these abnormalities may represent only assay artifacts.
- Some look at it as an adaptation to the sickness, NTIS resulting in slowing of metabolism and thereby preserving calories
- In low T3 state, it is possible that in pituitary the conversion of T4 to T3 may be normal and so it is only peripheral low T3 that is seen due to lack of central adaptation (as central levels of T3 are normal).
- NTIS may actually be a sickness-related change representing secondary hypothyroidism. It is possible that this may be the result of illness and may be actually disadvantageous to the patient. Some proponents of this theory have postulated that it may be advantageous to initiate thyroxine if T4 levels are below 4 µg/dL.

THE CHANGES IN THYROID HORMONE LEVELS AND THEIR EXPLANATIONS IN NTIS

There have been series of changes described as well as postulations/proofs for their occurrence in NTIS. The most commonly described change is of low T3 level. Majority of the serum T3 comes from liver deiodinase (D1) and this enzyme function is most commonly inhibited by the illness response. The free T3 levels are also low and this has been constant across assays including commercial assays as well as equilibrium dialysis. There has been evidence of activation of D3 deiodinase in NTIS and rT3 has been documented to be elevated in some but not all studies. In fact low, normal, and high levels of rT3 all have been documented in NTIS. One possible reason for low/normal rT3 can be due to reduction in substrate T4 also as it is usually seen in low T4 states (usually severe or prolonged underlying illness). Some small studies of T4 supplementation have yielded more increase in rT3 as compared to T3 further supporting D3 activation and D1 suppression in NTIS.

As compared to T3 then T4 levels have yielded mixed results. There have been reports of T4 levels being low and free T4 being normal and also reports of free T4 levels being read low by commercial assays but normal by equilibrium dialysis. This has been attributed to interfering substances. One interference has been seen in patients on heparin resulting in increased free fatty acid and elevated T4 (false elevation) due to same. These factors make realize the fact that it is important to take proper clinical history as well as use reliable free T4 assay, if possible, equilibrium dialysis before taking treatment decision.

The TSH level in NTIS is often low and at times even associated with low levels of other axes suppression [reduced follicle-stimulating hormone (FSH) and luteinizing hormone (LH) and testosterone levels, low growth hormone level but raised cortisol level as part of stress response]. Often there is low responsiveness to thyrotropin-releasing hormone (TRH) stimulation by pituitary indicating that there is at least some level of primary dysfunction at pituitary level in NTIS though variable level of hypothalamic dysfunction is also described in critical illness. Usually, recovery from illness is associated with normalization or rise in TSH level.

HYPOTHYROIDISM IN NTIS: CLINICAL OR ENIGMA: A CLINICIANS DILEMMA

Is hypothyroidism in nonthyroidal illness clinical is an enigma. The biggest confounder is the underlying illness itself which makes clinical diagnosis of hypothyroidism difficult, e.g., a febrile illness causing rise in temperature, pule rate, and basal metabolic rate. Starvation also alters the clinical picture. The underlying illness also causes alterations in the levels of thyroxine-binding globulin, creatinine kinase, liver enzymes, cholesterols, etc. which make relevance of these markers in diagnosis of hypothyroidism ambiguous.

MECHANISMS OF NONTHYROIDAL ILLNESS SYNDROME

Various mechanisms have been proposed for the changes seen in NTIS. One of them is reduced deiodinase I activity resulting in reduced T3 synthesis and thereby reduced levels. The other mechanism proposes selenium deficiency which thereby results in reduced function of deiodinase but supplementation of selenium has failed to reverse these changes. An interesting observation is reduced consumption of thyroid hormones seen in NTIS. This ideally should result in increase in hormone levels but the levels actually reduce indicating much stronger suppression of synthesis of hormones. There has been evidence of excessive consumption of thyroxine-binding globulin especially in patients with postcoronary artery bypass surgery. One hypothesis has been reduced TRH from the hypothalamus. This can be due to the cytokine effect. Also, it can be due to increased cortisol levels as seen in sickness or starvation. The reduced LH, FSH, and testosterone levels seen in NTIS also point to hypothalamic dysfunction. Van den Berghe and team proved that administration of TRH leads to increased TSH, T4, and T3 levels and this is the strongest evidence of the hypothalamic suppression hypothesis. Van den Berghe et al. also proposes the biphasic alterations in NTIS. The initial response may be a response to the organism and the next phase an adaptive response to the treatment given for the primary illness. This response can go maladaptive with insulin resistance and maladaptive wasting.

Various cytokines have been proposed as responsible for this NTIS. But the evidence for interferon-γ (IFN-γ) and tumor necrosis factor-α (TNF-α) is not concrete. The strongest evidence comes for interleukin 6 (IL-6). Miscellaneous factors have also been attributed to be responsible altering T4 supply in NTIS. One of them is altered central nervous system metabolism as seen in low T4 levels in subjects with asphyxia. The raised glucagon levels inhibit T4 to T3 conversion and dopamine infusion has been shown to reduce both TSH and T4 levels. Leptin levels have also been shown to suppress the TSH secretion through increasing production of pro-opiomelanocortin which acts on the arcuate nucleus thereby reducing TSH secretion. This adaption can be a part of the energy conserving mechanism in response to illness. Atrial natriuretic peptides have also been shown to reduce free T3 and free T4 levels due to inhibition of thyroid hormone release from the gland.

DIAGNOSIS OF NONTHYROIDAL ILLNESS SYNDROME

Typical presentation is of a sick patient with low T3 and free T3 levels. The T4 levels may vary and the ones below 4 ng/mL usually indicate poor prognosis. Also, the TSH levels may be variable and if elevated may help in diagnosis or point toward preexisting hypothyroidism. Estimation of antithyroid peroxidase antibody strengthens but not surely confirms the diagnosis of hypothyroidism. It is of utmost importance to estimate cortisol levels which are usually elevated above 30 µg/dL in stress. Levels below 20 µg/dL of cortisol should be followed up by adrenocorticotropic hormone (ACTH) testing in addition and if low levels are confirmed other pituitary hormones like FSH may be looked at. If all are pointing toward depressed pituitary function then an imaging of the pituitary gland may be considered. It is important to note the ongoing medications as some of them may interfere with the assay or have effect on the hypothalamic–pituitary–thyroid (HPT) axis.

COVID-19 AND NONTHYROIDAL ILLNESS SYNDROME

There are increasing reports suggesting increased prevalence of NTIS in coronavirus disease 2019 (COVID-19). Some studies did suggest that presence of NTIS predicted worse outcomes in COVID-19 infection.

TREATMENT OF NTIS WITH THYROID HORMONES

There is no clear evidence from human studies to suggest that treatment of NTIS with thyroid hormones is beneficial. The study by Brent and Harshman tried supplementing thyroxine 1.5 µg/kg in 12 critically ill patients and the outcomes were not different than controls. Another study tried giving 200 µg T3 in burn patients again failed to demonstrate the benefit of therapy. On the contrary, the hypermetabolic state induced by the intervention could be detrimental. The biggest caution came from the study of Acker et al. which showed that the mortality was less in control group as compared to the intervention group but the study was criticized for the fact that the mortality in control group was also less than the usual mortality in the ICU thereby implying possibility of selection bias.

The animal studies also failed to prove the benefit of thyroid hormone therapy except in cases of myocardial infarction or cardiogenic shock. Mainly the beneficial effect was of improved cardiac index implying the myocardial salvage may be better. But these results are too primitive to be applied to humans. Chapital et al. showed that T3 supplementation may reduce antithrombin levels and thereby may improve outcomes of disseminated intravascular coagulation but did not have a hard endpoint proof of same.

As regards specific settings then intervention of T3 supplementation in brain dead individuals failed to show a desired hemodynamic effect or myocardial salvage. But the results have been promising in setting of cardiac surgery in children. Haas et al. extensively reviewed the literature in this regard and concluded that this is at least a desirable intervention. Notivasky noted improvement in myocardial function in patients with reginal or global myocardial ischemia or hypoxia in brain dead patients. Many studies have shown contrary results with either no benefit or some benefit in soft and occasionally hard endpoints in postcardiac surgery patients in whom T3 supplementation was tried. However, the quality of evidence from this study was also weak. However most did not show any harm. Considering this more studies regards the aspect are needed.

Which thyroid hormone to consider in treatment?
Quite obvious that due to defective conversion of T4 to T3, the later should be considered in initial treatment in NTIS. Also, the best group to target is the one with T4 levels below 4 µg/dL as mortality is high and newer therapy is needed. The reassuring fact is that at least studies of supplementation have not shown any harm though benefit is also doubtful. It is important to look for cardiac arrhythmias before therapy as well as during therapy. Generally, 50–75 µg of T3 given in two divided doses is the intervention used most frequently with alternate day monitoring to keep T3 levels at least low normal range of 70–100 ng/dL. It is important to simultaneously start thyroxine replacement and if the prognosis improves and replacement is successful to gradually withdraw T3 and continue T4 under close supervision. However, if the severe illness persists then it may be prudent to continue T3 due to the conversion defect from T4 to T3. While considering thyroid hormone replacement in NTIS it is of utmost important to look at the nutrition and other hormone axis. Also, it is important to remember that this is merely adjunct therapy with unproven benefit in addition to ongoing measures.

CONCLUSION

After reviewing the available literature, it appears that NTIS is a common entity with prognostic implications depending on the picture seen. Treatment of this is not the mainstay of the whole illness but may be an adjunct. Current evidence though assures about no harm from the treatment but is far from proving the benefit which if proven later is likely to be modest and mainly in cardiac illness setting. The correct treatment strategy though currently focused on T3 supplementation is still ambiguous and may also involve multiple interventions based on hormonal deficiencies and also trophic hormone supplementations which we may realize only with time.

SUGGESTED READINGS

1. Fliers E, Boelen A. An update on non-thyroidal illness syndrome. J Endocrinol Invest. 2021;44(8):1597-607.
2. Van den Berghe G. Non-thyroidal illness in the ICU: a syndrome with different faces. Thyroid. 2014;24(10):1456-65.
3. DeGroot LJ. The Non-Thyroidal Illness Syndrome. (2015). In: Feingold KR, Anawalt B, Boyce A, Chrousos G, de Herder WW, Dhatariya K, et al. (Eds). Endotext [Internet]. South Dartmouth (MA): MDText.com, Inc.; 2000.
4. Wang B, Liu S, Li L, Yao Q, Song R, Shao X, et al. Non-thyroidal illness syndrome in patients with cardiovascular diseases: A systematic review and meta-analysis. Int J Cardiol. 2017;226:1-10.
5. Lui DTW, Lee CH, Chow WS, Lee ACH, Tam AR, Fong CHY, et al. Role of non-thyroidal illness syndrome in predicting adverse outcomes in COVID-19 patients predominantly of mild-to-moderate severity. Clin Endocrinol (Oxf). 2021;95(3):469-77.
6. De Vries EM, Fliers E, Boelen A. The molecular basis of the non-thyroidal illness syndrome. J Endocrinol. 2015;225(3):R67-81.
7. Fliers E, Bianco AC, Langouche L, Boelen A. Thyroid function in critically ill patients. Lancet Diabetes Endocrinol. 2015;3(10):816-25.

CHAPTER 31

Drugs and Other Substances Interfering with Thyroid Function

Kunal Thakkar, Tushar Bandgar

INTRODUCTION

There is an increasing list of medications and other substances that adversely affect thyroid function (anywhere in hypothalamopituitary-thyroid axis) or interfere in standard thyroid function laboratory tests. Some of these adverse effects are taken advantage of, i.e., inhibitory effects of lithium, perchlorate, iodine, and certain iodinated compounds used in treatment of hyperthyroidism in some uncommon scenarios. These drugs vary from over the counter supplements to advanced medical treatments and include biotin, glucocorticoids, antiarrhythmic, antiepileptic, and antineoplastic medicines. The unintended consequences of these drugs and substances on thyroid function vary from just laboratory test issues to severe thyroid dysfunction. Included in this chapter is a description of such drugs affecting thyroid function, with emphasis on clinically relevant interactions and on artifacts on laboratory assays.

CLASSIFICATION OF DRUGS INTERACTING WITH THYROID FUNCTION

There are drugs and substances which are likely to interfere with one or the other steps in thyroid hormone control, synthesis, transport and metabolism, while some may lead to interference with laboratory results in euthyroid individuals **(Table 1)**. On the other hand, some of the drug classes are known to interfere at multiple levels (glucocorticoids, amiodarone, and antiepileptics).

■ Drugs Affecting Hypothalamic-pituitary Control of Thyroid

Glucocorticoids

Corticosteroids are involved in regulating diurnal rhythm of thyroid-stimulating hormone (TSH) secretion. Glucocorticoids have multiple effects on thyroid functions at both physiologic and pharmacologic concentrations **(Table 2)**. They exert suppressive effect on TSH release without significantly affecting T4 release. Sudden or short-term exposure to even physiologic dose of glucocorticoids often results in TSH suppression while long-term exposure

TABLE 1: Classification of drugs affecting thyroid function.

Mechanism	Drugs
Drugs interfering with endogenous thyroid function	
Affecting hypothalamopituitary control of thyroid	Glucocorticoids, dopamine/agonists/antagonists, somatostatin/analogs, retinoids, ipilimumab, mitotane, and metformin
Decreased thyroid hormone synthesis or secretion	Iodine/iodinated compounds, lithium, thionamides, and amiodarone
Increased thyroid hormone synthesis	Iodine/iodinated compounds, and amiodarone
Enhanced thyroid autoimmunity	Interleukins, interferon, alemtuzumab, TCAs, and HAART
Destructive thyroiditis	Interleukins, interferon, nivolumab, sunitinib, and amiodarone
Changes in thyroid hormone binding proteins	Oral estrogen, androgens, fluorouracil, and SERMs
Inhibition of thyroid hormone activation (reduced T4 to T3 conversion)	Amiodarone, dexamethasone, and propranolol
Displacing thyroid hormones from binding proteins	Carbamazepine, furosemide, salsalate, salicylates, and heparin (in vitro)
Increased thyroid hormone metabolism or elimination	Phenobarbital, phenytoin, carbamazepine, sorafenib, and rifampin
Drugs interfering with thyroid hormone therapy	
	Proton pump inhibitors, antacids, ferrous sulfate, and calcium carbonate
Drugs interfering with laboratory tests in euthyroid individuals	
	Heparin, biotin, and amiodarone

(HAART: highly active antiretroviral therapy; SERM: selective estrogen receptor modulators; TCA: tricyclic antidepressants)

TABLE 2: Effects of glucocorticoids on thyroid functions.

	Effect	Mechanism
Physiologic doses	Suppression of TSH	Inhibition of TRH mRNA expression at paraventricular nucleus of hypothalamus
Pharmacologic doses		
All dose ranges	Suppression of TSH	Inhibition of TRH mRNA expression at paraventricular nucleus of hypothalamus
Relatively lower doses	Reduced T4 (with normal free T4)	Decreased TBG secretion from liver
Relatively higher doses	High normal T4 and reduced T3	Inhibition of 5'-monodeiodination and decreased hepatic uptake of T4

(mRNA: messenger ribonucleic acid; TBG: thyroxine binding globulin; TRH: thyrotropin releasing hormone; TSH: thyroid stimulating hormone)

to even high dose glucocorticoids or endogenous Cushing's syndrome does not lead to the same. Although TSH suppression in such cases is metabolically insignificant, it may be confused with subclinical hyperthyroidism. On the contrary serum TSH levels may be elevated in patients with adrenal insufficiency and normalize with physiologic glucocorticoid replacement. At pharmacologic concentrations, glucocorticoids for short duration also lead to inhibition of deiodinase type 1, decrease in thyroxine binding globulin (TBG), decreased hepatic uptake of T4 and increased renal clearance of iodine. In addition, immunosuppressive effects of pharmacologic doses of glucocorticoids may reduce levels of stimulating antibodies in patients with Graves' disease and reduce inflammation in various types of thyroiditis.

Dopamine/Dopamine Agonists and Dopamine Antagonists

Dopamine is one of the major regulators of HPT axis through D2 receptors. Dopamine infusion and agonists (bromocriptine and cabergoline) suppress TSH secretion while dopamine antagonists such as metoclopramide increase TSH secretion, in euthyroid as well as hypothyroid individuals.

Somatostatin/Somatostatin Analogs

Somatostatin reduces both frequency and amplitude of TSH secretion. These agents bind to five different receptors on pituitary cells and exert suppressive effects. The same effect makes somatostatin analogs clinically useful in TSH secreting pituitary adenomas.

Retinoids

Rexinoids, a subclass of retinoids bind to a specific nuclear hormone receptor involved in various cellular functions known as *retinoid X receptors (RXR)*. RXR binds with other nuclear transcription factors and these heterodimers influence transcription of many different genes, including the genes coding for TSH beta subunit. Accordingly, retinoids, including bexarotene (rexinoid used in treatment of T-cell lymphoma) induce central hypothyroidism.

Immune Check-point Inhibitors

Immune check-point inhibitors (ICIs) including those that inhibit cytotoxic T lymphocyte antigen 4 (CTLA4) and programmed cell death 1 (PD 1) receptor, lead to a variety of endocrine disruptions. CTLA4 inhibitors more frequently lead to hypophysitis while programmed death protein 1 (PD-1) inhibitors to primary thyroid dysfunctions. *Ipulimumab*, an anti-CTLA4 agent used in treatment of melanoma, has been linked to destructive hypophysitis in 3–10% of patients treated with this agent, leading to central hypothyroid, adrenal insufficiency, and hypogonadism. The effects ensue within 1–3 months of commencement of therapy and patients present with headache, fatigue, weight loss, cold intolerance, loss of libido. Magnetic resonance imaging (MRI) is useful in making diagnosis, showing typical picture of hypophysitis in many but not all. Thyroid and gonadal functions recover in approximately half of the patients after stopping therapy, while recovery of adrenal functions is rare.

Mitotane

Mitotane used in treatment of adrenocortical carcinoma causes central hypothyroidism in many patients (subnormal free T4 levels with low or inappropriately normal TSH levels). These thyroid function disturbances are apparent within 3 months of starting treatment with mitotane and require long term thyroxine replacement.

Metformin

Metformin, frequently used to treat diabetes and prediabetes, reduces TSH levels in those patients with coexisting hypothyroidism (irrespective of treatment status). The same effect has not been observed in euthyroid diabetic subjects. The mechanism of this metformin effect on TSH secretion remains unknown.

Drugs Affecting Thyroid Hormone Synthesis and/or Release

Iodine and Iodinated Compounds

Excess intrathyroidal iodine inhibits thyroid hormone release (Wolff–Chaikoff effect) as well as synthesis through inhibition of thyroid peroxidase. An escape from this effect usually occurs within 1–2 weeks in individuals with normal thyroid, but those with compromised gland because of lymphocytic infiltrates or other causes, may not escape from this effect until iodine is cleared. On the other hand, iodine excess has also been linked to thyrotoxicosis (Jod–Basedow phenomenon) particularly in patients with pre-existing autonomous thyroid functions. The common sources of excess iodine include *radiographic contrast dyes*, drugs with high iodine content such as *amiodarone, topical povidone iodine*, some *cough syrups and multivitamin preparations*. However, amiodarone-induced thyroid disturbances are described underneath owing to its multiple mechanisms.

Lithium

Long-term treatment with lithium (used for treatment of bipolar mood disorders) is associated with hypothyroidism in approximately 20% and goiter in 40%. In animal studies, lithium has been found to decrease the release of thyroidal iodine without affecting its uptake, resulting in an excess of intrathyroidal iodine. This inhibitory effect of lithium on thyroid functions makes this drug clinically useful as an adjuvant treatment of hyperthyroidism and to increase intrathyroidal levels of radioactive iodine, thereby enhancing its effectiveness in treating Graves' disease and thyroid carcinoma. Lithium-induced hypothyroidism warrants thyroxine replacement but not lithium withdrawal. Although thyrotoxicosis, mainly because of destructive thyroiditis is observed in some patients on lithium therapy, the incidence of this is much less common than that of hypothyroidism and goiter.

Some of the drugs are known to affect thyroid functions at multiple levels of HPT axis as well as thyroid hormone metabolism (amiodarone, phenytoin, cytokines, glucocorticoids, etc.), are discussed underneath.

Tricyclic Antidepressants and Selective Serotonin Reuptake Inhibitors

Tricyclic antidepressants (TCAs) (amitriptyline and nortriptyline) may variably interfere with hypothalamic-pituitary-thyroid (HPT) axis. These can decrease TSH response to TRH via noradrenergic or serotonergic systems. In addition, TCAs may promote autoimmunity and favor appearance of thyroid autoantibodies, by enhancing the expression of major histocompatibility complex antigens. Selective serotonin reuptake inhibitors (SSRIs) on the other hand, predominantly fluoxetine and sertraline have been known to lead to decrease in T3 and T4 levels (within their normal ranges) in patients without pre-existing thyroid disease. Overall observations suggest only minor changes in thyroid functions by SSRIs.

Drugs that Enhance Thyroid Autoimmunity

Newer antineoplastic agents designed to enhance immune system targeting of cancer cells, increase the risk of autoimmune disorders.

Immune Check-point Inhibitors

As is the case with immune check-point inhibitors (ICIs) increasingly being associated with hypophysitis, primary thyroid dysfunction is also observed in significant number of patients—5–10% of patients treated with anti-cytotoxic T-lymphocyte-associated antigen 4 (anti-CTLA4) (*ipilimumab*), 10–20% of patients treated with anti-PD-1 receptor (*pembrolizumab* and *nivolumab*) and anti-programmed death-ligand-1 (anti-PD-L1) (*atezolizumab*) and >20% of patients treated with combination therapy. Most patients manifesting primary thyroid dysfunction would have painless thyroiditis—transient thyrotoxicosis followed by hypothyroidism. Thyrotoxic phase starts between 2 and 18 weeks (4–6 weeks in most) after initiating therapy. Hypothyroidism ensues between 10 and 20 weeks after initiating therapy, and is usually irreversible. It is not advisable to stop ICI based therapy in such patients, thyroid dysfunction is managed conventionally. Antibodies against thyroid peroxidase antibodies (TPO) and/or thyroglobulin are present in approximately 50% of affected patients. Positive pretreatment antibodies increase the risk of thyroid dysfunction with ICI drugs.

Cytokines (Interleukin and Interferon)

These cytokines used in treatment of hepatitis, melanoma or metastatic renal cell carcinoma, lead to thyroid dysfunction in 15–50% of patients. The most common thyroid dysfunction is varying degrees of hypothyroidism, preceded by transient thyrotoxicosis and often with positive anti thyroid antibodies (painless thyroiditis), although some may develop Graves' disease. Positive pretreatment antibodies and female gender are associated with increased likelihood of developing thyroid dysfunction. Patients, who develop autoimmune thyroid dysfunction, can continue interferon, while treating hypothyroidism with levothyroxine.

Anti-CD52 Antibody–Alemtuzumab

Alemtuzumab is a monoclonal antibody against glycoprotein CD52 on B cells, used in treatment of multiple sclerosis (MS) and B cell chronic lymphocytic leukemia (CLL). Alemtuzumab therapy in MS has been associated with autoimmune thyroid dysfunction in approximately 30–40% of patients, most common being Graves' disease with positive antibodies against TSH receptor. Most patients have overt hyperthyroidism and are diagnosed within 3 years of start of therapy, but cases are reported even up to 9 years after starting therapy. Alemtuzumab-induced Graves' disease is associated with more than usual fluctuations in stimulating and blocking antibodies against TSH receptor and consequently periods of hyperthyroidism and hypothyroidism. Subacute thyroiditis and primary hypothyroidism are also seen with increased frequency in patients treated with alemtuzumab. It is interesting to note that Graves' disease is not associated with alemtuzumab use in patients with leukemia and rheumatoid arthritis in contrast to its use in MS, reasons being unknown.

Other Causes of Increased Thyroid Autoimmunity

Examples of thyroid autoimmunity occurring after recovery of immune system include, Graves' disease after highly active antiretroviral therapy (HAART) for advanced HIV infection, in children receiving stem cell transplantation for immunodeficiency states, after cure of endogenous Cushing's disease and in postpartum period.

Drugs Acting at Multiple Levels to Affect Thyroid Hormone Homeostasis

Amiodarone

This antiarrhythmic agent is rich in iodine content (standard 200 mg tablet containing 75 mg iodine), with long half-life of 40–60 days. Amiodarone inhibits DIO1 and DIO2 in a dose dependent manner. This leads to marked decrease in T3, increase in T4 and rT3. Thyroid-stimulating hormone levels increase slightly in early months of treatment. Because its structure resembles to that of thyroxine to some extent, amiodarone may interfere with entry of thyroxine into cells. It may also interfere with binding of thyroid hormone to its receptors, and may antagonize the effects of thyroid hormones at cellular levels. The effects of amiodarone on thyroid functions are summarized in **Table 3**.

Amiodarone-induced hypothyroidism (AIH) is directly related to its high iodine content, leading to suppression of synthesis and secretion of thyroid hormones, and inability to escape from Wolff–Chaikoff effect. It has been observed that AIH is more common in iodine replete areas, with prevalence varying from 2 to 10%. Development of hypothyroidism does not warrant withdrawal of amiodarone and is treated conventionally. Even when amiodarone is discontinued, it takes months for thyroid functions to recover, because of its prolonged half-life.

In contrast to AIH, amiodarone-induced thyrotoxicosis (AIT) is more prevalent in areas with relative iodine deficiency. Prevalence of AIT reported in various studies is different and varies from 5 to 22%. It can develop from few weeks to many months after starting amiodarone and even many months after stopping amiodarone because of its long residence time in body. Two forms of AIT have been described; type 1 AIT occurring in patients with pre-existing Graves' disease or nodular thyroid disease, while type 2 AIT occurring in apparently normal thyroids. Type 1 AIT represents excess synthesis of thyroid hormones due to iodine load in a pre-existing thyroid disease, while type 2 AIT is a form of drug-induced destructive thyroiditis due to cytotoxic effects of amiodarone. The uptake of ^{99m}Tc-sestamibi is very low in type 2 versus higher in type 1 AIT. Mixed forms of AIT have also been described where uptake is intermediate. Color flow Doppler on thyroid ultrasound is a useful tool to differentiate these two forms of AIT, flow being increased in type 1 and low to absent in type 2 AIT. Considering these issues, it is recommended that thyroid functions be checked prior to initiation of amiodarone and monitored every 6 months until 1 year after stopping the drug. Treatment differs between types of AIT. Type 1 AIT requires initiation of high dose thionamides while type 2 AIT responds well to glucocorticoids showing improvements within weeks. In severe cases or in cases with uncertain diagnosis between two types of AIT, it is prudent to start simultaneous treatment with thionamides as well as glucocorticoids. If there is a rapid improvement in thyroid functions within 7 days, type 2 AIT is more likely to be present. Thyroidectomy may be considered in patients not responding to conventional treatment, RAI ablation is option for some patients who show increased uptake.

Phenytoin

Phenytoin induces cytochrome (CYP450) activity, thus increasing hepatic metabolism of T4 and T3. At therapeutic doses, serum concentrations of phenytoin are high enough to displace some T4 from TBG binding sites, thus reducing serum levels of T4. Phenytoin also increases conversion of T4 to T3. So ultimately it leads to low T4, free thyroxine (fT4), and rT3 due to increased catabolism and normal T3 due to increased conversion from T4, despite its increased hepatic degradation. Thyroid-stimulating hormone levels are usually normal with low T4 and fT4, mimicking central hypothyroidism. However, both low as well as high TSH levels have been reported with its use, reflecting possible alterations in nuclear effects of thyroid hormones at hypothalamic or pituitary level.

Tyrosine Kinase Inhibitors

These agents are used in the treatment of various malignancies including renal cell carcinoma, gastrointestinal stromal tutors, hematologic malignancies, and advanced thyroid cancers. Targeted cancer therapy with tyrosine kinase inhibitors (TKIs) has been associated with increased risk of thyroiditis, manifesting as hypothyroidism, with preceding transient thyrotoxicosis in some patients. Most of the TKIs-induced thyroid dysfunctions are reported with the use of sunitinib. The frequency of such thyroid dysfunction in various studies is between 12 and 36%. The mechanism contributing to thyroiditis may be related to ischemia because of inhibition of vascular endothelial growth factor

TABLE 3: Effects of amiodarone on thyroid functions.		
	Changes in thyroid functions	Mechanism
Clinically euthyroid	Low T3, high T4, high rT3, and high TSH	Inhibition of deiodinase 2 and 3, interference with entry of T4 into cell
Clinically hypothyroid (AIH)	Low T3, low T4, and high TSH	High iodine content—Wolff–Chaikoff effect
Clinically thyrotoxic (AIT)	High T3, high T4 and low TSH	*Type 1 AIT*: Excess iodine load in a pre-existing thyroid condition
		Type 2 AIT: Destructive thyroiditis

(AIH: amiodarone-induced hypothyroidism; AIT: amiodarone-induced thyrotoxicosis)

receptors by these agents. Some patients show significant thyroid involution on ultrasound.

Additional effect of TKIs is increased thyroid hormone catabolism, requiring levothyroxine dose increments in previously hypothyroid patients. Tyrosine kinase inhibitors also have been noted to be associated with induction of DIO3, leading to low T4, rT3, and high T3. Given the increased frequency of thyroid dysfunctions, it is recommended to assess thyroid function tests prior to initiation of TKIs and at regular intervals thereafter.

Other Drugs Affecting Thyroid Functions at Multiple Levels

Glucocorticoids, cytokines, immune check point inhibitors (anti-CTLA4 and anti-PD-1), and iodinated radiographic contrast agents are some of the agents known to alter thyroid functions by disrupting multiple steps thyroid hormone synthesis, metabolism or action and have been described above.

■ Drugs Affecting Protein Binding of Thyroid Hormones

Drugs that Lead to Increase in Thyroxine Binding Globulin

Oral estrogen including oral contraceptive pills, *selective estrogen receptor modulators (tamoxifen and raloxifene), methadone, heroin, mitotane, and fluorouracil* lead to increases in TBG levels. As a consequence, there is increase in total T4 levels. Patients with functional thyroid will increase thyroid hormone synthesis and hence would have normal fT4 as well as TSH levels. On the other hand, patients who are dependent on exogenous thyroxine replacement would need dose increments to keep fT4 and TSH in normal range. Transdermal estradiol has minimal effects on TBG levels, because this route circumvents the hepatic first pass metabolism.

Drugs that Lead to Decrease in TBG

Androgens (including testosterone replacement in hypogonadal males), *glucocorticoids* and *niacin* are some of the drugs that reduce synthesis of TBG from liver. As a result, there may be low levels of total thyroid hormones while free hormones and TSH would be normal.

Drugs Displacing Thyroid Hormones from Binding Proteins

Antiepileptic agents such as *phenytoin and carbamazepine*, some nonsteroidal anti-inflammatory drugs especially *salicylates* and *salsalate*, high dose *furosemide* and *heparin* are some of the drugs that lead to displacement of thyroid hormones from protein binding sites in circulation. The clinical effects of these interactions are often negligible. In the case of phenytoin and heparin, which cause alterations of laboratory testing in euthyroid patients, are discussed underneath.

■ Drugs Affecting Thyroid Hormone Activation, Metabolism, and Excretion

Amiodarone, dexamethasone, high dose propranolol, cholecystographic agents, and propylthiouracil are some of the drugs that inhibit conversion of T4 to T3. The effect of propranolol on deiodinase is not clinically relevant in usual doses.

Phenobarbital, phenytoin, carbamazepine, rifampin, etc., induce hepatic glucuronidation enzymes and consequently necessitate increase in levothyroxine dose requirement in hypothyroid patients.

Bile acid sequestrants *cholestyramine, colestipol, and colesevelam* are known to interfere with recycling of thyroid hormones and consequently reduce thyroid hormone levels in patients with thyrotoxicosis.

■ Drugs Affecting Absorption of Thyroid Hormone Preparations

Levothyroxine tablets require acid milieu for dissolution, followed by its transportation to small intestine for absorption. Daily *proton pump inhibitors* use is associated with increased levothyroxine requirement. Drugs interfering with gastrointestinal absorption of thyroid hormones include *ferrous sulfate, calcium carbonate, aluminum hydroxide, sucralfate, raloxifene, and bile acid sequestrants*. It is recommended to take levothyroxine at least 4 hours before ingesting any of these medications.

■ Drugs Causing Abnormal Thyroid Tests in Euthyroid Patients

Several drugs are known to lead to abnormal results of laboratory tests in clinically euthyroid individuals **(Table 4)**. Knowledge of such interactions helps to distinguish these abnormalities from true thyroid dysfunction and thus preventing unnecessary diagnostic and therapeutic interventions.

Biotin

Biotin is a popular nutritional supplement used in treatment of alopecia as well as used therapeutically in treatment of neuromuscular disorders such as multiple sclerosis. In addition, biotinylated reagents are widely used in many commercial laboratories because of their strong binding to streptavidin, which is fixed to a solid phase such as magnetic beads or ELISA plates. Many commercial assays for fT4, T3, TSH, and TSH receptor antibody contain biotin-streptavidin detection systems, giving falsely high T3, T4, and falsely low TSH values in some patients. False positive results of TSH receptor antibody tests make exact biochemical resemblance

TABLE 4: Drugs causing laboratory tests interference in euthyroid individuals.

Drug	TSH	fT4	T3	Condition mimicked
Biotin	Low	High	High	Primary hyperthyroidism
Heparin	Normal	High	High	TSH secreting pituitary adenoma, thyroid hormone resistance
Amiodarone	High, high-normal	High	Low-normal	TSH secreting pituitary adenoma, thyroid hormone resistance
Carbamazepine, phenytoin, and salsalate	Normal	Low	Low-normal	Central hypothyroidism

(fT4: free thyroxine; TSH: thyroid stimulating hormone)

to Graves' disease. Although such cases often are associated with high biotin doses of 300 mg daily or more, lesser degrees of interference have been reported with doses as low as 10 mg/day. The direction and degree of interference depend on the assay platform; two site-sandwich methods used in most TSH assays show falsely low values, while competitive immunoassays utilized for thyroid hormone measurements give falsely high values. This interaction should be suspected in all patients showing incongruous biochemical test results, given the high prevalence of biotin supplements used for various reasons. Although interference resolves within 48 hours after drug discontinuation, repeat test should be ordered only after several days have elapsed after stopping biotin.

Amiodarone
In addition to causing AIH and AIT, amiodarone may also lead to predictable changes in thyroid laboratory test results in euthyroid persons. Amiodarone and its active metabolite desethylamiodarone lead to decreased peripheral and central conversion of T4 to T3, resulting in reductions in circulating and intrapituitary T3 levels, thereby stimulating TRH and TSH release. Increases in TSH prompt T4 release, which further accumulates because of reduced conversion to T3. The end result is elevated or high normal TSH with elevated T4 and fT4, with low T3 levels in a euthyroid patient. Elevations of TSH and fT4 can be confused with TSH secreting pituitary adenoma or thyroid hormone resistance, but normal values on tests performed before initiating amiodarone rule out these disorders, again highlighting the need to carry out thyroid function tests in all patients before initiating amiodarone therapy.

Heparin
Heparin releases lipoprotein lipase (LPL) from vascular endothelium. Blood samples from patients receiving heparin have increased LPL activity, which persists in vitro. Free fatty acids hence released by activity of lipase, displace T4 and T3 from protein binding sites, causing spuriously high values of free triiodothyronine (fT3) and fT4. Similar effects are also seen with low molecular weight heparin preparations. Assays with prolonged incubation periods such as measurements of free hormones by equilibrium dialysis, are most affected, while standard competitive free hormone assays and TSH assays are unaffected. Repeating tests with use of these assays or rechecking after stopping heparin for 24 hours would help in confirmation.

Other Substances Interfering with Thyroid Function

Thyroid Disruptors
A recent review of studies suggested onset of Hashimoto's thyroiditis or thyroid nodules following environmental or occupational exposure to some pollutants such as *polychlorinated biphenyls (PCB), polybrominated biphenyls (PBB), pesticides* [the most studied being *organochlorines*, including *dichlorodiphenyltrichloroethane (DDT), aldrin, heptachlor, chlordane, and lindane*], and *heavy metal. Sulfur dioxide and nitrogen dioxide* are possibly associated with increased prevalence of differentiated thyroid carcinoma as suggested by studies performed in urban population of Beijing and Guangzhou. *Smoke, PCB, solvents, metals*, and *other anthropogenic compounds* have been implicated in thyroid inflammation and autoimmunity. The mechanism involved may be disruption of immune tolerance by these substances, predisposing to autoimmune thyroid disorders. *Mercury* has been found to be associated with reductions in T3 and T4 and Cadmium linked to decreased TSH. A variety *of benzophenone UV screens* (*BP*2), when applied for 5 days in adult ovariectomized rats, led to a significant reduction of T4 and T3 plasma levels. The suggested mechanism was the inhibition of thyroid peroxidase. It is important to be aware that UV screens, besides being potent estrogen disruptors, may exert potential thyroid-disrupting activity within just a few days.

CONCLUSION
Various drugs and other substances, some of which are used very commonly for many ailments while others used infrequently, are known to lead to variable degree of thyroid dysfunction. On the other hand, there are some drugs known to be associated with only laboratory test results abnormalities in otherwise euthyroid individuals, creating confusion with and mimicking Graves' disease,

central hypothyroidism, central hyperthyroidism, etc. Drugs causing thyroid dysfunctions do so by affecting any one or more of the mechanisms controlling and maintaining thyroid hormone homeostasis. Awareness of these possible interactions allows clinicians to correctly diagnose them, intervene when appropriate and avoid unnecessary tests and treatment.

SUGGESTED READINGS

1. Ross DS, Burch HB, Cooper DS, Greenlee MC, Laurberg P, Maia AL, et al. 2016 American Thyroid Association guidelines for diagnosis and management of hyperthyroidism and other causes of thyrotoxicosis. Thyroid. 2016;26(10):1343-421.
2. Jonklaas J, Bianco AC, Bauer AJ, Burman KD, Cappola AR, Celi FS, et al. Guidelines for the treatment of hypothyroidism: prepared by the american thyroid association task force on thyroid hormone replacement. Thyroid. 2014;24(12):1670-751.
3. Haugen BR. Drugs that suppress TSH or cause central hypothyroidism. Best Pract Res Clin Endocrinol Metab. 2009;23(6):793-800.
4. Colao A, Merola B, Ferone D, Marzullo P, Cerbone G, Longobardi S, et al. Acute and chronic effects of octreotide on thyroid axis in growth hormone-secreting and clinically non-functioning pituitary adenomas. Eur J Endocrinol. 1995;133(2):189-94.
5. Russo M, Scollo C, Pellegriti G, Cotta OR, Squatrito S, Frasca F, et al. Mitotane treatment in patients with adrenocortical cancer causes central hypothyroidism. Clin Endocrinol. 2016;84(4):614-9.
6. Sherman SI, Gopal J, Haugen BR, Chiu AC, Whaley K, Nowlakha P, et al. Central hypothyroidism associated with retinoid X receptor–selective ligands. N Engl J Med. 1999;340(14):1075-9.
7. Chang LS, Barroso-Sousa R, Tolaney SM, Hodi FS, Kaiser UB, Min L. Endocrine toxicity of cancer immunotherapy targeting immune checkpoints. Endocr Rev. 2019;40(1):17-65.
8. Martino E, Bartalena L, Bogazzi F, Braverman LE. The effects of amiodarone on the thyroid. Endocr Rev. 2001;22(2):240-54.
9. Basaria S, Cooper DS. Amiodarone and the thyroid. Am J Med. 2005;118(7):706-14.
10. Lazarus JH. Lithium and thyroid. Best Pract Res Clin Endocrinol Metab. 2009;23(6):723-33.
11. Scott ES, Long GV, Guminski A, Clifton-Bligh RJ, Menzies AM, Tsang VH. The spectrum, incidence, kinetics and management of endocrinopathies with immune checkpoint inhibitors for metastatic melanoma. Eur J Endocrinol. 2018;178(2):173-80.
12. Pariani N, Willis M, Muller I, Healy S, Nasser T, McGowan A, et al. Alemtuzumab-induced thyroid dysfunction exhibits distinctive clinical and immunological features. J Clin Endocrinol Metab. 2018;103(8):3010-8.
13. Illouz F, Braun D, Briet C, Schweizer U, Rodien P. Endocrine Side-effects of Anticancer Drugs: Thyroid effects of tyrosine kinase inhibitors. Eur J Endocrinol. 2014;171:R91-9.
14. Curran PG, Degroot LJ. The effect of hepatic enzyme-inducing drugs on thyroid hormones and the thyroid gland. Endocr Rev. 1991;12(2):135-50.
15. Sachmechi I, Reich DM, Aninyei M, Wibowo F, Gupta G, Kim PJ. Effect of proton pump inhibitors on serum thyroid-stimulating hormone level in euthyroid patients treated with levothyroxine for hypothyroidism. Endocr Pract. 2007;13(4):345-9.
16. Kummer S, Hermsen D, Distelmaier F. Biotin treatment mimicking Graves' disease. N Engl J Med. 2016;375(7):704-6.
17. Oliveira KJ, Chiamolera MI, Giannocco G, Pazos-Moura CC, Ortiga-Carvalho TM. Thyroid function disruptors: from nature to chemicals. J Mol Endocrinol. 2018;JME-18-0081.
18. Benvenga S, Elia G, Ragusa F, Paparo SR, Sturniolo MM, Ferrari SM, et al. Endocrine disruptors and thyroid autoimmunity. Best Practice and Research Clinical Endocrinology and Metabolism. 2020;34(1):101377.
19. Burch HB. Drug effects on the thyroid. N Engl J Med. 2019;381(8):749-61.

32 CHAPTER

Thyroid Emergencies

A Mythili, Ch. Mounika Anitha

INTRODUCTION

Thyroid emergencies are rare, life-threatening endocrine emergencies. Myxedema coma results from severe deficiency of thyroid hormones and thyroid storm is a state of severe thyrotoxicosis with excess action of thyroxine (T4) and triiodothyronine (T3). Very severe sight-threatening Graves' orbitopathy (GO) with dysthyroid optic neuropathy (DON) and corneal breakdown constitutes an emergency (discussed in Graves' ophthalmopathy chapter). Hashimoto's encephalopathy (HE), an acute encephalopathy is now recognized to have an autoimmune basis and accompanied by elevated antithyroid antibodies. Understanding the pathophysiology, early diagnosis, and appropriate treatment of the above disorders is crucial in optimizing survival. The following emergencies shall be discussed here.
- Myxedema coma
- Thyroid storm
- Hashimoto's encephalopathy

MYXEDEMA COMA

Myxedema coma is a rare, severe presentation of long-standing untreated hypothyroidism. The reported incidence rate is 0.22/million/year and is considered an endocrine emergency with a high mortality rate (20–30%). It is commonly seen in elderly women, especially during the winter months.

The clinical features include symptoms of hypothyroidism for many months before the onset of stupor or coma. Myxedema coma is triggered by cold exposure, infection, drugs (e.g., sedatives, antidepressants, antipsychotics, anesthetics, and tranquilizers), trauma, stroke, heart failure, pulmonary embolism, respiratory failure, and gastrointestinal bleed. The typical features of severe hypothyroidism such as dry, coarse and scaly skin, sparse, coarse hair, nonpitting edema of periorbital regions, hands and feet, macroglossia, hoarseness, and delayed deep tendon reflexes are often apparent. The presence of a goiter or a thyroidectomy scar provides an important clue. Myxedema coma is characterized by an altered mental state, bradycardia, hypoventilation, and hypothermia. Other features include hypotension, hypoxia, hypercapnia, hyponatremia, hypoglycemia, and heart failure. Pericardial, pleural, and peritoneal effusions are often seen. Paralytic ileus is frequently found. Seizures, stupor, and coma are the usual central nervous system manifestations seen. Euthermia in myxedema coma patients suggests the presence of infection.

The diagnosis is made on clinical grounds and confirmed by laboratory testing with elevated serum thyroid-stimulating hormone (TSH) and decreased total and free thyroxine (T4) and triiodothyronine (T3). Laboratory abnormalities include anemia, hyponatremia, hypoglycemia, hypercholesterolemia, high serum lactate dehydrogenase (LDH) and creatine kinase concentrations. Arterial blood gases often reveal hypoxemia and hypercapnia. ECG shows sinus bradycardia, T wave flattening, and various degrees of heart block. The diagnostic scoring system for myxedema coma developed by Popoveniuc et al., is shown in **Table 1**.

The treatment of myxedema coma requires a multifaceted approach in a critical care setting. These include:
- *Ventilatory support*: Maintenance of airway and ventilation is of utmost importance as respiratory failure is associated with high mortality. Most patients need ventilatory support for 36–48 hours and some may require it for several weeks. Though the hypercapnia is relieved rapidly with mechanical ventilation, hypoxia persists due to shunting in nonaerated lung areas. Therefore, until full consciousness is attained, it is advisable not to extubate the patients prematurely.
- *Hyponatremia*: Severe hyponatremia (105–120 mmol/L) likely contributes to coma in these patients. Management includes administration of 50–100 mL hypertonic saline (3% sodium chloride), which increases sodium concentration by about 2 mmol/L. This is followed by an intravenous bolus dose of 40–120 mg furosemide

TABLE 1: Diagnostic scoring system for myxedema coma.[a]			
Thermoregulatory dysfunction (temperature, °C)		**Cardiovascular dysfunction**	
>35	0	Bradycardia	
32–35	10	Absent	0
<32	20	50–59	10
Central nervous system effects		40–49	20
Absent	0	<40	30
Somnolent/lethargic	10	Other EKG changes[b]	10
Obtunded	15	Pericardial/pleural effusions	10
Stupor	20	Pulmonary edema	15
Coma/seizures	30	Cardiomegaly	15
Gastrointestinal findings		Hypotension	20
Anorexia/abdominal Pain/constipation	5	*Metabolic disturbances*	
Decreased intestinal motility	15	Hyponatremia	10
Paralytic ileus	20	Hypoglycemia	10
Precipitating event		Hypoxemia	10
Absent	0	Hypercarbia	10
Present	10	Decrease in GFR	10

[a] Score of 60 or higher is highly suggestive/diagnostic of myxedema coma; a sore of 25–59 is suggestive of risk for myxedema coma, and a score below 25 is unlikely to indicate myxedema coma.

[b] Other EKG changes—QT prolongation, low voltage complexes, bundle branch blocks, nonspecific ST-T changes, or heart blocks.

(EKG: electrocardiogram; GFR: glomerular filtration rate)

Source: Popoveniuc G, Chandra T, Sud A, Sharma M, Blackman MR, Burman KD, et al. A diagnostic scoring system for myxedema coma. Endocr Pract. 2014;20(8):808-17.

to promote water diuresis. Rapid correction of severe hyponatremia can result in osmotic demyelination. Given elevated vasopressin levels seen in myxedema, therapy with vasopressin antagonists can also be considered. The recommended dose of conivaptan is a loading dose of 20 mg IV infusion over 30 minutes followed by continuous IV infusion at a rate of 20 mg/day for another 2–4 days but there are no reports of its use. Tolvaptan is administered at an oral dose of 15 mg initially.

- *Hypothermia*: Therapy with T4 and/or T3 itself restores body temperature to normal. Blankets or raising the room temperature can be used to keep the patient warm until the thyroid hormone effect is achieved. Avoid aggressive warming as it may result in peripheral vasodilatation leading to hypotension or shock.
- *Hypotension*: Hypotension should be corrected by cautious administration of IV fluids. Isotonic sodium chloride is used if there is hyponatremia. If hypoglycemia is present, either 5–10% dextrose in half-normal saline can be administered. Rarely patients may require vasopressor drug therapy to maintain blood pressure. Hydrocortisone is administered until the hypotension is corrected as there are chances of relative adrenal insufficiency.
- *Glucocorticoid therapy*: Adrenal reserve can be decreased in 5–10% of patients, due to hypopituitarism or primary adrenal failure accompanying Hashimoto's disease (Schmidt syndrome). The rationale for the treatment with corticosteroids is the potential risk of precipitation of acute adrenal insufficiency due to the accelerated metabolism of cortisol following T4 therapy. Signs and symptoms that signal the coexistence of adrenal insufficiency are hypotension, hypothermia, hypoglycemia, hyperkalemia, and hyponatremia. Hydrocortisone is given at a dose of 50–100 mg every 6–8 hours during the first 7–10 days, thereafter the dose is tapered based on the clinical response.
- *Thyroid hormone therapy*: The initial goal of treatment is to rapidly replace the depleted thyroid hormone pool. The normal extrathyroidal pool of T4 is 300–600 μg. Levothyroxine (T4), triiodothyronine (T3), or both can be used for the treatment. Impaired gastrointestinal absorption and paralytic ileus may reduce the effectiveness of oral levothyroxine; hence, intravenous T4 is preferred over oral administration of levothyroxine. However, some clinical studies have shown that outcomes are not influenced by the route of administration of levothyroxine (oral/intravenous). An intravenous bolus dose of 300–500 μg LT4 is given followed by 50–100 μg daily until initiation of oral medications. If intravenous preparations are not available, alternative option is to give a 500 μg oral loading dose of levothyroxine (by nasogastric tube) followed by 100 μg daily. Use of T4 is advised because it results in steady and smooth levels of serum T4, but the drawbacks of T4 are its slow onset of action and impaired conversion of T4 to T3 in critical illness. The use of T3 is suggested because it has greater biological activity and rapid onset of action; but, it is associated with wide fluctuations in serum levels and increased risk of cardiovascular events. If T3 is given alone, the recommended dosage is 20 μg IV bolus followed by 10 μg every 6 hours for 24–48 hours, by which time oral administration should be feasible and can be switched over to oral levothyroxine. In combination therapy, T4 is given at a dose of 4 μg/kg lean body weight (or about 200–300 μg) followed by 100 μg 24 hours later and then 50 μg daily either IV or orally as appropriate. As soon as the patient is conscious, approximately by the third day, daily maintenance dose of 50 μg, can be given by mouth. Along with the initial dose of T4, a bolus of 10 μg T3 is given intravenously and is continued at a dosage of 10 μg every 8–12 hours until the patient regains consciousness and takes maintenance dose T4 orally.
- *General supportive measures*: Treat the underlying precipitating conditions such as infection and congestive heart failure. There is need to modify the doses of

specific medications (e.g., digoxin for congestive heart failure) based on their altered distribution and slowed metabolism in myxedema coma.

Highlights: Myxedema Coma

- Hypothermia is a cardinal clinical finding and euthermia in myxedema can be a clue to an underlying infection.
- Empirical use of antibiotic therapy is justified in myxedema coma.
- IV/oral levothyroxine remains the treatment of choice.
- Ventilatory, cardiac support, and management of other associated conditions are of paramount importance.

THYROID STORM

Thyroid storm is an endocrine emergency characterized by severely exaggerated symptoms of thyrotoxicosis with multiorgan dysfunction. It is associated with a mortality rate of 20-30% and requires urgent medical attention. Thyroid storm generally occurs in Graves' disease (GD) or toxic multinodular goiter but may occur with subacute thyroiditis, hydatidiform mole, metastatic thyroid carcinoma, or factitious thyrotoxicosis. It is less common today than in the past due to early diagnosis and treatment of thyrotoxicosis. Nevertheless, it may occur in 1-2% of hospital admissions for thyrotoxicosis.

Thyroid storm is commonly precipitated by infections, trauma, surgeries, acute psychosis, acute emotional stress, acute medical illness, after radioiodine therapy, pregnancy, labor, exposure to neurotoxins, organophosphate poisoning, and abrupt discontinuation of antithyroid drugs. It is more common in those who are noncompliant to treatment than in treatment-naïve individuals. The cardinal manifestations are excessive diaphoresis with fever (temperature >102°F) out of proportion to an apparent infection, tachycardia out of proportion to fever, gastrointestinal dysfunction such as nausea, vomiting, diarrhea, and, in severe cases, jaundice. Central nervous system dysfunction ranges from marked hyperirritability and anxiety to confusion, paranoia, psychosis, and coma. In addition to marked sinus tachycardia, other cardiovascular manifestations are atrial fibrillation, supraventricular arrhythmias, and rarely ventricular tachyarrhythmias. Congestive heart failure or a reversible dilated cardiomyopathy can occur, even in those patients without known antecedent cardiac disease. Thyroid storm may present with acute abdomen, intestinal obstruction, and diffuse hepatosplenomegaly. **Table 2** depicts the diagnostic criteria of thyrotoxic storm proposed by Burch and Wartofsky in 1993.

The diagnosis is established on a clinical basis because the laboratory findings are much like those seen in uncomplicated hyperthyroidism. Indeed, serum total T3 levels may be normal in patients who have been sick for more than a few days, due to reduced conversion of T4 to T3 as seen in the sick euthyroid syndrome. Therefore, a semiquantitative scale has been developed to aid in the diagnosis by assessing the presence and severity of the most common signs and symptoms. Other laboratory abnormalities are leukocytosis, modest hyperglycemia, elevated serum lactate dehydrogenase, aspartate, alanine aminotransferase, and bilirubin levels. Serum alkaline phosphatase levels are also increased, because of increased osteoblastic bone activity and hepatic dysfunction. Mild hypercalcemia and renal failure may occur. Adrenal reserve in thyrotoxic crisis may be exceeded as the adrenal gland

TABLE 2: Diagnostic criteria of thyrotoxic crisis.

Thermoregulatory dysfunction		
Temperature (°F)	99–99.9	5
	100–100.9	10
	101–101.9	15
	102–102.9	20
	103–103.9	25
	≥104	30
Central nervous system effects		
Absent		0
Mild agitation		10
Delirium, psychosis, and lethargy		20
Seizure or coma		30
Gastrointestinal dysfunction		
Absent		0
Diarrhea, nausea, vomiting, or abdominal pain		10
Unexplained jaundice		20
Cardiovascular dysfunction		
Tachycardia (beats/min)	90–109	5
	110–119	10
	120–129	15
	130–139	20
	≥140	25
Congestive heart failure	Absent	
	Mild (edema)	
	Moderate (bibasilar rales)	
	Severe (pulmonary edema)	
Atrial fibrillation	Absent	0
	Present	10
History of precipitating event	Absent	0
	Present	10

Interpretation: Based on the total score, the likelihood of the diagnosis of a thyrotoxic storm is unlikely <25; impending 25–44; likely 45–60; highly likely >60.

Source: Burch HB, Wartofsky L. Life-threatening thyrotoxicosis. Thyroid storm. Endocrinol Metab Clin North Am. 1993;22(2):263-77.

cannot cope up with the increase in metabolic demands and augmented turnover of glucocorticoids. Moreover, there are well known coincidences of adrenal insufficiency with GD and the diagnosis of adrenal insufficiency should be considered when there is hypotension, hyponatremia, and hyperkalemia.

The components of treatment are as follows:

- *Therapy directed against the thyroid gland*: Thionamide antithyroid drugs—either propylthiouracil (PTU) or carbimazole, methimazole (MMI) are given orally or by a nasogastric tube to inhibit the new synthesis of thyroid hormones. PTU is preferred because it also inhibits the peripheral conversion of T4 to T3 and is given with a loading dose of 500–1,000 mg followed by 250 mg every 4 hours. MMZ is administered at a dose of 20 mg every 4 hours. As thionamides inhibit new hormone synthesis but not the release of already preformed glandular stores of the hormone, separate treatment must be administered to inhibit proteolysis of colloid and the continuous release of T4 and T3. Either inorganic iodine or lithium carbonate may be used for this purpose. Iodides may be given either orally as Lugol's solution (10 drops 3 times a day) or as a saturated solution of potassium iodide (five drops every 6 hours). It is essential that thionamide antithyroid drugs should be given about an hour before inorganic iodine is given as iodine alone will increase the thyroid hormone synthesis and exacerbates the thyrotoxic state. When iodine is administered in conjunction with full doses of antithyroid drugs, dramatic rapid decreases in serum T4 are seen, with values approaching the normal range within 5–7 days. Lithium carbonate may be used as an alternative drug if patients are allergic to iodine or who had serious toxic reactions (e.g., hepatitis or agranulocytosis) to MMI or PTU. Lithium is administered initially at a dose of 300 mg every 6 hours, with subsequent adjustments of dosage as necessary to maintain serum lithium levels at about 0.8–1.2 mEq/L. Oral cholecystographic agents such as ipodate and iopanoate can be used to treat severe thyrotoxicosis. They inhibit thyroid hormone release because of their large iodine content and are potent inhibitors of peripheral T4 to T3 conversion and may antagonize thyroid hormone binding to nuclear receptors. A loading dose of 2 g is given followed by 1g daily but should not be used without prior blockade with antithyroid drugs.
- *Therapy directed against peripheral actions of thyroid hormone*: The peripheral effects of thyroid hormones are targeted by diminishing the adrenergic manifestations, inhibiting the peripheral conversion of T4 to T3, and physically removing the thyroid hormones from the circulation. Beta-adrenergic blockers alleviate the manifestations of thyroid hormone excess. Propranolol is the most used β-blocker. Recommended doses are 60–80 mg of oral propranolol given every 6 hours or 0.5–1 mg intravenous dose given over 10 minutes with subsequent intravenous doses of 2–3 mg given over 10–15 minutes every several hours under constant cardiac rhythm monitoring. Propranolol is also a weak inhibitor of extrathyroidal conversion of T4 to T3, but this occurs over about a week and doesn't account for beneficial effects in thyroid storm. The use of β-blockers corrects the heart rate and diminishes the oxygen demand of the cardiac muscle, improves agitation, convulsions, psychotic behavior, tremor, diarrhea, fever, and diaphoresis. In patients with a history of bronchial asthma, treatment with selective β-1-blockers should be considered. A short-acting β-adrenergic blocker, esmolol, can be given intravenously with an initial loading dose of 0.25–0.5 mg/kg followed a by continuous infusion of 0.05–0.1 mg/kg/min. Alternatively, calcium channel blockers such as diltiazem can be used to control heart rate in those β-blockers are contraindicated.

  Inhibition of peripheral conversion of T4 to T3 is an important aspect of thyroid storm treatment and is accomplished as an additional effect of therapeutic agents such as PTU, propranolol, ipodate, and glucocorticoids. The physically circulating hormone in thyroid storm can be removed by plasmapheresis and charcoal plasma perfusion techniques. Plasmapheresis should be considered in patients who fail to respond rapidly to conventional therapy, have moderate hepatocellular dysfunction, have a history of agranulocytosis, and are being prepared for emergent thyroidectomy. Oral cholestyramine therapy at doses of 4 g four times daily help to interrupt the enterohepatic circulation of thyroid hormones by binding them in the gastrointestinal tract thereby decreasing the circulating levels of T3 and T4.
- *Therapy directed against systemic disturbances*: Hyperthermia, dehydration, and congestive heart failure are to be managed effectively. External cooling techniques such as tepid sponging, ice packs, and cooling blankets are used for the reversal of hyperthermia. Fluid losses due to fever, diaphoresis, vomiting, and diarrhea must be vigorously replaced to avoid vascular collapse and shock by isotonic saline containing 5–10% dextrose. Congestive cardiac failure should be treated with diuretics and if digoxin is used, a higher dose is needed because of its rapid clearance in thyrotoxicosis. Empirical use of glucocorticoids in thyroid storm is recommended because of postulated risk of relative adrenal insufficiency and high doses of glucocorticoids such as dexamethasone and hydrocortisone have an inhibitory effect on the extrathyroidal conversion of T4 to T3. Hydrocortisone is given intravenously at a loading dose of 300 mg followed by 100 mg every 8 hours during the initial stages of thyroid storm and subsequently, the dose is tapered and discontinued.

- *Therapy directed against precipitating illness*: All patients with thyroid storm should be evaluated for precipitating events. In some patients, it is obvious (surgery, trauma, and labor) and no added management is needed. However, when precipitating factors are not apparent, a careful search for underlying infection must be performed. Urine, blood, and sputum cultures should be obtained. Empirical broad-spectrum antibiotic coverage may be required initially while awaiting the results of cultures.

Clinical improvement is remarkable and is evident within the first 24 hours in most patients who survive thyrotoxic crisis. During recovery over next few days, based on patient status, oral intake of calories and fluids, vasomotor stability, and continuing improvement supportive therapy such as corticosteroids, antipyretics, and intravenous fluids may be tapered and gradually withdrawn. After resolution of thyroid storm definitive therapy with either surgery or radioactive iodine ablation is recommended to prevent a recurrent crisis.

Highlights: Thyroid Storm

- Evaluation for the presence of illness that precipitated thyroid storm is of paramount importance.
- Long-term definitive therapy is a must to prevent a recurrence of thyroid storm.

HASHIMOTO'S ENCEPHALOPATHY/STEROID-RESPONSIVE ENCEPHALOPATHY ASSOCIATED WITH AUTOIMMUNE THYROID DISEASE

The term "Hashimoto's encephalopathy" (HE) is now referred to as "steroid-responsive encephalopathy associated with autoimmune thyroid disease" (SREAAT). This is because of a better understanding of its pathophysiology and response to steroid therapy. SREAAT is an acute encephalopathy with variable clinical presentation. It presents with symptoms of impaired mental status, somnolence, and multiple stroke such as episodes, seizures, tremors, myoclonus, and ataxia. As affected patients have been found to have positive antithyroid antibodies [antithyroid peroxidase (anti-TPO) and antithyroglobulin] in the serum and the cerebrospinal fluid (CSF), it was believed that these antibodies might play a pathophysiological role in causing encephalopathy, possibly by promoting an antibody-mediated cerebritis. Patients can be either hypothyroid, euthyroid, or hyperthyroid during the presentation, and treatment of hypothyroid patients with thyroid hormone replacement has produced no beneficial effects on the encephalopathy. Magnetic resonance imaging (MRI) brain shows either normal or nonspecific findings. The electroencephalography (EEG) typically shows nonspecific slowing and epileptiform discharges. The diagnosis should be considered in patients with the above neurological symptoms, associated with either a euthyroid state or mild hypothyroidism with elevated serum anti-TPO antibodies, normal or nonspecific CSF, and MRI findings. There are no diagnostic laboratory tests, and this condition is a diagnosis of exclusion, where vasculitic, paraneoplastic, infectious, and psychiatric causes have been ruled out. Significant improvement is seen with intravenous or oral high-dose glucocorticoid therapy. Methylprednisolone IV 1 g daily for 3–5 days followed by oral steroids for a period of 6 months to 2 years is the regimen of choice. If no response to steroids, intravenous immunoglobulin, plasmapheresis, and immunosuppressive agents are considered and are reported to be efficacious.

Highlights: Hashimoto's Encephalopathy/Steroid-responsive Encephalopathy Associated with Autoimmune Thyroid Disease

- HE is a diagnosis of exclusion associated with elevation of serum anti-TPO antibodies.
- Corticosteroids are the treatment of choice.

CONCLUSION

A multifaceted aggressive approach and following the principles of management are important to reduce morbidity and mortality in myxedema coma and thyroid storm. Early diagnosis and treatment have reduced the occurrence of these disorders. A high index of suspicion is needed to diagnose HE in acute rapidly progressive encephalopathy. A better understanding of thyroid emergencies has improved the management of these disorders.

SUGGESTED READINGS

1. Warsofsky L. Myxedema coma. Endocrinol Metab Clin North Am. 2006;35(4):687-98, vii-viii.
2. Ono Y, Ono S, Yasunaga H, Matsui H, Fushimi K, Tanaka Y. Clinical characteristics and outcomes of myxedema coma: Analysis of a national inpatient database in Japan. J Epidemiol. 2017;27(3):117-22.
3. Klubo-Gwiezdzinska J, Wartofsky L. Myxedema coma. In: Wass J, Arlt W, Semple R (Eds). Oxford textbook of endocrinology and Diabetes, 2nd edition. Oxford: Oxford University Press; 2011. pp. 537-43.
4. Hline SS, Pham PT, Pham PT, Aung MH, Pham PM, Pham PC. Conivaptan: a step forward in the treatment of hyponatremia? Ther Clin Risk Manag. 2008;4(2):315-26.
5. Dutta P, Bhansali A, Masoodi SR, Bhadada S, Sharma N, Rajput R. Predictors of outcome in myxoedema coma: a study from a tertiary care centre. Crit Care. 2008;12(1):R1.

6. Klubo-Gwiezdzinska J, Wartofsky L. Thyrotoxic storm. In: Wass JAH, Stewart PM, Amiel SA, Davies MC (Eds). Oxford textbook of endocrinology and diabetes, 2nd edition. Oxford: Oxford University Press; 2011. pp. 454-61.
7. Bahn Chair RS, Burch HB, Cooper DS, Garber JR, Greenlee MC, Klein I, et al. Hyperthyroidism and other causes of thyrotoxicosis: management guidelines of the American Thyroid Association and American Association of Clinical Endocrinologists. Thyroid. 2011;21(6):593-646.
8. Wartofsky L, Ransil BJ, Ingbar SH. Inhibition by iodine of the release of thyroxine from the thyroid glands of patients with thyrotoxicosis. J Clin Invest. 1970;49(1):78-86.
9. Boehm TM, Burman KD, Barnes S, Wartofsky L. Lithium and iodine combination therapy for thyrotoxicosis. Acta Endocrinol (Copenh). 1980;94(2):174-83.
10. Feely J, Forrest A, Gunn A, Hamilton W, Stevenson I, Crooks J. Propranolol dosage in thyrotoxicosis. J Clin Endocrinol Metab. 1980;51(3):658-61.
11. Brunette DD, Rothong C. Emergency department management of thyrotoxic crisis with esmolol. Am J Emerg Med. 1991;9(3):232-4.
12. Solomon BL, Wartofsky L, Burman KD. Adjunctive cholestyramine therapy for thyrotoxicosis. Clin Endocrinol (Oxf). 1993;38(1):39-43.
13. Menon V, Subramanian K, Thamizh JS. Psychiatric Presentations Heralding Hashimoto's Encephalopathy: A Systematic Review and Analysis of Cases Reported in Literature. J Neurosci Rural Pract. 2017;8(2):261-7.
14. Zhou JY, Xu B, Lopes J, Blamoun J, Li L. Hashimoto encephalopathy: literature review. Acta Neurol. Scand. 2017;135(3):285-90.
15. Tamagno G, Celik Y, Simó R, Dihné M, Kimura K, Gelosa G, et al. Encephalopathy associated with autoimmune thyroid disease in patients with Graves' disease: clinical manifestations, follow-up, and outcomes. BMC Neurol. 2010;10:27.
16. Laurent C, Capron J, Quillerou B, Thomas G, Alamowitch S, Fain O, et al. Steroid-responsive encephalopathy associated with autoimmune thyroiditis (SREAT): Characteristics, treatment and outcome in 251 cases from the literature. Autoimmun Rev. 2016;15(12):1129-33.

SECTION 9

Miscellaneous Thyroid Disorders

CHAPTER 33

Thyroiditis

Subhankar Chatterjee, Deep Dutta

INTRODUCTION

Thyroiditis is one of the most frequent endocrinological problems which are encountered in day-to-day practice by adult physicians, pediatricians, and endocrinologists alike. Literally "thyroiditis" is defined by the inflammation of the thyroid gland caused by diverse etiologies. It is very important to recognize this disorder as the clinical manifestations may range from frank thyrotoxicosis to incidentally detected abnormalities in thyroid function test (TFT) and from painless goiter to life-threatening acute febrile illness with neck pain. This makes thyroiditis as one of the most commonly misdiagnosed and mistreated disorders. Not so uncommonly thyroiditis can masquerade as pyrexia of unknown origin (PUO) and befools the physicians until a simple thyroid function test is ordered. Proper history, minute clinical examination and few basic laboratory investigations can differentiate thyroiditis from its potential mimickers. In this chapter, we will discuss about the varied etiologies of thyroiditis, clinical pointers to its diagnosis, followed by biochemical, radiological, and pathological evaluation.

TYPES OF THYROIDITIS

Based on the duration of the disease, thyroiditis can be acute, subacute, or chronic. Some authors have divided it into painful and painless subtypes. Destruction-induced thyroiditis can be painful (such as subacute thyroiditis and acute suppurative thyroiditis) but more commonly painless (such as sporadic painless thyroiditis, sometimes Hashimoto's thyroiditis). Most drug-induced thyroiditis is painless (like those associated with immune checkpoint inhibitors and interferon-α), while amiodarone-induced thyroiditis can occasionally be painful. Radiation thyroiditis is usually painful. Thyroiditis can be divided most comprehensively when it is done etiologically **(Box 1)**.

BOX 1: Types of thyroiditis based on etiology.

- *Autoimmune*:
  - Hashimoto's thyroiditis
  - Sporadic painless thyroiditis
  - Postpartum thyroiditis
  - Subacute thyroiditis
  - Riedel's thyroiditis
- *Infectious*:
  - Viral
  - Bacterial
  - Mycobacterial
  - Fungal
  - Parasitic
  - Syphilis
- *Infiltrative*:
  - Amyloidosis
  - Sarcoidosis
- *Drugs*:
  - Amiodarone
  - Interferons
  - Interleukin-2
  - Tyrosine kinase inhibitors
  - Immune checkpoint inhibitors
- Radiation

Hashimoto's Thyroiditis

Hashimoto's thyroiditis is also known as chronic lymphocytic thyroiditis, chronic autoimmune thyroiditis, and lymphadenoid goiter. Although transient thyrotoxicosis is well-described at the onset of the disease process secondary to immune-mediated thyrocyte injury, the clinical picture is dominated by chronic hypothyroidism. The detailed description of this disease is beyond the scope of the chapter and has been described elsewhere in the treatise.

Painless Sporadic Thyroiditis

Painless sporadic thyroiditis is also known as silent sporadic thyroiditis or subacute lymphocytic thyroiditis among many other eponyms. Postpartum thyroiditis (occurs 4–12 months after delivery) is a special form of painless sporadic thyroiditis. It relapses more commonly (in subsequent pregnancy) than other forms of sporadic painless thyroiditis.

Epidemiology

Like Hashimoto's thyroiditis it is also autoimmune in nature with female predominance (M:F = 1:2). It can affect all ages peaking at 30–60 years, but usually spares children.

Clinical Features

Unlike subacute thyroiditis, there are no prodromal symptoms in painless sporadic thyroiditis. Clinical features depend upon the phase in which patient comes to the clinic. Although classically four phases are described in its natural history, all may not be distinctly present in the same patient. Painless goiter may be evident in all phases.

- *Phase-1 or thyrotoxic phase*: It occurs due to leakage of preformed thyroid hormones into systemic circulation giving rise to thyrotoxic signs and symptoms, but usually the stigmata of longstanding thyrotoxicosis such as weight loss, and muscle wasting are generally uncommon. This phase generally lasts for 1–3 months. Clinical clue to distinguish it from hyperthyroidism is sudden onset of "toxic" symptoms in comparison with insidious and progressive pattern of symptom evolution seen in Graves' disease. Patients generally remember the date when the malady started. The thyrotoxic phase sometimes can be so mild that it can be overlooked and patient directly presents during phase 3.
- *Phase-2 or euthyroid phase*: In this period the thyroid hormones come down to normal and result in a clinical and biochemical phase of euthyroidism. This phase goes frequently unnoticed in clinical practice.
- *Phase-3 or hypothyroid phase*: When the gland is depleted of the hormones, a hypothyroid phase develops and may persist up to a year or more. 54% patients can ultimately go on to develop permanent hypothyroidism, while rest regain the synthetic capability and come back to euthyroid state (phase-4).

Biochemical Investigations

Thyroid function test (TFT) evolves as the clinical course progresses as described. Serum thyroglobulin (Tg) is increased as seen in other types of destructive thyroiditis. Antithyroid peroxidase (TPO) and antithyroglobulin (Tg) antibodies may be significantly positive, although in lower titer than classical Hashimoto's thyroiditis. Sometimes thyrotoxic phase of painless thyroiditis can be difficult to distinguish from Graves' disease. T3 to T4 ratio is less than in Graves' disease. If it is still difficult to distinguish thyroiditis from Graves' disease, thyroid-stimulating hormone (TSH) receptor antibody (TRAb) can separate these two entities in most cases, if not all. White blood cell (WBC) count and inflammatory markers are generally normal with erythrocyte sedimentation rate (ESR) rarely >40 mm/h (difference with subacute thyroiditis). Common associated human leukocyte antigens (HLA) are HLA-DR3, -DR4, -DR5, -A1, and -B8.

Imaging

- *Ultrasonography*: Mostly normal with few showing bilateral heterogeneous hypoechogenicity as the phase of hypothyroidism ensues.
- *Color Doppler*: This modality can be helpful when toxic phase of the disease cannot be certainly distinguished from Graves' disease clinically and based on biochemical parameters. Flow is markedly decreased in toxic phase of silent painless thyroiditis, while it is much increased in patients with Graves' disease. During the recovery phase of euthyroidism the flow may again be increased.
- *Radioactive iodine uptake (RAIU) study*: This study is generally needed when there is still confusion to separate the entity of painless sporadic thyroiditis from Graves' disease. In marked contrast to the latter, 24 hours RAIU is <5% in thyrotoxic phase of painless sporadic thyroiditis. Both feedback suppression of TSH secretion and destruction of thyroid follicular cells are the reasons behind the decreased radioiodine uptake. When there is need to differentiate it from other close differentials with low RAIU in neck like thyrotoxicosis factitia, serum Tg estimation is a key test.

Pathology

Grossly there is diffuse involvement of both lobes. Microscopically there is lymphocytic infiltration (T-cell predominant), collapsed follicles, and degeneration of follicles. During the recovery phase follicular hyperplasia and disruption is noted. In opposition to the chronic pathological stigmata of Hashimoto's thyroiditis such as stromal fibrosis, oxyphilic changes and formation of germinal centers are usually absent in painless sporadic thyroiditis.

Treatment

It is important to pinpoint the diagnosis and separate it from hyperthyroidism. Failure to do so may lead to inadvertent use of antithyroid drugs which have no role in its management. To control the initial thyrotoxic symptoms β-adrenergic receptor antagonists should suffice. Sodium ipodate and iopanoic acid may also have a role in rapid control of thyrotoxic symptoms. When hypothyroidism develops, it is important to pick it up early and treat with levothyroxine. Withdrawal of levothyroxine should be tried after 6–9 months (depends on clinical and TFT evaluation case-by-case basis) in expectation of recovery of de novo synthesis of thyroid hormones.

Prognosis

Studies have shown that patients who comes to the clinical attention at phase-1 are less likely to be suffering from protracted course of hypothyroidism than those whose thyrotoxic phase remains unnoticed and directly present to the doctor with clinical complaints of hypothyroidism. Other risk factors of development of permanent hypothyroidism are persistent goiter, recurrent events of thyroiditis, severe degree of hypothyroidism, high titer of antibodies and persistent hypoechogenicity on ultrasound imaging.

■ Painful Subacute Thyroiditis

Subacute thyroiditis, the most common cause of painful thyroid, has also been described as De Quervain's thyroiditis or giant T-cell thyroiditis or subacute granulomatous thyroiditis or pseudogranulomatous thyroiditis or pseudo-tuberculous thyroiditis or migratory creeping thyroiditis in literature.

Etiology

Even after centuries of research the exact etiopathogenesis of subacute thyroiditis remains obscure. Infectious and autoimmune association with a background of genetic predisposition has been suggested. Its temporal association with a viral prodromal illness (mostly upper respiratory tract infection) and seasonal variation of incidence in accord with viral epidemics make a case for infectious etiology of the disease. Subacute thyroiditis has commonly been described in association with enteroviruses (most common-Coxsackie), mumps, measles, influenza, Epstein–Barr virus, parvovirus B19, echovirus, and adenovirus. Rare reports of subacute thyroiditis following dengue, hepatitis, encephalitis have been documented. Recently outbreak of subacute thyroiditis following COVID-19 infection has been reported. Interestingly, vaccination against influenza, hepatitis has also been reported to cause subacute thyroiditis. Rising antibody titers against above mentioned viruses amongst patients of subacute thyroiditis and its fall with resolution of the disease further suggests both viral and immunological etiologic role. However, failure to isolate cytopathic viruses from thyroid tissues of patient suffering from subacute thyroiditis in most of the studies has questioned the causative association. Nonviral infections such as malaria and Q fever have been described in association with the development of subacute thyroiditis. Subacute thyroiditis has been rarely reported in association with other autoimmune disorders such as temporal arteritis, Takayasu arteritis, and Sweet's syndrome. Although anti-TPO and anti-TG may be found in low titer and its level correlate with severity of hypothyroidism, the generation of antibodies in subacute thyroiditis is probably an epiphenomenon secondary to damage to thyrocytes rather than the primary immune response. Some studies have showed production of TRAb thus causing Graves' disease following thyroiditis; recent observations have refuted the idea. HLA Bw-35, DRw8, B15/62 have been shown to be associated with increased predisposition of subacute thyroiditis.

Epidemiology

It is female predominant disease with M:F = 1:5 and mostly affects in fourth to fifth decade. Subacute thyroiditis has been rarely described in children and pregnant women.

Clinical Features

More often than a viral prodrome is present before the actual disease is set in. Systemic symptoms such as fever, malaise, myalgia, arthralgia, and sore throat are usually there. Even high-grade febrile episodes may be present mimicking an infectious process instigating a search for a hidden focus. Goiter can be exquisitely painful, hard, and nodular on palpation, but the absence of pain does not rule out the diagnosis. In contrast to painless sporadic thyroiditis, goiter in subacute thyroiditis is usually transient. Thyroid pain may be focal or radiate to jaw, ear, anterior chest, and occiput. Pain may increase on the movement of head, swallowing or coughing. Unilateral involvement is not uncommon. Occasionally cervical lymph nodes may be enlarged. These clinical pictures closely mimic pharyngitis. Clinical phases follow the path of other destruction-induced thyroiditis as described previously under painless sporadic thyroiditis. Rarely the disease can manifest with dramatic presentation with acute obstructive features. Subacute thyroiditis presenting with nontender solitary nodule and histopathology masquerading a papillary thyroid neoplasm has been reported in literature.

Biochemical Investigations

Thyroid function test evolution over the disease course is similar to painless sporadic thyroiditis. Total T4:T3 ratio is much higher (generally 20:1) than Graves' disease. Serum fT3:fT4 ratio of 0.4 or less during the thyrotoxic phase helps to differentiate subacute thyroiditis from Graves' disease biochemically. Transient rise of thyroid autoantibodies may be seen, although in much low titer. Painful Hashimoto's thyroiditis, which may clinically present like De Quervain's thyroiditis, are associated with persistently high autoantibodies. High inflammatory markers, mild leukocytosis, and deranged liver enzymes may be present. High ESR is the hallmark of the disease and a normal ESR makes the diagnosis of De Quervain's thyroiditis very unlikely.

Imaging

- *Ultrasonography*: Generalized or focal areas of hypoechogenicity with nodular changes are frequently found.
- *Color Doppler*: Low vascular flow to the hypoechoic areas is frequently observed.
- *Nuclear scan*: 24 hours RAIU is <2% in thyrotoxic phase. During the recovery phase RAIU becomes greater than normal for a while as the gland tries to replete its

hormone stores. Another more easily available nuclear scan is Tc^{99} pertechnetate which also corroborate with the findings of iodine scan.

Pathology

Histopathological examination is generally not required to diagnose subacute thyroiditis, unless there is suspicion of infiltrating thyroid neoplasm. Disintegration and destruction of follicular epithelial architecture with degenerative changes in a background of cellular debris are commonly observed. Central core of colloid surrounded by multinucleated giant T-cell (foreign body type) with epithelioid granuloma formation is the characteristic for the disease. The giant T-cell in subacute thyroiditis is actually a conglomeration of a number of histiocytes. Large number of histiocytes in background of atypical follicular cells sometimes pretends as papillary carcinoma of thyroid. Reversibility of these pathologic features is the rule unless permanent hypothyroidism develops where complete destruction of thyroid parenchyma and stigmata of chronic inflammation such as fibrosis may occur.

Treatment

Similar to other destruction-induced thyroiditis, β-adrenergic blockers are sufficient to tackle the thyrotoxic symptoms. As thyroid pain is one of the chief concerns, aspirin and nonsteroidal anti-inflammatory drugs are often needed. Glucocorticoids are sometimes necessary to abate severe pain refractory to other measures. Prednisolone is usually started at 40 mg/day which is continued for a week and then tapered over next 4 weeks. Too rapid tapering of glucocorticoid may lead to recurrence. The diagnosis of subacute thyroiditis is to be questioned if the neck pain does not resolve within 48 hours of starting of glucocorticoid. Very rarely patients may suffer from relapse and repeated exacerbation even with multiple courses of glucocorticoid therapy. In these circumstances radical measures such as thyroidectomy or radioiodine ablation is needed.

Prognosis

Although transient hypothyroid is pretty common (30–50%), incidence of permanent hypothyroidism in subacute thyroiditis is much lower (5–15%) than painless sporadic thyroiditis. Both symptomatic transient hypothyroidism and permanent hypothyroidism should be treated with appropriate levothyroxine replacement therapy. Thyroid function test should be repeated after 6–9 months to assess the spontaneous recovery.

Infectious Thyroiditis

Infectious thyroiditis is exceedingly uncommon, but potentially life-threatening disease. Thyroid gland is inherently resistant to infections. Fibrous capsule completely surrounding the gland and tight fascial planes, separating it from the other neck structures forms strong anatomical barriers against the spread of infection from contiguous structures to the thyroid. High intrathyroidal iodine content, acts as bactericidal. Moreover, rich lymphatic drainage and blood supply of the thyroid gland helps in limiting the infection by rapid recruitment of WBC.

Unlike other forms of thyroiditis, infectious thyroiditis has an equal sex incidence. Children and immunosuppressed individuals are particularly susceptible. In children with bacterial thyroiditis the presence of piriform sinus fistula should be strongly suspected and closure of the fistulous tract is essential to prevent recurrence. Piriform sinus is the residual connection following the path of migration of ultimobranchial body from the fifth pharyngeal arch to thyroid gland. Although after birth right ultimobranchial body becomes progressively atrophic, the left one persists in many occasions. In repeated infection of the pyriform sinus, a fistulous tract is formed between the left lobe of thyroid and the sinus and extending the infection to the thyroid gland. This explains the reason behind the increased occurrence of infectious thyroiditis involving left lobe of thyroid, particularly in children. Neck trauma, esophageal rupture, extension from retro- and parapharyngeal abscess, infected branchial cyst, thyroglossal duct cyst or seeding of microorganisms after fine needle aspiration biopsy are the common routes of infection. More often than not preexisting thyroid disorders are prevalent among patients suffering from infective thyroiditis.

Infectious thyroiditis can be bacterial, fungal, mycobacterial, parasitic, or syphilitic in the descending order of incidence **(Box 2)**. Viral thyroiditis is traditionally described in the context of sporadic painless thyroiditis and painful subacute thyroiditis.

Clinical Features

Bacterial or suppurative or pyogenic thyroiditis is often heralded by a preceding event of apparently innocuous

---

BOX 2: Different types of infectious thyroiditis and causative microorganisms.

- *Bacteria*: Staphylococcus aureus and non-*aureus*, Streptococcus pyogenes, Escherichia coli, Haemophilus influenzae, Klebsiella species, Pseudomonas aeruginosa, Salmonella species, Actinomyces naeslundii, Actinobacillus actinomycetemcomitans, Arcanobacterium haemolyticum, Brucella melitensis, Clostridium septicum, Eikenella corrodens, Enterobacter, and Serratia marcescens
- *Mycobacteria*: Mycobacterium tuberculosis, Mycobacteroides chelonae, Mycobacterium avium intracellulare, and Mycobacterium leprae
- *Fungi*: Aspergillus species, Coccidioides immitis, Histoplasma capsulatum, Candida albicans, Alleschaeria boydii, Nocardia asteroides, and Nocardia brasiliensis
- *Parasites*: Echinococcus, Strongyloides stercoralis, Taenia solium, and Pneumocystis jiroveci
- Syphilis

upper respiratory tract infection. The clinical picture is predominated by features of systemic toxicity with fever, severe neck pain, cervical lymphadenopathy, and obstructive features such as dysphonia and dysphagia. Sometimes patient may not appreciate the anterior neck pain as the referred pain in pharynx and ears dominate. The thyroid is excruciatingly tender to touch associated with warmth and erythema of overlying skin. Fluctuant abscess can also be felt on palpation. Unlike bacterial thyroiditis, mycobacterial, fungal or parasitic thyroiditis does not have a dramatic onset and follow a chronic course with painless enlargement of thyroid nodules.

Biochemical Investigations

Majority of the patients remain euthyroid, although thyrotoxicosis in acute phase and hypothyroidism after resolution of infection has been reported in 5–10% cases. Sometimes it may be difficult to differentiate acute infectious thyroiditis from subacute thyroiditis clinically. Very high inflammatory markers and a greater degree of leukocytosis generally indicate an acute infectious cause.

Imaging

Ultrasonography usually shows hypoechoic lesion which more commonly affects left lobe. It is also an excellent modality to identify a thyroid abscess and plays an important role in diagnosis of fungal and parasitic thyroiditis. Barium swallow is helpful in locating the site and extension of piriform sinus fistula. Computed tomography (CT) or magnetic resonance imaging (MRI) studies are helpful in greater delineation of abscess, identification of soft tissues gases and piriform sinus fistula, if any.

Pathology and Microbiology

Fine needle aspiration biopsy followed by appropriate staining and culture is the most important and gold standard to diagnose infectious thyroiditis. Apart from routine Gram staining and acid-fast bacilli staining, fungal stain, and Gomori's silver methenamine stain for *Pneumocystis jiroveci* should be undertaken especially among immunocompromised patients.

Treatment

Acute bacterial thyroiditis is an emergency and must be managed as such. Prompt recognition and institution of treatment is the key, otherwise it leads to grave prognosis. If airway patency is threatened, urgent incision and drainage should be done after initial stabilization. Considering the virulence of the disease process, an early empiric broad-spectrum antibiotic therapy should be instituted followed by appropriate selection of antibiotics based on the culture/sensitivity reports. Fungal infections should be treated with combination of antifungals (amphotericin B, voriconazole, and caspofungin). Multidrug antitubercular therapy is to be started for mycobacterial thyroiditis according to protocol. On long-term to prevent further recurrence it is important to identify a potential treatable route of infection and operated (like piriform sinus fistula).

Riedel's Thyroiditis

Riedel's thyroiditis is also known as fibrous thyroiditis or chronic sclerosing thyroiditis. Although the first description of this disorder dates back to 1896, the etiopathogenesis is obscure. Of late, Riedel's thyroiditis is viewed as a thyroid-specific manifestation of a more generalized immunoglobulin G4 (IgG4)-related disease process.

Epidemiology

Riedel's thyroiditis is rare with estimated incidence of 1.06 cases per 100,000 population. Although classical cases have been described among middle aged women (M:F = 1:4).

Clinical Features

The thyroid is moderately enlarged with stony hard feeling on palpation (cast iron struma). Extension of the diffuse fibrotic process may involve the adjacent structures leading to their compression resulting in dysphagia, dysphonia. Thus, the clinical picture may closely mimic an advanced thyroid carcinoma. Lack of associated cervical lymphadenopathy generally favors the diagnoses of Riedel's thyroiditis in oppose to a malignancy. Systemic manifestations (salivary glands, lacrimal glands, pancreas, pituitary, hepatobiliary system, kidneys, aorta, mediastinum, and retroperitoneum) of fibrotic and sclerosing disease may be present and should be searched for.

Biochemical Investigations

Hypothyroidism may occur. Thyroid autoantibodies, if found, are present in much lower titer. Serum IgG4 is usually >135 mg/dL. Associated hypoparathyroidism has also been reported in literature.

Imaging

Ultrasonography shows diffuse low echogenicity with reduced vascular flow on color Doppler in the regions of fibrosis. Extent of fibrosis is best determined by neck computed tomography (CT) or magnetic resonance imaging (MRI). Thyroid nuclear scanning shows a heterogenous pattern with overall low uptake, cold areas reflecting areas of fibrosis. ^{18}Flurodeoxyglucose positron emission tomography-CT scan (showing intense uptake in the areas of inflammation) holds an important place while searching for extrathyroidal involvement.

Pathology

Open biopsy is the gold-standard for diagnosis. Some of the cases of Riedel's thyroiditis show classical histopathological features of IgG4-related disorders—dense lymphoplasmacellular inflammatory infiltrate consisting of IgG4-positive plasma cells with exuberant storiform fibrosis and obliterative phlebitis. But this characteristic description is not equivocally present in every case. Pathological diagnostic hallmark of Riedel's thyroiditis is complete destruction of involved thyroid tissues, with loss of normal lobulated architecture, lack of granulomatous reaction, presence of few foci of lymphocytes, plasma cells, eosinophils, and Hürthle cells and extension of the fibrosis to the adjacent neck structures.

Treatment

Tamoxifen with or without glucocorticoids have been tried with varying success. Tamoxifen probably acts by suppressing transforming growth factor-beta (TGF-β). Surgery (extensive or wedge resection) may be needed to relieve compressive features. Levothyroxine replacement is to be started if hypothyroidism develops.

Drug-induced Thyroiditis

Amiodarone is one of the most frequently implicated drugs causing thyroid abnormalities by causing both hypothyroidism and thyrotoxicosis. Amiodarone-induced thyrotoxicosis (AIT) is of two type—(1) AIT type 1 and (2) AIT type 2. While type 1 occurs due to iodine excess superimposed on pre-existing thyroid pathologies (such as Graves' disease and multinodular goiter) and causes true hyperthyroidism, type 2 is caused by cytotoxic effect of amiodarone itself on thyrocytes giving rise to similar picture of destruction induced thyroiditis. AIT type-2 is more common than type-1 and very rarely they can coexist. Type 2 AIT generally occurs after long-term use of amiodarone (median—30 months). AIT type 2 patients generally are nongoitrous and devoid of thyroid autoantibodies. On color flow Doppler sonography there is reduced vascularity with suppressed RAIU on thyroid scan. AIT type 2 is frequently self-limiting and only requires oral prednisolone therapy to mitigate the thyroid inflammation. In rare instances severe thyrotoxicosis unresponsive to medical therapy may occur, necessitating a total thyroidectomy. Following remission, it is possible to readminister amiodarone among these patients. 17% patients may develop permanent hypothyroidism. Similar to AIT type-2 lithium can rarely cause destruction-induced thyroiditis by its direct cytotoxic effect on the gland.

Interferons, interleukin-2, granulocyte/macrophage colony stimulating factor (GM-CSF) and newer immune checkpoint inhibitors [cytotoxic T-lymphocyte–associated antigen 4 (CTLA4) inhibitors and programmed cell death protein-1 (PD1) inhibitors] have been associated with thyroiditis by exacerbating the underlying autoimmune disease. Phases of evolution are nearly same as silent painless thyroiditis, but duration of phases generally brief (few weeks than months). Unique cytological features of immune checkpoint inhibitors are clusters of necrotic cells in abundance, lymphocytic proliferation and CD163 positive histiocytes.

Leuprolide, and small molecule kinase inhibitors (such as sunitinib and sorafenib) have been reported to cause initial thyrotoxicosis followed by hypothyroidism, but the mechanisms have still not been completely unveiled.

Radiation-induced thyroiditis is particularly noted following ^{131}I therapy for Graves' disease or thyroid cancer. It is generally painful. External beam radiotherapy for Hodgkin's or non-Hodgkin's lymphoma, breast cancer or other head-neck cancer has also been reported to cause radiation thyroiditis. Conservative management with glucocorticoid is the treatment of choice.

AN INDIAN PERSPECTIVE

The universal salt iodization program significantly improved the iodine status of the Indian population, and has had a major role in reducing the population prevalence of goiter and hypothyroidism secondary to iodine deficiency. As of today autoimmune hypothyroidism is the most common cause of hypothyroidism in India like the western world. Many of these patients have preceding history of thyroiditis. Vitamin-D deficiency is very rampant in India, and its deficiency has also been linked to impaired thyroid function and thyroid autoimmunity.

CONCLUSION

Hence, it is apparent that thyroiditis is a spectrum disorder with varied etiologies and presentations. Treatment is primarily symptomatic and determined by the underlying etiology. It can be considered as a great "endocrine mimic." As a rule of thumb, any patient with pyrexia of unknown origin where we are not able to establish the etiology, it may be a good clinical practice to check for thyroid profile to rule out biochemical hyperthyroidism due to an underlying thyroiditis. However, routine thyroid profile testing is discouraged in sick patients as thyroid reports are difficult to interpret in sick people due to the underlying "sick euthyroid syndrome."

SUGGESTED READINGS

1. Brent GA, Weetman AP. Hypothyroidism and Thyroiditis. In: Melmed S, Auchus RJ, Goldfine AB, Koenig RJ, Rosen CJ (Eds). Williams Textbook of Endocrinology, 14th edition. Philadelphia, PA: Elsevier; 2020. pp. 404-32.
2. Dutta D, Ahuja A, Selvan C. Immunoglobulin G4 related thyroid disorders: Diagnostic challenges and clinical outcomes. Endokrynol Pol. 2016;67(5):520-4.
3. Farwell AP, Pearce EN. Sporadic painless, painful subacute and acute infectious thyroiditis. In: Braverman LE, Cooper DS, Kopp P (Eds). Werner & Ingbar's the Thyroid: A fundamental and clinical text, 11th edition. New Delhi: Wolter Kluwer (India) Pvt Ltd; 2021. pp. 395-418.

4. Ghosh R, Dubey S, Sarkar A, Biswas D, Ray A, Roy D, et al. Antithyroid arthritis syndrome in a case of post-COVID-19 subacute thyroiditis. Diabetes Metab Syndr. 2021;15(3):683-6.
5. Guimarães VC. Subacute and Riedel's Thyroiditis. In: Jameson JJ, DeGroot LJ, deKretser DM, Giudice LC, Grossman AB, Melmed S, et al (Eds). Endocrinology: Adult and Pediatric, 7th edition. Philadelphia, PA: Elsevier; 2016. pp. 1528-39.
6. Kibirige D, Luzinda K, Ssekitoleko R. Spectrum of lithium induced thyroid abnormalities: a current perspective. Thyroid Res. 2013;6(1):3.
7. Pearce EN, Farwell AP. Thyroiditis. In: Wass JAH, Arlt W, Semple RK (Eds). Oxford Textbook of Endocrinology and Diabetes, 3rd edition. Oxford, UK: Oxford University Press; 2022. pp. 443-53.
8. Popescu M, Ghemigian A, Vasile CM, Costache A, Carsote M, Ghenea AE. The New Entity of Subacute Thyroiditis amid the COVID-19 Pandemic: From Infection to Vaccine. Diagnostics (Basel). 2022;12(4):960.

CHAPTER 34: Thyroid and Coronavirus Disease 2019

Vaishali Deshmukh, Paulami Deshmukh, Shashank R Joshi

INTRODUCTION

Severe acute respiratory syndrome coronavirus 2 (SARS-CoV-2) infection and the coronavirus disease 2019 (COVID-19) pandemic has posed a serious challenge to all aspects of clinical practice, with nearly all organs and biological systems being affected by the virus directly or indirectly. Endocrine system is no exception and some of the endocrine organs like the thyroid were found to be affected by COVID-19.

Coronavirus disease 2019 affects thyroid function and triggers inflammation of the thyroid which leads to thyroid-specific consequences. This chapter aims to review the associations between COVID-19 infection and thyroid disorders (**Fig. 1**).

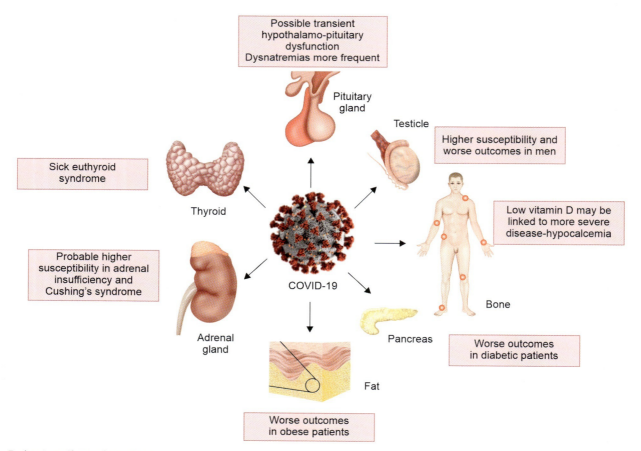

Fig. 1: Endocrine effects of COVID-19.
Source: Marazuela M, Giustina A, Puig-Domingo M. Endocrine and metabolic aspects of the COVID-19 pandemic. Rev Endocr. Metab Disord. 2020;21(4):495–507.

EFFECT OF PRE-EXISTING THYROID DISEASES ON COVID-19

There is no evidence that patients with existing autoimmune thyroid disease, thyroid dysfunction, thyroid nodules, or cancer are more susceptible to contracting SARS-CoV-2 viral infection, or at risk of developing more severe COVID-19 disease and baseline thyroid dysfunction does not foster a worse progression of COVID-19.

However, certain subsets of patients are likely to be at increased risk of developing severe coronavirus infection. Patients with thyroid ophthalmopathy receiving glucocorticoid and immunosuppressive therapy, are considered to be extremely vulnerable and are highly likely to aggravate the disease once infected with COVID-19. Conjunctivitis is a manifestation of COVID-19, and SARS-CoV-2 messenger ribonucleic acid (mRNA) can be detected in teardrops. Hence, patients with ophthalmopathy combined with COVID-19 may have a higher risk of infection transmission, especially when they have significant ocular soft-tissue involvement.

Coronavirus disease 2019 infection in hyperthyroid patients often activates an excessive immune-response and predispose to high risk of thyroid storm. Hence, patients with thyroid dysfunction should continue to take their antithyroid medications. However, patients on antithyroid drug treatment are at risk of developing agranulocytosis, (0.2–0.5% chances). Symptoms of agranulocytosis can overlap with flu-like symptoms of COVID-19, often making it difficult to differentiate one from the other clinically. The coexistence of these conditions contributes to a worse prognosis because both conditions are associated with impaired immunologic system. Therefore, it is recommended that patients on antithyroid drugs with symptoms suggestive of neutropenia immediately discontinue the drug and obtain an urgent full blood count to measure neutrophil count until symptoms have resolved. Uncontrolled thyrotoxicosis may be associated with more severe complications from COVID-19. Urgent surgery or 131-I may be undertaken in selected cases of uncontrolled thyrotoxicosis. COVID-19 has been suggested to trigger the activation of pre-existing thyroid disease or autoimmunity.

Hypothyroid patients on replacement treatment with thyroid hormones should continue their medicine and monitoring as usual and many were and could be managed through virtual clinics to reduce the risks associated with hospital exposure. High-risk thyroid nodules require a fine-needle aspiration without relevant delay, whereas other nonurgent diagnostic procedures and therapeutic interventions should be postponed.

HOW DID THE PANDEMIC AFFECT THYROID MANAGEMENT? IMPACT ON QOL

A survey by the British Thyroid Foundation (BTF) done by Maria G Pavlatou et al., was conducted to see how COVID-19 had affected 633 patients. Of the 633 respondents, the average age was 49 years and 93.6% were female. The majority of respondents (82%) lived in England and included subjects with hypothyroidism (54%) and hyperthyroidism (34%). 57% had at least one other medical condition most commonly depression affecting nearly 30% of these. Six respondents (1%) had tested positive for COVID-19 at the time of the survey and another 108 (18%) had symptoms suggestive of COVID-19 but had not been tested. When asked to rate on a scale of 0–10 (0 = no concern, 10 = very concerned) concern about your thyroid disease predisposing you to COVID-19, the average score was 4.6. When asked to score quality of life before and after the pandemic, average score before COVID-19 of 7/10. This dropped to 5.6/10 during the pandemic. 58% felt that anxiety and depression had increased during the pandemic. 52% had gained weight during the pandemic. 65% required medical advice for thyroid during the pandemic; 12% were unable to get to their general physician (GP) or thyroid specialist. 7.6% had had their thyroid treatment [surgery, radioiodine or treatment for thyroid eye disease (TED)] postponed. 83% desired to have telephone or video consultations with thyroid experts in different parts of the country. The level of satisfaction with GP services for patients with thyroid diseases during the pandemic had average rating of 4.3/10. About 9.6% encountered difficulties obtaining repeat thyroid prescriptions during the pandemic.

EFFECT OF SARS-COV-2 ON THYROID GLAND: PATHOPHYSIOLOGIC AND MOLECULAR MECHANISMS OF THYROID AFFECTION IN COVID-19

Angiotensin-converting enzyme 2 (ACE2) is the receptor for cellular entry of SARS-CoV-2. Viral ribonucleic acid (RNA) has also been detected in blood, stool, and urine samples of patients with COVID-19. In study done by Rotondi et al., it showed that the mRNA encoding for the ACE2 receptor is expressed in thyroid follicular cells, making them a potential target for SARS-COV-2 entry, thereby suggesting a mechanism for thyroiditis in patients with COVID-19 infection. Similar expression was also seen in the pancreas, testis, ovary, adrenal gland, pituitary gland along with thyroid gland. The serum ACE level was positively correlated with 3,5,3′-triiodothyronine (T3) and thyroxine (T4). Association with endocrine diseases may worsen the adverse prognosis of COVID-19.

Thyroid dysfunction secondary to SARS CoV-2 infection is likely a mixture of several mechanisms. Various hypotheses have been postulated as follows:
- There is a direct influence on the thyroid gland by SARS-CoV-2, which invades through the wall of trachea and the upper respiratory tract. However, no significant abnormalities in thyroid follicular morphology were found in postmortem examination of COVID-19

- patients, and no SARS-CoV-2 was found in thyroid tissues by immunohistochemistry and polymerase chain reaction analysis.
- Possibility of underlying nonthyroidal illness syndrome (NTIS) caused by critical illness. Patients have normal or low serum thyroid-stimulating hormone (TSH) concentration and low T3 concentration, accompanied by a low concentration of T4 in more severe or prolonged illness. A study by Khoo et al., detected that patients with COVID-19 had lower admission TSH and free thyroxine (FT4) levels compared to those without COVID-19 after eliminating the potential interference of cortisol on TSH and none had thyrotoxicosis clinically.
- Ten patients with COVID-19 in a study by Lui et al. were found to have isolated low free triiodothyronine (FT3), with normal TSH and FT4 levels, suggesting a possible NTIS; FT3 in the study showed a decreasing trend with worsening clinical severity of COVID-19. Furthermore, an independent inverse correlation between erythrocyte sedimentation rate and FT3/FT4 ratio was also demonstrated, which suggested the potential effect of systemic inflammation on deiodinase activity.
- Dysfunction of the HPT axis causes a diminished level of serum TSH. Severe acute respiratory syndrome coronavirus 2 infection can affect the nervous system and cranial nerves of smell and taste. Due to lack of pathological evidence of SARS-CoV-2 invading the hypothalamus or pituitary cells, and data on pituitary hormones, more comprehensive data are needed to prove this hypothesis.
- Indirect effects of immune-mediated postviral inflammatory reaction caused by COVID-19 infection. The second stage of COVID-19 is characterized by pulmonary inflammation and coagulation disorders, usually combined with innate immune activation and accompanied by triggering of proinflammatory responses, including cytokines interleukin-1-beta (IL-1β), interleukin 6 (IL-6), tumor necrosis factor α, and adaptive T-cell-mediated immune response, while the postviral inflammatory reaction may be the inducing factor of thyroid dysfunction. A retrospective study by Lania et al., found that the thyroid function evaluated at hospitalization correlated with some inflammatory parameters. This study included 287 noncritical patients hospitalized for COVID-19. Of all patients, 20.2% had thyrotoxicosis, and 5.2% had hypothyroidism. Increased IL-6 levels in this study indicated high risk of thyrotoxicosis related to systemic immune activation induced by the SARS-CoV-2 infection.
- Thyroid function abnormalities may also be a result of anti-COVID-19 drugs and the iodine load due to examination with computed tomography scan may also influence euthyroid status of the patients.

All said, thyroid assays should be performed in patients with severe infection/at acute phase of COVID-19 in order to detect thyrotoxicosis.

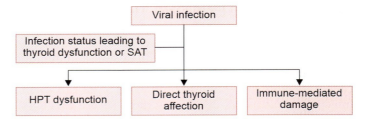

Flowchart 1: Potential mechanisms for effects of severe acute respiratory syndrome coronavirus-2 (SARS-CoV-2) infections on thyroid.
(HPT: hypothalamic–pituitary–thyroid; SAT: subacute thyroiditis)

- The etiopathogenesis of subacute thyroiditis (SAT) is not completely understood, but is known to follow a viral infection or a postviral inflammatory reaction, especially in genetically predisposed individuals. Individuals carrying some human leukocyte antigen (HLA) haplotypes (such as HLA-Bw35, HLA-B67, HLA-B15/62, and HLA-Drw8) were susceptible to SAT. Other viruses associated with SAT include echovirus and coxsackievirus, Epstein–Barr virus, orthomyxovirus, hepatitis E, mumps, adenovirus, rubella, human immunodeficiency virus (HIV), and *Cytomegalovirus* **(Flowchart 1)**.

CLINICAL AND BIOCHEMICAL PRESENTATIONS OF THYROID AFFECTION IN COVID-19

A retrospective study of thyroid function in 50 patients of COVID-19 without a history of thyroid disease done by Chen et al., looked at clinical manifestations, laboratory results, and chest computed tomography scans who underwent thyroid function testing during their course of COVID-19 and after recovery. TSH lower than the normal range was present in 56% (28/50) and overall TSH and serum total triiodothyronine (TT3) of the patients were significantly lower than those of healthy control and non-COVID-19 pneumonia patients while total thyroxine (TT4) level was not different in the groups. 34% (17/50) of the patients showed lower-than-normal values only for TSH during the course of their COVID-19 infection that may not be fully explained by NTIS. The degree of the decreases in TSH and TT3 levels was positively correlated with the severity of the disease. After recovery, no significant differences in TSH, TT3, TT4, fT3, and fT4 levels were found between the COVID-19 and control groups.

In addition, in the subgroup analysis of patients with COVID-19 according to disease severity, the degree of the decrease in TSH and TT3 correlated positively with the severity of the disease; the more severe the COVID-19 infection was, the lower the TSH and TT3 levels were. The observed decrease in TSH level in patients with COVID-19 could be induced by direct viral affection or chronic stress from hypoxemia and the glucocorticoids with which most patients (31/50) were treated, though the dosage was low (57.3 mg methylprednisolone/day).

Subacute Thyroiditis in COVID-19 Patients

In a review by Speer et al., Subacute thyroiditis, autoimmune thyroiditis and an atypical form of thyroiditis were reported complications of COVID-19. Patients with the coronavirus may be at risk of developing SAT during the acute phase of COVID-19 infection or a few weeks post infection. It presents as reversible, subclinical and atypical thyroiditis. In a review 19 papers (17 case reports and two case series) were included, describing 27 patients, 74.1% females, and aged 18–69 years. Coronavirus disease 2019 was diagnosed by nasopharyngeal swab in 66.7% cases and required hospitalization in 11.1%. In 83.3% cases, SAT occurred after COVID-19. Neck pain was present in 92.6% cases and fever in 74.1%. Median TSH, fT3, and fT4 were 0.01 mU/L, 10.79 pmol/L, and 27.2 pmol/L, respectively. C-reactive-protein and erythrocyte sedimentation rate were elevated in 96% of cases. Typical ultrasonographic characteristics of SAT were observed in 83.3% of cases. Steroids were the most frequent SAT therapy. Complete remission of SAT was recorded in most cases.

It is usually a temporary, painful and associated with tenderness in the thyroid gland, sore throat, flu-like symptoms and/or fever. There is a thyrotoxic phase during which patient may experience nervousness, tremor, palpitations, insomnia, and may feel feverish. This may be followed by a hypothyroid phase when patient may experience slowness, fatigue, and feeling colder than usual. In some patients, subacute thyroiditis resolves itself without treatment, or with the help of anti-inflammatory drugs like steroids. Complete recovery usually occurs in 2–5 months although 5–20% may land in permanent hypothyroidism. It differs from "nonthyroidal illness," which occurs in very sick patients and T4, T3, and TSH all go down as the body attempts to conserve energy and divert it toward survival and restores to normal when acute illness subsides.

In study by Muller et al., the investigators looked at the prevalence of thyrotoxicosis (suggestive of subacute thyroiditis) in COVID-19 patients admitted to the high intensity of care unit (HICU) in Milan's main public hospital and found that critically ill COVID-19 patients may be prone to subacute thyroiditis. They studied 85 patients in the COVID-19 group and 78 in the control group. All subjects had serum thyroid function measured within the first 2 days after intensive care unit (ICU) admission: Serum thyroid function (TSH, fT4, and fT3) and C-reactive protein (CRP) was measured and those with TSH concentrations below the reference range and/or free T4 concentrations above the reference range were deemed "thyrotoxic." In the COVID-19 group, 13 of 85 (15%) patients were biochemically thyrotoxic, as compared with 1 of 78 (1%) in the control group ($p = 0.002$). (64% were men and 36% women). The authors believed that COVID-19 induced an atypical form of subacute thyroiditis as there was no neck pain, and did not affect predominantly women, as seen in a typical case of SAT.

A study by Bahcecioglu et al., showed that total number of SAT cases during the pandemic period was comparable to prepandemic period. Out of 64 patients, 18.8% had coronavirus (CoV)-associated SAT, 9.3% had vaccine associated SAT and 71.9% had non-CoV related SAT. Coronavirus severe acute respiratory syndrome (CoV-SAT) and non-CoV-SAT groups were similar in terms of clinical, laboratory, and treatment characteristics. Coronavirus disease 19 presented with SAT, as the first manifestation in three cases. Vaccine-related cases developed in a shorter time period, clinical presentation was milder, and only a few required corticosteroids.

Review of five retrospective studies of 10 COVID-19 patients (nine women and one man), aged 18–68 years; 7 Italian, 3 Burmese, Turkish, and Mexican was done by Chen et al. Symptoms were nonserious and all had only mild fever and upper respiratory symptoms, and no one had been treated in ICUs. The time from diagnosis of COVID-19 infection to typical symptoms of SAT was from 5 to 42 days. The symptoms of SAT in all patients were classic, including fever, anterior neck pain, fatigue, tremors, anosmia, sweating, and palpitations **(Table 1)**.

Our Experience of Subacute Thyroiditis Cases

In contrast to the reported literature, five of our patients presented with subacute thyroiditis nearly 12 weeks after COVID-19 **(Table 2)**. All these five subjects were males with average age of 38.6 years (32–53 years) and presented with neck pain (5/5), low grade fever (4/5) of an average duration of 4 weeks. Goiter was present in 2/5. Diabetes and hypertension were present in 1/5. Thyroid tenderness was present in all, even in absence of goiter. Fatigue and weakness were present in 4/5 and two of them had significant weight loss. One patient had heat intolerance. None of them had TPO positivity. All had history of COVID-19 prior to the above symptoms and had raised serum T3 and serum T4 with low S. TSH (average: 0.029 μIU/mL), raised erythrocyte sedimentation rate (ESR) (average: 26.4 mm/h) and CRP (average: 49.8 mg/L). Average duration between detection of COVID-19 infection and presentation with above symptoms was 12.8 weeks. COVID-19 was mild in one case (required home-care), and moderate (hospitalized without oxygen or ventilatory support) in remaining 4/5. All patients responded well to oral prednisolone and thyrotoxicosis management. Average duration of prednisolone therapy was 2 months and average dose of prednisolone required was 6.8 mg/day. All recovered to euthyroid state with normalization of ESR and CRP in 2 months time without any long-term thyroid sequalae.

TABLE 1: Subacute thyroiditis patient's characteristics, symptoms, radiographic findings, laboratory findings, and treatment measures.

Author, years	Country	Number of patients, sex	Symptoms of COVID-19	Time from symptom onset to recovery, days	Time from diagnosis of COVID-19 to SAT, days	Symptoms of SAT	Laboratory indexes	Imaging examination	Treatment of SAT	Time from diagnosis of SAT to recovery, days
Brancatella et al. (2020)	Italy	18, F	Rhinorrhea and cough	14	15	Fever, palpitations, fatigue, and neck pain	TSH(↓), FT4 (↑), FT3 (↑), TgAb(↑), Tg(-), TPOAb(-), TRAb(-), ESR(↑), CRP(↑), and WBC(↑)	Ultrasound—multiple diffuse hypoechoic areas	Prednisone	40
Brancatella et al. (2020)	Italy	38, F	Fever, rhinorrhea, anosmia, and asthenia	4	16	Fever, asthenia, neck pain, and anorexia	TSH (↓), FT4 (↑), FT3 (↑), TgAb(-), Tg(↑), TPOAb(-), TRAb(-), ESR(↑), and CRP(↑)	Ultrasound: enlarged thyroid, multiple, diffuse hypoechoic areas, decreased vascularity	Prednisone	53
		29, F	Rhinorrhea	3	30	Neck pain, fever, palpitations, asthenia, and sweating	TSH(↓), FT4 (↑), FT3 (↑), TgAb(↑), Tg(↑), TPOAb(-), TRAb(-), ESR(↑), and CRP(↑)	Ultrasound: multiple diffuse hypoechoic areas, decreased vascularity. Thyroid scan: no uptake of Tc-99m	Prednisone	46 (asymptomatic with subclinical hypothyroidism)
		29, F	Fever, cough, rhinorrhea, anosmia, and diarrhea	14	36	Neck pain, palpitations, and sweating		Ultrasound—enlarged thyroid, multiple diffuse hypoechoic areas, and decreased vascularity	Ibuprofen	47 (asymptomatic with subclinical hypothyroidism)

Continued

CHAPTER 34

Thyroid and Coronavirus Disease 2019

Continued

Author, years	Country	Number of patients, sex	Symptoms of COVID-19	Time from symptom onset to recovery, days	Time from diagnosis of COVID-19 to SAT, days	Symptoms of SAT	Laboratory indexes	Imaging examination	Treatment of SAT	Time from diagnosis of SAT to recovery, days
		46, F	Fever, cough, rhinorrhea, anosmia, and asthenia	£	20	Neck pain, fever, palpitations, asthenia, insomnia, anxiety, and weight loss	TSH(↓), FT4(↑), FT3(↑), TRAb(-), and CRP(↑)	Ultrasound: enlarged thyroid, multiple diffuse hypoechoic areas	Prednisone	44
Ippolito et al. (2020)	Italy	68, F	Mild fever, cough, and dyspnea	60	5	Palpitations, insomnia, and agitation	TSH(↓), FT4(↑), FT3(↑), TgAb(-), Tg(↑), TPOAb(-), and TRAb(-)	Ultrasound—enlarged hypoechoic thyroid, decreased vascularity. Thyroid scan: no uptake of Tc-99m	Methylprednisolone, prednisone	28
Asfuroglu, Katkan, Ates (2020)	Turkey	41, F	Fever	5	NA	Fever and neck pain	TSH(↓), FT4(↑), FT3(↑), TgAb(↑), TPOAb(-), ESR(↑), CRP(↑), and WBC(↑)	Ultrasound: diffuse hypoechoic areas, decreased vascularity	Prednisolone	28
Ruggeri et al. (2020)	Italy	43, F	Fever, rhinorrhea, cough, and hoarseness	14	42	Fever, neck pain, fatigue, tremors, and palpitations	TSH(↓), FT4(↑), FT3(↑), TgAb(-), Tg(↑), TPOAb(-), TRAb(-), ESR(↑), CRP(↑), and WBC(↑)	Ultrasound: diffuse hypoechoic areas. Thyroid scan: reduced uptake of Tc-99m	Prednisone	
Mattar et al. (2020)	Singapore	34, M	Fever, cough, headache, and anosmia	NA	9	Fever, neck pain, and tachycardia	TSH(↓), FT4(↑), FT3(↑), TPOAb(-), TRAb(-), CRP(↑), and WBC(↑)	Ultrasound: enlarged hypoechoic thyroid, decreased vascularity.	Prednisolone and atenolol	70

Continued

Continued

Author, years	Country	Number of patients, sex	Symptoms of COVID-19	Time from symptom onset to recovery, days	Time from diagnosis of COVID-19 to SAT, days	Symptoms of SAT	Laboratory indexes	Imaging examination	Treatment of SAT	Time from diagnosis of SAT to recovery, days
Campos-Barrera et al. (2020)	Mexico	37, F	Odynophagia and anosmia	NA	30	Neck pain and fatigue	TSH(↓), FT4 (↑), TT3 (↑), TgAb(-), TPOAb(-), TRAb(-), ESR(↑), CRP(↑), and WBC(-)	Thyroid scan: no uptake of Tc-99m	-	-

(COVID-19: coronavirus disease 2019; CRP: C-reactive protein; ESR: erythrocyte sedimentation rate; F: female; FT3: free 3,3,5'-triiodothyronine; FT4: free thyroxine; NA: not available; SAT: subacute thyroiditis; TgAb: thyroglobulin antibody; Tg: thyroglobulin; TPOAb: thyroid peroxidase antibody; TRAb: thyroid stimulating hormone receptor antibody; TSH: thyroid-stimulating hormone; WBC: white blood cell count)

Source: Chen W, Tian Y, Li Z, Zhu J, Wei T, Lei J. Potential Interaction Between SARS-CoV-2 and Thyroid: A Review. Endocrinology. 2021;162(3):bqab004.

TABLE 2: Characteristics of our COVID-19 patients presenting with SAT.

Name	Age in years	Sex	COVID-19 recovery weeks	COVID severity	Fever at presentation	Fever duration	Nature of fever	Pain in throat	Duration of pain	Goiter/Swelling	Thyroid tenderness	ESR mm/h	CRP mg/L	TSH mIU/mL
MG	36	M	12	Moderate	Present	4 weeks	Mild	Yes	1 month	Yes	Yes	38	89	0.05
SB	33	M	14	Moderate	Absent	NA	Na	Yes	3 months	No	Yes	23	16	0.06
RS	39	M	12	Mild	Present	4 weeks	Mild	Yes	1 month	No	Yes	27	55	0.01
ST	32	M	16	Moderate	Present	4 weeks	Mild	Yes	1 month	No	Yes	21	44	0.02
RN	53	M	10	Moderate	Present	4 weeks	Mild	Yes	1 month	Yes	Yes	23	45	0.005

(COVID-19: coronavirus disease 2019; CRP: C-reactive protein; ESR: erythrocyte sedimentation rate; TSH: thyroid-stimulating hormone)

Also, the remaining 16 patients of SAT who did not suffer from COVID-19 still had close contact with at least one COVID-19 positive individual in their proximity.

Our study therefore concluded that, it is imperative to monitor thyroid function in COVID-19 affected patients or their close contacts, especially those presenting with throat pain or unexplained fever or long COVID symptoms much after occurrence of COVID-19 **(Table 2)**.

Silent Thyroiditis

Asymptomatic silent thyroiditis has been reported in COVID-19 and in post vaccination studies. Nearly 50% and more had ultrasonography (USG) evidence of thyroiditis and areas of thyroiditis within the thyroid gland persist for months after the infection. The thyroid function is promptly restored and no apparent increase of thyroid autoimmunity need to be observed though there is a need to monitor for development of primary hypothyroidism in future years.

Treatment of Subacute Thyroiditis

Benefit of glucocorticoids for the treatment of SAT is debated, however administration of glucocorticoids is beneficial for relieving symptoms quickly and significantly reducing the recurrence rate.

Impact of Medical Management of COVID-19 on Thyroid Function

More than 100 different drugs or experimental therapies have been used to treat COVID-19. Glucocorticoids and heparin may affect thyroid hormone secretion and measurement, respectively, leading to possible misdiagnosis of thyroid dysfunction in severe cases of COVID-19 **(Flowchart 2)**.

Based on the results of the RECOVERY Collaborative Group UK study the latest World Health Organization guideline on drugs for COVID-19 recommended use of systemic corticosteroids in patients with severe and critical disease. Glucocorticoids affect serum TSH levels by inhibiting TSH-releasing factor (TRH) in the hypothalamus directly. Dexamethasone appears to suppress the release of TSH from thyrotropes in a protein kinase C-dependent manner through the protein annexin. There are direct evidences that high-dose glucocorticoids could decrease TRH mRNA expression in the paraventricular nucleus of the human hypothalamus.

Low-molecular-weight heparin used in the second stage of COVID-19 illness interferes with the measurement of serum free thyroid hormone, which was first reported in a study by Schatz et al. A prompt increase was found within 2–15 minutes and up to fivefold increase in FT4 concentrations was found in this cohort. Previous studies have proven that this phenomenon is due to the significant increase of serum nonesterified fatty acid (NEFA) concentration induced by heparin-induced endothelial lipoprotein lipase activation. When the concentration of NEFA exceeds the normal serum-binding capacity, NEFA will directly compete for T4 and T3 binding sites on thyroxine-binding globulin. Therefore, patients treated with heparin should generally avoid having FT4 and FT3 measured. Meanwhile, when indicated, measurement of total thyroid hormone levels, together with TSH and thyroxine-binding globulin, can help confirm the patient's euthyroid status **(Flowchart 2)**.

COVID VACCINE AND THYROID DYSFUNCTION

Iremli et al., reported that autoimmune/inflammatory syndrome induced by adjuvants (ASIA syndrome) can be seen as a postvaccination phenomenon that occurs after exposure to adjuvants in vaccines that increase the immune responses. Three cases of subacute thyroiditis after inactivated SARS-CoV-2 vaccine (CoronaVac®). Three female healthcare workers presented with anterior neck pain and fatigue 4–7 days after SARS-CoV-2 vaccination. Two of them were in the breastfeeding period. They were negative for thyroid antibodies, and there was no previous history of thyroid disease, upper respiratory tract infection, or COVID-19. Laboratory test results and imaging findings were consistent with subacute thyroiditis. Severe acute respiratory syndrome coronavirus 2 vaccination can lead to subacute thyroiditis as a phenomenon of ASIA syndrome. Subacute thyroiditis may develop within a few days after the SARS-CoV-2 vaccination. Being in the postpartum period may be a facilitating factor for the development of ASIA syndrome after the SARS-CoV-2 vaccination.

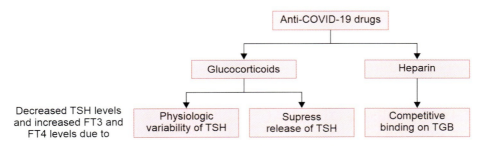

Flowchart 2: Medications that may cause thyroid damage or affect its metabolism.
(COVID-19: coronavirus disease 2019; FT3: free triiodothyronine; FT4: free thyroxine; TGB: thyroxine binding globulin; TSH: thyroid-stimulating hormone)

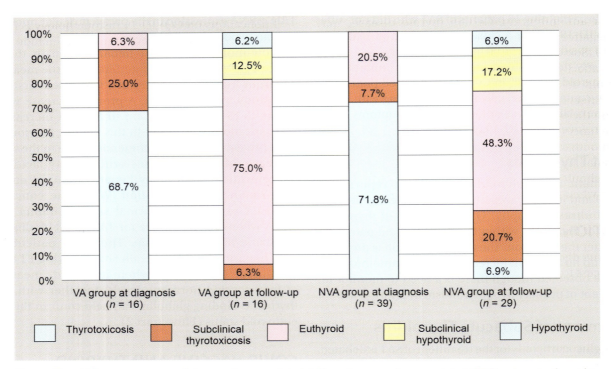

Fig. 2: Thyroid hormone status of the vaccine-associated (VA) and nonvaccine associated (NVA) subacute thyroiditis (SAT) patient groups at the time of diagnosis and at follow-up.

Bostan et al., evaluated the diagnostic features and clinical course of COVID-19 vaccine-associated subacute thyroiditis. A total of 55 patients diagnosed with SAT. Of the study population, 16 (29.1%) were diagnosed with COVID-19 vaccine-associated SAT (10 with CoronaVac® and six with Pfizer-BioNTech® vaccine), with a median time to onset of symptoms after vaccination of 6.5 (range; 2–20) days. There was no statistically significant difference between the vaccine-associated (VA) and nonvaccine associated (NVA) groups in terms of age, gender, time to diagnosis, thyroid volumes, thyroid function tests, and acute phase reactants. Seven (43.8%) and 25 (64.1%) patients were treated with methylprednisolone in the VA group and NVA group, respectively ($p = 0.16$). Follow-up data of 45 patients (16/16 for VA and 29/39 for NVA) were available. The mean follow-up of these patients was 47.4 ± 19.4 days, and the follow-up periods of the VA group and NVA group were comparable ($p = 0.24$). There was no difference between the two groups in terms of the frequency of euthyroidism at the follow-up visit (12/16 vs. 14/29, $p = 0.08$). Most patients with VA SAT had a mild clinical course that improved with nonsteroidal anti-inflammatory drugs. The frequency of euthyroid status during the follow-up of VA SAT cases was similar to that of the NVA group **(Fig. 2)**.

3,5,3′-TRIIODOTHYRONINE: A POTENTIAL MEDICATION FOR SEVERE COVID-19

A trial conducted by Pantos et al., has been registered (ClinicalTrials.gov ID: NCT04348513) to investigate the efficacy and safety of intravenous high-dose T3 for critically ill patients with COVID-19. Patients with severe/critical illness such as sepsis, trauma, and myocardial infarction, may present with thyroid dysfunction secondary to NTIS or specific thyroid damage (direct, indirect, or both), and low circulating T3 has been proven to be associated with increased mortality. T3 does, however, have some potential mechanisms for the treatment of COVID-19, such as increasing the tolerance of cells to hypoxia by inhibiting p38 mitogen activated protein kinase activation, promoting tissue repair by regulating *Akt* activity, and inhibiting lung fibrosis by improving epithelial mitochondrial function. The decreased and low concentration of T3 present in patients with severe extrathyroidal diseases is a component of NITS, which is an adaptive phenomenon to severity of infection, and this low T3 syndrome should not be treated with T3 in most patients. Therefore, in view of the lack of strong arguments, the effect of T3 in COVID-19 is questionable.

CONCLUSION

The thyroid gland and the entire hypothalamic-pituitary-thyroid (HPT) axis may represent key targets of SARS-CoV-2. Most of the thyroid disorders, including Graves' disease, euthyroid sick syndrome, Hashimoto's thyroiditis and subacute thyroiditis, have been documented as sequelae to COVID-19, and the SARS-CoV-2 virus has been implicated in the etiology of each. Coronavirus disease 2019 has been suggested to trigger the activation of pre-existing thyroid disease or autoimmunity. Certain thyroid diseases may have a negative impact on the prevention and control of COVID-19. Some anti-COVID-19 agents may cause thyroid injury or affect its metabolism. Coronavirus disease 2019 and thyroid disease may mutually aggravate the disease burden. Effects of SARS-CoV-2 infection and COVID-19 disease on thyroid function seem mild and transient. Most cases the function of the thyroid gland returned to normal after 12 months and residual functional abnormalities were seen in small number of people. Patients with SARS-CoV-2 infection should not ignore the effect on thyroid function, especially when there are obvious related symptoms.

LIMITATIONS OF THE REVIEW

Coronavirus disease 2019 is a relatively new disease with limited access to public information.

Publications on COVID-19 histopathology is increasing almost every day, hence review may not include all up-to-date publications.

Second, the conclusion of the effect of SARS-CoV-2 on thyroid morphological and pathological changes has been mainly from autopsy reports containing only a limited number of cases; hence more focused cytology/histology studies are needed to understand the pathophysiology of thyroid gland affection by SARS-CoV-2. Whether newer vaccines will interact with the thyroid gland is yet to be understood. Is thyroid dysfunction one of the reasons for the "long COVID 19" symptoms is still being investigated.

Meanwhile, periodic thyroid function should be assessed in all patients who have recovered from COVID-19.

Disclosure: None

Conflict of interest: None

SUGGESTED READINGS

1. Marazuela M, Giustina A, Puig-Domingo M. Endocrine and metabolic aspects of the COVID-19 pandemic. Rev Endocr. Metab Disord. 2020;21(4):495-507.
2. Boelaert K, Visser WE, Taylor PN, Moran C, Léger J, Persani L. Endocrinology in the time of COVID-19: management of hyperthyroidism and hypothyroidism. Eur J Endocrinol. 2020;183(1):G33-9.
3. Taylor PN, Zhang L, Lee RWJ, Muller I, Ezra DG, Dayan CM, et al. New insights into the pathogenesis and nonsurgical management of Graves orbitopathy. Nat Rev Endocrinol. 2020;(2):104-16.
4. Durán CS, Mayorga GDC. The eye: "an organ that must not be forgotten in coronavirus disease 2019 (COVID-2019) pandemic." J Optom. 2021;14(2):114-9.
5. Xia J, Tong J, Liu M, Shen Y, Guo D. Evaluation of coronavirus in tears and conjunctival secretions of patients with SARS-CoV-2 infection. J Med Virol. 2020;92(6):589-94.
6. De Leo S, Lee SY, Braverman LE. Hyperthyroidism. Lancet. 2016;388(10047):906-18.
7. Naguib R. Potential relationships between COVID-19 and the thyroid gland: an update. J Int Med Res. 2022;50(2):3000605221082898.
8. Pavlatou MG, Priestley J, McMullan C, Perros P. (2019). BTF survey on the impact of COVID-19 on people with thyroid disorders. [Online] Available from https://www.btf-thyroid.org/btf-survey-on-the-impact-of-COVID-19-on-people-with-thyroid-disorders [Last accessed December, 2022].
9. Wang W, Xu Y, Gao R, Lu R, Han K, Wu G, et al. Detection of SARS-CoV-2 in different types of clinical specimens. JAMA. 2020;323(18):1843-4.
10. Rotondi M, Coperchini F, Ricci G, Denegri M, Croce L, Ngnitejeu ST, et al. Detection of SARS-COV-2 receptor ACE-2 mRNA in thyroid cells: a clue for COVID-19-related subacute thyroiditis. J Endocrinol Invest. 2021;44(5):1085-90.
11. Lazartigues E, Qadir MMF, Mauvais-Jarvis F. Endocrine significance of SARS-CoV-2's reliance on ACE2. Endocrinology. 2020;161(9):bqaa108.
12. Li MY, Li L, Zhang Y, Wang XS. Expression of the SARS-CoV-2 cell receptor gene ACE2 in a wide variety of human tissues. Infect Dis Poverty. 2020;9(1):45.
13. Smallridge RC, Rogers J, Verma PS. Serum angiotensin-converting enzyme. Alterations in hyperthyroidism, hypothyroidism, and subacute thyroiditis. JAMA. 1983;250(18):2489-93.
14. Rubino F, Amiel SA, Zimmet P, Alberti G, Bornstein S, Eckel RH, et al. New-onset diabetes in COVID-19. N Engl J Med. 2020;383(8):789-90.
15. Kim BW. Critically Ill COVID-19 patients may be prone to subacute thyroiditis. Clin Thyroidol. 2020;32(9):412-4.
16. Chen W, Tian Y, Li Z, Zhu J, Wei T, Lei J. Potential Interaction Between SARS-CoV-2 and Thyroid: A Review. Endocrinology. 2021;162(3):bqab004.
17. Ohsako N, Tamai H, Sudo T, Mukuta T, Tanaka H, Kuma K, et al. Clinical characteristics of subacute thyroiditis classified according to human leukocyte antigen typing. J Clin Endocrinol Metab. 1995;80(12):3653-6.
18. Desailloud R, Hober D. Viruses and thyroiditis: an update. Virol J. 2009;6:5.
19. Bradley BT, Maioli H, Johnston R, Chaudhry I, Fink SL, Xu H, et al. Histopathology and ultrastructural findings of fatal COVID-19 infections in Washington State: a case series. Lancet. 2020;396(10247):320-32.
20. Lisco G, De Tullio A, Jirillo E, Giagulli VA, De Pergola G, Guastamacchia E, et al. Thyroid and COVID-19: a review on pathophysiological, clinical and organizational aspects. J Endocrinol Invest. 2021;44(9):1801-14.
21. Fliers E, Bianco AC, Langouche L, Boelen A. Thyroid function in critically ill patients. Lancet Diabetes Endocrinol. 2015;3(10):816-25.
22. Khoo B, Tan T, Clarke SA, Mills EG, Patel B, Modi M, et al. Thyroid function before, during, and after COVID-19. J Clin Endocrinol Metab. 2021;106(2):e803-11.
23. Lui DTW, Lee CH, Chow WS, Lee ACH, Tam AR, Fong CHY, et al. Thyroid dysfunction in relation to immune profile, disease status, and outcome in 191 patients with COVID-19. J Clin Endocrinol Metab. 2021;106(2):e926-35.
24. Lechien JR, Chiesa-Estomba CM, De Siati DR, Horoi M, Le Bon SD, Rodriguez A, et al. Olfactory and gustatory dysfunctions as a clinical presentation of mild-to-moderate forms of the coronavirus disease (COVID-19): a multicenter European study. Eur Arch Otorhinolaryngol. 2020;277(8):2251-61.
25. Zhou F, Yu T, Du R, Fan G, Liu Y, Liu Z, et al. Clinical course and risk factors for mortality of adult inpatients with COVID-19 in Wuhan, China: a retrospective cohort study. Lancet. 2020;395(10229):1054-62.

26. Lania A, Sandri MT, Cellini M, Mirani M, Lavezzi E, Mazziotti G. Thyrotoxicosis in patients with COVID-19: the THYRCOV study. Eur J Endocrinol. 2020;183(4):381-7.
27. Chen M, Zhou WB, Xu WW. Thyroid function analysis in 50 patients with COVID-19: a retrospective study. Thyroid. 2021;31(1):8-11.
28. Muller I, Cannavaro D, Dazzi D, Covelli D, Mantovani G, Muscatello A, et al. SARS-CoV-2-related atypical thyroiditis. Lancet Diabetes Endocrinol. 2020;8(9):739-41.
29. Li T, Wang L, Wang H, Gao Y, Hu X, Li X, et al. Characteristics of laboratory indexes in COVID-19 patients with non-severe symptoms in Hefei City, China: diagnostic value in organ injuries. Eur J Clin Microbiol Infect Dis. 2020;39(12):2447-55.
30. Speer G, Somogyi P. Thyroid complications of SARS and coronavirus disease 2019 (COVID-19). Endocr J. 2021;68(2):129-36.
31. Bahçecioğlu AB, Karahan ZC, Aydoğan BI, Kalkan IA, Azap A, Erdoğan MF. Subacute thyroiditis during the COVID-19 pandemic: a prospective study. J Endocrinol Invest. 2022;45(4):865-74.
32. Trimboli P, Cappelli C, Croce L, Scappaticcio L, Chiovato L, Rotondi M. COVID-19-associated subacute thyroiditis: evidence-based Data from a systematic review. Front Endocrinol (Lausanne). 2021;12:707726.
33. Deshmukh P, Deshmukh V. Case series of subacute thyroiditis presenting as a late complication of COVID-19. VideoEndocrinology. 2022;9(2):44-5.
34. Quaytman J, Gollamudi U, Bass N, Suresh S. Reactive arthritis and silent thyroiditis following SARS-CoV-2 infection: case report and review of the literature. Clin Case Rep. 2022;10(2):e05430.
35. Fatourechi V, Aniszewski JP, Fatourechi GZ, Atkinson EJ, Jacobsen SJ. Clinical features and outcome of subacute thyroiditis in an incidence cohort: Olmsted County, Minnesota, study. J Clin Endocrinol Metab. 2003;88(5):2100-5.
36. Arao T, Okada Y, Torimoto K, Kurozumi A, Narisawa M, Yamamoto S, et al. Prednisolone dosing regimen for treatment of subacute thyroiditis. J UOEH. 2015;37(2):103-10.
37. Sanders JM, Monogue ML, Jodlowski TZ, Cutrell JB. Pharmacologic treatments for coronavirus disease 2019 (COVID-19): a review. JAMA. 2020;323(18):1824-36.
38. RECOVERY Collaborative Group; Horby P, Lim WS, Emberson JR, Mafham M, Bell JL, et al. Dexamethasone in hospitalized patients with COVID-19—preliminary report. N Engl J Med. 2021;384(8):693-704.
39. Alkemade A, Unmehopa UA, Wiersinga WM, Swaab DF, Fliers E. Glucocorticoids decrease thyrotropin-releasing hormone messenger ribonucleic acid expression in the paraventricular nucleus of the human hypothalamus. J Clin Endocrinol Metab. 2005;90(1):323-7.
40. Schatz DL, Sheppard RH, Steiner G, Chandarlapaty CS, de Veber GA. Influence of heparin on serum free thyroxine. J Clin Endocrinol Metab. 1969;29(8):1015-22.
41. Mendel CM, Frost PH, Cavalieri RR. Effect of free fatty acids on the concentration of free thyroxine in human serum: the role of albumin. J Clin Endocrinol Metab. 1986;63(6):1394-9.
42. İremli BG, Şendur SN, Ünlütürk U. Three cases of subacute thyroiditis following SARS-CoV-2 vaccine: postvaccination ASIA Syndrome. J Clin Endocrinol Metab. 2021;106(9):2600-5.
43. Bostan H, Kayihan S, Calapkulu M, Hepsen S, Gul U, Ozturk Unsal I, et al. Evaluation of the diagnostic features and clinical course of COVID-19 vaccine-associated subacute thyroiditis. Hormones (Athens). 2022;21(3):447-55.
44. Pantos C, Tseti I, Mourouzis I. Use of triiodothyronine to treat critically ill COVID-19 patients: a new clinical trial. Crit Care. 2020;24(1):209.

CHAPTER 35

Sustaining Elimination of Iodine Deficiency Disorders in India

Kapil Yadav, Surabhi Puri, Girish Jeer, Garima Gautam, Chandrakant S Pandav

INTRODUCTION

Iodine is an essential micronutrient, required for the production of hormones by the thyroid gland—triiodothyronine (T3) and thyroxine (T4). These hormones are vital for the optimal physical and mental development of an individual. They also regulate body metabolism, generate heat and maintain body temperature. Deficiency of iodine is the leading cause of preventable brain damage worldwide. Leaching from glaciation, flooding, and erosion deplete the surface soil of iodide. Iodine deficient soils are common in mountainous areas (like the Himalayas) and areas of frequent flooding (e.g., Ganges river plane). Consumption of food grown in these soils makes people susceptible to iodine deficiency. Historically, the outcome of iodine deficiency was thought to be limited to goiter, primarily a cosmetic concern. However, further research shed light on the spectrum of functional and developmental abnormalities caused by deficiency of iodine, grouped under the term—iodine deficiency disorders (IDDs). India was one of the earliest adopters of salt iodization to prevent IDDs after its success in the Kangra Valley study, with the launch of the National Goiter Control Programme in 1962.

IODINE AND THYROID METABOLISM

Iodide is almost completely absorbed (>90%) from the stomach and duodenum. A healthy adult body contains around 15–20 mg of iodine, 70–80% of which is in the thyroid. Thyroid gland epithelium actively accumulates iodide ion, mediated by Na^+/I^- symporter (NIS). Iodide is then oxidized by thyroperoxidase (TPO) and hydrogen peroxide enzymes, and attached to tyrosyl residues on thyroglobulin producing monoiodotyrosine and diiodotyrosine. Coupling of these molecules occurs catalyzed by TPO to produce thyroid hormones—triiodothyronine (T3) and thyroxine (T4) **(Fig. 1)**. Iodide is cleared from circulation by the thyroid and kidney. Thyroid clearance depends upon iodine intake. Iodine uptake by the thyroid gland can increase up to 80% in chronic iodine deficiency. Iodine is also concentrated in mammary glands. During lactation, iodine is secreted into breast milk. More than 90% of ingested iodine is excreted in the urine.

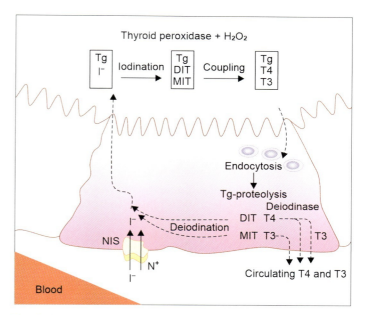

Fig. 1: Iodine pathway in the thyroid cell.

Note: Iodide (I^-) is transported into the thyrocyte by the sodium/iodide symporter (NIS) at the basal membrane and migrates to the apical membrane. I^- is oxidized by the enzymes thyroperoxidase (TPO) and hydrogen peroxidase (H_2O_2) and attached to tyrosyl residues in thyroglobulin (Tg) to produce the hormone precursors iodotyrosine (MIT) and diiodotyrosine (DIT). Residues then couple to form thyroxine (T4) and triiodothyronine (T3) within the Tg molecule in the follicular lumen. Tg enters the cell by endocytosis and is digested. T4 and T3 are released into the circulation, and iodine on MIT and DIT is recycled within the thyrocyte.

> Major source of iodine in Indian population is—*adequately iodized salt.*

Dietary Intake of Iodine

The major source of iodine in the Indian population is iodized salt. Marine food (especially seaweed), and food

TABLE 1: Recommended dietary intake of Iodine in different population groups.				
Age group	EAR (µg/day)	RDA (µg/day)	TUL (µg/day)	WHO (µg/day)
Infants	-	-	-	90
Children				
1–3 years	65	90	200	90
4–6 years	65	90	300	90
7–9 years	65	90	400	120
10–12 years	70	100	600	120
13–15 years	100	140	900	150
16–18 years	100	140	1,100	150
>18 years	95	140	1,100	150
Pregnant woman	160	220	1,100	250
Lactating woman	200	280	1,100	250

(EAR: estimated average requirement; RDA: recommended dietary allowance; TUL: tolerable upper intake level; WHO: World Health Organization)

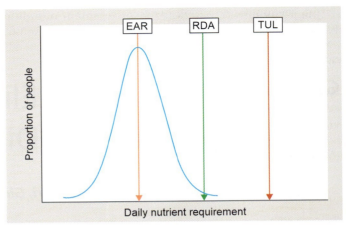

Fig. 2: Distribution of the requirement of a nutrient in a population.
(EAR: estimated average intake; RDA: recommended daily allowance; TUL: tolerable upper limit)

grown in iodine sufficient soil are other contributors to iodine intake. Cooking processes during the addition of iodized salt might cause about 40% loss of iodine content. Considering this loss, along with an estimated iodized salt intake among Indians of about 10 g, the usual diet in India is sufficient to fulfil the physiological needs of the body. The recommended daily iodine intake by the National Institute of Nutrition (NIN), Hyderabad is tabulated in **Table 1**.

A newer concept of estimated average requirement (EAR) has come up, which would be the daily iodine intake that meets the requirement of half of the healthy individuals in a particular life stage. *The EAR can be used for groups, but it is not meant to be used in the assessment of intake in individuals.* While the recommended dietary allowance (RDA) for iodine is the average daily intake sufficient to meet the iodine requirement of 97–98% of healthy individuals in a life stage. RDA can be used as a goal for daily iodine intake by individuals. The RDA is derived from the EAR, considering the estimated variability in individual requirements. Tolerable upper level refers to the highest average daily nutrient intake level that is likely to pose no risk of adverse health effects to almost all individuals in the general population **(Fig. 2)**.

Goitrogens

Dietary iodine intake is also influenced by the intake of goitrogens. Goitrogens are dietary substances and environmental substances interfering with thyroid metabolism. Metabolites of lima beans, sorghum, and cassava might contain thiocyanates competing with iodine for uptake by NIS. Thiocyanates in serum are also elevated by cigarette smoking. Metabolites of cruciferous vegetables (cabbage, kale, and cauliflower) also compete with iodine for uptake by the thyroid gland. Flavonoids in soy and millets might impair TPO activity. These may lead to iodine deficiency in people with marginal iodine status. Selenium, iron, and vitamin A deficiency might exacerbate IDDs. Selenium is required for adequate enzyme functioning (glutathione peroxidase and deiodinase) in thyroid metabolism. Deficiency of iron impairs heme-dependent TPO activity. It is also known to reduce the efficacy of iodine supplementation. Vitamin A deficiency stimulates TSH production and raises the risk of goiter due to the inability of vitamin A-mediated suppression of the *TSH-β* gene.

Iodine Deficiency

Iodine deficiency has been a global public health problem with only a few countries being iodine sufficient before 1990. About 2 billion people are at risk of developing iodine deficiency disorders due to insufficient iodine intake. International efforts have dramatically reduced the burden of iodine deficiency across the globe. However, identification of groups at risk of inadequate iodine status is crucial to devising an effective control strategy.

Groups at risk of iodine insufficiency:
- *People living in areas with soil deficient in iodine*: Initially, iodine deficiency disorders were thought to be a concern in the Himalayan area with surrounding plains extending to the northeast, called the "goiter belt." However, with evidence from surveys over the years it was realized that iodine deficiency disorders were a public health problem across districts all over the country.
- *Pregnant women*: Iodine requirement in pregnancy increases by up to 50% due to an increase in T4 production to transfer to the fetus before the fetal thyroid is functional, iodine transfer to the fetus, and increased renal clearance.
- *People using noniodized salt*: Even after years of adoption of salt iodization, according to the India Iodine Survey (IIS) (2018–2019), only 76.3% of the population was found to consume adequately iodized salt in the country. While the use of iodized salt according to the National Family Health Survey (NFHS-5), was reported to be 94.3%.

The recommended methods for assessment of iodine nutrition in a population are urinary iodine concentration, serum thyroglobulin, goiter rate and serum TSH. They are tabulated in **Table 2**.

Iodine Deficiency Disorders

Iodine deficiency adversely affects the health of humans across the whole life cycle. The spectrum of diseases caused by deficiency of iodine is termed iodine deficiency disorders **(Table 3)**.

Burden of IDD in India

Iodine deficiency disorders are diseases of public health significance. A total of 350 million people in India are estimated to be at risk for IDDs. With prevalence >10%, 263 districts out of the 325 districts surveyed were found to be IDD endemic.

- *Pregnancy*: Thyroid iodine stores are utilized to meet the increase in iodine demand during pregnancy. The cases of chronic iodine deficiency already run low in iodine stores, hence, a rise in demand is followed by

TABLE 2: Methods of assessment of iodine nutrition in a population.

Assessment method	Iodine status	Measurement	Interpretation/Remarks
Urinary iodine concentration	Recent (days)	• 24 urine iodine • Spot urine iodine (not for individual assessment, day-to-day variability)	School-aged children: Iodine level (µg/L): • <20 — Iodine intake: Insufficient — Iodine nutrition: Severe deficiency • 20–49 — Insufficient — Moderate • 50–99 — Insufficient — Mild • 100–199 — Adequate — Optimum • 200–299 — More than adequate — Risk of adverse health outcomes • >300 — Excessive — Risk of adverse health outcomes Pregnant women: • <150 — Insufficient • 150–249 — Adequate • 250–499 — More than adequate • >500 — Excessive Lactating women: • <100 — Insufficient • ≥100 — Adequate Children <2 years of age: • <100 — Insufficient • ≥100 — Adequate
Serum thyroglobulin	Intermediate (weeks to months)	• Serology • Dried blot spot	• <10 µg/L—normal • Fall in raised thyroglobulin—sensitive indicator of iodine repletion

Goiter rate	Long-term (months to years)	Inspection and palpation	• Grade 0—thyroid not palpable (lateral lobe volume greater than terminal phalanx of thumb) or visible
			• Grade 1—palpable but not visible
			• Grade 2—visible thyroid enlargement
			• Degree of IDD by goiter rate:
			  ○ 0–4.9% (none)
			  ○ 5–19.9% (mild)
			  ○ 20–29.9% (moderate)
			  ○ ≥30% (severe)
			• Low sensitivity and specificity

		Thyroid ultrasonography	• Degree of IDD by goiter rate:
			  ○ 0–4.9% (none)
			  ○ 5–19.9% (mild)
			  ○ 20–29.9% (moderate)
			  ○ ≥30% (severe)
			• Requires expertise and appropriate equipment

Serum TSH		• Dried blood spot • Serology	• Sensitive indicator of iodine deficiency in the neonatal period—neonatal screening for congenital hypothyroidism • Not a sensitive indicator in adults

TABLE 3: Health consequences of iodine deficiency across different age groups.	
Age group	Health consequences
All ages	• Goiter • Increased susceptibility of the thyroid gland to nuclear radiation
Fetus	• Abortion • Stillbirth • Congenital anomalies • Perinatal mortality
Neonate	• Infant mortality • Endemic cretinism
Child and adolescent	• Impaired mental function • Delayed physical development
Adult	• Impaired mental function • Reduced work productivity • Toxic nodular goiter • Iodine-induced hyperthyroidism • Increased occurrence of hypothyroidism in moderate-to-severe iodine deficiency • Decreased occurrence of hypothyroidism in mild-to-moderate iodine deficiency

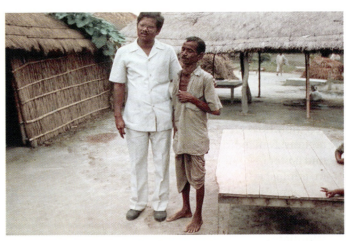

Fig. 3: Dr Pandav with Nakeshawar, cretin with goiter, resident of Katarashahwajpur, Colonelganj PHC, Gonda district, Uttar Pradesh, 1980 (left to right).

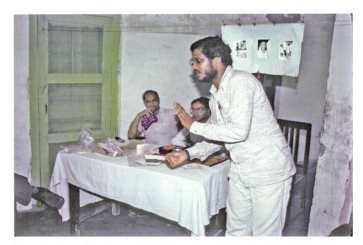

Fig. 4: Late Professor MG Karmakar (sitting); Dr Chandrakant S Pandav (standing) conducting training course of traditional birth attendants on how to collect umbilical cord blood on filter paper strip (Colonelganj, Gonda district, Uttar Pradesh, 1980).

compensatory pathological changes in the thyroid gland (such as goiter and hypothyroidism). Iodine deficiency in pregnancy is detrimental to both maternal and fetal health. Maternal thyroid hormone transferred transplacentally to the fetus is crucial for normal neuronal migration and myelination of the brain in the fetal and postnatal period. Hypothyroxemia during this critical phase might lead to irreversible brain damage. It also leads to poor pregnancy outcomes such as stillbirths, abortions, congenital malformations, and perinatal and infant mortality.

- *Infancy and early childhood*: Most consequences of IDD are invisible and irreversible. At the same time, they are preventable. IDDs are the most common cause of mental retardation. The World Health Organization (WHO) describes iodine deficiency as "the single most important preventable cause of brain damage."

Iodine deficiency in neonates affects the functioning of the thyroid gland leading to neonatal goiter and hypothyroidism. The infant brain at birth has only reached about one-third of its usual size and continues to grow rapidly until the end of the second year. The thyroid hormone, essential for normal brain development at this critical time, is dependent on iodine. Neonatal hypothyroidism persists into infancy and childhood if the deficiency is not corrected and results in retardation of physical and mental development.

In McCarrison's original description of cretinism in northern India, he delineated two forms—(1) a neurological form, with predominantly neuromotor defects, and a myxedematous form, marked by severe hypothyroidism and short stature **(Fig. 3)**. Higher burden of neonatal hypothyroidism was observed in areas with environmental iodine deficiency as compared to nondeficient ones **(Fig. 4)**. In the fully developed form of neurological cretinism, the three characteristic features are severe mental retardation with squint, deaf-mutism, and motor spasticity. The mental deficiency is characterized by a marked impairment of abstract thought, whereas autonomic and vegetative functions and memory are relatively well preserved, except in the most severe cases. Vision is unaffected, whereas deafness is characteristic. This may be complete in as many as 50% of cretins, as confirmed by studies of auditory brainstem-evoked potentials. The motor disorder shows proximal rigidity of both lower and upper extremities and the trunk, and corresponding proximal spasticity with exaggerated deep tendon reflexes at the knees, adductors, and biceps.

However, to achieve the best mental prognosis, iodine deficiency-related cretinism must be diagnosed early, preferably before the third month of life.

- *Late childhood and adolescence*: Moderate-to-severe iodine deficient children were found to have impaired cognitive function. On average, the children born in iodine-deficient regions have 13.5 intelligence quotient (IQ) points lesser than children born in iodine-sufficient regions. Deficiency of iodine also caused hypothyroidism and goiter in children and adolescents. Iodine deficiency in adolescent girls is of concern, since on entering pregnancy in an iodine deficient state in future raises the risk of neurological effects on the fetus.
- *Adulthood*: Mild-to-moderate iodine deficiency stimulates a compensatory increase in the activity of the thyroid gland to maintain euthyroidism. However, a chronic deficiency might cause hyperthyroidism and toxic multinodular goiter. Severe iodine deficiency leads to goiter and hypothyroidism in adults. Since there is a reduced intake of iodine, as a compensatory mechanism, the gland increases in size. Iodine deficiency stimulates an increase in the production of TSH, which is a thyroproliferative hormone causing thyroid hypertrophy and hyperplasia. As a result, goiter appears. Fluctuations in the stimulation of gland lead to the development of multinodular goiter. Hypothyroidism in adults leads to lethargy, reduced work output, menstrual abnormalities, and infertility among adults.

Treatment and Prevention of Iodine Deficiency Disorders

India has been at the forefront from research to policy to program against IDDs globally. After the release of preliminary findings from the milestone Kangra Valley Study, India launched the National Goiter Control Programme (NGCP) in 1962 with the key strategy of adequate iodization of salt in endemic areas. Further research on the consequences of iodine deficiency beyond goiter brought about the evolution of the program from the National Goiter Control Programme to the National IDDs Control Programme in 1992 to be implemented in all states and Union Territories (UTs). The program aimed to reduce the prevalence of IDDs to <5% in the country, and ensure 100% consumption of adequately iodized salt, ≥15 parts per million (ppm) at the household level.

- *Fortification of iodine*: Salt iodization has been found to be one of the most cost-effective interventions to prevent iodine deficiency. Universal salt iodization is the key strategy for control of IDDs worldwide. Salt proves to be a good vehicle for iodine fortification due to the following reasons:
    - Universally consumed by the population
    - Fairly consistent intake throughout the year
    - Simple and inexpensive iodization technology
    - Fortification without alteration of color or taste
    - Ease of monitoring at production, retail, and household levels
    - Affordable, available, and acceptable

The addition of 20–40 mg iodine per kg salt is recommended by WHO/ United Nations International Children's Emergency Fund (UNICEF)/International Council for the Control of Iodine Deficiency Disorders Global Network (ICCIDD), depending on local salt intake. Revised Food Safety and Standards (Fortification of Foods) Regulations released in 2019 fixed the adequate iodine level required at the manufacturer level to be 20–30 ppm, while at the distribution level, they should be 15–30 ppm based on the dry weight. Fortification can be done by one of the two techniques:

1. *Wet method*: Solution of potassium iodate (KIO_3) sprayed at a regular rate to salt passing on a conveyor belt
2. *Dry method*: Potassium iodide (KI) or KIO_3 powder sprinkled over dry salt

- *Iodine supplementation*: In areas where the iodization of salt is not possible, supplementation with iodine formulations could be adopted to reduce iodine deficiency **(Table 4)**. However, in mild-to-moderate iodine deficiency, iodine supplementation did not conclusively show a beneficial effect.

TABLE 4: Recommendation for iodine supplementation in pregnancy and infancy.

Target group	Dose
Women of childbearing age	One yearly oral dose of 400 mg of iodine as iodized oil, or a daily oral dose of iodine as potassium iodide should be given, so that the total iodine intake meets the recommended nutrient intake (RNI) of 150 µg/day of iodine
Women who are pregnant or lactating	• One yearly oral dose of 400 mg of iodine as iodized oil, or a daily oral dose of iodine as potassium iodide should be given, so that the total iodine intake meets the new RNI of 250 µg/day of iodine • Iodine supplements should not be given to a woman who has already been given iodized oil during her pregnancy or up to 3 months before her pregnancy started
Children aged 0–6 months	• One oral dose of 100 mg of iodine as iodized oil or a daily oral dose of iodine as potassium iodide should be given so that the total iodine intake meets the 90 µg/day requirement of iodine • They should be given iodine supplements only if the mother was not supplemented during pregnancy or if the child is not being breastfed
Children 7–24 months	One yearly oral dose of 200 mg of iodine as iodized oil as soon as possible after the child is 7 months old, or a daily oral dose of iodine as potassium iodide should be given so that the total iodine intake meets the RNI of 90 µg/day of iodine

Note: In areas where <90% of households use iodized salt and the median urinary iodine concentration is <100 µg/L in school children.

Risk versus Benefits of Iodine Supplementation

Evidence from the Kangra Valley study unequivocally provided the evidence for the effectiveness of iodine supplementation by salt iodization to prevent goiter. Further studies over the years highlighted the potential of iodine deficiency to irreversibly impact the neurological development and growth of an individual, if left uncorrected.

Iodine intake has been postulated to be determining the occurrence of some thyroid-related disorders such as:
- *Iodine induced hyperthyroidism (IIH)*: Occurrence of IIH had been reported subsequent to iodine supplementation. However, these instances were minimal and transient, mostly occurring in people above 40 years of age, when large doses of iodine are given over a short duration in severely iodine-deficient areas. Also, IIH was believed to unmask underlying thyrotoxicosis, affecting those with latent Grave's disease or pre-existing nodular goiter.
- *Autoimmune thyroiditis (AIT)*: The existing evidence does not prove this hypothesis equivocally. High iodine intake can be one of the multiple risk factors for the development of AIT.
- *Thyroid carcinoma*: The incidence of thyroid cancer has not been proven to increase with iodine supplementation. However, there has been an increase in the ratio of less malignant papillary cancer to a more malignant follicular cancer.

Iodine deficiency disorders affect a larger population with the potential to cause serious irreversible effects in comparison to the smaller population affected with mostly treatable thyroid disorders seen with high iodine supplementation. On assessing the risk versus benefits of iodine supplementation, the benefits far outweigh the risks.

Iodine Deficiency Disorders Control in India: Current Status and the Way Forward

The milestone Kangra Valley study paved the way for the National Goiter Control Programme (NGCP) in India in 1962 **(Fig. 5)**. The program had the objectives of identification of goiter endemic districts in India and Iodine supplementation in those areas. With repeated surveys over the years, the endemicity of IDDs was found to be spread all over India instead of the earlier identified Goiter belt of the Himalayan and Tarai region. Moreover, the scope of IDDs expanded from goiter to include the spectrum of diseases as tabulated in **Table 1**.

The salt iodization program in India evolved through the following phases:
- *Phase 1*: Scientific research leading to program (1956–1983)
- *Phase 2*: From goiter to IDD (1983–2000)

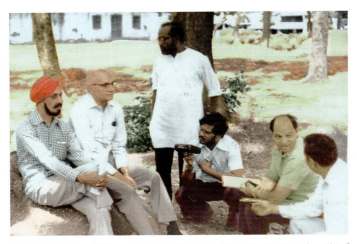

Fig. 5: Kangra Valley study (left to right): Dr SS Sooch, Chief Medical Officer, Kangra; Late Professor V Ramalingaswami, Director, AIIMS, New Delhi; Dr N Kochupillai, Professor of Endocrinology (standing); Dr Chandrakant S Pandav (sitting), former HOD, Centre for Community Medicine, AIIMS, New Delhi; Late Dr MG Karmakar, Professor and Head, Department of Laboratory Medicine, AIIMS, New Delhi, Kangra Valley, 1981.

- *Phase 3*: Lifting the ban on sale of noniodized salt (2000–2005)
- *Phase 4*: Reinstatement of ban on sale of noniodized salt and consolidation of sustainable elimination of IDD (since 2005)

Universal salt iodization (USI) was implemented in a phased manner in India in 1986. NGCP was revamped to launch the National Iodine Deficiency Disorders Control Programme (NIDDCP) in 1992, with the objectives to conduct surveys to assess the magnitude of the IDD, supply of iodized salt in place of common salt, and resurvey after every 5 years to assess the extent of IDD and the impact of iodized salt, laboratory monitoring of iodized salt and urinary iodine excretion and health education and advocacy. Universal salt iodization continued to be the face of the program. India adopted the iodization of salt strategy in endemic districts after the success of the Kangra valley study. This was followed by a ban on noniodized salt under the Prevention of Food Adulteration Act in 1997 accompanied by an expansion of the salt industry. The ban on mandatory iodization was lifted in 2000 leading to a drop in the percentage of population consuming adequately iodized salt from 49 to 30%. The ban was reinstated in 2005 on recommendation by The Core Advisory Group on Public Health and Human Rights of National Human Rights Commission, realizing the status of IDDs in India to be of public health significance **(Flowchart 1)**. The National Coalition for Sustained Optimal Iodine Intake (NCSOII), established in 2006, brought together the key stakeholders of universal salt iodization program, from government agencies, Salt Commissioner of India, academic

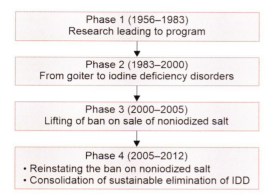

Flowchart 1: Phases in the evolution of iodine deficiency disorders (IDD) control program in India.

institutions, salt producers and traders, to bilateral and multilateral development agencies and civil society. This coalition was instrumental in providing continued efforts for elimination of IDDs in India by sustained advocacy.

In the recent National Iodine Survey of India (2018–19), 92.4% of the population was consuming iodized salt, while 76.3 were consuming adequately iodized salt. Household coverage of adequately iodized salt was lowest in Tamil Nadu (61.9%), Andhra Pradesh (63.9%), Rajasthan (65.5%), and Odisha (65.8%), Jharkhand (68.8%), and Puducherry (69.9%). The median urinary iodine concentration (UIC) for pregnant women was 173.4 µg/L, for lactating women was 172.8 µg/L and for nonpregnant nonlactating women was 178.0 µg/L. These were higher in urban areas as compared to rural areas.

Moving forward, the program needs to evolve to not only maintain the success of the interventions but also to reach the "last mile" to ensure the elimination of IDDs. Strengthening state and district IDD cells to tailor the control strategy to tackle IDDs in the area. Capacity building of salt manufacturing industries extending to the private sector, to ensure adequate production of iodized salt in the country would be essential. There is also a need to progress from quantity to quality ensuring adequate salt iodization at different levels. This could be achieved by strict vigilance by public health laboratories. The program should aim to achieve equitable distribution of iodized salt to the vulnerable population. Linkages with Public Distribution Scheme, integrated.

Child Development Services (ICDS) scheme and Midday meal (MDM) program might serve as an opportunity to reach vulnerable population. Moreover, with the rising intake of junk food, expanding salt iodization to fast food industries would improve the coverage of iodine supplementation. All these are to be coupled with intensified behavior change and communication for demand generation in the population. Regular monitoring and evaluation of the program are keys to identifying challenges and modifying the control approach to achieve elimination.

THREATS TO CONTROL OF IODINE DEFICIENCY DISORDERS

Continued efforts over the past decades have turned the control of iodine disorders into a success story. However, there is a need to be cautious about the arising threats slowing the progression to cover the "last mile."

- *Increase in thyroid disorders on iodine supplementation*: Studies showed risk of an increase in the incidence of thyroid disorders on supplementation with iodine in an iodine-deficient population. However, it is usually transient. This paved the need for the concept of a tolerable upper level (TUL) which was addressed in the latest dietary guidelines released by NIN. Food Safety and Standards Authority of India (FSSAI) also set an upper limit to the recommended level of iodine in salt to 30 ppm/kg.
- *Change in pattern of dietary consumption*: With the shift in dietary patterns, the proportion of salt consumption by intake of processed foods is on the rise. Regulating the iodization of salt at the production level of processed food could be an opportunity to tackle this threat. The consumption pattern of the population needs to be studied frequently as was previously done by National Nutritional Monitoring Bureau (NNMB).
- *Salt reduction for noncommunicable disease (NCD) control*: Reduction of salt intake to <5 g/day is advised to reduce the prevalence of NCDs. The current diet prepared using iodized salt is considered adequate to fulfil the daily requirement, considering the salt intake to be 10 g/day. Hence, adoption of salt reduction might pose a threat to iodine deficiency control. Other vehicles or iodine supplementation might be required to bridge this gap.

CONCLUSION

Iodine is a trace element essential for thyroid hormone synthesis, crucial for the growth and development of an individual. The deficiency of iodine can cause a spectrum of disorders, from abortion and stillbirth to goiter, and cretinism. Universal salt iodization is the key intervention that has driven the success of IDDs control in the country. Moving forward, the "end-game" strategy should be focused on research, advocacy and innovation to achieve the elimination of IDDs from the country and globally.

SUGGESTED READINGS

1. World Health Organization. Assessment of iodine deficiency disorders and monitoring their elimination: A guide for programme managers, 3rd edition. Geneva Institutional Repository for Information Sharing; 2007.
2. Zimmermann M, Trumbo PR. Iodine. Adv Nutr. 2013;4(2):262-4.
3. Sooch SS, Ramalingaswami V. Preliminary report of an experiment in the Kangra valley for the prevention of Himalayan endemic goitre with iodized salt. Bull World Health Organ. 1965;32(3):299-315.
4. Eskandari S, Loo DDF, Dai G, Levy O, Wright EM, Carrasco N. Thyroid Na$^+$/I$^-$ Symporter. Mechanism, stoichiometry, and specificity. J Biol Chem. 1997;272(43):27230-8.
5. Sayyed A. (2020). Nutrient Requirement for Indians. [Online] Available from https://www.metabolichealthdigest.com/nutrient-requirements-for-indians-icmr-nin-2020/ [Last accessed January, 2022].
6. McLaren EH, Alexander WD. Goitrogens. Clin Endocrinol Metab. 1979;8(1):129-44.
7. de Benoist B, McLean E, Andersson M, Rogers L. Iodine Deficiency in 2007: Global Progress since 2003. Food Nutr Bull. 2008;29(3):195-202.
8. Pandav CS, Kochupillai N. Endemic goitre in India: Prevalence, etiology, attendant disabilities and control measures. Indian J Pediatr. 1982;49(2):259-71.
9. Pandav CS, Yadav K, Srivastava R, Pandav R, Karmarkar MG. Iodine deficiency disorders (IDD) control in India. Indian J Med Res. 2013;138(3):418-33.
10. Zimmermann MB. Iodine deficiency in pregnancy and the effects of maternal iodine supplementation on the offspring: a review. Am J Clin Nutr. 2009;89(2):668S-672S.
11. Glinoer D. The regulation of thyroid function in pregnancy: pathways of endocrine adaptation from physiology to pathology. Endocr Rev. 1997;18(3):404-33.
12. Zimmermann MB. Assessing iodine status and monitoring progress of iodized salt programs. J Nutr. 2004;134(7):1673-7.
13. Sack J. Thyroid function in pregnancy—maternal-fetal relationship in health and disease. Pediatr Endocrinol Rev PER. 2003;1 (Suppl 2):170-6; discussion 176.
14. McCarrison R. Observations on Endemic Cretinism in the Chitral and Gilgit Valleys. Proc R Soc Med. 1909;2(Med Sect):1-36.
15. Kochupillai N, Pandav CS, Godbole MM, Mehta M, Ahuja MMS. Iodine deficiency and neonatal hypothyroidism. Bull World Health Organ. 1986;64(4):547-51.
16. Delange F, Heidemann P, Bourdoux P, Larsson A, Vigneri R, Klett M, et al. Regional variations of iodine nutrition and thyroid function during the neonatal period in Europe. Biol Neonate. 1986;49(6):322-30.
17. Bleichrodt N, Born MP, Stanbury JB. Work and Organizational Psychology. A metaanalysis of research on iodine and its relationship to cognitive development. In: The damaged Brain of Iodine Deficiency. New York: Cognizant Communication Corporation; 1996. pp. 195-200.
18. World Health Organization/International Council for the Control of the Iodine Deficiency Disorders/United Nations Childrens Fund (WHO/ICCIDD/UNICEF). (2001). Assessment of the iodine deficiency disorders and monitoring their elimination. [Online] Available from http://apps.who.int/iris/bitstream/handle/10665/43781/9789241595827_eng.pdf?sequence=1 [Last accessed January, 2023].
19. Pandav CS, Yadav K, Ansari MA, Sundaresan S, Karmarkar MG. Salt for Freedom and Iodized Salt for Freedom from Preventable Brain Damage, 7th edition. New Delhi: Indian Coalition for Control of Iodine deficiency Disorders (ICCIDD); 2012.
20. FSSAI. (2019). Minutes of meeting with salt manufacturers on iodine levels in salt. [Online] Available from https://ffrc.fssai.gov.in/assets/news/file/mom-with-salt-manufacturer-iodine-100519.pdf [Last accessed January, 2023].
21. Dineva M, Fishpool H, Rayman MP, Mendis J, Bath SC. Systematic review and meta-analysis of the effects of iodine supplementation on thyroid function and child neurodevelopment in mildly-to-moderately iodine-deficient pregnant women. Am J Clin Nutr. 2020;112(2):389-412.
22. Pandav CS. Evolution of iodine deficiency disorders control program in India: a journey of 5,000 years. Indian J Public Health. 2013;57(3):126-32.
23. Yadav K, Chakrabarty A, Rah JH, Kumar R, Aguayo V, Ansari MA, et al. The National Coalition for Sustained Optimal Iodine intake (NSOI): a case study of a successful experience from India. Asia Pac J Clin Nutr. 2014;23 (Suppl 1):S38-45.
24. Todd CH, Allain T, Gomo ZA, Hasler JA, Ndiweni M, Oken E. Increase in thyrotoxicosis associated with iodine supplements in Zimbabwe. Lancet. 1995;346(8989):1563-4.
25. Shi X, Han C, Li C, Mao J, Wang W, Xie X, et al. Optimal and safe upper limits of iodine intake for early pregnancy in iodine-sufficient regions: a cross-sectional study of 7190 pregnant women in China. J Clin Endocrinol Metab. 2015;100(4):1630-8.
26. Laurberg P, Cerqueira C, Ovesen L, Rasmussen LB, Perrild H, Andersen S, et al. Iodine intake as a determinant of thyroid disorders in populations. Best Pract Res Clin Endocrinol Metab. 2010;24(1):13-27.
27. World Health Organization. Guideline: Sodium intake for adults and children. Geneva: World Health Organization; 2012.
28. WHO Secretariat, Andersson M, de Benoist B, Delange F, Zupan J. Prevention and control of iodine deficiency in pregnant and lactating women and in children less than 2-years-old: conclusions and recommendations of the Technical Consultation. Public Health Nutr. 2007;10(12A):1606-11.
29. Zimmermann MB, Jooste PL, Pandav CS. Iodine-deficiency disorders. Lancet. 2008;372(9645):1251-62.

Thyroid and Bone

Sanjay K Bhadada, Rajat Gupta

INTRODUCTION

Thyroid hormones are crucial for skeletal development and growth in children and bone preservation in adults. Thyroid hormone skeletal activities are mediated by binding of triiodothyronine (T3) to its nuclear receptor thyroid hormone receptor α1 (TRα1) **(Flowchart 1)**. Circulating thyroid hormone levels are kept in euthyroid range by the hypothalamic–pituitary–thyroid (HPT) axis. Any deviation from euthyroid state, in childhood or adult, affects bone metabolism. This chapter explains in detail the complex relationship of thyroid hormone and bone.

MOLECULAR MECHANISM OF THYROID HORMONES ACTION

The action of thyroid hormone is mediated by nuclear thyroid hormone receptor (TR). There are four subtypes of TR—TRα1, TRα2, TRβ1, and TRβ2. TRs heterodimerize with retinoid X receptor (RXR) before binding to deoxyribonucleic acid (DNA). TR/RXR binds to particular DNA sequences (thyroid hormone response element, TREs) located in the regulatory region of target gene. In the absence of ligand, TR recruits corepressor and represses the target gene. T3, a biologically active form of thyroid hormone upon entering the nucleus of the target cell disrupts corepressor binding and recruits steroid receptor coactivator 1 and other related transcriptional coactivators, leading on to activation of target gene.

In skeletal tissue, chondrocytes (reserve, proliferative and prehypertrophic zone but not hypertrophic zone of epiphyseal growth plate), osteoblastic bone marrow stromal cells, and osteoblasts predominantly express TR. It is unclear whether osteoclasts also express TRs. TRα1 is the main subtype expressed in skeletal tissue, at least 10-fold higher than TRβ1. Thyroid hormone is pivotal for endochondral as well as intramembranous ossification. Final chondrocytes differentiation followed by vascular incursion of cartilage is dependent on thyroid hormone. Thyroid hormones also stimulate osteoblast proliferation and differentiation, bone matrix creation, and bone mineralization. Paradoxically, excess in thyroid hormone leads to increased osteoclast number and activity causing bone resorption. This may be facilitated by direct nongenomic actions of T3 on osteoclasts or indirect effect through cells of osteoblast lineage.

OVERT HYPERTHYROIDISM AND BONE

Friedrich von Recklinghausen was first to recognize the relationship between thyroid hormones and adult skeleton, while reporting multiple fractures in a patient with thyrotoxicosis in 1891. Hyperthyroidism truncates the bone remodeling cycle resulting in a high bone turnover state. The duration of bone formation is reduced to a greater extent than that of bone resorption, resulting in 10% bone loss per remodeling cycle and this leads to osteoporosis. Markers of both bone formation and resorption are raised and also correlate with disease severity. Further, various studies have shown association of hyperthyroidism with increased fracture risk. Vestergaard et al. in meta-analysis of 20 studies

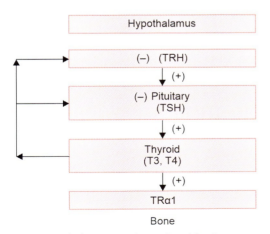

Flowchart 1: Hypothalamic–pituitary–thyroid axis.
(TRα1: thyroid hormone receptor α1; TRH: thyrotropin-releasing hormone; TSH: thyroid-stimulating hormone)

TABLE 1: Effect of thyroid disorders on bone health in adults.

	BMD	Bone formation markers	Bone resorption markers	Fracture risk
Overt hyperthyroidism	↓	↑	↑↑	↑
Subclinical hyperthyroidism	↓	↑	↑↑	↑ (postmenopausal females)
Overt hypothyroidism	↔	↔	↔	↑
Subclinical hypothyroidism	↔	↔	↔	↔
(BMD: bone mineral density)				

of patients with thyrotoxicosis concluded that bone mineral density (BMD) was reduced at the time of diagnosis and there was an increased risk of hip fracture **(Table 1)**. Enhanced mobilization of bone minerals in hyperthyroid state leads to increased urinary excretion of calcium and phosphorus. Baxter and Bondy reported increased serum concentration of calcium in 19 of their 77 hyperthyroid subjects. Manicourt et al. reported increase in free serum calcium levels in 50% of their study subjects with hyperthyroidism. Serum parathyroid hormone levels are inversely related to serum calcium levels and generally low normal in most individuals with hyperthyroidism.

SUBCLINICAL HYPERTHYROIDISM AND BONE

Data showing effect of subclinical hyperthyroidism on bone health is conflicting. However, majority of cohort studies and meta-analyses have found reduced BMD and increased fracture risk with subclinical hyperthyroidism. Blum et al. in a recent meta-analysis including nearly 70 thousand subjects showed that a thyroid-stimulating hormone (TSH) value <0.01 mU/L was associated with a 2- and 3.5-fold increased risk of hip and spine fractures, respectively. As a whole, bone loss is more often seen with endogenous TSH suppression, postmenopausal females and in patients with long duration of disease.

OVERT HYPOTHYROIDISM AND BONE

Histomorphometric studies have shown that hypothyroidism prolongs the bone remodeling cycle resulting in a low bone turnover state. Both osteoclastic and osteoblastic activity is reduced. There is net increase in bone mineralization and mass without any change in bone volume. These changes are very time consuming and hence long-term prospective clinical study of untreated hypothyroid patients is difficult to accumulate. Studies available to date have shown normal BMD in newly diagnosed patients of hypothyroidism. Despite of normal BMD, fracture risk was found to be increased in patients with hypothyroidism at the time of diagnosis, possibly due to poor bone quality in hypothyroid patients. In a recent study, this increase in risk of fracture in hypothyroid patients was attributed to hyperthyroidism due to accumulated periods of over-replacement with thyroxine.

SUBCLINICAL HYPOTHYROIDISM AND BONE

Subclinical hypothyroidism was not found to be associated with changes in BMD or increase in fracture risk.

CHILDHOOD HYPOTHYROIDISM AND BONE

Congenital hypothyroidism is the most common congenital endocrine disorder. Untreated congenital and juvenile acquired hypothyroidism can profoundly affect skeletal growth. It may lead to deficient bone maturation and growth arrest in the affected child. Typical clinical features include broad flat nasal bridge, hypertelorism, wide patent fontanels, flat vertebral bodies, scoliosis, and congenital hip dislocation. Abnormal epiphyseal development and irregular ossification results in stippled epiphyseal dysgenesis; typically seen on X-rays. Thyroid hormone treatment results in rapid catch-up in bone age and consequent height gain. However, predicted adult height may not be reached, mainly relating to the length and severity of hypothyroidism before diagnosis and treatment.

CHILDHOOD HYPERTHYROIDISM AND BONE

The most common cause of thyrotoxicosis in children is Graves' disease. Juvenile thyrotoxicosis results in rapid skeletal development and height gain early on, but premature closure of growth plates due to advance bone age finally leads to short height. Early closure of the cranial sutures resulting in craniosynostosis can happen in severe cases of childhood hyperthyroidism.

THYROID-STIMULATING HORMONE SUPPRESSION THERAPY FOR THYROID CARCINOMA AND BONE

There is no adverse effect of TSH suppressive therapy on BMD in premenopausal women. Although fracture data is not available in this group. In postmenopausal women, data from systematic reviews is inconsistent with regard to effect of suppressive thyroxine therapy on BMD. Meta-analyses however showed reduction in lumbar spine BMD by 7% [confidence interval (CI) 4–10%] and at the femur by 5%

(CI 2–8%). No prospective fracture data are available in this age group also. In a study done by Flynn et al., they showed 2.5-fold higher fracture rate in admitted patients with TSH <0.05 mU/L. Collectively available data suggest increased risk of bone loss and osteoporosis in postmenopausal women on suppression therapy with thyroxine.

CONCLUSION

Thyroid hormones are essential for human skeletal development and linear growth. In adults, thyrotoxicosis is an accepted cause of secondary osteoporosis and increase in fracture risk. TSH suppressive therapy in thyroid carcinoma can lead to increase bone loss and consequent increase fracture risk in postmenopausal women. Congenital and juvenile hypothyroidism results in delayed bone maturation and skeletal development. Typical clinical features are short stature and dysmorphic facial features; depending on the age of onset and severity of disease. Overall, thyroid hormones have anabolic actions in the childhood and catabolic effects in adults.

SUGGESTED READINGS

1. Braverman LE, Cooper DS. Werner and Ingbar's the Thyroid: a Fundamental and Clinical Text, 11th edition. Philadelphia, PA: Lippincott Williams Wilkins; 2021.
2. Bassett JH, Williams GR. Role of thyroid hormones in skeletal development and bone maintenance. Endocr Rev. 2016;37(2):135-87.
3. von Recklinghausen F. Festschrift Rudolf Virchow. Berlin: Dietrich Reimer Verlag GmbH; 1891. p. 20.
4. Mosekilde L, Eriksen EF, Charles P. Effects of thyroid hormones on bone and mineral metabolism. Endocrinol Metab Clin N Am. 1990;19(1):35-63.
5. Mosekilde L, Melsen F. Effect of antithyroid treatment on calcium-phosphorus metabolism in hyperthyroidism. II: Bone histomorphometry. Acta Endocrinol (Cph). 1978;87(4):751-8.
6. Vestergaard P, Mosekilde L. Hyperthyroidism, bone mineral, and fracture risk: a meta-analysis. Thyroid. 2003;13:585-93.
7. Baxter JD, Bondy PK. Hypercalcemia of thyrotoxicosis. Ann Intern Med. 1966;65:429-42.
8. Manicourt D, Detester Mirking N, Brauman H, Corvilain J. Disturbed mineral metabolism in hyperthyroidism: Good correlation with triiodothyronine. Clin Endocrinol (Oxf). 1979;10:407-12.
9. Blum MR, Bauer DC, Collet TH, Fink HA, Cappola AR, da Costa BR, et al. Subclinical thyroid dysfunction and fracture risk: a meta-analysis. JAMA. 2015;313(20):2055-65.
10. Vestergaard P, Mosekilde L. Fractures in patients with hyperthyroidism and hypothyroidism: a nationwide follow-up study in 16,249 patients. Thyroid. 2002;12:411-9.
11. Abrahamsen B, Jorgensen HL, Laulund AS, Nybo M, Brix TH, Hegedus L. The excess risk of major osteoporotic fractures in hypothyroidism is driven by cumulative hyperthyroid as opposed to hypothyroid time: an observational register-based time-resolved cohort analysis. J Bone Miner Res. 2015;30(5):898-905.
12. Hüffmeier U, Tietze HU, Rauch A. Severe skeletal dysplasia caused by undiagnosed hypothyroidism. Eur J Med Genet. 2007;50:209-15.
13. Murphy E, Williams GR. The thyroid and the skeleton. Clin Endocrinol (Oxf). 2004;61(3):285-98.
14. Uzzan B, Campos J, Cucherat M, Nony P, Boissel JP, Perret GY. Effects on bone mass of long term treatment with thyroid hormones: a meta-analysis. J Clin Endocrinol Metab. 1996;81(12):4278-89.
15. Quan ML, Pasieka JL, Rorstad O. Bone mineral density in well-differentiated thyroid cancer patients treated with suppressive thyroxine: a systematic overview of the literature. J Surg Oncol. 2002;79(1):62-9.
16. Heemstra KA, Hamdy NA, Romijn JA, Smit JW. The effects of thyrotropin-suppressive therapy on bone metabolism in patients with well-differentiated thyroid carcinoma. Thyroid. 2006;16(6):583-91.
17. Faber J, Galloe AM. Changes in bone mass during prolonged subclinical hyperthyroidism due to l-thyroxine treatment: a meta-analysis. Eur J Endocrinol. 1994;130(4):350-6.
18. Flynn RW, Bonellie SR, Jung RT, MacDonald TM, Morris AD, Leese GP. Serum thyroid-stimulating hormone concentration and morbidity from cardiovascular disease and fractures in patients on long-term thyroxine therapy. J Clin Endocrinol Metab. 2010;95(1):186-93.

37 CHAPTER

Thyroid Hormone Resistance

Kripa Elizabeth Cherian, Thomas V Paul

INTRODUCTION

First described in 1967 by Refetoff, thyroid hormone resistance refers to the clinical syndrome of decreased sensitivity to the action of thyroid hormones. Classically, there is reduced clinical manifestations of thyroid hormone action, relative to the circulating levels of thyroid hormones, and an inappropriately nonsuppressed thyroid-stimulating hormone (TSH). Previously it was considered to be synonymous with mutations in the thyroid hormone resistance β (*THRβ*) gene. In the last decade, however, various genetic defects involving the *THRα* gene, thyroid hormone transport, and metabolism have also been included in this category of impaired thyroid hormone sensitivity. The nomenclature for this inherited condition has also undergone changes; from "reduced sensitivity to thyroid hormone (RSTH)" in 2005 to "impaired sensitivity to thyroid hormone" at the 10th international conference on resistance to thyroid hormone and action held in Quebec city in Canada in 2012. This chapter focuses on the classical syndrome of thyroid hormone resistance as exemplified by mutations in the β subunit of the thyroid hormone receptor (TR).

EPIDEMIOLOGY

The earliest report of resistance to the action of thyroid hormones was reported in a pair of siblings who were born of a consanguineous marriage and had features of deaf-mutism, stippled epiphyses, delayed bone age, and high levels of protein-bound iodine. As most neonatal screening programs measure TSH in dried blood spot samples, the exact prevalence of thyroid hormone resistance is not known. Recent surveys, however, have estimated the prevalence to be about 1 in 40,000 to 1 in 19,000 live births. The frequency is reported to be equal in both genders, while it might differ across various ethnic groups. A cursory search has revealed that the number of cases reported so far exceeds 1,000 and the inheritance is noted to follow an autosomal dominant pattern.

NORMAL PHYSIOLOGY

The optimal action of thyroid hormones requires the following: (1) the availability of intact thyroid hormone, (2) its appropriate transfer across cell membrane, (3) intracellular metabolism and activation, (4) cytosolic and nuclear processing, (5) binding to receptors, and (6) interaction with coregulators and other postreceptor modifications that are required for the normal expression of thyroid hormone action. A constant circulating concentration of thyroid hormone is ensured by a feedback system involving the hypothalamic-pituitary unit and the thyroid gland. A decrease in the circulating concentration of thyroid hormone induces a hypothalamus-stimulated release of TSH from the pituitary thyrotrophs, which in turn act on the thyroid follicular cells to synthesize and secrete more thyroid hormone. On the other hand, an excess of thyroid hormones shuts down the system, using the same pathway. In order to cater to local thyroid hormone requirements, additional systems are in place. These include the control of thyroid hormone entry into the cell through active transmembrane transporters as well as the activation of the thyroxine (T4) to form triiodothyronine (T3) by removal of the outer ring iodine (5′-deiodination). Moreover, T4 is inactivated by removal of iodine from the inner ring (5-deiodination) to form reverse T3 (rT3) and T2. Thus, differing concentrations of deiodinases in various cells ensures additional local regulation of hormone availability. The presence and number of TRs, through which thyroid hormone action is mediated, determines the type and degree of hormonal response. Thyroid hormone action takes place in the cytosol and the nucleus; the action in the nucleus is known as the genomic effect. TRs are transcription factors that are found to be in close association with the deoxyribonucleic acid (DNA) of genes whose expression they regulate.

Thyroid hormone receptors: The human TRs are transcribed separately from two genes namely (1) *THRα* and (2) *THRβ*. From the *THRα* gene (located on chromosome 17) is transcribed three distinct mRNA THRα1, THRα2, and

THRα3. While THRα1 binds T3 and is capable of forming dimers, THRα2 and THRα3 cannot bind the hormone. The *THRβ* gene is located on chromosome 3, and is expressed either as THRβ1 or THRβ2 which are T3-binding isoforms. In mice, it was found that THRα1 and THRβ1 were expressed in all tissues although THRα1 mRNA was predominantly expressed in the heart and brain, while THRβ1 mRNA was greatly expressed in skeletal muscle, kidney, and liver as compared to other tissues. As far as the expression of THRβ2 mRNA is concerned, it is found to be higher in the brain, pituitary gland, retina, and inner ear than in other tissues. Data for the tissue distributions of expression of the THRα and THRβ isoforms in human tissues are limited; THRα1 and THRβ1 are well expressed in the trophoblast and stromal cells of the placenta.

CLASSIFICATION OF THYROID HORMONE RESISTANCE SYNDROMES

The classification of thyroid hormone resistance may be biased by practical constraints and the paucity of methods available to determine the responsiveness to thyroid hormones in different tissues. However, the currently used classification system categorizes this condition as follows:

- *Generalized resistance to thyroid hormone (GRTH)*: This encompasses most of the cases of resistance to thyroid hormone. Affected individuals are usually eumetabolic at the expense of high circulating levels of thyroid hormone maintained by the secretion of normal TSH in response to hypothalamic thyrotropin-releasing hormone (TRH).
- *Pituitary resistance to thyroid hormone (PRTH)*: Also referred to as non-neoplastic inappropriate TSH secretion or non-neoplastic central hyperthyroidism, this syndrome differs from GRTH in that the clinical manifestations of thyrotoxicosis are apparent. PRTH also encompasses other conditions that include non-neoplastic pituitary hyperplasia, defective pituitary deiodinase type II, and cases of GRTH with more severe hyposensitivity of the thyroid hormone.
- *Peripheral tissue resistance to thyroid hormone (PTRTH)*: The resistance to thyroid hormone is confined to peripheral tissues and was described in detail in one individual who required high doses of triiodothyronine (T3) to main normal metabolic state. Due to lack of resistance at the level of the pituitary, affected individuals maintain normal TSH and thyroid hormone levels. Due to lack of compensatory mechanism to increase the TSH and thyroid hormone levels, these patients manifest features of hypothyroidism. Due to the lack of specific tests to detect hyposensitivity in peripheral tissues, the likelihood of detecting this syndrome remains low.

ETIOPATHOGENESIS AND MOLECULAR BASIS

It has been reported that most cases of resistance to thyroid hormone β (RTHβ) are caused by point mutations in the isoforms of the *TRβ* gene, although the exact molecular mechanism remains unknown. Most commonly, RTHβ is caused by a minor defect in one of the arms of the *TRβ* gene. RTHβ is not merely due to a decrease in the functional TRs, but is likely related to an interaction between the mutant and the wild type TRβ. Majority of the mutations described are reported to occur in two "hot spots" which are separated by a highly conserved region of 80 amino acids known as the "cold zone" from codons 349 to 429. Recently, a new mutation has been discovered, and the range of hot spots has been extended to include the codons that extend between 309–353 and 374–461. In addition, a third mutation cluster has been confirmed with the range of codons 234–282. There are >100 mutations that have been reported to date.

CLINICAL FEATURES

RTHβ: Clinical features of RTHβ are variable and depend on the extent of tissue responsiveness to elevated thyroid hormone levels in an individual. The same mutation could manifest with differing phenotypes in different patients, even within the same family. Usually, patients with mutations in THRβ have an autosomal dominant inheritance and present with RTHβ, typically characterized by elevated thyroid hormone levels, with TSH being normal or mildly elevated, goiter, and the absence of symptoms of thyrotoxicosis. Homozygous mutations involving THRβ on the other hand have been reported in few patients wherein the affected patient presents with goiter, elevated levels of T4 and TSH with delay in both growth and bone development, tachycardia, structural abnormalities of the heart, hearing and visual loss, as well as intellectual disabilities. These patients lack a wild copy of the *THRβ* gene, and it has been suggested that severe phenotypes in these individuals might be due to a dominant-negative effect of mutant THRβ on wild-type THR. Similarly, members of a family in which RTHβ was inherited as an autosomal recessive disease had a mutation that resulted in deletion of the entire coding region. Family members that were homozygous for this mutation presented with hearing impairment, color blindness, epiphyseal stippling, and growth delay but had a normal IQ.

RTHα: In the last decade, human THRα mutations have now been identified in a few families with hypothyroid features and thyroid hormone resistance in target tissues, but associated paradoxically with near-normal thyroid function

TABLE 1: Clinical manifestations of RTHα.	
Appearance	Flattened nasal bridge, broad face, thickened lips, macroglossia, coarse facies, skin tags, and moles
Skeletal	Disproportionate short stature, macrocephaly, delayed tooth eruption
Gastrointestinal	Constipation
Cardiovascular	Bradycardia, low blood pressure
Neurological and cognitive	Delayed developmental milestones, slow, dysarthric speech, slow initiation of movement, ataxic gait, dysdiadochokinesis, fine and gross motor incoordination (dyspraxia), seizures, autism spectrum disorder
Hematological	Mild anemia

(RTHα: resistance to thyroid hormone α)

tests. A summary of the clinical features encountered in RTHα are depicted in **Table 1**. Usually, these subjects have a low to low normal free T4 and a high T3, a low free T4:free T3 ratio and a normal TSH.

COURSE OF THE DISEASE

The course of the disease may be as variable as its presentation itself. While most of the subjects have normal growth and development and are capable of leading a normal life at the expense of high thyroid hormone levels and a small goiter, others may present with differing degrees of mental and growth retardation. It has been shown that symptoms of hyperactivity tend to improve with age. Goiter usually recurs after surgery and some individuals with RTH have been submitted to several thyroidectomy surgeries or repeated sessions of treatment with radioiodine.

LABORATORY FINDINGS

Resistance to thyroid hormone β is characterized by a high serum free T4 concentration in the presence of a nonsuppressed (normal or slightly elevated) TSH. These features are essential requirements for the diagnosis of the same. Serum levels of T3 and reverse T3 (rT3), if measured, are usually also high. The concentration of thyroglobulin is also high reflecting the extent of TSH-mediated thyroid gland hyperactivity. If these abnormalities are found, they should be confirmed by repeat measurements several weeks later. In contrast, RTHα is characterized by low to low-normal free T4 and a high free T3, a low free T4: free T3 ratio and a normal TSH. Confirmation requires demonstration of mutations in the TR gene by direct sequencing.

DIFFERENTIAL DIAGNOSES

All conditions that present with high serum T4 and T3 concentrations in association with a normal to high TSH levels should be considered in the differential diagnosis. These are shown in **Table 2**.

Non-TR-RTH

In 15% of families with RTHβ and THRβ gene mutations are not detected and this is condition is known as "non-TR-RTH." With respect to clinical and biochemical features it is indistinguishable from RTHβ with THRβ gene mutations. In such cases mosaicism should be excluded by sequencing the receptor in DNA obtained from different tissues or by in-depth sequencing. Mutations in some of the cofactors that interact with the receptor cannot be excluded and may be responsible for the resistance in some of these families.

TREATMENT

RTHβ: The underlying defect cannot be fully corrected with treatment. Care should be taken not to intervene for the sole purpose of normalizing TSH levels. Symptomatic palpitation and sinus tachycardia can be treated with β-blockers. Usually, in most individuals with RTH, the partial tissue resistance to thyroid hormone is adequately compensated

TABLE 2: Differential diagnoses of resistance to thyroid hormone β (RTHβ).							
	Thyroid function tests						
Defect	T4	T3	rT3	TSH	fT4 (direct)	fT4 (dialysis)	Prevalence
Increased thyroid-binding globulin	↑	↑	↑	N	N	N	Common
Increased transthyretin	↑	N	↑	N	N	N	Rare
Familial dysalbuminemic hyperthyroxinemia	↑	↑ or N	↑	N	↑	N	Common or rare depending on ethnicity
RTH	↑	↑ or N	↑	↑ or N	↑	↑	Uncommon
TSH-producing pituitary adenoma	↑	↑	↑	↑ or N	↑	↑	Rare
SBP2/SECISBP2 (selenocysteine insertion sequence binding protein 2 mutation) (causes a thyroid hormone metabolic defect)	↑	↓	↑	↑ or N	↑	↑	Unknown
Acute nonthyroidal illness syndrome	↑	↓↓	↑	N	↑ or N	N	Common

(↑: increased; ↓: decreased; N: normal)

for by an increase in the TSH-mediated increase in thyroid hormone and treatment is not required. However, in patients with limited reserve due to prior radioiodine ablation of the thyroid gland, thyroid hormone replacement is required and, in these patients, the serum TSH level may be used to guide hormone therapy. When the compensation is incomplete, judicious administration of supraphysiologic doses of the hormone may be required. In particular, in children, attention must be paid to growth, bone maturation, and mental development. The development of a catabolic state is an indication of overtreatment.

Prenatal diagnosis and counseling may be required in families whose affected members show evidence of growth or mental retardation. Rarely, infants may present with failure to thrive. This is often associated with features of hypermetabolism and severe tachycardia that may be refractory to β-blockers. Frameshift mutations producing a TRβ with an extended nonsense carboxyl terminal sequence may account for the severity of the disease. Such cases might warrant abrupt reduction of the thyroid hormone level with somatostatin analogs. If this proves ineffective, administration of antithyroid drugs or triiodothyroacetic acid may be required.

Pregnancy: Management of RTH during gestation in a pregnant woman may be complicated. Interestingly, a fetus with a *THRβ* gene mutation carried by a woman with RTHβ is protected from adverse effects of the high maternal thyroid hormone levels while in offspring that do not carry the mutation, features of fetal thyrotoxicosis may be apparent.

Mothers with RTH carrying unaffected fetus: Antithyroid drugs may be indicated, depending on the well-being of the fetus. In such women, the free T4 should be maintained not >50% above the upper limit of normal. This can be achieved by the administration of propylthiouracil (PTU) taking extreme caution to avoid hypothyroidism.

Mothers with RTH who are carrying affected fetus (as determined by prenatal genetic analysis): There is no basis for regular treatment of normal mothers carrying affected fetus unless the fetus is found to have a large goiter or is in distress, in which case, intra-amniotic infusion of levothyroxine is indicated to reduce the size of the goiter.

RTHα: Clinical experience in the treatment of this condition is limited and it is uncertain as to whether levothyroxine therapy offers any benefit in affected subjects. Treatment with levothyroxine in few cases showed that the hypothalamic-pituitary axis responded to exogenous thyroid hormone, but the skeletal, gastrointestinal, and myocardial tissues were resistant. This response is consistent with the differential tissue expression of the TRα subtype. In another instance liothyronine was given, which reduced the TSH and consequently the T4 level at the expense of an increase in the heart rate. At present, the experience concerning treatment of RTHα is minimal, precluding definitive recommendations to be made in this regard.

CONCLUSION

Resistance to thyroid hormone is an uncommon disorder and in the classical syndrome of RTHβ, affected individuals present with goiter, normal to high normal levels of thyroid hormone, and a normal or nonsuppressed TSH. Usually, levothyroxine treatment to suppress TSH is not warranted except in instances where the individual has undergone thyroidectomy or ablative therapy. Symptomatic patients who manifest with tachycardia respond to β-blockers. In the last decade, few cases of RTHα have been reported, where patients present with clinical features of hypothyroidism which is poorly responsive to levothyroxine therapy. Pregnant women with RTH may be managed depending on whether the fetus is affected or not. Other conditions that may present with the biochemical features of RTH include familial dysalbuminemic hyperthyroxinemia, TSH-secreting pituitary adenoma, and an acute nonthyroidal illness syndrome, all of which may be distinguished from RTH by appropriate tests.

SUGGESTED READINGS

1. Refetoff S, Weiss RE, Usala SJ. The syndromes of resistance to thyroid hormone. Endocr Rev. 1993;14(3):348-99.
2. Pappa T, Refetoff S. Resistance to Thyroid Hormone Beta: A Focused Review. Front Endocrinol (Lausanne). 2021;12:656551.
3. Refetoff S, Bassett JHD, Beck-Peccoz P, Bernal J, Brent G, Chatterjee K, et al. Classification and proposed nomenclature for inherited defects of thyroid hormone action, cell transport, and metabolism. J Clin Endocrinol Metab. 2014;99(3):768-70.
4. Refetoff S, DeWind LT, DeGroot LJ. Familial syndrome combining deaf-mutism, stuppled epiphyses, goiter and abnormally high PBI: possible target organ refractoriness to thyroid hormone. J Clin Endocrinol Metab. 1967;27(2):279-94.
5. Lafranchi SH, Snyder DB, Sesser DE, Skeels MR, Singh N, Brent GA, et al. Follow-up of newborns with elevated screening T4 concentrations. J Pediatr. 2003;143(3):296-301.
6. Vela A, Pérez-Nanclares G, Ríos I, Rica I, Portillo N, Castaño L, et al. Thyroid hormone resistance from newborns to adults: a Spanish experience. J Endocrinol Invest. 2019;42(8):941-9.
7. Refetoff S, Dumitrescu AM. Syndromes of reduced sensitivity to thyroid hormone: genetic defects in hormone receptors, cell transporters and deiodination. Best Pract Res Clin Endocrinol Metab. 2007;21(2):277-305.
8. Ortiga-Carvalho TM, Sidhaye AR, Wondisford FE. Thyroid hormone receptors and resistance to thyroid hormone disorders. Nat Rev Endocrinol. 2014;10(10):582-91.
9. Sun H, Cao L, Zheng R, Xie S, Liu C. Update on resistance to thyroid hormone syndrome β. Ital J Pediatr. 2020;46(1):168.
10. Moran C, Chatterjee K. Resistance to thyroid hormone due to defective thyroid receptor alpha. Best Pract Res Clin Endocrinol Metab. 2015;29(4):647-57.

11. Reutrakul S, Sadow PM, Pannain S, Pohlenz J, Carvalho GA, Macchia PE, et al. Search for abnormalities of nuclear corepressors, coactivators, and a coregulator in families with resistance to thyroid hormone without mutations in thyroid hormone receptor beta or alpha genes. J Clin Endocrinol Metab. 2000;85(10):3609-17.
12. Weiss RE, Hayashi Y, Nagaya T, Petty KJ, Murata Y, Tunca H, et al. Dominant inheritance of resistance to thyroid hormone not linked to defects in the thyroid hormone receptor alpha or beta genes may be due to a defective cofactor. J Clin Endocrinol Metab. 1996;81(12):4196-203.
13. Weiss RE, Dumitrescu A, Refetoff S. Approach to the patient with resistance to thyroid hormone and pregnancy. J Clin Endocrinol Metab. 2010;95(7):3094-102.
14. Pappa T, Anselmo J, Mamanasiri S, Dumitrescu AM, Weiss RE, Refetoff S. Prenatal Diagnosis of Resistance to Thyroid Hormone and its Clinical Implications. J Clin Endocrinol Metab. 2017;102(10):3775-82.
15. Sakurai A, Takeda K, Ain K, Ceccarelli P, Nakai A, Seino S, et al. Generalized resistance to thyroid hormone associated with a mutation in the ligand-binding domain of the human thyroid hormone receptor beta. Proc Natl Acad Sci USA. 1989;86(22):8977-81.
16. Bochukova E, Schoenmakers N, Agostini M, Schoenmakers E, Rajanayagam O, Keogh JM, et al. A mutation in the thyroid hormone receptor alpha gene. N Engl J Med. 2012;366(3):243-9.
17. Espiard S, Savagner F, Flamant F, Vlaeminck-Guillem V, Guyot R, Munier M, et al. A Novel Mutation in THRA Gene Associated with an Atypical Phenotype of Resistance to Thyroid Hormone. J Clin Endocrinol Metab. 2015;100(8):2841-8.

CHAPTER 38

Environmental Thyroid Disruptors

Uma Kaimal Saikia, Sanjay Kalra, Gopinath N

INTRODUCTION

Endocrine disruptors (EDs) are exogenous chemical agents which can alter the function of hormones. Studies in invertebrates, vertebrates, mammals, nonhuman primates as well as in humans have shown a disturbing trend of increasing endocrine dysfunction. Their role in the pathogenesis of various endocrine conditions has gained interest in recent years as they are widely available in commodities of daily life and in the environment and hence a wide exposure exists. The US Environment Protection Agency (EPA) defines an ED as "an exogenous agent that interferes with the production, release, transport, metabolism, binding, action, or elimination of natural hormones in the body responsible for the maintenance of homeostasis and the regulation of developmental processes". In 2012, the Endocrine Society put forward a more simplified definition as "an exogenous chemical or mixture of chemicals that can interfere with any aspect of hormone action". The thyroid is very sensitive to the action of disruptors and considering the importance of thyroid hormones on various metabolic processes, it is to be expected that thyroid disruptors may lead to significant changes in physical and cognitive functioning. Problems in evaluating the effect of an ED on a particular system include differences in age of exposure, duration, involvement of multiple chemicals, variable latency, differences in elimination of the compound, and the dose-effect relationship which may not be linear. Hence, considerable caution should be exercised in extrapolating data from animal studies or from small human studies to the general population.

IMPACT OF ENDOCRINE DISRUPTORS

It is not necessary to experience exposure to an ED in adulthood to suffer a detrimental effect. Exposure in critical times during antenatal or postnatal life sometimes leads to irreversible effects on the endocrine system. This happens if exposure happens when programming of the endocrine system is in progress. This is particularly dangerous because normal development in mammals and other vertebrates is highly dependent on a normal euthyroid hormonal milieu. Exposure to the same level of an endocrine signal at different stages in the life history or in different seasons may produce different effects.

CLASSIFICATION OF THYROID DISRUPTORS

Environmental thyroid disruptors may be classified based on their chemical structure or on their mechanism of action.

Sources and categorization of industrial chemicals causing thyroid disruption:
- *Plasticizers*: Bisphenol A (BPA), phthalates
- *Pesticides*: Dichlorodiphenyltrichloroethane (DDT), hexachlorobenzene (HCB), chlorpyrifos
- *Flame retardants*: Polybrominated diphenyl ethers (PBDEs)
- Polychlorinated biphenyls
- Perfluoroalkyl substances
- *Heavy metals*: Mercury
- *Other compounds*: Resorcinol, perfluorooctane sulfonate
- *Radiation*: Iatrogenic, environmental manmade disasters

Classification based on mechanism of disruption:
- *Hypothalamus and pituitary-related effects*: Phthalates, BPA
- *Effect on sodium iodide symporter (NIS)*: Perchlorates, thiocyanates, nitrates
- *Effect on thyroid hormone synthesis*: Pesticides
- *Effect on thyroid hormone transport*: Polychlorinated biphenyls (PCB), phthalates, polychlorinated dibenzo-dioxins, perfluoroalkyl substances (PFAS)
- *Effect on thyroid hormone action and metabolism*: Polybrominated diphenyl ethers, phthalates, and pesticides

Plasticizers (Bisphenol A and Phthalates)

These chemicals are seen in abundance as components of toys, cosmetics, food packaging, building appliances, and also in some detergents. They are found in unbound form in environment and are widely used; hence, exposure of the population is immense and diffuse. Both BPA and phthalates cause hypothalamo-pituitary axis disruption. BPA interferes with the binding of T3 to its receptor and also suppresses its transcriptional activity in a dose-dependent manner. BPA and its structural analogs cause dysregulation of thyroid receptor gene expression in pituitary and thyroid gland by suppressing the expression of the gene encoding retinoid X receptor (RXR) gamma which forms heterodimers to thyroid hormone receptors. Phthalate compounds are known to downregulate messenger ribonucleic acid (mRNA) expression of thyroid-stimulating hormone (TSH) receptor in thyroid and also of transthyretin (TTR) involved in thyroid hormone transport. Phthalate metabolites can also interfere with the regulation of the NIS and thus affect iodine uptake. Epidemiological studies have shown controversial results between exposure and effects on thyroid hormone levels.

In a fertility center at Massachusetts general hospital among 408 men who attended this clinic from 2000 to 2004, an inverse relationship was found between urinary monophthalate and serum T3 levels. The NHANES survey data (2007–2008) studied urinary samples of 1,346 adults and 329 adolescents and found urinary concentrations of phthalate metabolites was associated with lower T4 levels in males or high TSH values suggesting that there may be sex-based differences in the response to phthalates. The Taiwan Environmental Study for Toxicants showed a negative association between phthalate metabolites and T4 levels in adults but a positive association with free T4 levels in children. Studies in pregnancy have shown a negative correlation between several metabolites and thyroid hormones and positive correlation with TSH levels which however, may depend on the timing of exposure during gestation. Phthalates have also been postulated to induce oxidative stress with changes in levels of thyroid-binding globulin (TBG) and interleukin-7 and exacerbate chronic lymphocytic thyroiditis.

Pesticides

This group includes mainly chemicals such as DDT, HCB, and chlorpyrifos. Long-term studies on contamination of these chemicals have been shown to disrupt thyroid hormone transport and have histomorphometrical effects on the thyroid gland. Though a wide number of thyroid disruptors have been identified among pesticides, studies are needed to identify the toxicity levels and duration of exposure. Chlorpyrifos can cross the placental barrier and acts by inhibiting acetylcholinesterase. Its exposure has resulted in neurodevelopmental defects, low IQ scores, and impaired memory skill in children. DDT exposure inhibits TSH release by affecting postreceptor cyclic adenosine monophosphate (AMP) production and inhibits its activity at the TSH receptor. Prenatal HCB exposure was found to be associated with lower maternal T3 levels and lower thyroid hormone levels in the newborn and defective neurodevelopment.

Organochlorine pesticides like DDT have structure similar to T3 and T4 and might mimic their activity by binding to thyroid receptors. In an animal study, exposure to low doses of DDT in rats for 4 weeks, showed decrease in T4 levels and size of follicles. On histopathology thyroid follicle epithelial cells showed decrease in length and amount of microvilli. A cross-sectional study carried out in rural areas of Brazil studied 19 organochlorine pesticides and its effect on thyroid hormones, TSH and thyroid peroxidase (TPO) antibodies. Total T3 levels were associated with lower concentrations of endosulfan 2 in men and with higher endosulfan 2 and methoxychlor in women. Levels of free T4 showed inverse association with β-hexachlorocyclohexane (HCH) and p,p'-DDT in men, and were positively associated with HCB and DDT in women. Serum TSH levels were associated with higher β-HCH in men. This study showed pesticides affect thyroid gland by gender-specific mechanisms, which differ among various compounds. Glyphosate-based herbicides (GBHs) are widely used and have shown to cause disruption of the hypothalamo-pituitary axis. A reduction in the hypothalamic genes encoding for deiodinase 2 and 3 and thyroid hormone transporters has been reported. Exposure has been shown to lead to decreased TSH levels and normal thyroid hormone levels. Fipronil, an insecticide used in crops such as rice and corn, has been shown in vitro to cause anti-thyroid-stimulating hormone receptor-α (anti-TSHR α) activity.

Polychlorinated biphenyls (PCBs) were widely used as pesticides before the 1970s. Though banned exposure still exists through the food chain. PCBs and their metabolites bind to thyroid transporters as TTR and interfere with their transport. Action of PCBs at the level of thyroid receptors is both agonistic and antagonistic depending on PCB congeners and target tissue. PCBs concentrations as commonly observed in humans, interfere with Thyroid hormone receptor β complex and disturb oligodendrocyte differentiation and white matter maturation during early development.

In a study on toxin exposure, PCB was measured in maternal milk where high concentrations of PCB was associated with reduced levels of maternal TT3 and TT4 and higher values of TSH in newborns. However, a recent study among electronic waste recycling workers did not show any corelation between thyroid hormones and serum concentrations of PCBs. Contradicting this many studies have showed positive association between PCBs and TSH, negative association with T3 and T4 levels.

Flame Retardants

Polybrominated diphenyl ether compounds are found in building materials, electronics, furnishing materials, and textiles. PBDEs are highly resistant to degradation process. These compounds have structure similar to thyroid hormones hence bind to thyroid hormone receptors, inhibiting the binding of T3 and hence suppressing its action. They also have other proposed actions like competitive binding for serum transporters such as TTR, TBG, upregulation of clearance enzymes (like glucuronidases), and liver metabolism and inhibition of thyroid deiodinase activity.

There are conflicting results as >200 different PBDE compounds are in use. Its effect depends on specific chemical administration, timing, and dosage as well. Majority of studies have found decrease in T4 levels and TT3, FT3 levels in relation to concentrations of PBDEs. However, other few studies showed an increase in thyroid hormone levels and some have shown no correlation. Exposure to high dose can cause histological changes in thyroid gland with degeneration or attenuation of follicular epithelium. The presence of PBDEs in pregnant women and transfer across the placenta has been a matter of concern. Some compounds have been found to be inversely associated with first trimester total T3 and TSH levels. Maternal PBDE exposure in early pregnancy has been reported to cause decreased cord blood fT4 levels and maternal TT4 and fT3 at delivery. Hence, prenatal PBDE exposure may be associated with neuropsychological and cognitive dysfunction in children.

Perfluoroalkyl Compounds

These compounds are mainly used in surface coating in industries like textiles, food packaging, cosmetics and cookware. Perfluoroalkyl substances (PFAS) interfere with binding of thyroid hormone to TTR and upregulate deiodinase in the thyroid gland. Several human studies have been conducted to assess effects of exposure to these compounds which have shown varying results depending on age and sex of exposure. The chemicals, health and pregnancy study conducted in Canada among 152 euthyroid pregnant women, showed PFAS to be positively associated with TSH along with weak negative association with FT4 levels, in a subset of pregnant women who were positive for thyroid peroxidase antibodies. The Northern Norway Mother-and-Child Contaminant Cohort Study studied PFA levels in the maternal blood in the second trimester of pregnancy and 3 and 6 days after delivery. A positive association was seen with serum TSH levels along with reduced free T4 levels in women in the highest quartile of PFA levels. The results of effects of PFAS on neurocognitive development in children have been inconsistent.

Effects of Radiation

The thyroid gland is exquisitely sensitive to irradiation. Thyroid cancers especially papillary carcinomas and follicular tumors which are >1.5 cm in diameter, multicentric with local invasion and distant metastasis are common in patients with exposure to irradiation. Children are at higher risk as reported from Belarus after the Chernobyl disaster.

Benign abnormalities such as focal hyperplasia, single or multiple adenomas, chronic lymphocytic thyroiditis, colloid nodules and fibrosis may occur in up to 20–30% of an irradiated population.

CHILD NEURODEVELOPMENT AND ENDOCRINE DISRUPTORS

The necessity of thyroid hormones for normal brain development is well known with even mild thyroid hormone insufficiency in pregnancy leading to IQ score loss in the offspring. Although iodine deficiency is the most common cause of thyroid hormone insufficiency, the effects of EDs has also come to the forefront. Adverse effects of PCBs and PBDEs on neurogenesis, neural migration, and neural connectivity have been described with imaging studies showing cortical thinning. Fetal exposure may occur due to crossing of the placenta and blood-brain barrier and neonatal exposure may occur due to secretion in breast milk. However, results of effects of EDs on developmental milestones, cognition, behavior, and academic function have been inconsistent stressing the need for multidisciplinary studies on health outcomes in children.

THYROID CANCER

The incidence of thyroid cancer has been increasing steadily all over the world. Although this increase may partly be due to improved methods of detection, environmental disruptors are also thought to play a role. Studies on the association have been sporadic and results are conflicting. Flame retardants such as PBDEs, phthalates, and pesticides have all been incriminated. Mechanisms proposed include the creation of deoxyribonucleic acid (DNA) adducts and disruptions in thyroid homeostasis for polyphosphodiesters (PPDEs), or activation of key oncogenic transcription factors like the aryl hydrocarbon receptor (AHR) for PCBs. Phthalates especially di(2-ethylhexyl) phthalate (DEHP) metabolites have been shown to induce carcinogenesis by the production of reactive oxygen species (ROS) and has been stated to be a human carcinogen by the Centers for Disease Control and Prevention (CDC) and the US Department of Health and Human Services. A higher risk of differentiated thyroid cancer (DTC) has been reported with exposure to DEHP. Bisphenol A activates nuclear factor kappa B (NF-κB) which is a known transcription factor in thyroid tumorigenesis and also inhibits the expression of DNA damage response enzymes.

Longitudinal population-based studies are however needed to establish the potential role of EDs on thyroid carcinogenesis.

NEWER MODELS TO ASSESS EFFECTS OF ENDOCRINE DISRUPTORS

The emerging data on the effects of environmental disruptors on the thyroid underscores the need for good research methodology both in vivo and in vitro. As water is a route for distribution of pollutants, levels of EDs in aquatic animals may be considered as an indicator of contamination. The zebra fish is one such model which has been studied by seeing the expression of enhanced green fluorescent protein (EGFP) which is controlled by TSH-β on exposure to thyroid agonists or antagonists.

Another rapidly advancing technology called "omics" which are used to define the adverse molecular effects due to exposure to environmental chemicals. This can quantify a variety of ribonucleic acid (RNA), protein, and many other biological molecules in tissues or cell cultures. Such omics technologies include measuring changes in gene expression (transcriptomics), protein (proteomics), and metabolism (metabolomics).

The total exposure to a substance from internal and external sources over a lifetime has been termed as the "exposome". Integrating this with adverse outcomes would lead to an understanding of the risk assessment from multiple exposures on human health.

CONCLUSION

Although the concept of environmental pollutants causing disruption of the endocrine system has been known for decades, it is only in recent years that this has been recognized as a major public health problem. Most studies have been in small populations of different areas with varying exposure making it difficult to arrive at a definite conclusion. Factors to be considered in evaluating the effect of an ED include the age and duration of exposure as well as a possible latency period between exposure and response. Also effects of exposure to a single compound may be different from exposure to the same compound contaminated with other pollutants. As the thyroid gland is unique in its need for iodine, response to an ED may also depend on the iodine status of the population. As normal thyroid function is crucial during pregnancy especially for fetal neurodevelopment as well as in every stage of life for cardiovascular, neuromuscular, and cognitive and reproductive functions, larger longitudinal multidisciplinary studies are the need of the hour. It is to be hoped that newer technological advances will provide solid conclusions on thyroid disruptors thus paving the way for guidelines on their identification and prevention of adverse health outcomes.

SUGGESTED READINGS

1. Kavlock RJ, Daston GP, De Rosa C, Fenner-Crisp P, Gray LE, Kaattari S, et al. Research works for the risk assessment of health and environmental effects of endocrine disruptors: a report of the US EPA sponsored workshop. Environ Health Perspect. 1996;104 (Suppl 4):715-40.
2. Zoeller RT, Brown TR, Doan LL, Gore AC, Skakkebaek NE, Soto AM, et al. Endocrine-Disrupting Chemicals and Public Health Protection: A statement of principles from the Endocrine Society. Endocrinology. 2012;153(9):4097-110.
3. Calsolaro V, Pasqualetti G, Niccolai F, Caraccio N, Monzani F. Thyroid Disrupting Chemicals. Int J Mol Sci. 2017;18(12):2583.
4. Oliveira KJ, Chiamolera MI, Giannocco G, Pazos-Moura CC, Ortiga-Carvalho TM. Thyroid function disruptors: from nature to chemicals. J Mol Endocrinol. 2019;62:R1-R19.
5. Ghassabian A, Trasande L. Disruption in Thyroid Signalling Pathway: A Mechanism for the effect of Endocrine-disrupting Chemicals on Child Neurodevelopment. Front Endocrinol. 2018;9:1-7.
6. Meeker JD, Ferguson KK. Relationship between urinary phthalate and Bisphenol A concentrations and serum Thyroid Hormone measures in US adults and adolescents from the National Health and Nutrition Examination Survey (NHANES) 2007-2008. Environ Health Perspect. 2011;119(10):1396-402.
7. Huang H, Huang P. Does exposure to phthalates influence thyroid function and growth hormone homeostasis? Environ Res. 2017;153:63-72.
8. Webster GM, Venners SA, Mattman A, Martin JW. Associations between perfluoroalkyl acids (PFASs) and maternal thyroid hormones in early pregnancy: a population-based cohort study. Environ Res. 2014;133:338-47.
9. Berg V, Nost TH, Hansen S, Elverland A, Veyhe A, Jorde R, et al. Assessing the relationship between perfluoroalkyl substances, thyroid hormones and binding proteins in pregnant women; a longitudinal mixed effects approach. Environ Int. 2015;77:63-9.
10. Alsen M, Sinclair C, Cooke P, Ziadkhanpour K, Genden E, Van Gerwen M. Endocrine disrupting chemicals and Thyroid Cancer: an overview. Toxics. 2021;9:14.
11. Barton-Maclaren TS, Wade M, Basu N, Bayen S, Grundy J, Marlatte V, et al. Innovation in regulatory approaches for endocrine disrupting chemicals: The journey to risk assessment modernization in Canada. Environ Res. 2022;204(Part C):112225.

INDEX

Page numbers followed by *b* refer to box, *f* refer to figure, *fc* refer to flowchart, and *t* refer to table.

A

Abortion 302
Abundant granular eosinophilic cytoplasm 69*f*
Actinobacillus actinomycetemcomitans 284*b*
Actinomyces naeslundii 284*b*
Acute thyroxine
    ingestion 240
    overdose 239
Adenomas 155
Adenosine monophosphate 316
Adenovirus 115, 283, 290
Adipocyte 140*f*
Agenesis 49, 90
Alemtuzumab 116, 267
Alimentary system 117
Aluminum hydroxide 269
American College of Radiology 58, 183
American Joint Committee on Cancer 173, 174, 184
American Thyroid Association 35, 35*t*, 105, 176, 208, 254
Aminoglutethimide 90, 91, 230
Aminosalicylic acid 230
Amiodarone 20, 27, 62, 90, 91, 115, 119, 267-270, 286
    effects of 268*t*
    therapy 27
Amitriptyline 267
Amyloid goiter 63
Amyloidosis 64*f*, 90
Anaplastic carcinoma 59, 77*f*, 78*f*
Anaplastic follicular cell-derived thyroid carcinoma 66, 76, 78*f*
Anaplastic lymphoma kinase 191, 192
Anaplastic thyroid cancer 173, 175, 175*t*, 180, 188, 190*t*, 191
    management of 189*b*
    treatment of 177
Anaplastic thyroid carcinoma 135, 188, 189, 190*t*, 193
Ancillary tests 81
Androgens 269
Angioinvasive follicular thyroid carcinoma 71*f*
Angiotensin-converting enzyme 2 289
Antiepileptics 230
    drugs 230
Anti-Müllerian hormone 204
Antineutrophil cytoplasmic antibody 124
Anti-thyroglobulin 24
    antibodies 22, 182, 203
Antithyroid drugs 27, 82, 83*t*, 90, 123-126, 130, 212, 213, 230, 236, 237, 237*b*, 240
    adverse effects of 236
    therapy, monitoring of 236, 236*b*
Antithyroid peroxidase 24, 276, 282
    antibodies 22
Arcanobacterium haemolyticum 284*b*
Arnold–Chiari malformations 220
Artificial reproductive techniques 254
Aryl hydrocarbon receptor 317
Assisted reproductive technology 203, 204
Atenolol 124
Atezolizumab 135, 267
Atherosclerotic cardiovascular disease 105, 105*f*
Athyreosis 30
Atrial fibrillation 26, 100, 117
Attention deficit hyperactivity disorder 131
Auscultation 21
Autoantibodies 140*f*
Autoimmune thyroid
    diseases 207, 260, 276
Autoimmunity 258
Autonomous thyroid
    hormone synthesis 119
    nodule 247
Avelumab 135

B

Bacteria 284
Basal metabolic rate 93, 251, 257, 259
B-cell chronic lymphocytic leukemia 267
Benign thyroid
    disorders 45
    nodules 57
Beta-blockers 124, 124*t*, 237
Bethesda scoring system 163*t*
    cytology diagnostic categories of 174*t*
Bethesda terminology 60, 61*t*
Bexarotene 91
Bile acid sequestrants 269
Binding
    fraction of 14
    inhibitory immunoglobulins 84
Biotin 28, 269, 270
    effect 121
Biphasic growth pattern 74*f*
Bipolar disorder 27
Bisphenol A 316
Blood pressure 103
    diastolic 103
    systolic 103
Body mass index 93, 208, 258, 259*t*
Bone 307, 308
    loss, accelerated 100
    mineral density 308
Borderline follicular tumors 172
Brain 90, 252
Breast cancer 286
British Thyroid Foundation 289
Bronchial asthma 124
Brown adipose tissue 108, 257
Brucella melitensis 284*b*

C

Café au lait spots 136*f*
Calcitonin 26, 159, 245
Calcium carbonate 269
Cancer 260
    immunotherapy 62
    risk of 158
    vaccines 62
Candida albicans 284*b*
Carbamazepine 91, 269, 270
Carbimazole 82, 123, 236, 275
Carcinoembryonic antigen 78, 182
Carcinoma, malignant 172
Cardio-ankle vascular index 252
Cardiovascular disease 252
Cardiovascular dysfunction 273
Cardiovascular system 117, 254
Carotid artery 29
C-cell hyperplasia 64
Cell
    higher magnification of 76*f*
    membrane thyroid hormone transporter defect 133
    multiple clusters of 76*f*
Cemiplimab 135
Central compartment lymph node
    dissection 182
Central neck dissection 246
    role of 246

Central nervous system 131, 219, 229, 273
Chemosis 113f, 120f
Chemotherapy 192
Chernobyl disaster 243
Childhood hyperthyroidism 308
   etiology of 230b
Childhood papillary thyroid carcinoma 243
Chlordane 270
Cholecystographic agents 269
Cholestatic liver dysfunction 237
Cholesterol ester transport protein 252
Cholestyramine 269
Chronic obstructive pulmonary disease 124
Cirrhosis 98
Clostridium septicum 284b
Coagulative necrosis, foci of 188f
Coccidioides immitis 284b
Colesevelam 269
Colestipol 269
Colloid 59
   background of 65f
   goiter 59, 60f, 65f
Color Doppler 122, 282, 283
Comparative genomic hybridization 221
Complete blood count 191
Computed tomography 29, 38, 40, 45, 49f, 51-55, 135, 153, 159, 177, 183, 191, 285
   scan 45f
Congenital hypothyroidism 8, 23, 30f, 31f, 219, 222t, 224fc, 225, 226fc, 308
   etiology of 219b
   late onset 229, 230
   syndromic associations of 221t
Congo red stain 64f
Conjunctival redness 120f, 113f
Conservative management 245
Contrast-enhanced computed tomography 179, 182, 189
Controlled ovarian hyperstimulation 200, 203
Cord blood 241
   sample 222
Coronary artery disease 105, 108
Coronavirus disease 2019 (COVID-19) 91, 194, 263, 288-291, 294, 296, 297
   disease 297
   endocrine effects of 288f
   infection 263, 283, 288, 289
   pandemic 288
   symptoms of 292-294
   vaccine 296
Cough syrups 267
Coxsackievirus 115, 290
Craniopharyngioma 230b
C-reactive protein 115, 123, 252, 291, 294
Cribriform morular thyroid carcinoma 66, 81
Cuboidal cells, benign 66f
Cuboidal epithelial cells 61f
Cushing's syndrome 266
Cystic adenoma 5
Cystic degeneration 59
Cystinosis 90, 230

Cytokine 267
   based therapy 116
Cytology 59, 64, 162
   benign 165
Cytomegalovirus 290
Cytopathology guidelines 59

D

De Quervain's thyroiditis 91, 283
Decreased libido 197
Deiodinase 14, 219
Dengue 115
Deoxyribonucleic acid 156, 307
Dermopathy 114
Dexamethasone 269
Diabetes mellitus 24, 26, 104, 114, 208, 257
Dichlorodiphenyltrichloroethane 270, 315
Differentiated thyroid
   cancer 173, 175, 180, 188f, 189
   carcinoma 84, 128, 243
Diffuse thyroid enlargement 57f
Diffuse toxic goiter 65
DiGeorge syndrome 260
Diiodotyrosine 13, 220
Dopamine 90, 230, 266
   agonists 266
   antagonists 266
Down syndrome 27, 260
Drugs affecting thyroid hormone
   activation 269
   synthesis 266
Dry eye 143
Dual oxidase maturation factor A2 31
Durvalumab 135
Dysgenesis 219
Dyshormonogenesis 31, 31f, 225
   etiology of 31fc
Dyshormonogenetic goiter 64
Dyslipidemia 105, 254
   management of 260
Dyspnea 158
Dysthyroid optic neuropathy 140, 142f

E

Echovirus 115, 283
Ectopic adrenocorticotropic hormone 186
Ectopic thymoma 81
Ectopic thyroid 30
   gland 49f
Eikenella corrodens 284b
Electrocardiogram 273
Electroencephalography 276
Electrolyte balance 117
Elevated thyroid-stimulating hormone 251
Embryo 197
Embryonal thyroid neoplasms 66, 81
Encephalopathy, steroid responsive 276
Endemic cretinism 225, 302
Endemic goiter 64, 90
Endocrine disruptors 315
   impact of 315

Endocrine system 288
Enhanced green fluorescent protein 318
Enteropathy, infiltrative 98
Enzyme linked immunosorbent assay 25, 222
Eosinophilic cytoplasm, moderate 67f
Epithelial origin, differentiated thyroid carcinoma of 84
Epithelial tumors, primary 172
Epithelioid cell granulomas 63f
Eprotirome 101
Epstein-Barr virus 115, 283, 290
Erectile dysfunction 197
Erythema 113f
Erythrocyte sedimentation rate 91, 115, 123, 282, 294
Escherichia coli 284b
Esophagus 29
Ethionamide 90, 91
European Group of Graves' orbitopathy 20
European Society for Endocrinology 222
European Thyroid Association 254
Euthyroid hyperthyroxinemia 121, 128
   causes of 121t
Exogenous thyroid hormone excess 134
Exophthalmos, bilateral severe 120f
External beam radiotherapy 189, 192
Extraocular muscle 138
   enlargement of 142f
Extrathyroidal extension 174, 176
Extrathyroidal origin, thyrotoxicosis of 116, 126
Eye 117
   disease 145
   examination 20
Eyelid
   retraction 140f, 238
   unilateral 141f
   swelling 113f

F

F fluorodeoxyglucose 5, 53
Familial isolated pituitary adenoma 128
Fasciitis 74f
Fatty acids, nonesterified 136
Fatty liver disease, nonalcoholic 106, 107
Female reproductive
   health 201f
   tract 197t
Female sexual function index 198
Ferrous sulfate 269
Fertility 198, 200, 202, 253
   outcomes 260
Fibroblasts 140f
Fibromatosis 74f
Fibrosis 61f
Fibrous thyroiditis 63
Fine-needle aspiration 35, 160, 161t, 162, 174, 183
   biopsy 115, 153, 244, 245
   cytology 23, 55, 59, 83, 114, 153, 166, 173, 183, 189

Follicular neoplasm 65, 67f, 164, 167
Follicular thyroid
    cancer 34, 160, 185
    carcinoma 58f, 66, 70, 243, 246
Follicular tumor 70
Food Safety and Standards Authority of India 305
Food, fortification of 303
Fractures 100
Free thyroxine 22, 24, 84, 204, 251, 270, 294
Free triiodothyronine 22
Functional metastatic thyroid carcinoma 134
Fungi 284
Furosemide 269

G

Gamma camera planar scanner 44
Gamma scintillation probe 44
Gene sequencing classifier 164
Genetics 172
    disease 244
    syndromes 260t
    testing, role of 221
Germ cells 204
Gestational age 240
Gestational thyrotoxicosis 119, 126, 135, 211, 212
Giant cell collection 65f
Glioma 230
Glomerular filtration rate 206, 273
Glucocorticoids 143, 230, 265, 269
    effects of 266t
    therapy 273
Goiter 3, 19, 57f, 63, 114, 114f, 147, 149, 150, 155, 254, 302
    radioiodine ablation of 153
Goitrogens 90, 155, 230, 300
    large quantities of 229
Gomori's silver methenamine stain 285
Gonadotropin releasing hormone 197, 199, 205
Granular amphophilic cytoplasm 80f
Graves' dermopathy 114f
Graves' disease 20, 25, 33, 34, 34f, 35f, 47, 47f, 65, 82, 83, 113-115, 121, 122f, 128, 138, 157, 159, 202, 211, 212, 235, 236, 237b, 238t, 240, 243, 267, 270, 274, 282, 286, 296, 304, 308
    management of 82, 123
    medical management of 236
    neonatal 25
    radioactive iodine treatment of 238
    surgical management of 237
    ultrasonographic appearance of 33f
Graves' hyperthyroidism 26, 83t, 125t, 138
Graves' ophthalmic involvement 113
Graves' ophthalmopathy 20, 113, 120f, 138, 238
Graves' orbitopathy 20, 113f, 144fc, 145fc
Growth 251
    hormone 129

H

Haemophilus influenza 284b
Hashimoto's disease 273
Hashimoto's encephalopathy 231, 272-276
Hashimoto's thyroiditis 24, 25, 31, 32, 33f, 62, 63, 63f, 90, 228, 230, 235, 243, 251, 281, 296
Hashitoxicosis 114, 239
Head
    and neck tumors, external irradiation for 230
    injury 230
Heart disease 106
    cardiovascular 254
    coronary 100
    ischemic 106, 254
Heart failure 100, 106, 254
    chronic 125
    congestive 202
    pathogenesis of 106f
Helicobacter pylori 99t
Hemangiomas, congenital hepatic 219
Hematopoietic system 117
Hemochromatosis 90, 230
Hemorrhage 59, 230
Heparin 269, 270
    releases lipoprotein lipase 270
Hepatic lipase 252
Hepatitis E 115, 290
Heptachlor 270
Heroin 269
Heterophile
    antibodies 99
    antigens 27
Hexachlorobenzene 315
Hexachlorocyclohexane 316
High serum lactate dehydrogenase 272
High-density lipoprotein-cholesterol 105
Highly active antiretroviral therapy 265, 267
Histoplasma capsulatum 284b
Hodgkin's disease 152
Hodgkin's lymphoma 286
Hormonal alterations 198, 202
Hormone, adrenocorticotropic 263
Horner's syndrome 159, 189
Human antimouse antibodies 27
Human chorionic gonadotropin 115, 126, 128, 135, 197, 205
    molecule 135
Human immunodeficiency virus 99, 115, 290
Human leukocyte antigen 84, 290
Human placental lactogen 197
Hürthle cell 52, 59, 60f, 62, 62f, 63f, 68f, 75f, 163, 185
    carcinoma 38f, 185
    thyroid 55f
    neoplasm 62, 173
Hydrocortisone 275
Hydrogen peroxide generation 219
Hydroxymethylglutaryl coenzyme A 105
Hyoid bone 43f
Hypercholesterolemia 272
Hypercoagulation 253
Hyperechoic thyroid gland 33f
Hyperlipidemia 26
Hyperparathyroidism 186
Hyperplasia 64, 157
    congenital adrenal 222
Hypertension 103, 125
    pregnancy-induced 197, 211
Hyperthyroid 240
    disorders 33
Hyperthyroidism 20, 22, 33, 60, 115, 119, 137, 202, 205, 211, 212, 234, 239, 240fc, 241, 252
    causes of 33, 211, 234t
    clinical features of 235b
    diagnosis of 93fc, 212
    exogenous 234
    familial gestational 119
    incidence of 234
    iodine induced 304
    management of 235
    maternal 219
    mild 239
    neonatal 239, 240
    pathological 212
    physiological 212, 213
    primary 234
    signs of 20t
    subclinical 239, 308
    symptoms of 100
    thyrotropin induced 116
Hyperthyrotropinemia 259
Hypocalcemia 237
Hypoechogenicity 58f, 244
Hypoglycemia 272
Hyponatremia 272
Hypophysitis, lymphocytic 90
Hypoplasia 8, 30, 90
Hypotension 273
Hypothalamic disease 90
Hypothalamic disorders 230

Hypothalamic–pituitary–thyroid axis 12, 12f, 15, 43f, 90f, 129, 265, 307, 307fc
Hypothalamic thyrotropin-releasing hormone 89, 311
Hypothalamus 90, 197, 315
Hypothermia 273
Hypothyroid ophthalmopathy 231
Hypothyroidism 19, 20, 20t, 22, 25, 60, 87, 89, 94b, 95, 96b, 103-105, 105f, 106, 106f, 107, 107f, 108, 137, 198, 200, 205, 206, 208, 208b, 213, 228, 230f, 232, 257, 258b, 259f, 260, 263
   acquired 90
   amiodarone-induced 268
   autoimmune 230
   central 90, 120, 219, 220, 229, 230, 234, 260
   congenital 8, 23, 30, 30f, 31f, 90, 219, 222t, 224fc, 226fc, 229, 308
   consumptive 90, 229, 230
   drug-induced 91
   effects of 199f, 206
   etiology of 230
   iatrogenic 91
   management of 94fc
   maternal 198, 206
   moderate 106
   permanent congenital 220
   presentation of 92
   prevalence of 96, 105, 257
   primary 25, 89, 90, 228, 231f
   screening of 95b
   secondary 94, 220
   severe 106
   subclinical 103, 106, 199, 228, 230, 251-254, 257, 308
   system wise clinical manifestations of 92t
   tertiary 94
   transient 25, 90, 220
   treatment of 203t, 207

I

Imatinib 91
Immune checkpoint inhibitors 91, 229, 230, 266, 267
Immunocytochemistry 59, 81, 188, 191
Immunoglobulins, intravenous 201
Immunometric assay 26
Immunomodulatory drugs 62
In vitro fertilization 200, 203
Indian Society for Pediatric and Adolescent Endocrinology 222
Infections 115, 230
Infectious thyroiditis 61, 284
   types of 284b
Infertility 26, 254
Inflammatory bowel disease 98
Influenza viruses 115
Insulin
   like growth factor-1 157
   resistance 253, 257
Intact parathyroid hormone 186, 246

Intensity modulated radiation therapy 191, 192
Intercellular adhesion molecule-1 140
Interferon 267
   alpha 90, 91, 119, 230
Interleukin 91, 123, 140, 267
International Council for Control of Iodine Deficiency Disorders Global Network 303
International Society for Pediatric and Adolescent Diabetes 104
Intracytoplasmic sperm injection 202, 203
Intrauterine insemination 202
Invasive encapsulated follicular variant papillary carcinoma 66, 70
Invasive follicular thyroid carcinoma 71f
Iodide 299
   transport 90
Iodine 31, 44, 90, 266, 299, 305
   deficiency 90, 155, 182, 229, 230, 243, 251, 300
      disorders 299, 301, 303-305, 305fc
      health consequences of 302t
   dietary intake of 299
   fortification of 303
   insufficiency, risk of 300
   isotopes 44
   nutrition, assessment of 301t
   organification
      abnormalities 50
      defect 31
   pathway 299f
   sufficient areas 155, 157
   supplementation 153, 303, 303t, 305
      benefits of 304
      risk of 304
   transport defect 31
   uptake of 13
Iodotyrosine dehalogenase 31
   deficiency 90
Iodotyrosine deiodinase 150, 156
Ipilimumab 91, 267
Irradiation 230
Isolated thyroid-stimulating hormone 229
Isthmus 29

J

Janus kinase 104
Jod–Basedow effect 14
Jod–Basedow phenomenon 266
Joint susceptibility 104

K

Kangra valley study 304f
Klinefelter syndrome 260
Kocher–Debre–Semelaigne syndrome 231

L

Langerhans cell histiocytosis 230
Laryngeal nerve, recurrent 10
Larynx 43f

Laser thermal ablation 166
Lateral neck dissection, role of 246
Lecithin-cholesterol acyltransferase 252
Left ventricular ejection fraction 106
Leptin 258
Lesions, benign 245
Leukemia inhibitory factor 197
Leuprolide 286
Levothyroxine 104, 128, 202, 204, 206, 208, 253, 254, 269
   suppression therapy 153, 245
   therapy 105
Leydig cells 204
Lid retraction 140
Lindane 270
Liothyronine 104
Lipoprotein lipase 252
Liquid chromatography-mass spectrometry 28
Lithium 27, 62, 90, 91, 230, 267
   therapy 251
Live birth rate 200
Liver 197
   diseases 98
   function test 123
   hemangioma 230
      presence of 230f
Low birth weight 197, 222
Low molecular weight keratin 59
Low-density lipoprotein 117, 252
   cholesterol 105
Lugol's solution 241
Luteinizing hormone 197, 199, 204, 205, 263
Lymph node metastasis 39, 80f, 73f
Lymphadenoid goiter 281
Lymphocytes, background of 62
Lymphomas, malignant 172

M

Magnetic resonance imaging 29, 38, 121, 152, 159, 191, 266, 276, 285
Malabsorption, evaluation of 100fc
Malignancy 183t
   risk of 35
   suspicious for 167
Malignant follicular neoplasms 156
Marine–Lenhart syndrome 33, 35f
Maturation defects 219
Maximum intensity projection 5, 53-55
McCune–Albright syndrome 119, 128, 136, 136f
Measles virus 115
Medullary thyroid
   cancer 38f, 39, 173, 175t, 180, 182
      treatment of 178
   carcinoma 41f, 66, 78, 79f-81f, 175, 185, 244, 246
Megabecquerel 44t
Meningioma 230b
Menorrhagia 198
Menstrual disturbances 198

Mental function 302
Mental health 254
Mercury 315
Messenger ribonucleic acid 258, 266, 289
Metabolite 236
Metaplastic cells 65f
Metastasis 182, 230
Metastatic disease 192
Metastatic functioning thyroid carcinoma 126
Metastatic lymph nodes, mapping of 41f
Metastatic medullary thyroid carcinoma, management of 186
Metformin 266
Methadone 269
Methimazole 82, 83t, 123, 124, 213, 236, 275
Methoxyisobutylisonitrile 50
Metoprolol 124
Microcalcification 244
Microfollicles, abundant 67f
Microfollicular growth patterns 79f
Mid-day meal program 305
Minimally invasive follicular thyroid carcinoma 71f
Miscarriage, recurrent 197
Mitogen activated protein kinase pathway 182
Mitotane 266, 269
Mixed medullary-papillary carcinoma 81f
Molecular genetic
  role of 245
  studies 245
Molecular tests 81, 163
Monocyte chemoattractant protein 140
Monoiodotyrosine 13
Monomorphic nuclei 60f
Mood disturbances 254
Multifocal granulomatous folliculitis 63
Multinodular goiter 48, 65, 66f, 114, 156, 157, 182
  management of 84, 167
Multinucleated giant cells 62f-64f
Multiple endocrine neoplasia 173, 244
Multiple metastatic cervical lymph nodes 50f
Multiple thyroid follicle 62f
Mumps 115, 290
Muscle 29, 117
  cells 140f
  hypertrophy 232f
Mycobacterium
  avium intracellulare 284b
  leprae 284b
  tuberculosis 284b
Mycobacteroides chelonae 284b
Myxedema coma 272, 273t, 274

N

Nadolol 124t
National Family Health Survey 257, 300
National Goiter Control Programme 303, 304
National Health and Nutrition Examination Survey 253
National Institute of Nutrition 300
National Iodine Deficiency Disorders Control Programme 304
National Iodine Survey of India 305
National Nutritional Monitoring Bureau 305
Neck, examination of 20
Necrosis, background of 77f
Negative predictive value 164
Neonatal hyperthyroidism 239, 240
  clinical features of 240
  evaluation of 241
  management of 241
Neoplasms, malignant 66, 70
Nephrotic syndrome 98
Nervous system 117, 252
Neuroendocrine C-cell derived thyroid cancer 173
Neurofibromatosis 260
Neuron-specific enolase 78
Neurotrophic tyrosine receptor kinase gene fusion 191, 192
Neutropenia 237
Next-generation sequencing 221
Niacin 269
Nitrates 315
Nitrogen dioxide 270
Nivolumab 91, 135, 267
Nocardia asteroides 284
Nocardia brasiliensis 284
Nodular goiter 57f, 114f, 240
Nodular thyroid
  disease 155, 156, 158, 164t, 166fc, 169, 243
  goiter 34-36, 38
  swelling 58f
Nodule 245
  growth of 157
  sonographic pattern of 35
Nonalcoholic fatty liver disease 106, 107
  prevalence of 106
Nonalcoholic steatohepatitis 106
  management of 260
Noncommunicable disease control 305
Nonepithelial tumors, primary 172
Non-Hodgkin's lymphoma 62, 286
Noninvasive follicular thyroid neoplasm 66, 69, 69f
Non-necrotizing epithelioid cell granulomas 64f
Nonsteroidal anti-inflammatory drugs 136
Nonthyroidal illness syndrome 25, 120, 262, 263, 290
  diagnosis of 263
  mechanisms of 263
Nontoxic goiter 149
Noonan syndrome 260
Normal thyroid
  function 204
  imaging 29, 47
Nortriptyline 267

Nuclear
  factor kappa B 140f
  pleomorphism, severe 78f
  radiation 302
  scan 283
  thyroid hormone receptor 307

O

Obesity 107, 108, 251, 257, 259f, 260, 260t
  management of 260
  mechanisms of 258fc
  prevalence of 257
Obstructive liver disease 98
Oncocytic adenoma 65, 68, 68f, 69f
Ophthalmopathy 114
  thyroid associated 26
Opioids 90
Oral contraceptive pills 269
Oral estrogen 269
Oral tyrosine kinase inhibitors 91
Orbit 140f
  computed tomography of 142, 142f
Orbital fibroblasts, activation of 140f
Orbital radiotherapy 144
Orbitopathy, thyroid associated 138, 140, 140f, 141t, 144f, 144fc, 145fc
Organ system 20
Organic anion-transporting polypeptide 133
Organification disorders 90
Organochlorines 270
Orthomyxovirus 115, 290
Osteoporosis 26, 27, 100
Ovaries 197
Overt hyperthyroidism 307, 308
Overt hypothyroidism 198, 228, 251, 308
Oxidation 13

P

P-aminosalicylic acid 91
Papanicolaou stain 68f
Papillary carcinoma 59, 71f-75f
  nuclear features of 75f
Papillary thyroid
  cancer 160, 178, 186
  carcinoma 37f, 53f, 66, 70, 81, 156, 160, 182, 184, 246
  microcarcinoma 185
Parasites 284
Parathyroid
  glands 10
  neoplasm 67f
Parenchyma 29f
Parvovirus B19 115, 283
Pediatric thyroid nodules, majority of 247
Pemberton's maneuver 159
Pemberton's sign 20
Pembrolizumab 91, 135, 267
Pendred syndrome 50, 155
Pendrin mutations 90, 219
Perchlorate discharge test 31

Periodic acid–Schiff 70
Peroxidase
　antibody 208
　deficiency 50
Pesticides 270, 315, 316
Phenobarbital 91, 269
Phenylketonuria 222t
Phenytoin 91, 268-270
Pheochromocytoma 186
Phosphatidylinositol-3-kinase 173
Phthalates 315, 316
Pituitary adenoma 90, 230
Pituitary vasoactive intestinal peptide 198
Pizzillo method 152
Placenta 197
Plasma cell free DNA 165
Plasticizers 315, 316
Pneumocystis jiroveci 284b, 285
Polybrominated biphenyls 270
Polybrominated diphenyl ethers 315
Polychlorinated biphenyl 270, 315, 316
Polychlorinated dibenzodioxins 315
Polycystic ovary syndrome 198
Polyethylene glycol 99, 230
Polygonal tumor cells 80f
Polyphosphodiesters 317
Poorly differentiated thyroid carcinoma 66, 76f, 77f, 180
Positive predictive value 164
Positron emission tomography 35, 45, 45f, 52-55, 182, 183
Postpartum thyroiditis 91, 115, 126, 197, 208, 209, 281
　high-risk for 209b
Postradioactive iodine ablation 251
Post-therapy hypothyroidism 229
Post-thyroidectomy 230
Potassium
　iodide, saturated solution of 241
　perchlorate test 50
Povidone iodine 267
Prader–Willi syndrome 260
Prednisone 90
Pre-existing thyroid disease 243
Pregnancy 115, 122, 206, 207, 208b, 211, 212, 254, 301, 313
　first trimester of 120
　nausea of 136
　outcomes study 202, 212
　toxemia of 136
　vomiting of 136
Premature menarche 231f
Premature ovarian failure 200
Primary hypothyroidism 25, 89, 90, 228, 231f
　atypical manifestations of 231b
Propaylthiouracil 82
Propranolol 124
　high-dose 269
Propylthiouracil 123, 124, 133, 213, 236, 269
Proton pump inhibitors 269
Pruritic rash 237
Psammoma body 72f

Psammomatous calcification 73f
Pseudomonas aeruginosa 284b
Pseudotumor cerebri 231
Pyrexia of unknown origin 281

R

Radiation 180, 192, 315
　effects of 317
　exposure 243
　thyroiditis 63
Radioactive iodine 125, 126, 143, 176-178, 182, 237, 238, 240, 247
　ablation 176, 246
　therapy 123
　uptake study 121, 282
Radioimmunoassay 24
Radioiodine 125, 168, 203
　therapy 203
　treatment 90, 153
　whole-body scan 50
Radionucleotides 30
Radionuclide scan 235
Radiopharmaceuticals 43
Rainbow pills 107
Raloxifene 269
Reactive lymphoid follicles 63f
Recombinant human thyroid-stimulating hormone 51
Refractory hypothyroidism 98, 100, 100fc
　causes of 98, 98t
　management of 101
　treatment of 101
Regional lymph node 175
Reproductive health 197, 202
Reproductive system 117, 252
Respiratory system 117
Retinoid 266
　X receptor 266, 307, 316
Ribonucleic acid 289, 318
Riedel's struma 63
Riedel's thyroiditis 32, 63, 90, 91, 281, 285, 286
Rifampin 91, 269
Rituximab 144
Roux-en-y duodenal diversion 99
Rubella 290
　viruses 115

S

Salicylates 269
Salivary gland 34f, 48f, 66
　secretory carcinoma of 66
Salpingo-oophorectomy 135
Salsalate 270
Salt reduction 305
Sarcoidosis 90
Sarcomas 172
Schmidt syndrome 273
Scleroderma 90
Sclerosing mucoepidermoid carcinoma with eosinophilia 66, 81

Sclerosis, multiple 267
Selective estrogen receptor modulators 265, 269
Selective lymph node dissection 182
Selective serotonin reuptake inhibitors 267
Selective thyroid receptor beta agonists 260
Serratia marcescens 284
Sertoli cells 204
Serum antithyroid antibodies 93
Serum binding proteins 14, 121t
Seven-point clinical activity score 20
Severe acute respiratory syndrome coronavirus 2 115, 288
Sex hormone binding globulin 130, 197, 202, 205
Sexual dysfunction 198, 202
Shear wave elastography 162
Sheehan's syndrome 90
Short bowel syndrome 98
Silent thyroiditis 32, 34
Simon's triangle 10
Simple goiter 149, 153
　pathogenesis of 150f
Single-photon emission computerized tomography 39, 45f, 49f, 51, 53
Skeletal system 117
Slipped capital femoral epiphyses 231
Small solitary thyroid nodule 151f
Sobetirome 101
Sodium iodide symporter 30, 44, 45, 134, 315
Solitary thyroid nodule 47, 157, 182
Somatostatin receptor scintigraphy 41
Sperm cells 204
Spindle cell morphology 80f
Spindle epithelial tumor 81
Sporadic thyroiditis, painless 282
Staphylococcus aureus 115, 284b
Stavudine 91
Steatohepatitis, nonalcoholic 106
Steroid receptor coactivator 14
Stillbirth 302
Streptococcus pyogenes 284b
Strongyloides stercoralis 284b
Struma ovarii 34t, 127, 128, 135
Subacute granulomatous thyroiditis 63, 63f, 64f, 91, 229
Subclinical hypothyroidism 103, 106, 199, 228, 230, 251-254, 257, 308
　etiology of 251, 251b
Sucralfate 269
Sulfisoxazole 91
Sulfonamide 90
Sulfur dioxide 270
Sunitinib 91
Superior laryngeal nerve, external branch of 10
Suppression thyroid scintigraphy 49
Suppurative inflammation 59
Surgery 82, 123, 125, 153, 168, 180, 245, 246
　complications of 246
Surgical therapy 145
Synaptophysin 78

Syphilis 284
Systemic lupus erythematosus 91, 124

T

Taenia solium 284b
Takayasu arteritis 283
Tamoxifen 269
Technetium-99 scan 122f, 123f
Teprotumumab 144
Tetraiodothyronine 22, 43, 89
Thalassemia 230
Thalidomide 91, 116
Thermoregulatory dysfunction 273, 274
Thiocyanates 315
Thionamides 236
Thygenext 165
Thymic tumors 66, 81
ThyraMIR 165
Thyroblastoma 66, 81
Thyrocyte function 12
Thyrocyte structure 12
Thyroglobulin 25, 26, 78, 122, 150, 177, 178, 182, 190, 191, 198, 219, 220
   antibodies 25, 178, 240, 294
   elevated negative iodine scintigraphy 13, 52-54
   levels 26
   serum 221
Thyroglossal cyst 61f
Thyroglossal duct 50f
   carcinoma 60, 61f
   cyst 60, 61f, 65
Thyroid 3, 29, 66, 81, 152, 197, 202, 257, 288, 307
   ablation 237
   abnormalities, congenital 65
   agenesis 30f
   antibodies 235
   autoimmunity 197, 200, 201, 201f, 202, 203, 203t, 228, 267
   autonomy 34f, 157
   binding globulin 14, 206, 316
   biochemical presentations of 290
   blocking antibody 26
   bud 8
   cancer 40f, 85t, 147, 158, 172, 175t, 178, 180, 181t, 188, 188f, 254, 317
   carcinoma 158, 172, 178, 304, 308
      management 52
   carrier proteins 14, 14t
   C-cell derived carcinoma 66, 78
   cell 299f
   clinical evaluation of 19
   cork phenomenon 159
   cytopathology 184t
   deficiency 95
   dermopathy 114
   destruction of 119
   diseases 289
      surgical treatment of 6
   disorders 28, 89, 113, 195, 217, 249, 260t, 288, 305
      diagnosis of 17
      effects of 308t
      miscellaneous 279
      nuclear imaging in 43
   disruption 315
      classification of 315
   drugs affecting hypothalamic-pituitary control of 265
   dysfunction 141f, 200t, 202, 289
      effects of 205t
   dysgenesis 49, 90, 219, 220
   dyshormonogenesis 30, 219, 220
   emergencies 272
   endocrine abnormalities 60
   enlargement 19
   examination 20
   excess 211
   eye disease 138, 289
      mild 141f
   follicles 61f, 62f, 63f
   follicular
      carcinoma of 52
      cells 59, 60f, 65f, 71f
      nodular disease 65
   folliculogenesis 8
   function 223t, 236, 265, 265t, 266t, 268, 268t, 270
      laboratory evaluation of 22
      test 22, 22t, 25t, 26, 28, 103, 121, 128, 178, 207, 234, 236, 240, 241, 244, 245, 281, 282, 312
   gland 6, 8, 9, 9f, 10, 12, 12f, 13, 29, 33f, 34t, 43, 48f, 49f, 225, 275, 289
      abnormal growth of 155
      anatomical relation of 43f
      anatomy of 8
      arterial supply of 9f
      congenital anomalies of 8
      ectopic sublingual 31f
      embryogenesis of 8f
      embryology of 8
      examination of 21f
      increased susceptibility of 302
      infections of 115
      lymphatic drainage of 10
      normal 99mtc scan of 30f
      physiology of 12
      shape 8
      size 8
      vascular anatomy of 9
      venous drainage of 10f
   hormone 13, 14, 46, 34, 90, 90f, 105-107, 116, 119-121, 128, 129, 131, 197, 202, 251-253, 257-259, 264, 269, 275, 296f, 307, 310, 311, 312
      action 14, 307
      alpha 307, 312
      beta 107, 229, 312t
      drug-induced 115
      drugs affecting protein binding of 269
      effects of 197t, 204t
      excess 111, 113, 117t, 119, 123, 125, 128, 129t, 211
      factitious ingestion of 34
      homeostasis 268
      levels 262
      measurement 22
      metabolism defect 133
      optimal action of 310
      physiology of 257
      preparations 269
      receptor 14, 15, 15t, 197, 230, 310
      resistance syndromes, classification of 311
      secretion of 90fc
      structure 13f
      suppression 168, 177
      synthesis 13, 13f, 15, 315
      transport 219, 315
   huge multinodular swelling of 58f
   imaging 29, 30, 41
      reporting and data system 174, 183
   infiltration 90
   inflammation of 119
   lobectomy 125
   malignancy 34, 36, 38, 50
   management 289
   medullary
      cancer 158
      carcinoma of 84
   metabolism 299
   molecular mechanism of 289
   mucoepidermoid carcinoma of 66
   multinodular swelling of 57f
   neoplasm 156
      classification of 172, 180fc
   nodule 34, 35t, 49f, 57, 147, 158t, 160t, 173, 180, 243, 244, 260
      assessment of 57, 173
      autonomously functioning 45, 156
      classification of 155t
      hypoechogenicity of 58f
      imaging of 34
      liquid biopsy of 153
      malignant 57
      management of 84
      prevalence of 57, 243
      principal causes of 155
      treatment of 173
      ultrasound of 35
   nuclear scanning 285
   oncocytic
      adenoma of 65, 68
      carcinoma of 66, 74, 75f
   palpation 20
   papillary carcinoma of 58f, 71f-75f
   parenchyma 64f
   peroxidase 13, 59, 89, 198, 206, 219, 220, 240
      antibody 24, 203, 204, 207, 235, 257, 267
   planar scintigraphy 49f
   post-radioablation of 230
   receptor antibodies 211
   scan 45, 244
      interpretation, principles of 46

scintigraphy 30, 33, 36, 46, 47f-49f, 224fc
specific autoantibodies 24
spindle epithelial tumor 82f
status, management of 204fc
stimulating hormone 6, 12, 22-25, 34, 43, 46, 83, 84, 89, 94t, 107, 113, 120, 128, 149, 155, 159, 166, 176, 197, 203, 208, 219, 223, 226, 231, 234, 240, 244, 258, 262, 265, 266, 270, 272, 282, 290, 294, 307, 316
   binding inhibitory immunoglobulins 122
   concentrations 23t
   deficiency 25
   dependent hyperthyroidism 25
   levels 103, 232
   receptor 25, 107, 119, 122, 138, 140f
   secreting pituitary adenoma 34
   suppressive therapy 247, 308
storm 239, 272, 274, 276
suppression 166
surgery 6
swelling 83fc
transcription factor 1 59, 190
tumors 66, 70, 81, 82t
ultrasonography 159, 235
Thyroidal reference radioactive iodine uptake 47f
Thyroidea ima 9
Thyroidectomy 41f, 85, 184, 237
   subtotal 90
Thyroiditis 31, 34f, 47, 48f, 61, 122f, 126, 240, 281, 282
   acute 32, 32f, 34, 61, 119, 230
      bacterial 285
      infectious 115, 126
   amiodarone-induced 34
   autoimmune 61, 228, 304
   chronic
      autoimmune 90, 281
      lymphocytic 90, 228, 230, 281
   cytokine-induced 230
   destructive 135
   drug-induced 62, 286
   invasive 63
   lymphocytic 61, 62f, 63f, 65
   painful subacute 283
   painless 32, 34, 119
   palpation 63
   radiation-induced 286
   sporadic painless 126, 281
   subacute 25, 32, 32f, 34, 91, 114, 115, 119, 126, 281, 290, 291, 292t, 294, 296, 296f
   treatment of 126t
   types of 32, 32t, 126, 281, 281b
Thyromimetics 101, 133
Thyroperoxidase 299

Thyrotoxic crisis, diagnostic criteria of 274t
Thyrotoxicosis 19, 20, 27, 113, 119, 120fc, 126, 134, 135, 152, 202
   amiodarone-induced 116, 122, 127, 268, 286
   clinical features of 117
   diagnosis of 119
   differential diagnosis of 121t
   etiology of 121
   iatrogenic 34, 126
   juvenile 308
   management of 124t
   treatment of 27
   typical symptoms of 19
Thyrotrophic receptor 150
Thyrotropin
   binding inhibiting immunoglobulin 26
   hormone stimulation test 130
   receptor
      antibody 235, 240, 241
      hormone 12, 22, 43, 90, 197-199, 229, 258, 263, 266, 307
Thyrotropinoma 121
Thyroxine 12, 22, 23, 25, 89, 94t, 251, 258, 272, 289, 299
   absorption test, protocol for 100b
   binding globulin 25, 130, 201, 211, 257, 266, 269
   stimulating hormone 98
   supratherapeutic doses of 100
   therapy 27
Tissue distribution 15
Toxic adenoma 34, 119, 121, 125, 126
Toxic autonomous nodule 48
Toxic multinodular goiter 34, 48, 114, 119, 121, 123f, 125, 126
   development of 157
Toxic thyroid
   hyperplasia, hereditary 136
   nodule 239, 240
Trachea 29, 43f
Transforming growth factor-beta 140, 157
Transthyretin 14
Trauma 230
Tricyclic antidepressants 265, 267
Triiodothyroacetic acid 101
Triiodothyronine 12, 22, 25, 34, 43, 89, 107, 128, 251, 258, 270, 272, 289, 290, 294, 296, 299, 307
   suppression test 130
Trophoblastic disease 34, 119
Trophoblastic tumors 135
Truncal hypotonia 133
Tubercular thyroiditis 32
Tumors 82, 176, 188f, 230
   benign 65, 66

   cells 73f, 80f
      cohesive cluster of 67f
      loose clusters of 75f
   cuboidal 67f
   malignant 155
   necrosis factor-alpha 263
   node, metastasis 173, 184
   secondary 172
Turner's syndrome 27, 260
Tyrosine kinase inhibitors 20, 90, 116, 119, 229, 230, 268

U

Ultrasonography 29, 83, 122, 178, 182, 225, 244, 282, 283
Ultrasound 159
   elastography 36, 162
   guided fine needle aspiration 57
United Nations International Children's Emergency Fund 303
Urinary iodine concentration 305
Urticaria 237
Uterus 197

V

Van Wyk–Grumbach syndrome 231, 231f
Vasoactive intestinal peptide 199
Vitamin
   A deficiency 300
   B7 28

W

Wet method 303
White blood cell 123, 282
Whole body
   radioiodine scan 50f, 51-53
   scan 37, 50, 55
   scintigraphy 176
Whole exome sequencing 221
Williams syndrome 260
Wolff–Chaikoff effect 13, 266, 268
World Health Organization 188, 300
   Classification of Thyroid Neoplasms 65

X

X-chromosome inactivation 150
X-ray neck 183

Y

Yersinia enterocolitica 113

Z

Zuckerkandl tubercle 9